To Carol Monson ḊꞒ,
friend and colleague.

Don Waters MPH

ENVIRONMENTAL

HEALTH

HAZARDS

Also by Dr. Waite

Your Environment, Your Health and You

ENVIRONMENTAL

HEALTH

HAZARDS

RECOGNITION AND AVOIDANCE

Revised and updated

DONALD E. WAITE, D.O., M.P.H.
Professor Emeritus
Department of Family Medicine
Michigan State University
East Lansing, Michigan

ENVIRONMENTAL HEALTH CONSULTANTS   Columbus, Ohio

Published by Environmental Health Consultants
933 South High Street
Columbus, Ohio 43206

Publisher's Cataloging–in–Publication Data
Waite, Donald E.
Environmental Health Hazards; Recognition and Avoidance/revised and updated.
Donald E. Waite, DO, MPH.

> Includes bibliographical references.
> Includes glossary
> Includes index.

ISBN: 0-9640831-1-6

RA565.W35 2002

Printed in the United States of America
Printed on acid-free paper

Dedication

To the families of America, and especially to my own family; that institution of scorn by the elitist, the pompous and the perverse miscreants of our society. To my children, who have been the greatest source of pride and joy to me, while sparing me the heartaches delivered by many of their contemporaries. To my brothers and sisters, companions and friends throughout childhood and during my adult years. I am grateful for the hundreds of occasions when we have gathered and communed. Finally, to my parents, who spawned and nurtured it all. I give thanks to God for them all, and for the blessings that He has bestowed upon us, for sparing us all of the afflictions and mishaps that might have befallen us.

CONTENTS

PREFACE

The goal of this book is to provide, to the extent possible in a single volume, all of the information and references that the average individual or family needs to guide them in preserving the good health entrusted to them by God. In undertaking such a project I fully understand the broad scope of the task, and the fact that the information is constantly changing. This is well exemplified by the emergence of the hantavirus respiratory disease in the Southwest in 1993, the importation of the Asian tiger mosquito in 1985 and the sudden appearance of the West Nile virus in 2001. Prior to that it was Lyme disease, which first appeared in 1977, with the spirochaete being identified in 1982. The most dramatic of all new diseases of course is AIDS, first reported in 1981. It has since reached epidemic proportions with no resolution in sight. All of these events have served to humble the author, if not the victims.

In recognition of the increasing volume of travel by United States citizens to various parts of the world, and the corresponding visitation to the United States by individuals from those foreign lands, I have included in this volume coverage of some of the medical problems encountered in other parts of the world. Perhaps the most dramatic of these is the epidemic of cholera that began in Peru in 1991 and subsequently has spread to other countries in South and Central America and to Mexico. More than 100 cases of cholera have resulted in U.S. citizens as a result of travel to these regions, including 31 cases aboard an airline flight from Argentina to Los Angeles during February, 1992.

Similarly cases of the recently discovered hepatitis E have occurred in travelers to India. The occurrence of leishmaniasis and sandfly fever among the troops deployed to the Middle East during Desert Storm reminded us of the health risks of travel to that region.

The subsequent deployment of U.S. troops to Somalia presented us with reminders of the vast array of serious tropical diseases encountered during travel to Africa. To cover all of the diseases that are encountered in Africa alone would require a volume much larger than this work.

The explosive growth of the sexually transmitted diseases in the United States since the 1960s indicates an unmet need for a massive effort to enlighten the public regarding these serious diseases. As disgraceful as this chapter in the history of our society is, the AIDS epidemic and its management by the bureaucrats and politicians has been even more appalling. The deliberate subversion and distortion of known facts regarding this greatest plague since the fourteenth century has left the public totally unaware of the crisis that they face for an interminable period. In the chapter on sexually transmitted diseases I have attempted to present the facts as currently known, to serve as a reference and to fill this void.

Although drug abuse is at the same time a symptom of the social and moral sickness of our society, and a contribution to it, it is a major factor in the explosion of sexually transmitted diseases, including AIDS. There have been massive efforts by government and the authorities to control this problem, but much of the education has been misinformation designed to promote a social agenda. After the expenditure of billions of tax dollars and police state tactics that have snared many innocent citizens, the problem remains unsolved. The lessons of the prohibition era of the 1930s have been forgotten. In chapter XII I have presented the facts regarding the drugs commonly abused to serve as a reference to the serious risks thus entertained. The social and moral issues, just as relevant, perhaps are better addressed in a separate volume.

This book addresses many medical problems and potential problems, but only in a very general manner. The individual's personal physician should always be consulted for all medical needs. Only a well trained physician, dedicated to remaining current, can accurately assess an individual's complaints and medical problems. It is not the intention of this book to attempt to circumvent that absolute necessity. I admonish the reader to not attempt to substitute this book for the family physician. To do so would be much like deciding to take the controls of a Boeing 757 aircraft and attempting to do your own piloting. The captain had to read more than one book to occupy that seat. So it is with the diagnosis and treatment of illness.

The role of this book is to provide the education and references that will permit the individual to preserve health and prevent illness. This is not a difficult task but it does require knowledge and self discipline. For every disease prevention is far preferable to the best of treatments. Many illnesses leave residual damage to the vital organs of the body. Some illnesses are not curable by any means.

Donald E. Waite, DO, MPH
Professor Emeritus

INTRODUCTION

Quod enim mavult homo verum esse, id potius credit. For what a man would like to be true, that he more readily believes.
—— Francis Bacon 1561–1626

The above observation by Bacon contributes much toward an understanding of why politicians and other hucksters are so successful in misleading the public. It does not explain, however, why the quacks of "environmental protection" are so successful in beguiling the American people, and even extracting great sums of money from them. Their repeated extreme, frantic warnings of apocalypse invariably have no scientific basis, and eventually are exposed as a fraud. Their alarming warnings and predictions always make the headlines. If the truth and facts are indeed ever reported subsequently, they are buried in the back pages.

A classic example of such efforts to spread panic among the public is Al Gore's 1992 book, *Earth in the Balance: Ecology and the Human Spirit*, which is a collection of dire predictions such as that global warming is "the most serious crisis we have ever faced," and that an ozone hole would open over the Northern hemisphere in the spring of 1992 (it didn't). The global warming scare has had a long run, in spite of the return of the ice age in 1992-1993. The same National Academy of Sciences that is currently lending credence to the global warming alarmists warned in 1977 that a new ice age "is upon us."

One of those alarmists, who is currently widely quoted as an authority on global warming is Stephen Schneider, who in his 1976 book, *The Genesis Strategy*, was warning that the world might be facing a new ice age, "perhaps one akin to the Little Ice Age of 1500-1850," and should take steps to prepare for it.[1] He told *Discover* magazine in October 1989 that scientists should exaggerate the extent of the climate issue in order to attract attention and get public support for funding. In the July 1975 issue of *National Wildlife*, Nigel Calder warned that "the threat of a new ice age must now stand alongside nuclear war as a likely source of wholesale death and misery for mankind." In the same issue, C.C. Wallen of the World Meteorological Organization warned, "The cooling since

1940 has been large enough and consistent enough that it will not soon be reversed."[2]

The predictions of a melt of the polar ice cap as a result of a "greenhouse effect" has been repudiated by the majority of honest, knowledgeable scientists. The hoax is perpetuated by a few scientists who receive large government grants to study the "problem" and thus have a vested interest in producing reports of a pending catastrophe. The lies are also promoted by private groups whose fund raising depends upon maintaining the hysteria. If indeed the polar ice caps did melt, the sea levels would fall, not rise and flood the coastal areas as these hucksters would have you believe. To prove this to yourself fill a glass half full of ice cubes, then fill with water. As the ice cubes melt you will observe that the water level falls, not rises, because ice occupies more space than the comparable quantity of water.

Natural sources on earth emit 700 billion tons of carbon dioxide into the atmosphere each year, whereas industry produces about six billion tons, an infinitesimal quantity in comparison. Any increase in atmospheric carbon dioxide results in an increase in the growth of plant life, which results in the consumption of an increased amount of carbon dioxide. These natural processes far outweigh the capacity of even the most arrogant and egotistical of scientists to alter the balance. Nevertheless the alarmists have succeeded in eliminating Freon, the most efficient and safest refrigerant known. It has been replaced by a more expensive, more toxic and less efficient chemical, and billions of dollars have been wasted designing, building and replacing refrigeration and air conditioning units.

Gore is also convinced that the world is running out of renewable resources and food, when in fact both are more plentiful than ever before. He supported the wild claim in Paul Ehrlich's book, *The Population Bomb*, (1968) that "The battle to feed humanity is over. In the 1970s and 1980s hundreds of millions of people will starve to death in spite of any crash programs embarked upon now."[3] Two years later Ehrlich predicted that four billion people would starve to death between 1980 and 1989. In reality the millions of people who did starve to death were the result of the great famines produced by Mao's "Great Leap Forward" and Stalin's collectivization program.

When Ehrlich's predictions didn't come to pass he postponed the deaths until the next century. In 1976 Paul and Anne Ehrlich, in *The End of Affluence*, predicted that "before 1985 mankind will enter a genuine age of scarcity...in which the accessible supplies of many key minerals will be facing depletion." In 1980 Ehrlich accepted a bet from Julian Simon, professor of economics at the University of Maryland and author of *The Ultimate Resource*, who challenged him to select any five raw materials of his choosing. Simon bet that they would be more plentiful and thus cheaper ten years hence. Ten years later in 1990 the prices of all five that Ehrlich had picked had dropped and he was forced to write a check for $576.07 to Simon.

Paul Ehrlich,[4] who has been described as a "butterfly specialist,"[5] made many ignorant, irresponsible and unscientific claims. He claimed that DDT running off into the seas would kill all of the algae and thereby deprive the earth of 40 percent of its oxygen. In 1976 he stated that "giving society cheap, abundant energy would be the equivalent of giving an idiot child a machine gun." In retrospect, all of these predictions and alarms, including those of Al Gore, make the alarmists look very foolish, but the attention span and memories of the public are short indeed. It is only because of such short memories on the part of the public that the 450 odd environmental extremist organizations in the United States are able to stay in business and prey on the public. The majority of the news media, publishing houses and educational institutions have come under the control of left wing zealots, who have learned the techniques of propaganda well from their Marxist and Communist forefathers. The primary and secondary schools as well as the colleges and universities utilize the dishonest and inaccurate works of these individuals, such as Malthusian disciple Lester Brown's *State of the World*, to indoctrinate the emerging generation with their flawed ideology.

In the late 1970s Gore was so panicked by the Love Canal, New York "catastrophe" that he sponsored the Superfund law. The Superfund law has cost hundreds of billions of dollars without any benefit to anyone except trial lawyers, who have collected 80 percent of the money spent (Rand Corporation). Meanwhile the New York Department of Health has found no evidence that anyone's health was harmed at Love Canal. After having bought out and evacuated 3,500 residents, the Federal Government is now selling the houses to new residents; your tax dollars at work.

The Alar fiasco in 1989 (see chapter XIII) was another disgraceful and disgusting example of a doomsday propaganda barrage being unleashed on the public. The Environmental Protection Agency's (EPA) panel of scientific experts, in disagreement with the EPA's position, had concluded that Alar presented no hazard. The Natural Resources Defense Council (NRDC) nevertheless paid Fenton Communications more than $180,000 a year to convince the public that the Alar on apples caused cancer. Fenton had a long history of promoting radical groups and Marxist governments. Ed Bradley on *60 Minutes* told the public that Alar on apples was the most potent cancer-causing agent in our food supply, an unequivocal lie. Aflatoxin in our peanut butter holds this honor, and it is a naturally produced substance (see chapters V and XIII).

Alar in fact does not cause cancer. In retaliation against its council of scientific advisors, the EPA gave active support to the campaign of the NRDC, even though that organization had absolutely no scientific credentials. The Congress then scheduled televised hearings, complete with Hollywood celebrities, to further advance the smear campaign. The fact that the NRDC had no scientific credentials was known to *60 Minutes*, the EPA and the Congress. They did have deep pockets, however. As is the case with the global warming scam, the American people were deliberately lied to by the news media, the special interest groups and their representatives in Congress.

We do face some serious threats to our health from the environment, both as a society and as individuals. Most of these hazards, such as the toxic and infectious illnesses from food and water, have been clearly delineated. They do not provide sensational headlines that contribute to fund raising by extremist groups, however. The members of our society need to become better educated regarding these threats and the simple measures that they can take to protect themselves. Such information is outlined in each chapter of this book. The chapters on food and on recreation, for example, should be reviewed prior to planning any trip or vacation. The chapter on sex describes the epidemics, including AIDS, that have resulted from the promiscuity that has been promoted by government and the public schools, and gives the lie to their multibillion dollar campaign to promote "safe sex." With the mania for pets in the United States, everyone should review the chapter on zoonoses, and heed the advice given there.

Finally, the hazards that occur naturally in our environment should not be forgotten. Some of the health hazards that accompany herbal or folk medicines are reviewed in chapter XV. These have produced permanent brain and liver damage in unsuspecting victims. All of the laws that Congress has imposed upon us and all of the restrictive regulations that the bureaucrats have promulgated deal only with man-made substances. These actions invariably do nothing to resolve any perceived problem, and usually introduce new, more troubling problems. Our diet includes far more natural carcinogens than man-made ones, but these have been almost completely ignored. They should be subjected to the same study and evaluation as the synthetic substances. This issue is explored further in chapter XIII.

In responding to environmental hazards that are real, we need to be guided by facts, reason and logic, not by hysteria. We must constantly guard against being diverted from the facts and the true risks by sensational and inaccurate hype. Many of the environmental extremists are disciples of the New Age gospel that rejects God and all of His scriptures. The New Age Movement worships Lucifer instead of God, and teaches that each individual is his own god, free to establish his own moral, ethical and behavioral code. This removes all barriers to even the most abhorrent behavior and theoretically opens the door to endless pleasure and fulfillment. Once opened, that door also permits entry by evil forces of unimaginable horror. Members of this cult have reverted to the practice of sorcery and idol worship characterized by hedonistic societies of previous eras. An example is their worship of Gaea (also Gaia), the earth goddess of ancient Greek mythology. One might rationalize that such mythical gods and goddesses are at least cheaper to worship than a golden lamb.

The confused thinking of these individuals explains their fanaticism and the irrationality of their proposals and theories. The recent incoherent, illiterate babbling of one of these disciples who holds a Ph.D. degree reveals the depth of their ignorance and confusion. Zealous missionaries of this disastrous New Age

Movement are widely disseminated in alarming numbers in the news and entertainment media, in the universities and public schools and even in otherwise respectable businesses. Their activities and influence have contributed materially to the alarming disintegration of our society during the past fifty years.

The survival of our free society depends upon the recognition of the insidious schemes of these plotters, whether they are satanic in motivation, Marxists ideologues, or simply ignorant of the facts and misguided. We need to redirect some of the public funds and programs that are being wasted on social engineering endeavors in the schools and by public health organizations. These funds should be invested in educational and monitoring programs regarding the real threats, rather than the imagined ones. Food handling, a subject far less glamorous than sex, is a classic example where negligence results in many thousands of unnecessary illnesses each year. The American public of today is abysmally ignorant of the simple principles of disease transmission and the importance of hand washing, all of which used to be taught by parents and in elementary school.

Previously unknown hazards are discovered occasionally. Sometimes these discoveries are accidental, and sometimes they result from technological advancement. In the latter part of the 1960s for instance, technological advancements in analytical instruments made possible the detection of chemical substances at the level of parts per billion, one thousand times the sensitivity that was previously possible. In other words substances that would escape detection previously could now be recognized readily. While this advancement was a great achievement for the scientific community, it has delivered enormous mischief to society as a whole. When it was discovered that we were exposed to some of these substances, they were assumed to be a serious threat by the alarmists.

Before spreading the alarm, no consideration was given to the fact that we had been exposed to these for a long time without any ill effects, or to the fact that the exposures were to very minute quantities. The human organism includes many systems and processes which protect against invasion by harmful organisms and which detoxify harmful chemicals. We are on the threshold of further scientific advancements that will permit the measurement of even more minute quantities of substances. We need to greet this advancement rationally and intelligently, rather than hysterically.

In addition to their toxicity, some of the substances identified through the new technology were claimed to cause cancer, a claim that has proved to be not true. Nevertheless, the environmental extremists who make a living from alarming the public have had a field day with these "new discoveries." Congress and the bureaucrats never have to be persuaded to spend money on new agencies and more government controls. A classic example is the establishment of the Environmental Protection Agency (EPA) and the passage of the Toxic Substances Control Act and the Superfund bill in the 1970s. These newly created bureaucratic imbeciles have bankrupted and destroyed countless numbers of innocent citizens and extorted hundreds of millions of dollars from businesses as well as individuals. This money drained from the economy flows down the Washington D.C. black hole, lost forever, with serious economic consequences for us all.

One of the most glaring examples of the resulting bureaucratic stupidity squandering millions of dollars is the fiasco at *Times Beach*, Missouri, a small town of about 2,000 residents. In the mid-1970s, 2,000 gallons of a combination of oil and industrial wastes, contaminated by dioxin, were sprayed on unpaved roads near the town. In 1982, heavy rains caused flooding in the area, spreading the contamination. The EPA ordered a complete evacuation of the town. The federal government eventually shut down the town and paid the residents some $33 million in compensation, some of which was later recovered from private defendants.

Former town residents sued various companies connected with the dioxin, claiming that the exposure harmed their health and increased their risk of cancer. Four residents of nearby Lincoln County settled for $2.68 million in 1983; in another suit 128 plaintiffs eventually settled for $19 million in 1986. Two chemical companies settled another suit out of court for $14.5 million to avoid prolonged litigation. Many other lawsuits and settlements resulted from this irresponsible and unwarranted action by the EPA. Many millions of dollars have been paid out to individuals who suffered no damage whatsoever from dioxin. The television news media made their customary contribution to public hysteria by broadcasting a sensationalized misinformation show titled "A Plague on Our Children." This script was to provide a pattern for the subsequent show creating unfounded hysteria over Alar.

The action that had been taken by the bureaucrats in the *Times Beach* incident was without any scientific basis. The Centers for Disease Control had arbitrarily decided that 1 ppb of dioxin (tetrachlorodibenzodioxin, TCDD) in the soil was harmful. This was seven years after the massive TCDD poisoning of thousands of residents of Seveso, Italy. There were no fatalities and no serious ill effects apparent in the 36,000 residents who were medically monitored during the intervening nine years in that incident. A similar exposure of a much smaller number of workers in Nitro, West Virginia in 1949 similarly demonstrated no serious health consequences during follow-up. In other words we were not without data; the data suggested that no health risk existed in *Times Beach*. After many years and countless studies, many prompted by the Agent Orange controversy, the consensus of the majority of reputable experts is that dioxin exposure has not caused any illness in humans, except for chloracne at high levels of exposure. In spite of all of these facts, the Environmental Protection Agency spent millions of dollars each year for more than fifteen years demolishing houses and sanitizing dirt in Times Beach, for no reason whatsoever.

Although it is known to be a potent promoter, all of the abundant scientific data on dioxin (TCDD) to date has failed to show that it causes cancer in humans. That misconception continues to be fostered by the EPA and other bureaucracies. These agencies are wed to a common misconception of the 1970s that any substance that is a mutagen is also a carcinogen. This has long since been disproved, but government regulatory agencies dogmatically refuse to accept the new data. One of the most consistent characteristic of bureaucrats is their adamant refusal to ever admit that they were wrong about anything. Almost without exception when Congress passes a law to solve a problem, they create more problems than existed prior to their action. When a substance or process is banned it is usually replaced with one that is less efficient, more toxic and invariably more costly.

The government mandate that oxygenated gasoline be used resulted in the corrosion of fuel system components on automobiles, and a great increase in malfunctions due to vapor lock. The substitution of methyl tertiary butyl ether (MTBE) for tetraethyl lead as an additive to gasoline, mandated by the Clean Air Act of 1990, has now been related to numerous incidents of human illness. It has been found to be a possible carcinogen, and has contaminated bodies of water in virtually every state, partially from boaters. In some instances this contamination has destroyed the source of public drinking water. MTBE is very stable, is hard to break down, and there is no way to eliminate it from the environment. Finally in the year 2000 the EPA asked Congress to amend the Clean Air Act. The adverse reactions and catastrophes caused by this substance became so massive and obvious that they could no longer be ignored.

In 1972 the Consumer Product Safety Commission (CPSC) decreed that children's sleepwear would have to be fire resistant. In order to comply with this mandate manufacturers began treating the fabric in children's pajamas with Tris (tris-[2,3-dibromopropyl] phosphate). Garments treated with this chemical were even placed on newborn infants in hospital nurseries, certainly not a high-risk environment for fire. Recognizing the brilliance of their decision, and calculating the number of lives that could be saved (through whatever magic bureaucrats use in making such calculations) the CPSC made plans to extend the flammability standards to adult sleepwear, tents, sleeping bags, curtains, upholstered furniture, carpeting and automobile upholstery. Millions of automobiles manufactured by Ford, General Motors, Chrysler and American Motors between 1972 and 1977 contained upholstery treated with Tris.

Shortly after Tris was introduced physicians witnessed a nationwide epidemic of skin rashes that were ultimately discovered to be caused by the agent. The Consumer Product Safety Commission reassured mothers that the problem could be solved easily by three consecutive launderings of the pajamas, which would eliminate the sensitizing agent. Many parents questioned the value of the flame-retardant treatment (and associated cost) if it would be so readily removed in the laundry. Even more ominous was the discovery that Tris is a mutagen and carcinogen,[6,7] and that it is readily absorbed through the skin.[8] Subsequent studies found that the content of Tris in pajamas was reduced only from 5.8% to 5.1%

after fifty washings.[9] In reporting these findings McCann and Ames expressed concern that Tris posed a serious hazard to the millions of children wearing treated pajamas.[10] In April 1977 the Consumer Product Safety Commission, being finally persuaded by these studies, banned the use of Tris in children's sleepwear. Well over 50 million children were exposed to prolonged skin contact before this action was taken. General Motors began phasing out its use of the product in automobiles shortly thereafter.[11]

The federally mandated inclusion of air bags in automobiles is another example of a bureaucratic fiasco. Aside from the $800 to $1,000 that a single airbag added to the price of every automobile, at least 87 people, including 31 children, were killed by these devices from the time they were introduced in 1990 through March 1998. As of November 1999 the National Highway Transportation and Safety Board admitted to 140 confirmed deaths from air bags, including 84 children who had their necks broken in minor accidents that they would have otherwise survived. Many other injuries have resulted from the explosive deployment of air bags including eye injuries and loss of vision. The propellant in air bags, sodium azide, has caused serious skin irritation and infections. This substance also causes dilation of the blood vessels and inhibits blood clotting.

Some children have been decapitated by air bags even at low speeds. In one case which resulted from a minor bump in a parking lot a one-year-old child was decapitated with the head passing through the window and landing on the pavement. Simply working on an automobile can cause deployment of airbags. General Motors had given the National Highway Traffic Safety Admisnistration (NHTSA) the results of its crash testing that demonstrated the lethal potential of airbags, but Joan Claybrook, who was head of NHTSA chose to ignore those warnings.

The casualty list at long last has forced the officials to consider some modification and refinement of the device. These fascist bureaucrats steadfastly refuse to admit that airbags were a mistake, however, and continue to waste tax dollars in an attempt to develope a "safe" airbag. They continue to mandate that this lethal device be installed in all automobiles. Studies that revealed that mandatory seat belt laws not only did not save lives but may have resulted in an increase in fatalities were suppressed by the government.[12] The same mentality and deceit is being exhibited regarding air bags. May God save us from these brainless bureaucrats. A partial list of the injuries that have been reported in medical journals from airbags is included at the end of this chapter.

Another example of blind obedience to fanaticism is the mandated installation of expensive scrubbers on the smokestacks of every powerplant in the United States in the 1980s for the purpose of reducing sulfur emissions. This law was enacted even after Congress had received the report of a team of scientists who spent $540 million over a ten-year period studying the acid rain accusations. In their National Acid Rain Precipitation Assessment Project (NAPAP) report they found no evidence of harm to lakes, streams, fish, crops, forests or people from acid rain. They reported that the acidity of the lakes and streams reflected the acidity or alkalinity of the soil and rocks through which ground water had passed, not precipitation. Similar studies carried out in Europe between 1980 and 1990 reached the same conclusions, and demonstrated that there had been an actual increase in the total forest area since 1950, continuing through 1990. The same increase has been noted in the United States following the period of deforestation between 1850 and 1910. The NAPAP study found that the Great Lakes were four times cleaner than they had been in 1970. Those of us who used those bodies of water for recreation during that period had witnessed this cleanup first hand. Congress enacted the legislation in spite of having received the report.

This expenditure, which costs us over $4 billion every year, was required even of those powerplants that burned coal that contained no sulfur. The fact that this retrofit resulted in a reduction of thermodynamic efficiency that actually increased carbon dioxide emissions per kilowatt-hour by 10 percent was totally ignored. At the same time there has been a hysterical clamor to eliminate carbon dioxide emissions before they destroy the ozone layer. Another example of the right hand not knowing what the left hand was doing. In the meantime huge deposits of sulfur free coal have been discovered, and the acid rain theory has been completely disproved.[13] The hysteria that the environmentalists and news media cultivated over tree damage that was supposedly caused by SO_2 from smokestacks was allowed to quietly fade away after the damage was revealed to be caused by diseases and pests.

After the government and the environmental extremists had squandered billions of dollars on the smokestack fiasco, they undertook a campaign to eliminate coal fired generating plants completely. A virtual moratorium was placed on the construction of any new coal generating plants, and many existing plants were converted to natural gas, a fuel that is far less abundant. The great increase in the demand for natural gas gradually outstripped supply, and during the winter season of 2000-2001 the price of natural gas supplied to homes for heat skyrocketed. During this same period the failure to build new generating capacity to match increased industrial demand and population growth over the preceding decade resulted in power failures and periods of interrupted supply to homes and industry, most dramatic in California. This is just the beginning of woes. The inadequacy of power supplies is growing, and it takes years to build new generating plants, even if the extremists permitted such construction.

In the same Clean Air Act amendments of 1990[14] that mandated the oxygenated gasoline, Congress also required that auto manufacturers install on-board canisters to capture the gasoline vapors that normally escape into the atmosphere during refueling. The logic seemed to be that it was safer for the automobiles to carry this bomb, rather than have the vapors dissipated into the atmosphere where they produced no harm. Even the National Transportation Safety Board admits that these canisters of gasoline vapors present a serious safety hazard. They also cause gasoline to be spit out on the ground during the refueling process, and cause vapor locks during driving. As of the New Year 2001, after almost ten years of discussion of the hazards, the canisters are still required by law. Ralph Nader's Center for Auto Safety assures us that they do not present a hazard. His team of lawyers will benefit greatly from the injuries and deaths that ensue. Such complications of legislation and regulations, even though they almost always occur, are never anticipated and are never acknowledged by the culprits.

The Clean Air Act amendments of 1990 forced the reformulation of many aerosol products in order to save the world from the so called ozone-depleting solvents such as 1,1,1 trichloroethane, and carbon dioxide as a propellant because of its supposed contribution to the "greenhouse" effect. The result has been at least 198 reported cases of acute respiratory illness from shoe sprays that had been reformulated to comply with the new laws.[15] It does not take a Nobel laureate to recognize that carbon dioxide is a far more innocuous propellant than isobutane.

The lunacy continues; the EPA is currently spending many more millions of dollars to remove and replace soil at several former mining sites, ostensibly because of high lead levels. In fact their measurements have been shown to be faulty. Furthermore experts state that the type of lead present is not a threat and is safer left in place. A review of the subject that was published in *Regulatory Toxicology and Pharmacology* states that these mining wastes present little health hazard because of the form that the lead content is in. The low lead levels in the local residents has confirmed this. The advice of the experts is to treat the soil containing the lead, if any action must be taken. This is a repeat of the *Times Beach* circus, and it is being duplicated at several former mining sites in Colorado and in Pennsylvania.

The examples of a Congress and bureaucratic monsters out of control are too numerous to enumerate in this brief discussion. I highly recommend that everyone who is concerned with the issue read and study *Phantom Risk*,[16] *Galileo's Revenge;junk science in the courtroom*,[17] *EcoScam: The False Prophets of Ecological Apocalypse*,[18] *The True State of the Planet*[19] and *Earth Report 2000*.[20] The first book contains assessments of the true risk of many of the items and substances that have found their way into court to reward the trial lawyers. It includes the works of 23 imminent and reputable scientists and is based upon an analysis of all of the available scientific data. This data is tabulated for the reader. Also documented are the hundreds of millions of dollars that have been wasted in false claims of damage.

The latter three books by Ronald Bailey expose the hoaxes that are perpetrated on the public by the extremist groups, and explains their motives. Time alone has proved all of these wild predictions wrong. Huber's book on junk science details the deceit and dishonesty in the courts and legal system that permits huge settlements where there is indeed no blame or basis for liability. The philosophy of the trial lawyers is that the money comes out of the magical deep pockets of a corporation; in effect a money tree. The reality is that the loss of these enormous sums from our economic system means fewer jobs, higher prices for goods and a lower standard of living for our posterity. A significant portion of the price that the U.S. consumer pays for virtually every product and service represents a hidden tax to cover liability costs. In short this is nothing other than judicially sanctioned extortion.

It is ironic that the environmental extremists and the news media have been so successful in promulgating vast new government bureaucracies, with the concomitant tyranny, persecution and squandering of billions of dollars, during the very period when so much had been accomplished in cleaning up the lakes, streams and air. This progress was obvious to anyone who visited and enjoyed these natural resources. Nowhere was it more impressive than in the Great Lakes. It is fortunate that this progress was accomplished before the diversion of enormous sums of money by the EPA and the courts to non-productive judgements and legal fees.

H.L. Menken (1880-1956) observed that "The whole aim of practical politics is to keep the populace alarmed (and hence clamorous to be led to safety) by menacing it with an endless series of hobglobins, all of them imaginary." This tactic has been developed to a new level of perfection by government in recent years, cultivating a new "plantation system." In this system the politicians and the bureaucrats are the masters, while all of the working masses serve as their slaves. The challenge to the taxpaying public is to recognize this ploy and to attempt to make judgements based upon scientific fact about each "crises" thus presented. This is very difficult to do because the news media chooses to be a party to the fraud. They remain enchanted with the concept of a "people's paradise" and view themselves as members of the elite ruling class, the "self-annointed" as Thomas Sowell so aptly puts it. They fail to remember the history of the media's fate in previous totalitarian regimes, and as George Santayana[21] observed, are destined to repeat the past. The deception has also been successful because too few of the honest and legitimate scientific community have stepped forward in public forum to set the record straight. Fortunately more and more of these individuals, alarmed and disturbed by the lies and distortion of data by their colleages, are speaking out in protest.

This book attempts to present the facts regarding the various environmental risks that the public faces, with emphasis on those areas where a genuine hazard exists. The sensible precautions that can prevent exposure to these hazards are then described. These are usually simple, common sense actions that require only knowledge and awareness. It is late in the season, but if a large enough segment of the voting public becomes concerned and educated, the lunacy of the government and extremist self-serving organizations can be countered. If not, economic disaster and great violence await further down the road.

AIR BAG INJURIES REPORTED BY PHYSICIANS, 1998 & 1999*

Fracture of forearm (several cases reported).
Eye injuries, chemical and physical
Rupture of the diaphragm
Fatal brain injury at 12 miles per hour
Hearing loss at low speed
Traumatic dissection of the nerves in the heart
Alkali burns of face and neck
Contusion of the globe of the eye
Retinal detachment
Rupture of the choroid of the eye with permanent loss of vision
Laceration of the cornea of the eye from glasses
Corneal abraisions
Hemorrhage into the eye, frequently seen, many cases reported
Quadriplegia
Severed cervical spinal cord in the neck, fatal.
Subarachnoid (brain) hemorrhage
Dislocation of vertebra at base of skull d/t torn ligament
Fracture of fourth cervical vertebra, dislocation at base of skull, subarachnoid hemorrhage, multiple fractures of skull in 3½ year old at less than 30 mph.
Dislocation of jaw (two cases)
Eye injury with retinal tear
Bilateral pneumothorax
Eye injuries (over one hundred in this report).
Hemorrhage in the eye, retinal tear, retinal detachment.
Avulsion (tearing away) of occipital bone (base of skull).
Perilymphatic fistula
Retinitis sclopetaria
Fatal separation of spinal cord from dislocation at base of skull.
Primary enulceation (removal of the eyeball).

Placental abruptio and fetal death.
Permanent hearing loss, persistent tinnitus, dizziness (several cases).
Lower extremity burns in a child.
Dental injuries (several cases reported).
Fatal dislocation of spine at base of skull
Open fractures of forearm at low speed, two cases reported
Reflex sympathetic dystrophy
Forearm fracture
Dysequilibrium (10 cases), tympanic membrane perforation (four cases)
Full thickness chemical burn of hand from sodium azide propellent
Decapitation
Tricuspid (heart) valve injury
Persistent corneal edema requiring corneal transplant.
Tear of ascending aorta.
Fatal rupture of aortic isthmus
Dislocated pelvic fracture
Rupture of right atrium (heart).
Retinal detachment
Rupture of the sclera of the eye
Dislocation of the lens of the eye
Fatal cranio-cervical dislocation in a 5 year-old in 1996
Fatal basilar skull fracture at low speed
Perforation of eyeball by a pipe stem
Rupture of the lens of the eye requiring intraocular lens implant in ten-year-old, minor accident.
Laceration of cornea and sclera with significant permanent loss of vision, at low speed.
Rupture of eyeball and retinal detachment
Bilateral displacement of lens of eye and anterior chamber hemorrhage resulting in blindness.
Rupture of azygos vein
Blow out rupture of the orbit into the nasal cavity.
Twenty-five cases ranging from mild corneal abraision to retinal detachment.
Bilateral hyphema (hemorrhage into anterior chamber of eye).
Traumatic hearing loss
Fatal transection of ascending aorta
Facial nerve paralysis
Fatal injury to descending thoracic aorta
Rupture of the right atrium of the heart
Bilateral Smith fracture of the radius
Acute asthmatic attack from inhalation of air bag propellent.

Bilateral corneal contusion and angle recession
Fatal ventral rupture of medulla and diffuse axonal injury of brain.

    * These represent only some of the cases that were published in the medical literature during 1998 and 1999. Many injuries, probably the majority, thus are not listed here.

1. Schneider S H. *The Genesis Strategy*. New York: Plenum Press, 1976. pp. 84-92.

2. Walter Williams. *The Washington Times*, August 31, 2001.

3. Paul R. Ehrlich. The Population Bomb. Rivercity, Mass: Rivercity Press, 1975.

4. The current Paul Ehrlich, a professor at Stanford, should not be confused with the distinguished Dr. Paul Ehrlich of the Koch Institute in Germany (1854-1915) who was awarded the Nobel Prize in 1908. He made many contributions to science including the discovery of "compound 606", Salvarsan, for the treatent of syphilis, as well as insights into the function of the immune system.

5. Ray D L, Guzzo L. *Trashing the Planet*. Washington D.C.: Regnery Gateway, 1990.

6. Blum A, Ames BN. Flame-retardant additives as possible cancer hazards. Science **195**:17-23, Jan 7, 1977.

7. Gold MD, Blum A, Ames BN. Another flame retardant, Tris-(1,3-Dichloro-2-Propyl)Phosphate, and its expected metabolites are Mutagens. *Science* **200**:785-787 (May 19, 1978).

8. Blum A, Gold MD, Ames BN et al. Children absorb Tris-BP flame retardant from sleepwear: Urine contains the mutagenic metabolite, 2,3-Dibromopropanol. *Science* **201**, 1020-1023 (September 15, 1978).

9. Op cit.

10. McCann J, Ames BN. The *Salmonella*/microsome mutagenicity test: predictive value for animal carcinogenicity. In: Hiatt HH, Watson JD, Winsten JA eds. *Origins of Human Cancer*. New York: Cold Spring Harbor Laboratory, 1977: 1431-1450.

11. Ullman O. Carmakers dropping Tris. Associated Press, June 23, 1977.

12. Richens J, Imrie J, Copas A. Condoms and seat belts: the parallels and the lessons. *Lancet* 2000;**355**:400-403.

13. The Spring 1986 issue of *Amicus* stated that "acid rain is destroying our soil, forests and lakes — the basis of the earth's life-support system — and damage is

occurring coast to coast." The National Acid Rain Precipitation Assessment Project was established by the federal government to scientifically assess the issue. After five years of extensive study and research by the most eminent scientists, at a cost of $500 million, they concluded that the wild claims of damage from acid rain were totally without any foundation. The mandated expenditure of billions of dollars to install equipment to decrease sulfur dioxide emissions had no justification.

14. Public Law no. 101-549.

15. CDC. Severe acute respiratory illness linked to use of shoe sprays—Colorado, November 1993. *MMWR* 1993;**42**:885-887.

16. Foster KR, Bernstein DE and Huber, PW eds. *Phantom Risk; Scientific inference and the law*. Cambridge Mass: MIT Press, 1993.

17. Huber P. *Galileo's revenge: Junk science in the courtroom*. New York: Basic Books, 1991.

18. Bailey R. *EcoScam: The false prophets of ecological apocalypse*. New York: St. Martin's Press, 1993.

19. Bailey R. Ed. *The True State of the Planet*. The Free Press: New York, 1995.

20. Bailey, Ronald, ed. *Earth Report 2000*. New York: McGraw-Hill, 2000.

21. *Those who cannot remember the past are condemned to repeat it.* — George Santayana, Spanish-American philosopher

I

HAZARDS OF THE HOUSEHOLD

Whenever in doubt, tell the truth   — Mark Twain

ACCIDENTS
More than 20,000 people die as a result of accidents in or around the home each year in the United States. More than 6,000 of these deaths result from falls, many on stairs, ladders and in bathtubs. Most of these tragedies could be prevented by such simple measures as placement of nonskid mats in tubs, keeping stairs free of all toys and other materials, and more careful placement of ladders to assure a secure and firm base. If the ladder is constructed of wood, the rungs and steps should be inspected for cracks or other defects. Proper placement of the top of the ladder against a firm and secure surface is as important as having a secure platform at the bottom. Leaning too far out from the ladder is a sure recipe for a fall. Hand rails on stairways and in bathtubs are essential for the elderly and for those with arthritis or other afflictions that affect stability of footing.

About 160 people die in the home each year as a result of electrocution. This hazard has been greatly reduced by the modern electrical codes. Children remain at great risk, however, and solutions to this problem are discussed in Chapter III. Accidents of an unusual nature continue to occur each year, such as dropping a hair dryer in the bathtub while standing or sitting in water. No electrical appliance should ever be brought near or placed in the proximity of the bathtub or washbasin. This has been a repeated source of electrocution over the years.

The risk of electrocution while flying kites should have had enough publicity by now to eliminate this accident, but it continues to occur each year. The same can be said about the use of aluminum ladders and the erection of radio, television and CB antennas. Other aluminum or steel devices that are brought into contact with overhead power lines are cleaning devices for outdoor swimming pools and masts for sailboats. Digging into an underground power line can be just as deadly. When cleaning up fallen trees and branches following a storm, fallen power lines must be observed and avoided.

Approximately 700 people in the United States drown at home each year, in swimming pools and in bathtubs. Swimming pools are a particular hazard for children. An adequate fence and secure gate reduces this risk, but small children must still be kept under constant vigilance. Even small plastic pools for children present an opportunity for disaster, particularly when very young children are left unattended. Play equipment at home is another hazard for children. The surface beneath the equipment that they are likely to fall from should be a forgiving material such as wood mulch, rather than asphalt or cement. Equipment made from treated lumber should be sealed with varnish to prevent arsenic containing splinters from gaining entrance to the skin.

Outdoor power equipment causes many injuries each year. More than 60,000 people are treated each year in U. S. hospital emergency rooms for injuries received from power lawn mowers. Many of these injuries are severe, including loss of fingers and toes. The most common injury results from contact with the rotating blade, either with fingers or toes. This often happens on slopes where control is either lost or the mower rolls backwards over the feet. It is safer to mow perpendicularly across slopes than up or down. Sturdy shoes will offer more protection than bare feet or sandals. Attempts to lift the mower or adjust the height while it is running present an obvious risk to fingers. Few people wear a necktie while mowing the lawn, but loose clothing becoming entangled in power equipment has brought serious injury to many people. Loose, long hair can be just as hazardous, and it cannot be left hanging in the closet during the project.

Refilling the mower while the engine is hot invites the obvious fire hazard. The mower should be started outdoors; not only do you want to avoid carbon monoxide fumes, but also if the mower catches fire, you don't want the house and garage to go up in flames with it. Smoking during this task is a pretty obvious risk, but I still see people refueling automobiles while smoking. Projectiles such as stones, nails, dog bones and toys can be lethal when they evolve from the discharge chute of a mower. The many windows that they smash are perturbing, but if they hit your child's head it will be a greater jolt to your emotions and your pocketbook.

Children should be indoors when this job is underway.

Knives, razors, scissors and all similar sharp and pointed objects throughout the house should be locked up or placed securely out of the reach of children. Many such hazards are housed in the household sewing box. This should be kept in either a room or a closet that is securely locked.

Farm households are responsible for a disproportionate percentage of injuries reported. This is due in part because the hazards of the workplace are combined with the home, and the workplace is an inherently dangerous one. Traumatic amputations of fingers, hands and arms occur every year from farm machinery such as corn pickers and harvesters.

Particularly tragic are the incidents where women have had their scalp ripped off by hay balers when their hair became entangled in the drive train. One woman had her right ear ripped off along with her scalp. Hair has a long history of entanglement in machinery on the job. On average 16 workers per year are killed by entanglement in rotating drivelines on farm machinery in the United States. Approximately 150 non-fatal injuries from such equipment are treated in emergency rooms each year.

FIRE

More than 4,000 Americans die each year in residential fires and some 20,000 additional individuals suffer injuries. The financial loss amounts to about 8.6 billion dollars per year. Approximately three fourths of all fire related deaths occur in the home. It is safe to say that the thought of a fire in the home, especially during the night when the family is asleep, evokes fear in just about everyone.

The first step to take to minimize the risk of this personal and financial disaster in your home is to methodically tour the entire residence room by room, then the basement and garage, and remove all obvious risks. Matches, candles and cigarette lighters, with their fuel, should not be stored where children can get their hands on them. Simply placing these items on a shelf that is high off the floor will not safeguard them, as has been proven on many occasions. These items, along with medications, cleaning agents and harmful chemicals, need to be stored under lock and key. It is neither difficult nor expensive to have an effective lock installed on a closet or storage cabinet door. This may seem inconvenient but it is one of the necessary sacrifices that must be made for the privilege of having children.

Moving to the garage, inventory all combustible items such as solvents (naphtha, paint and lacquer thinner), gasoline for mowers, and Coleman fuel. These items should never be stored in the basement, and never in the garage if any pilot lights exist there. It is far safer to store gasoline and flammable liquids in a storage shed, removed from the house. The quantity of these items that are kept on hand should be limited. They tend to accumulate, and need to be inventoried and disposed of periodically. Stores of gasoline should be limited to the smallest practical volume. Gasoline is a highly flammable and dangerous substance.

Aluminum wiring is another fire hazard that exists, particularly in homes built between 1965 and 1973. During this period aluminum wiring was used in approximately 1.5 million homes in the United States. Aluminum wiring was approved by the National Electrical Code during that period. This approval was rescinded after fires occurred as a result of overheating at connections between the aluminum wire and switches and outlets. The overheating resulted from oxidation of the aluminum wire with a resultant increase in the electrical resistance at the connection with the terminals on the switch or appliance.

If your home was built during this period, the wiring should be inspected for this possibility. The type of wiring (aluminum or copper) can be readily ascertained by removing the cover plates of the wall outlets and switches and observing the wire where it connects. The same observation can be made at the entrance box where the fuses or breakers are located. It is possible that in a house built prior to 1965 aluminum wiring was used when additional circuits were installed. It is also still possible to purchase aluminum wiring for some applications such as cables to outlying buildings. The difference in the cost of the two materials makes the choice of aluminum attractive, particularly with the great increase in copper prices since about 1989. It is a bad bargain however.

In the event that you find aluminum wiring in your home, it is not necessary to rip it out and replace it. If the switches, outlets, light fixtures and appliances (dryers, ranges) are unmarked, or are marked AL/CU, they can be replaced by units that are marked

CO/ALR, indicating that they are safe for use with aluminum wire. Alternately you can attach a six to eight inch length of copper wire to the switch or outlet, and then connect this to the aluminum wire with connectors especially designed for this purpose. This connection requires a special crimping tool and a special technique. Sealing of this connection to prevent oxidation is also essential. A breach in the proper technique at any one of these connections may result in a house fire. It is also essential that all junction boxes be examined to assure that no copper to aluminum connection goes undetected. Contracting the services of an electrician who is trained and skilled in this technique is the best way to assure that this risk is properly dealt with.

Perhaps the next step to take is the installation of effective smoke detectors in strategic locations. One should be placed near the kitchen, one near the bedrooms and one near any room with a wood-burning fireplace or stove. Notice that I say near. If a smoke detector is installed in the kitchen, it will sound the alarm every time a meal is prepared. It will prove more peaceful to install the detector in a room next to the kitchen. If properly located, it will still detect a fire early, but will not be set off by cooking a meal. An exhaust fan in the kitchen, used when cooking, will also help to eliminate false alarms. Similarly the exhaust from an automobile may set off a smoke detector placed in the garage. A detector placed in a room with a furnace may be set off by combustion ions from the furnace. Trial and error may be necessary to determine a location where this is not a problem.

In two-story homes detectors should be placed on each level. One unit on the second level should be sufficient to protect the bedrooms in most homes. If you are unfortunate enough to have a smoker in the house, a detector should be placed in that bedroom. One should also be placed in the basement, although it must be located far enough away from the furnace to avoid false alarms. In locating detectors near sources of combustion such as in the kitchen, and near fireplaces and furnaces it may be wise to try a temporary placement long enough to assure that a false alarm will not be a problem before drilling holes in the ceiling.

After the smoke detectors have been installed, it is important to check their operation periodically. Most have a test button, but this may not test for dirt accumulation. All of the units should be vacuumed regularly to prevent dust buildup and blockage by insects. One positive way to test the units is to light a match underneath each unit, blow it out and allow the smoke to drift into the detector. Blowing fresh air across the detector with a small fan can shorten the length of the alarm thus evoked.

The nine volt batteries that power these units will last about one year, if they are fresh and of good quality. Most detectors emit periodic beeps for about a week when the battery needs replacement. This warning can easily be missed if it occurs while the family is away on vacation. The match test provides a more positive indication of battery integrity. Remember that a detector installed in the ceiling is nothing but an eyesore if it is inoperative.

After you have completed the installation of the smoke detectors, it is time to turn your attention to fire extinguishers. Better yet these should be purchased at the same time as the smoke detectors. This selection is more complex, because there are different types of extinguishers for different types of fires. The decision can be simplified by buying all-purpose extinguishers that are effective against all three classes of fires, A, B and C. If price is no object, you can select one of the halon models, which have the added advantage of not leaving a corrosive residue that will damage whatever items you save from the fire. If you choose a less expensive all-purpose unit, it will contain a chemical such as ammonium phosphate, which does leave a corrosive residue.

The most important location for a fire extinguisher is in the kitchen, for about three-fourths of all home fires occur there. One should also be accessible from any wood-burning fireplace or stove. One unit may serve this purpose as well as for the kitchen if they are not widely separated. A unit should be located in the basement, particularly if a workshop is located there, and one in the garage. These should also be all-purpose types.

If you have a spare three or four thousands dollars left over after the above purchases, you can consider having a sprinkler system installed. New technology in recent years has resulted in sprinkler systems for private residences that are effective, if costly. In new construction such units add about two thousand dollars to the cost. Some fire officials are pressing to have these units included in building codes as required items. In making such an argument the cost of a human life invariably surfaces.

While it is difficult to argue against saving lives, the cost of a new home already includes several thousand dollars mandated by building codes, licenses, plan inspection, foundation inspection, framework inspections, plumbing inspections, electrical inspections, final inspection, termite inspections, appraisal fees, credit checks, title searches, application charges, filing charges, realtor commission, and of course lawyer's fees. Mandatory radon inspection is on the horizon. Impact fees (road, sewers, water etc) currently add $24,000 to the cost of new homes in the San Diego area. And your irreplaceable, tenured congressman is complaining that houses are priced beyond the reach of the "average American," so more government subsidies are needed. Subsidies, of course, always mean picking the pocket of taxpayers.

THE KITCHEN

One of the most common hazards in the kitchen is that of burns. Most burns that are acquired during cooking or baking are not life threatening. More tragic are burns to children. These frequently occur as a result of the child pulling a pan of boiling water or hot food off of the stove as a matter of curiosity. Keeping the handles turned inward helps to reduce this risk. The inquisitive and exploring nature of young children is the major cause of accidents and injuries in this age group. Young children need constant supervision. Thousands are injured each year simply because they had a few minutes of unsupervised time.

These thermal burns have had wide publicity, and most people are at least aware that they are a risk. Not so well known is the risk of chemical burns, and the many substances in the household that can cause them. There are several very potent substances found in the kitchen that are not encountered in most other walks of life, other than in chemistry laboratories.

One of these hazardous substances, and one that is a threat to adults and children alike, is household ammonia (ammonium hydroxide). This substance penetrates the eye particularly rapidly when accidentally splashed in it, and can produce severe, permanent eye damage after as short a time as three minutes. This can occur even if copious irrigation is undertaken immediately. Household ammonia should never be mixed with household bleach of the chlorine type, or with any household cleaner including wall and tile cleaner, and toilet bowl cleaner. Mixing these two substances causes a chemical reaction that releases hazardous gases. Mixing household bleach, or any cleaner containing it, with any acid cleaner such as phosphoric acid, releases chlorine gas and other noxious chemicals. Many of the laundry and cleaning preparations have been reformulated to include chlorine bleach, sodium hypochlorite. Similarly ammonia is incorporated in some common cleaning solutions such as window cleaners.

It has become very important to study the contents on the labels of household cleaning substances. When substances of this nature are poured from a container in an occupational setting, eye protection such as a face shield is required, and the operation is undertaken in a ventilated hood. Mixing of these chemicals is usually done in systems that prevent human exposure. One does not often see such precautions taken at home.

Oven cleaners and drain cleaners are strong alkali substances that can produce severe chemical burns of both the skin and the eye. They contain sodium hydroxide, a very caustic substance. Durable rubber or plastic gloves must be worn when handling these materials, and the fumes must not be inhaled. A ventilating fan, **DUCTED TO THE OUTSIDE**, is helpful in minimizing inhalation of these irritating fumes. Many kitchen fans are not ducted to the outside, but merely recirculate the air through a filter. These are cheaper to install but they are of very limited usefulness. They do nothing to remove noxious or hazardous fumes. Strong alkali substances also can cause destruction of vision, and great care must be taken not to splash or spray this caustic in the eye. Particular care should be taken with the aerosol sprays to make certain that they are directed away from the body.

A properly installed ventilating fan can also help to reduce the risk of inhaling oil fumes from cooking. Oil inhaled into the lung interferes with the ciliary action that works to remove inhaled particles. It also can invoke a chronic inflammatory reaction in the lungs that may progress to lipoid pneumonia with fibrosis, and destruction of lung function. The ventilating fan should always be employed when cooking with oil, and when using aerosol cooking oil sprays. Lipoid pneumonia was more common in the past when mineral oil was commonly used as a vehicle for nose drops. Inhalation of mineral oil fumes remains an occupational risk for machinists and mechanics where adequate protective measures are not provided.

Drain cleaners are among the most heavily promoted household items encountered. A generous and diverse supply is available. One reason for this is that the members of households permit substances that will not readily flow through the drainpipes to enter the drains with remarkable frequency. In some instances inadequate or faulty plumbing contributes to the problem. Drains and sewers were basically designed to carry liquids for the most part, however. Another reason for the heavy promotion is that there is no magic bullet. None of the products produce a miracle in clearing plugged drains. Prevention remains the best solution.

The chemicals that are available to unclog drains are very strong substances, either a strong alkali or a potent acid. These obviously are hazardous to handle, and hazardous to store under your sink, where the children play. These substances can cause severe burns to the mouth, throat and esophagus. If the child survives, he will require some serious surgery. In pouring these substances into the drain the dangers of splashing them on the skin or in the eye are as severe as with ammonia discussed above. They should not be used without adequate protection, including eye protection. They should not be stored under the sink. If they are kept around the home, they should be stored under lock and key.

A safer and more direct approach to clogged plumbing is to use one of the mechanical devices available. The first tool to use should be a plunger or the hand auger. These will unclog most of the simple plugged drains. An electric auger can be rented at any of the rental agencies if the manual tool does not do the job. Various devices that apply pressure or a vacuum, or that attach to a hose and faucet for more pressure, have been introduced to deal with this ubiquitous household problem. Extreme caution should be taken in any instance where one of the strong chemicals has been tried first. It is far wiser to not get into that predicament.

In some instances, such as where the doll has been flushed down the toilet, there is no alternative to simply uncoupling the bowl and removing the culprit manually. In the case of the kitchen sink or bathroom basin, it is usually a simple chore to remove the trap and pour out the assortment of jewelry, beads, buttons and contact lenses. If the clog resides in the main sewer line it may well require a professional service. Consult the yellow pages.

Automatic dishwasher detergents are another strong alkali substance that has caused loss of vision. When one of the small particles is accidentally splashed in the eye it adheres, produces a burn and penetrates the eye. Alkali substances such as this are much more damaging than acids. If the detergent powder has been spilled, you should never blow on it. With the new liquid preparations, the risk of splashing it into the eye is present, as when pouring any liquid.

Another source of eye damage and loss of vision that is present in the kitchen, that one would not ordinarily think of, is the garbage disposal. Eye damage occurs when an object is ejected from the disposal. It is natural to look into the disposal during operation, but this temptation should be resisted. Objects sent into orbit from this appliance should strike the ceiling, not your eye.

Hand dishwashing detergents generally contain surfactants, not strong alkali substances, and are less damaging to the skin. They are effective at removing the protective oils from the skin, nonetheless, and produce dryness, irritation and cracking. Secondary infections are always a risk when the skin defensive barrier is thus disrupted. This problem can be dealt with by wearing latex or vinyl gloves when prolonged or repeated immersion of the hands is necessary. Frequent applications of a good hand cream such as Lanolor® will help to restore the protective oils to the skin. Hydrocortisone creams should NOT be used as a hand cream for this purpose. They contribute nothing that a plain hand cream does not, and carry the added risk of encouraging the spread of an infection if one occurs. Additionally, some absorption into the systemic circulation will occur with chronic application of hydrocortisone to the skin, especially with cracks and abrasions. This would be tantamount to taking a small oral dose daily, which could have a suppressive effect on the adrenal glands.

The use of aerosol cooking oils can present a risk of developing lipoid pneumonia, for which there is no cure, if oil particles are inhaled. These oil particles can remain suspended in the air for at least fifteen minutes, and can be inhaled during that period. An exhaust fan will help to clear the air, and the duration of spraying should be kept to a minimum. Working in the area should be avoided during the period of risk.

THE LAUNDRY

The effectiveness of laundry detergents has been greatly improved by the addition of enzymes to facilitate the removal of stains and soil. The enzyme commonly used is alcalase, which is produced by the fermentation of the bacterium, *Bacillus subtilis*. Many people become sensitized to this enzyme, and allergic reactions are common. The reaction may vary from sneezing and coughing to a severe asthmatic reaction. The latter is more likely to occur in individuals who have a history of asthma. This hazard can be minimized by exercising care when pouring the detergent to avoid disseminating the powder into the room air. Using the liquid forms of the detergents eliminates the dust problem, but skin contact still should be avoided if sensitization has developed. In fact skin contact with the enzyme detergents should be avoided to prevent the development of skin sensitivity to the enzyme.

TSP: Trisodium phosphate was formerly incorporated into all laundry detergents, greatly enhancing their cleaning ability. Many states and municipalities banned its use to lessen the phosphate buildup in lakes and streams, and it was subsequently eliminated from all laundry detergents in the United States. Nothing has been developed that cleans as well without the phosphates. It also was incorporated into other cleaners and sold separately as a powder for the cleaning of walls, floors and decks. It has been eliminated recently from even these products, although the label of some would have you believe that they still contain TSP. TSP is a strong irritant to the skin, and whenever these cleaning substances are used, latex or vinyl gloves should be worn to protect the skin. It should never be permitted to come in contact with the skin. Care should be taken also to avoid letting the solution run down the arm when cleaning overhead.

The goal of most people in doing laundry is to have the clothes come out looking clean. Many whiteners and bleaches have been marketed to make the laundry more pleasing to the eye. An equally important objective should be to destroy the many microbial agents, the bacteria, fungi, viruses and protozoa that go along with the dirt. Good laundry detergents, used in adequate concentration, are effective in accomplishing this goal, but the temperature of the water has much to do with the level of success. The higher the temperature of the wash water, the more effective is the laundry process in killing microbial agents.

Many spores, such as those that cause botulism and tetanus, are relatively resistant to destruction by high temperatures. High temperatures in conjunction with the surface-acting agents found in laundry detergents greatly increase the destruction of these disease-causing agents. The addition of household bleach of the chlorine type will increase the destruction of microorganisms to an even greater degree, where the fabric permits. It is also important to use an adequate quantity of detergent, and the instructions on the package are only a guide. More will be required where the water is hard (high mineral content) and where the clothing is heavily soiled. The proper amount must be determined for each load if the laundry is to be truly cleansed and sanitized.

It has become popular to lower the temperature of the water in laundry and dish washing operations in an effort to save energy. Laundry products are widely advertised for their cleaning ability in cold water. It is clear that clothes and linens can be made to appear bright and clean in cold water. There is no simple way to determine how many of the disease-producing agents have survived, however. The small amount of money saved by such false economy could better be saved by economies elsewhere in the household. This is especially true in the dishwasher.

Nowhere in the household is cleanliness more important than in the kitchen. Certainly one wants to destroy the *Salmonella* and other organisms that can produce diarrheal disease, and the virus that can transmit hepatitis, to mention only two. The temperature in the dishwasher should ideally be at least 160 degrees Fahrenheit, not the 120 degrees that some advocate. The practice of producing and marketing water heaters that deliver water at such low temperatures should not only be condemned, but should be banned as a public health measure. Outbreaks of Legionnaires' disease in hospitals has been traced to low temperature water heaters; the organism cannot thrive when the temperature in these is above 140° F.

The development of odors in towels and washcloths shortly after laundering is a clear sign that the level of cleaning was less than desirable. The addition of chlorine bleach, sodium hypochlorite, is effective in solving this problem for the reasons mentioned above. It must be used in accordance with the instructions on the package, however. These agents cannot be used on some fabrics. The so-called non-chlorine bleaches may be substituted to enhance cleaning in those fabrics that will not tolerate chlorine, but keep in mind that they do not possess the disease-killing power of chlorine bleach. Very hot water becomes all the more urgent in those circumstances.

Fabric softeners contain substances that neutralize the electrostatic charge on clothing. These substances do not carry a significant toxicity in normal use. The cloth fabric softeners produced a skin irritation in many people nationwide a few years ago, but this problem seems to have lessened. Presumably this irritation was due to a fiber in the cloth, since the irritation was similar to that produced by fiberglass. The perfumes in these fabric softeners may present a problem to some individual who are sensitive to them. Those individuals should use the unscented packages that are available.

THE BATHROOM

Toilet bowel cleaners contain the same strong alkali substances that are used in oven cleaners and drain cleaners. Great care must be taken to avoid splashing them into the eye. If they are accidentally spilled on the skin, it should be washed immediately, flushing with water first, then washing thoroughly with soap and water. These products should not be mixed with ammonia for the reasons discussed previously.

Electrocution has been an age-old hazard in the bathroom. This has resulted from tuning radios while in the bathtub, or dropping a hair dryer or other electrical appliance into water in the tub or basin. Caution must be exercised with any electrical appliance in the bathroom. Children in particular must be monitored to prevent these tragedies from claiming their lives. Hair curling irons left unattended in the bathroom brings about 6,400 children under the age of five years into emergency rooms each year. These same hot irons bring approximately 1,700 young adults into emergency rooms each year with accidental burns to the eyes while they are using them.

Several different aerosol sprays that present a health hazard are used in the bathroom. The propellant in all of these is a hazard. Freon was used in the past, and it was removed to satisfy the unwarranted concern over the ozone layer in the atmosphere. Then vinyl chloride was used until it was discovered that it produces cancer. Following that, methylene chloride was substituted, until it was discovered that it caused cancer in laboratory animals. This substance, more accurately identified as dichloromethane, is very toxic to the liver and the brain, in addition to its carcinogenicity. Butane is used in some products as a replacement for Freon, but environmentalists now complain that butane is as troublesome as was Freon. Carbon dioxide has been used recently as a propellant in some aerosol sprays, and does not present a toxic hazard. It also presents no hazard to the environment. It is a safe and effective substitute, and it should be the universal propellant today, but the bureaucrats and environmental extremists are obsessed with an unwarranted fear of a "greenhouse effect" crisis.

Of particular concern is the use of these toxic and hazardous substances in a small confined space such as a bathroom, where significant inhalation is assured. It has been demonstrated that these aerosols remain suspended in the air in bathrooms for at least fifteen minutes. Ideally, when these materials are used, one should have the exhaust fan on, should spray the hair as quickly as possible, and should vacate the bathroom as soon as possible. It should remain vacant for at least fifteen to twenty minutes.

In 1992 and 1993 at least 195 individuals were treated for an acute respiratory illness that resulted from using shoe spray leather conditioners.[1] These products had been reformulated to comply with the Clean Air Act amendments of 1990. While the new law had made them more "environmentally friendly," it had rendered them less consumer friendly; 23 persons were hospitalized. With our government protecting us with their usual zeal, it will be ever more urgent to be alert to new hazards. All chemicals and sprays should be used only where adequate ventilation is available. This is not provided in the bathroom.

In addition to the propellants in hair spray, other risks have been identified with components such as polyvinylpyrrolidone, the active ingredient in virtually all hair sprays. Thesaurosis, or storage disease in the lungs, was first described in 1958. It has been the subject of some controversy since that time. Some investigators have not been able to substantiate the existence of this disorder as a separate entity. There is no question that a lung condition similar to sarcoidosis has developed in some individuals, many of them beauticians. Some authorities feel that the disease is indeed sarcoidosis, and not a separate entity. The role of hair sprays in producing this problem is unclear at present. It would be prudent, however, to avoid inhalation of this or any other spray.

An additional problem with hair spray is contact lenses. Contact lenses should not be present in the bathroom, either in the eyes or in a container, unless it is closed, when hair spray, or any of the aerosol conditioners, are used. Once contact lenses have been contaminated with any substance, they should be taken to the optometrist or ophthalmologist for examination and purging, if that is possible.

A new hazard has been introduced into the bathroom by the ever-increasing heavy hand of government bureaucrats. The low flush toilets that use only 1.5 gallons of water per flush, as contrasted to the previous conventional units that used 3.5 gallons, have produced widespread outrage. They do not flush adequately, having to be repeatedly flushed, and have been responsible for clogged plumbing. In order to solve this government induced problem, toilet manufacturers have developed hydraulically assisted units that increase the force of the flush by compressing air. Although some aerosol is produced when any toilet is flushed, these pressure flush toilets produce much more. This increases greatly the volume of bacteria and other microorganisms that are dispersed into the bathroom air that you breathe. It is wise to close the cover on any toilet before flushing, but it is essential with these new units.

MERCURY

With all of the other exposures in the home that evolve from the ambient environment, we should not have to face hazards that are normally only a part of the workplace. There are many occupational exposures to mercury in the workplace, as discussed in Chapter X, and much concern has been expressed about the amounts found in various foods (Chapter V). Periodically other exposures surface in unexpected places. In August 1989 a physician in Michigan saw a four-year-old boy with symptoms of acute mercury poisoning. These included marked personality changes and advanced nerve damage that resulted in muscle weakness and dysfunction in the hips and legs. He also had leg cramps, fever, sweating, rash with itching, and peeling of the skin of the hands and feet.[2]

The other four members of the family also were found to have elevated levels of mercury in their bodies. Muscle weakness was found in one of the other children. After 4 months of hospitalization, including repeated chelation treatments, most of the symptoms subsided, and the boy was able to walk. Muscle weakness persisted, however. Mercury is a very potent nerve poison.

The interior of the house had been painted about one month previously with 17 gallons of a latex paint that contained 3 times the amount of phenylmercuric acetate that was recommended by the Environmental Protection Agency. The house was air-conditioned and the windows had been kept closed. Mercury compounds were added to water based (latex) paints to prevent bacterial and mold growth during storage. Neither this presence of mercury nor its concentration were required to be on the label. It had already been banned from oil based paint in 1976 because of its toxicity. Many people, including some members of Congress, had been under the impression that the previous ban had applied to all interior paints. The addition of mercury compounds was banned for all interior paints effective August 20, 1990. It is still permitted in outdoor paint, and skin contact with this should be avoided.

Families in 19 other homes that had been painted with the same paint were examined and found to have elevated blood levels of mercury also. Pregnant women were found to be living in four of these homes. A developing fetus should never be exposed to any level of mercury. The home environment also demonstrated elevated mercury levels. Mercury will continue to be released into the air in these homes for as long as 7 years.[3,4]

Four adults in Michigan died from acute mercury poisoning in 1989 as a result of attempts to recover the silver in dental amalgam. The amalgam had been smelted in a casting furnace in the basement of the home where the four individuals lived. Mercury fumes were distributed throughout the house through the heating ducts. All four of these people died in spite of the fact that the diagnosis of the mercury poisoning was made and intensive medical treatment was instituted.[5]

Mercury is extremely toxic to the nervous system and is disastrous during pregnancy. This was graphically demonstrated in a large population in Minamata, Japan in 1953 when hundreds of men, women and children suffered acute mercury poisoning. A nearby company had been dumping mercury waste into streams that emptied into Minamata Bay, the source of the fish that was the staple in the diet of the people. Fifty-two people died, and many more suffered severe nerve and brain damage. (See Chapter V)

GARBAGE AND WASTE

Proper management of garbage and waste is essential to the control of flies and rodents. Flies are the most common insect transmitters of disease in the United States. The habit of the fly of seeking out fecal material, manure or other rotting organic material to feed on and to lay its eggs on brings it in contact with a diverse array of microorganisms capable of causing disease in humans. In feeding, the hairy body and sticky feet of the fly literally soak up these organisms. A single fly may carry over six million of them. The fly can also carry bacteria in its digestive system for the duration of its one-month life span, and can pass them on to subsequent generations through its eggs.

The fly that has fed on manure and sewage may next alight on the food in your household, or on your baby. Here it regurgitates its previous meal, and drops its feces, both of which contain the disease-causing organisms. It also leaves behind some of the abundant supply of organisms from its body and feet. The black specks that are sometimes seen on the walls of restaurant kitchens represent dried vomit and fecal material from flies. The diseases that are transmitted through this process include typhoid, paratyphoid and other salmonella infections (the most common food borne infections), polio, cholera, typhus and diarrhea from a host of different organisms including bacteria, viruses and amoeba. (See Chapter V for a discussion of foodborne illnesses.)

Flies are attracted to the odor of food, garbage and other rotting organic matter. The most effective means that we have of controlling their growth and reproduction is to deny them food and breeding places. This can be done effectively in the city by adequate control of garbage, and by using screens. Screen doors should open outward, so that the flies are not swept into the house when they are opened. Garbage control has been rendered much easier and much more effective by the advent of the plastic garbage bag. These are very effective in denying access to breeding materials by flies.

The garbage bag still needs to be placed in a tight fitting, impervious container to deny access by rats (and dogs). Rodents are another important vector for the transmission of disease, and it is equally important to control them. Most people find them abhorrent, and accept this dictum of public health more readily than the control of flies, that are viewed, mistakenly, more as a nuisance. It has been amply demonstrated over the years that by denying access to food, garbage and grain stores to rats they can be effectively controlled. They thrive and multiply in neighborhoods where food is abundantly available, a situation commonly found in far too many cities.

The purist in public health would like to see twice-weekly pickup of garbage, but this is impractical and costly. Once weekly pickup is very effective in controlling flies. The fly eggs hatch in twenty-four to thirty-six hours. The larval stage exists for an additional five to eight days, and the pupal stage lasts for four to six days. The entire cycle takes about ten to fourteen days. If garbage is picked up once weekly, it is obvious that no flies will be hatching at your home from that batch. It is equally important, however, that no fly eggs or garbage fragments that have eggs implanted in them be left adhering to the garbage can. The plastic bags, again, are invaluable in preventing this. If garbage is dumped into the can loose (which it should not be), the can must be scrubbed sufficiently each week to remove the residue and destroy any remaining eggs.

In the context of fly propagation, garbage includes all food scraps and residue, cooked or uncooked, including meat, fruit and vegetable. Dead animals are a prime incubator for flies, and these should be buried promptly. Most garbage pickup services refuse to handle this form of refuse. In that event prompt burial provides a safe means of denying flies access to the carcass, as well as removing it from sight and smell.

Flies generally travel no more than about two miles, so effective control of garbage and waste at your site should markedly reduce the population, assuming cooperation from your neighbors. Pesticides can be used, judiciously, to further enhance control. This is especially important on the farm, where control of all organic material such as manure, or the animal droppings in the field, is impossible. In this setting, pesticides in residual sprays and in flytraps assist in controlling the population. These pesticides must be kept away from food and out of the house, for the agents commonly used for this purpose on the farm are organophosphates. Only the pyrethroids should be used in the home. (See pesticides, Chapter XIV.) Flies have proven adept at developing strains that are resistant to a given pesticide, so one must be alert to the need to switch to a different agent when such resistance develops.

SEPTIC SYSTEMS

Over one-half of the households in North America utilize underground septic tanks as their sewage disposal system. A properly installed and maintained septic system performs this service efficiently and presents no health hazard. For this we owe thanks to the public health departments and sanitary engineers that have designed safe, efficient and functional systems.[6] Building departments and local health departments of the state and local governments exercise their authority to approve designs for and supervise construction of these systems to safeguard our health. This protection breaks down when individuals violate the system, and the laws, and dump inadequately treated effluent into a stream or other body of water. Contamination also occurs when a drainage bed is installed too close to the surface on a hill so that the effluent seeps to the surface. In purchasing a used home with a sewage system, this is one of the many items to check out carefully.

A serious threat to health exists in communities where shallow wells (forty to sixty feet deep) have been installed in proximity to septic systems. This is particularly hazardous in sandy soil and in communities where residences are placed on lots of less than one acre. Such wells are almost certain to be contaminated by the effluent of the septic systems with the resultant danger of disease transmission. If nitrates are found in a test of the water from shallow wells, contamination from the septic system is virtually confirmed. Positive confirmation can be made by a culture of the water, performing the classic coliform count. The presence of coliform bacteria is clear evidence of fecal contamination of the water supply.

In some communities such as in southwestern Virginia the effluent from septic tanks percolates through the sandy soil efficiently, and into the porous limestone rock that forms the underlying geologic strata. The effluent continues to percolate through this porous rock and into the underground aquifers that provide the water supply for the residents of the area. When the residents complained of the foul taste of their water supplies, coliform counts as high as 1,600 were found (two is the maximum permissible). This same risk exists in many other parts of the U.S. where large deposits of limestone are found.

In households where such fecal contamination of water supplies are found, the water should not be used except for cooking and other uses where heating will destroy the bacteria, protozoa and viruses. The most satisfactory remedy is to establish a deeper well at a level that is proven to be free of contamination. This remedy may not be available in those areas where the deep underground aquifers are contaminated. All wells in these regions, no matter how deep, should be tested for contamination.

The most common disease risk from well water that is contaminated by effluent from a septic system is that of hepatitis A. Whereas this illness used to appear only periodically it is now with us year in and year out. It results only from eating or drinking food or liquids that have been contaminated by human feces. Giardiasis is another disease, an infectious diarrhea caused by a microorganism, which has moved from the realm of the uncommon to that of a common infection in the United States today. It too is acquired from contaminated food or drink, frequently from wells that contain the organism. More recently *Cryptosporidium*, a coccidian protozoan parasite that is passed in the stool of man has caused outbreaks of diarrhea from contaminated water supplies. It was first reported in humans in 1976, and has since become very common in AIDS patients (see Chapters V and XI).

Wells should always be drilled deep enough to assure against such contamination. This requires a depth of three hundred-fifty to four hundred feet in some localities. More commonly seventy to one hundred-sixty feet is adequate. This depends on the particular geologic strata in a given locality. The key is to reach a water source that is protected by an overlaying bed of impervious clay that prevents seepage of contaminants into the water table. The well must be drilled and sealed in such a manner as to prevent contaminants from being carried to the deep water source. Here again standards for wells are set by health departments in order to assure safe water supplies. The health officials in your area will know the depth required for an adequate and safe water supply. They also issue the permits and license the well drillers to assure that safe standards are maintained.

Most people do not appreciate that septic systems do require maintenance. Neglect results in a clogged drainage bed, which necessitates replacement at a considerable cost. Common sense and maintenance can prevent this. First, it must be remembered that all that goes into the septic system does not disappear by magic. The system is capable of "digesting" most organic material. Cellulose fiber, on the other hand, is not reduced to an effluent that can be disposed of in the drainage bed. Sanitary napkins, toilet tissue, facial tissue, vegetable fibers, eggshells, coffee grounds, seeds, pits and cigarette filters are examples of other materials that are not digested and accumulate in the tank. Once a sufficient quantity of this non-digestible residue has accumulated, these substances move out into your drain field and clog it up. Prudence would dictate that these substances be sent to the septic tank in limited quantities if at all. It is also important that very limited quantities of chlorine bleaches be drained into the septic systems, for they will interfere with the bacterial action that is essential to proper function.

An aerobic system that pumps air (oxygen) into the sewage tank and stirs the mixture on a preset schedule is far more efficient than a plain septic tank. The effluent from a properly operating aerobic system is pure enough to discharge directly into streams. These systems must be properly maintained however. As with any system, the more working parts there are, the more there is to break down. The most frequent part to fail is the pump that supplies the oxygen and agitation. This occurs more frequently if the pump is installed in the tank where it is exposed to the corrosive atmosphere (hydrogen sulfide gas). The timing mechanism must also be checked periodically, but a well-designed and properly constructed unit should render years of service. If the discharge from the system develops a distinct odor you can be certain that something has failed.

The septic tank should be pumped out every two to three years, depending on the number of residents and on the quantity of such nondegradable materials that is dumped into it. If all of the leftovers from the table are processed through the garbage disposal, this time frame should be shortened, perhaps to once a year or less. At any rate, the clean out must be done before there is any evidence of backup in the plumbing. Once this occurs, the filter bed has become clogged by the overflow of nondegradable material, and it must be dug up and replaced. That is a costly procedure.

Septic systems also have a limited liquid capacity. The leach bed relies upon not only percolation into the soil, but evaporation of water through absorption by plant life overlying the bed. The excessive use of laundry or any other heavy water use can overwhelm the septic system. Laundry should be limited to two loads per day in general, and not more than five loads per week. Even safer is to install a dry well to accommodate the wastewater from the laundry.

HEATING

The recent skyrocketing cost of petroleum based fuel products has prompted many people to turn to alternate fuel sources for home heating. Wood burning has been resurrected as a result, and new stove designs that offer greater efficiency than the fireplace have been introduced. One of the hazards associated with this means of heating is a chimney fire that results from creosote build up in the chimney. Such buildup occurs to a much greater extent in the airtight stoves that are designed to burn slowly in an oxygen starved atmosphere. Once this buildup of creosote ignites, it burns at 2,000 degrees F., threatening the integrity of the chimney and risking the spread of fire to the house. This event is best prevented by monitoring the creosote buildup, and removing it from the chimney before it accumulates to a dangerous level.

In a single-story home, it is a reasonably simple matter to look down the chimney with a powerful flashlight from the roof. Brushes to remove the buildup are widely available at hardware stores, but the creosote must be removed after it is brushed loose. It may be possible to do this from below in some instances, but it requires access to the chimney. This is frequently not possible with the fireplace inserts.

Chimney sweeps as a business have responded to this demand, and this service is available in most communities. More recently, catalytic burners have become available, both as add-ons and as integral units on new stoves. These burners increase the efficiency of combustion and reduce the quantity of creosote that is sent up the chimney. Secondary combustion chambers have also been added to new stoves recently in order to increase the efficiency of combustion.

TREATED LUMBER

Lumber that has been treated with any preservative should not be used as fuel in any wood-burning device, nor in a campfire. The newer treated products (Wolmanized® and all similar products) contain chemicals such as arsenic that have caused serious illness and death when burned in fireplaces. These products also have been used commonly to construct flower boxes, stairs, porches, decks, lawn furniture and playground equipment. A splinter from any of these products is a serious matter, and they should be removed promptly. Skin contact of the arms and hands, and walking barefoot on decks constructed with treated lumber results in significant absorption of arsenic. Arsenic has long been known to cause skin cancer, and it a substance that should not be injected into the skin by splinters.

All playground equipment, furniture, porches and decks constructed from treated lumber should be sealed with varnish or some other effective sealant to protect against splinters. This cannot be done until a sufficient amount of the moisture content of the preservative has evaporated and the wood has dried some. This will mean at least one season of unprotected use, during which period caution must be exercised. Having to seal these products defeats the purpose of the treatment to a degree, but the benefits of increased longevity of the lumber are still realized.

Timbers, fence posts and railroad ties that have been treated with creosote or pentachlorophenol release very toxic chemicals when burned. These are hazardous when inhaled and upon contact with the skin. They also can cause damage to the cornea of the eye. Great care should be taken to avoid the smoke and fumes when these products are burned outdoors. They should never be burned in home heating devices, or in campfires. Boy Scouts beware!

ALLERGIES

One of the side effects of wood burning has been the extension of the allergy season. Individuals who in the past suffered allergic rhinitis, cough and itching eyes when the trees started to bud in April have found that these symptoms are now with them throughout the year. These individuals have found that whereas they could discontinue their allergy injections in the fall in the past, they now must continue them through the winter. Allergic reactions of the nose, throat and lungs are made worse by the dry atmosphere present in virtually all heated homes. This can be relieved some by adequate humidification. More frequent vacuuming will be needed also to remove the debris from the wood and the ash that escapes from the appliance.

CANCER

A further concern has been expressed over the fact that cancer-causing agents are produced when wood is burned. The main culprit is *benzo-a-pyrene*, which is a known carcinogen, and is a byproduct of wood combustion. Studies have revealed that the use of a wood-burning stove in homes increases the level of *benzo-a-pyrene* five fold. Nitrogen oxides also are produced by wood-burning stoves, and increased levels of these have also been measured. The oxides of nitrogen do not cause cancer, but they do cause respiratory problems through irritation.

In some neighborhoods, where wood burning is common, ambient air levels of all of these combustion products reaches intolerably levels. Some communities, such as Missoula, Montana, with a population of 33,000, have enacted ordinances controlling or banning wood burning when ambient air levels reach a certain level. This problem is more common in geographic locations where air movement is restricted by mountains or other topography.

Periodically individuals will be seen with rhus dermatitis (poison ivy, oak, and sumac) in the winter as a result of contact with the vines that adhere to wood that has been cut for fuel. Obviously smoke from burning these vines should not be inhaled or allowed to come in contact with the skin.

The presence of radon in homes is not a new phenomenon, but it is a recent discovery. Concern has been expressed about the cancer risk from this radioactive gas, especially among cigarette smokers. This risk is present only in certain parts of the United States where characteristic underlying geologic strata releases the gas. It is also a problem where homes have been built over tailings from uranium or phosphate mining, or where these materials have been used in the construction of the home. You should first check with your local health department to find out if these conditions exist in your area. If they do, a simple radon screening test can be done for about $35. If the screening test is positive, then a more definitive test can be done, and remedial measures taken. (See Chapter VI)

SPACE HEATERS

Kerosene heaters that are not vented have become very popular as an alternate heating appliance. These units also have been the object of engineering improvements to provide a cleaner burn. In spite of these changes, kerosene heaters produce significant volumes of carbon monoxide, carbon dioxide, nitrogen dioxide and sulfur dioxide, the quantity of the latter being in direct relationship to the sulfur content of the fuel. Good quality K-1 kerosene contains less than 0.05 percent sulfur and poses no problem. K-2 fuel contains a higher level of sulfur, produces a hazardous level of sulfur dioxide, and gums up the wick. Any kerosene fuel turns yellow due to oxidation from one season to the next, and this also causes the wick to gum up, producing smoke and contaminants.

Even under the best of circumstances, with clean fuel and a clean, properly adjusted wick, all of the above listed gases are produced at levels that pose a hazard to health. Carbon dioxide in the room air where these units are operating is measured at levels well beyond what is considered to be safe. Carbon monoxide has been found to be eight to ten times above safe levels, especially if the wick is less than perfect (and it usually is).

Approximately 700 people in the United States die in their homes each year as the result of carbon monoxide poisoning. These air contaminants cause greater problems in individuals with asthma or bronchitis, in children and older people, in individuals with emphysema or chronic obstructive lung disease, and in individuals with heart disease. Pregnancy presents a particular risk, and this is not the ideal atmosphere in which to cultivate a healthy, normally developed baby.

GAS COOKING STOVES

Some studies have shown that residents of homes where gas stoves are used for cooking suffer a significantly higher incidence of respiratory problems. Nitrogen dioxide levels in these homes have been measured at two to three times the level of that in homes where electric stoves are used. Elevated levels of carbon monoxide have also been measured. Both hazards can readily be removed by the installation of a range hood that exhausts to the outside. It has become popular to install hoods over the kitchen range in new homes that merely recirculate the air through a charcoal filter. This practice is done presumably to save the minuscule cost of installing ductwork to the outside. The charcoal filters do not accomplish what would be done by ducting to the outside, especially once the charcoal is exhausted.

ASBESTOS

Many homes built in the fifties, and prior to that, contain furnaces and ductwork that are insulated with asbestos. Asbestos coated the exterior of the old gravity feed furnaces, and was wrapped around the ducts. This material has a tendency to flake off, particularly where some object has struck it. Remodeling also poses the risk of disseminating asbestos fibers into the air. Asbestos fibers were routinely incorporated into spackling compound and drywall materials until 1975. In remodeling, tearing this material out or sanding materials applied in that era exposes one to asbestos fibers.

Asbestos is a significant cancer hazard. Workers exposed to it develop lung cancer eight times as frequently as do nonexposed workers. Workers who are exposed to asbestos who also smoke cigarettes can multiply this by a factor of at least ten, meaning that their risk is increased to eighty times or more. Prolonged exposure is not needed to face this risk. A latency period of twenty to thirty years makes it difficult to make the connection between the exposure and the development of the cancer. Individuals who worked in the shipyards of Philadelphia, Pennsylvania and Oakland and Richmond, California during World War II began showing up with lung cancer as a result of their asbestos exposure in about 1978. Many women joined the work force in these shipyards, and this was about the time when smoking also became popular among women. Working in the presence of asbestos increased their odds of getting lung cancer by a factor of six to eight, but smoking plus the asbestos increased the odds by eighty to ninety times.

Mesothelioma is a cancer of the lining of the lung, and is a very rare tumor. It has been seen with alarming frequency in workers exposed to asbestos. A single exposure to asbestos may be adequate to produce this incurable disease thirty years later. (See Chapter X for more on asbestos.)

EXPLOSIONS

Volatile solvents (lacquer thinner, toluene, acetone, paint thinners) and fuels such as gasoline should not be stored in the house, basement or garage.   This risk is increased when wood-burning appliances are used. Fumes from these agents are easily ignited and may be explosive. Removal of ashes that contain hot coals can be disastrous if they are set in the garage alongside any of these volatile substances. Smoking in the workshop or basement where these are stored is risky business. Smoking while using flammable solvents, or with open containers nearby, is foolhardy. Smoking while one has one's head planted under the hood of an automobile is not wise either since both gasoline and hydrogen (from the battery) are present.

HAZARDOUS WASTE

While there has been much attention to the problem of hazardous waste in our environment, especially as it applies to plants and businesses, we do not consider that which exists in our own homes. These include left over paints and solvents, cleaning solutions and used motor oil. These cannot be simply dumped down the drain but must be disposed of properly. Public officials have been very slow to respond to this very public problem that is certainly the responsibility of government.

Many private service stations accept used motor oil, solving one of these disposal problems. Similarly most business that sell lead acid batteries will accept the depleted battery for recycling. Some local governments have jumped into the recycling business, attempting to collect and deal with substances such as glass that pose no threat to the environment. The greater need is for the proper and responsible disposal of the substances that should not end up in our underground aquifers. Some of these items and substances that accumulate in the home are listed below.

HAZARDOUS WASTE IN THE HOME

paints, varnishes	aerosol cans
solvents, thinners	photographic chemicals
wood preservatives	gasoline, diesel fuel
pesticides	charcoal lighter
weed killers	glues, adhesives
ant & rodent poisons	asphalt cement, tar
cleaners & polishes	used motor oil
drain cleaners	depleted batteries
oven cleaners	

1. CDC. Severe acute respiratory illness linked to use of shoe sprays — Colorado, November 1993. *MMWR* 1993;**42**:885-887.

2. CDC. Mercury exposure from interior latex paint — Michigan. *MMWR* 1990;**39**(8):125-126.

3. Agocs MM, Etzel RA, Pattish RG, et al. Mercury exposure from interior latex paint. *N Engl J Med* 1990;**323**:1096-1101.

4. CDC. Mercury exposure from interior latex paint — Michigan. *MMWR* 1990;**38**:125-126.

5. CDC. Acute and chronic poisoning from residential exposures to elemental mercury — Michigan, 1989-1990. *MMWR* 1991;**40**(23):393-395.

6. Public Health Service. Manual of Septic Tank Practice. PHS publication No. 526, 1963.

II

HAZARDS OF THE HOME WORKSHOP

A man's legs must be long enough to reach the ground.
— Abraham Lincoln

In this chapter is included all of those activities around the home or farm that involve the use of tools. These include the myriad do-it-yourself projects that have become an important element in our society and economy. A whole industry has evolved around the do-it-yourself concept, and this has provided a great deal of gratification and recreation to thousands of individuals. The furniture, home improvement and the recreational equipment that result from these projects also enrich the lives of families and provide items that might not otherwise be available. Since the labor involved is not assigned an hourly wage rate, the greater investment in time and care frequently yield a more durable product of higher quality. As my parents always said, *if you want a job done right, do it yourself.*

The increase in the use of the many power tools now available has also added another dimension to the potential for accidents around the home, however. It has become more important than ever to become acquainted with the risks associated with the use of these tools, and the prophylactic measures required in order to retain life and limb.

EYE PROTECTION

One of the most serious risks involved in most of the activities in the home workshop is eye injury. Although the United States has the lowest incidence of blindness of all of the major nations of the world, far too much loss of vision results from injuries at home or on the job. Virtually all of these injuries could be prevented by the simple expedient of wearing proper eye protection. Such protection may range from a simple plastic face shield when grinding or working under the auto to prescription ground safety glasses.

All prescription glasses in the United States are made from

impact resistant materials, by law, but a greater impact protection may be advisable for some projects. Safety glasses provide protection around the periphery of the eyes that regular glasses do not. Information on eye protection routinely accompanies all power tools, such as saws, grinders, routers, drills, lathes and jointers, when they are purchased. This information should be read carefully and all of the recommendations followed.

The most common injury sustained to the eye from these activities is the deposition in the eye of a foreign body, usually a fleck of wood or some other particulate material, or a metal fragment. The majority of these are removed at home with no complications. Far too often, however, a simple problem is converted to a more serious one when abrasion of the surface of the eye results from efforts to remove a foreign body at home. Such an event always raises the risk of infection in the eye, and should always be seen and cared for by a physician.

An even more serious complication occurs when the object is forced through the surface of the eye. Such penetrating wounds must always be managed by a competent ophthalmologist, for it will require surgical removal. It must be kept in mind that a particle from a grinding wheel may be so imbedded, either from the force of impact or from the heat of the particle, that removal at home is impossible and often difficult even for the physician. Removal is a task that should be undertaken by someone with experience and the proper equipment, in an appropriate environment.

In any event where pain in the eye is present examination by a physician is imperative. A variety of bacteria or viruses may gain entry to the eye through an abrasion or injury. This is the usual source of infection to the cornea. Such an infection can result in the loss of an eye when medical attention is delayed for as little as twenty-four hours. This risk has increased as a result of the emergence of bacterial strains that are resistant to antibiotics. Furthermore, there is no antibiotic that is effective against *Acantha-moeba* infections.

WELDING

Welding, whether at home or on the job, carries two main risks. The first is to the eyes, from a "flash burn." This is a burn of the surface of the eye resulting from ultraviolet ray exposure. It frequently results from viewing the arc produced by an electrode before the face shield is put in place, or as a result of a bystander looking at the arc. It does not require a prolonged exposure. Flash burns have also resulted when welders have used a face shield that had a fine crack in the lens that was not detected. The same type of burn can occur with exposure to the sun, especially on snow, or to a sunlamp.

No change is noticed after such an exposure for several hours. Pain in the eye then evolves; severe enough to prevent sleep, perhaps for two nights. The eye feels as though it has sand in it. Light sensitivity and the production of tears are usually present. Healing generally takes place with no permanent damage, but the degree of pain usually requires medication. Ophthalmic antibiotics should be used to prevent infection. Topical anesthetics give significant relief of the discomfort, but these should NOT be used. The cornea will not heal when it is anesthetized and this increases the risk of infection as well as delaying healing. Pain relief must come from oral medications provided by a physician.

This painful affliction can be prevented by always wearing adequate eye protection while welding. One cannot see through the lens of an electric welding helmet before the arc has been struck, but the practice of delaying placement of the hood until the arc is struck runs the risk of this burn. The glasses designed for an acetylene torch do not provide adequate light protection for electric welding. Bystanders or passers-by should always be protected from viewing the arc produced by welding. Welding in the open with no protection for passers-by is an all too common sight. Effective sunglasses will protect the eyes from the reflection of ultraviolet rays from snow. These are needed especially when at higher altitudes, such as when skiing, for the sun's rays are filtered less by the atmosphere at high altitudes.

The ultraviolet radiation that is produced by an electric welding arc can also produce a burn of the skin, just as exposure to the sun can. If a reflective surface such as polished aluminum is being welded, as much as 90 percent of the ultraviolet radiation can be reflected from its surface. The body should be fully covered during welding to protect against this risk, as well as sparks.

The second risk associated with welding involves the lungs. Welding produces fume particles that are much smaller than the particles that are produced by grinding or other mechanical means. As a consequence, these particles are not filtered out by the nasopharynx and thus have access to the deepest reaches of the lungs. Some of the components of this fume, such as iron oxide, do not by themselves produce serious harm. Any dust inhaled over a period of time, however, can produce bronchitis, and the risk is much greater in cigarette smokers. Cigarette smoke tends to paralyze the defense mechanisms that remove dust particles from the lungs, thus resulting in the deposition and retention of these materials. Smoking also increases the production of mucus, further interfering with clearance from the lungs. The result is that welders who also smoke have twice the incidence of emphysema and chronic obstructive lung disease as do non-smoking welders.

During the process of welding, both the welding rod and the material being welded are vaporized, producing the fume mentioned above. If the material in both of these sources is pure iron, little risk is involved. The significant risk comes from other substances in the metal being welded or in the rod. The presence of cadmium, either as an alloy or more commonly as a rust protective coating of the material being welded, produces a serious risk for the development of emphysema. Cadmium is often present in the coating on the rod, alloyed with copper or nickel. Cadmium is also virtually always present in the alloy of wire used for silver solder, and many disabling cases of emphysema have resulted from this process.

Silica has also been incorporated in the coating on the rod, and inhalation of this substance produces one of the most serious and most disabling of all lung disorders, silicosis. Nitrogen oxides (the villain in auto exhaust pollution) and ozone are also produced during electric welding and are present in the fume inhaled by the welder. Both of these produce irritation of the throat and lungs, and may lead to spasm, cough and bronchitis.

Adequate ventilation is essential in all welding, brazing and silver soldering operations. This means a properly designed booth with adequate exhaust and air replacement. Such a facility is never present at home, and all too often not on the job. Welding in the open results in significant inhalation of particles. Occasional welding of a pure iron based material with an electrode that does not contain silica or cadmium probably carries little risk. This ideal set of circumstances is rarely seen, however. One should avoid vaporizing materials that contain or are coated with cadmium (galvanized steel and plated screws) or spring brass that invariably contains beryllium. These exposures and these risks continue to be present at many worksites. They are a clear and common hazard on farms.

SOLDERING

Commercial solder sold for home use normally contains a mixture of tin and lead, usually 50 to 60 percent tin and 40 to 50 percent lead. This is the mixture that flows the best, provides the strongest joint and lasts the longest. Concerns regarding the risk of lead leaching into the water supply have prompted federal authorities to mandate the use of lead free solder in residential plumbing. The degree to which lead is leached from the joints is related to the acidity of the water supply. The problem has been found to be present in a few isolated regions.

One solder marketed to meet this new requirement contains 95 percent tin and 5 percent antimony. A more recent one contains zinc, silver and antimony in addition to the tin base. It is claimed that the latter product flows better. A eutectic mixture (that mixture which melts at the lowest temperature) of 63 percent tin, 37 percent lead melts at 361° Fahrenheit (183° Celsius). The lead free solders melt at 464° and 473° Fahrenheit respectively (240° and 245° Celsius). A significantly higher temperature will be needed in order to substitute these newer solders. This may not be easy to achieve during many soldering operations, and certainly will be difficult on three-inch copper plumbing joints.

The new solder alloys cost about twice as much as conventional solder, and it remains to be seen how effective they are. For most of the soldering jobs, the conventional solder will continue to provide a stronger joint and will be easier to work with. Judging from past experience, however, I suspect that the bureaucrats on high will eventually deny us access to them. If this transition proves to be a needed improvement it will be worth the added cost. It will also be a first for the federal bureaucracy.

WOODWORKING

One of the most common activities in the home workshop, and one of the most widely enjoyed, is woodworking. These projects carry several risks. The most obvious risk when operating various power tools is the loss of fingers or other personal injury. I have seen individuals who have passed one to three fingers through a bench saw along with the wood being processed. This tragedy can be avoided by using blocks of wood rather than fingers to feed the work, and by keeping the hands well away from the blade. These projects also should not be undertaken when you are tired. Safe operation, avoiding personal injury, requires that the operator be alert and attentive at all times. Eye injury, as previously discussed, must also be guarded against. The use of adequate eye protection when using power saws and the use of the anti-kickback device while ripping, are imperative.

A dust mask should be worn at all times when sawdust is being produced. The disposable paper masks are probably adequate for this purpose for most people, but every effort should be made to achieve a good fit. An efficient, well fit-respirator is preferable, and is essential for asthmatics and individuals with a proclivity toward bronchitis. Inhalation of so called benign dust over a period of time can produce a bronchitis even in healthy individuals. Those who have a family history of bronchitis (parents, grandparents, aunts or uncles) should avoid inhaling dust at all times. Individuals who inherit a deficiency of the enzyme *alpha-1-antitrypsin* develop bronchitis as a result of dust exposure much more readily (see Chapter IV). A respirator, like safety glasses, is a nuisance when working, but the discomfort of advanced lung disease is more than a nuisance.

Asthmatics must face the added risk of an attack due to sensitization to certain woods, particularly western red cedar, mahogany and oak. Aside from bronchitis and asthma, inhalation of the sawdust of hardwoods and western red cedar can produce cancer of the nose and sinuses. Hardwoods carry five times the risk of producing cancer as do softwoods. Sawdust from treated lumber should never be allowed to come in contact with the skin. Precautions should be taken also to avoid inhaling or ingesting any of this material. Lumber that has been treated with pentachlorophenol or creosote provides the potential for absorption of these very toxic chemicals through the skin (see pentachlorophenol and creosote in Chapter XIV). Treated lumber that is popularly sold for decks contains copper and arsenic compounds that can cause serious illness and cancer. Death has resulted from burning these products in a fireplace.

Even more dangerous than bench saws and radial saws are chain saws. Numerous serious injuries have occurred, including massive destruction of the face and jaw requiring extensive reconstructive surgery. Newer anti-kickback devices have lessened this risk some, but serious injuries still occur all too frequently. Regardless of any safety device currently in place or developed in the future, these will continue to be a very dangerous tool. It is essential to have secure footing and a firm grip on the saw at all times. This is not always easy to achieve in a tree or on a ladder. Eye protection always should be worn, and hearing protection from noise is important here (see Hearing in Chapter VIII).

Some general safety rules should be adhered to strictly in the workshop, and whenever power tools are being used. These are included in abundance in the instruction sheets that accompany all power tools. These warnings are so voluminous at times that it is difficult to locate the instructions, and we thus tend to disregard them as superfluous. A few common sense precautions, however, may prevent the loss of a finger or hand and considerable suffering.

The worker in the home workshop should not wear loose jewelry or clothing such as a necktie, loose sleeves or any gloves while operating power tools. I have seen a finger pulled into a bench saw by a glove that became entangled. Hair should be covered and secured so that it cannot be caught in power tools. Power cords should be disconnected before changing blades on power saws. All guards should be put back in place after servicing power tools and before operating them. Remove all clutter, keep the work area clear to avoid stumbling and falling into a moving blade. Adequate lighting is important, and it seems that more is required as we age.

No one should ever operate an electrical appliance while standing in water or on a damp surface. Dry rubber soled shoes give an added measure of protection against electrical shock. In this same vein, all grounding devices should be retained. This means not cutting the grounding prong on a three pronged plug simply because an adapter is not at hand. Some of the newer double insulated tools do not require grounding.

Children should be kept out of the workshop and away from

all power tools (and soldering irons). The workshop should be locked when not in use to prevent exploring by young children. Switches that permit locking or disabling of saws and other tools are very desirable. When children are old enough to be taught the use of power tools, this should be done under strict supervision. As proficiency and maturity progress, a watchful eye can replace strict supervision.

An additional risk from vibrating tools is Raynaud's phenomenon, a spasm of the small arteries in the fingers that results in a diminished circulation of blood. After prolonged use this can become permanent, and in the extreme it can result in the loss of fingers. This problem develops more readily at some resonating frequencies than at others, and work is underway to redesign tools to lessen this risk. Some individuals seem more prone to develop this problem than others do. There appears to be some inherited predisposition. Once the disease has developed, certain medications for blood pressure and certain eyedrops for glaucoma may make the symptoms worse.

SOLVENTS

Organic solvents are used in the workshop and around the home and farm for many purposes. Cleaning of auto, tractor and machinery parts and removing grease, paint and other residues are but a few of the uses. Some, such as acetone, naphtha and lacquer thinner, are highly flammable. An explosion may result from a nearby water heater or from a spark from the battery of a car while using these solvents. Even static electricity or a dropped tool can produce a spark that can ignite the vapors (see Fire, Chapter I). Inhalation of and skin contact with these solvents can produce damage to the liver, kidney and brain, with irritability, memory loss and personality changes. They may also produce a weakness of the skeletal muscles (solvent myopathy).

Other solvents, notably carbon tetrachloride, trichloroethylene, trichloroethane and methylene chloride, are neither flammable nor explosive, but they are toxic to the liver, kidney and nervous system (brain) when the fumes are inhaled. They are just as toxic when absorbed through the skin. Methylene chloride is also known to produce cancer. Lead in gasoline is readily absorbed through the intact skin and causes damage to the nervous system and other organs. Commercially available gasolines no longer contain lead.

Gasoline also contains considerable benzene (up to 38 percent of alkylbenzenes) which should not be inhaled or absorbed through the skin. It has been associated with the development of leukemia and serious connective tissue disorders. Kerosene is a much safer cleaning agent and is less flammable than gasoline. Kerosene does not contain the additives that are present in diesel fuel. These additives may present some risk to health when applied to the skin.

In addition to their use in cleaning operations around the house, organic solvents are commonly encountered in glues and adhesives, paints and lacquer, and dyes. Adequate ventilation is essential when using any of these substances in order to minimize the risk. Ordinary respirators provide no protection against vapors. An appropriate charcoal canister filter does offer protection, if it is well fitted and properly maintained, but these are not commonly available in the home workshop. All skin contact should be avoided unless special solvent resistant gloves and aprons are available. These solvents penetrate most gloves, but materials such as Viton® provide some protection. These cost in excess of $35.00 however, and again are not likely to be available at home.

Methylene chloride (dichloromethane) is an organic solvent that is widely used in industry in a variety of products. It is often included in products such as furniture strippers because it does not present a fire or explosive risk. It does causes damage to the central nervous system as do most of the organic solvents. It produces "fatty liver" changes but does not cause the death of liver cells that is seen in such solvents as carbon tetrachloride and chloroform.

Inhalation of any of these solvents may cause problems in patients with heart conditions. The greater risk with methylene chloride may relate to the findings that it causes cancer in rats and mice. All consumer products that contain this solvent must now include a warning about the possible cancer risk on the label. This concern prompted OSHA in early 1992 to propose a marked reduction in the allowable exposure level for workers exposed to this chemical. You should provide equally safe conditions in your home workshop. (See also Chapters X and XIII.)

FURNITURE REFINISHING

Another very popular home workshop activity, one frequently undertaken by women, is the refinishing of furniture. Many of the solvents listed in the previous discussion are also used in these projects. Furniture strippers and sanding liquids usually contain such volatile and flammable agents as acetone, toluol, xylol and methyl ethyl ketone. These are the common constituents in lacquer thinner, and while they are effective in softening paint and varnish, they carry a serious explosive risk. This risk particularly is present when these substances are used in a basement with a gas furnace and water heater. Methylene chloride is also incorporated in strippers and sanding solutions, sometimes without the other solvents, since a mixture that is not explosive can thus be marketed. Methylene chloride, even though it is not explosive, carries its own serious risks as mentioned above. None of these solutions should be permitted to come in contact with the skin. Methylene chloride should be used only outdoors where good ventilation is present. It should not be used in the basement.

Applying these agents and at the same time avoiding all skin contact is difficult. The use of a paintbrush to spread the solution over the surface helps to avoid skin exposure during application. Heavy-duty vinyl gloves offer some protection, but these are not impervious to organic solvents. Reliance upon this protection should be limited to short periods at best. Only special gloves provide adequate protection against these solvents, and their cost renders them impractical for most home projects.

In refinishing furniture without the use of the solvents mentioned above, sanding may expose the worker to the inhalation of older paint pigments that contain lead or cadmium. Arsenic and mercury compounds have been used commonly as wood preservatives in outdoor lumber and furniture. Sanding or scraping these also carries the risk of inhalation of these very poisonous substances into the body. All four are metals that are absorbed after ingestion. Inhalation of their dust thus may result in toxicity after absorption in the stomach as well as in the lung. The use of an effective well-fit respirator and showering afterward can help to protect from this hazard. Getting a good fit is impossible with a beard, however. In industry on jobs where respirators are required, beards are prohibited.

Needless to say none of the substances discussed above should be inhaled or applied to the skin during pregnancy. This is a particular problem during early pregnancy, when uncertainty as to status still exists. The first three months of pregnancy is the period of most rapid development of the fetus and the most sensitive for the development of abnormalities. Some fetal abnormalities that are caused by exposures or deficiencies develop in the first month of gestation. No one should be painting a room or refinishing furniture during pregnancy, or when pregnancy is a possibility.

PRODUCTS THAT MAY CONTAIN METHYLENE CHLORIDE

Adhesives and glues	Paint thinners
Adhesive removers	Paint strippers
Aerosol spray paints	Spray paints
Automobile spray primers	Water repellents
Cleaning fluids and degreasers	Wood stains and varnishes.

SANDBLASTING

This activity requires eye protection, but of equal importance is protection of the lungs. Most sandblasting in the United States is still done with silica sand, although other safer materials are available. Carborundum (silicon carbide) and aluminum oxide are not readily available from paint stores and builder supplies but they can be purchased in most cities at suppliers of sandblasting equipment. They are considerable more expensive, especially where they are used in systems that do not recover the abrasive. They are much safer than silica sand, however.

Silica sand carries the risk of development of silicosis when inhaled. The silica particle, when deposited in the lung, provokes a destructive process in the lung that leads to a very disabling and very unpleasant disease, silicosis and chronic pulmonary fibrosis. A high-quality respirator, not a simple dust mask, is required to filter out silica and proper fit is critical. It is futile to spend the money for a quality respirator if it leaks around the seal. The presence of a beard makes it virtually impossible to obtain a good fit, as discussed above.

There is no cure, no treatment, for silicosis and it may not make its presence known for many years. (See silicosis in Chapter X for a complete discussion of this risk.)

PAINT SPRAYING

Projects that involve spraying of paint present a dual hazard of inhalation of the particulates and pigments as well as the solvents. Paint pigments have commonly contained such toxic elements as lead, cadmium and chromium. The solvents are toxic to the brain and nervous system in general, as well as to the liver. A good, well-fit respirator protects against the inhalation of particulates and pigments, but gives no protection against inhalation of the solvent vapors. Respirators with charcoal canisters that do provide protection for this hazard are available, but are not frequently used outside of industry, and seldom around the home.

THE WEEKEND MECHANIC

One of the most serious hazards associated with this activity is that of carbon monoxide. About 700 people die at home each year from this poison. Sources that produce carbon monoxide includes furnaces, cooking stoves, charcoal grills and internal combustion engines (automobiles, lawn mowers). The hazards of carbon monoxide are widely known, but its presence is virtually never recognized or suspected because it is invisible and has no odor. The most obvious risk is from leaving the engine of an auto-mobile or tractor running in a garage, shed or other enclosed space. Flexible extensions are available to carry the exhaust outdoors, and these should be installed wherever these vehicles must be left running indoors.

The onset of a headache during or after working in these cir-cumstances should always prompt immediate suspicion of carbon monoxide toxicity. This does not occur early, and headache is such a common occurrence that it usually is ascribed to "sinus trouble" or some other everyday cause. Kerosene heaters in closed work-places also produce significant levels of carbon monoxide. These heaters present the additional risk of fire or explosion in such settings, since gasoline is frequently present.

The hazards associated with the use of gasoline as a solvent to wash parts in has been discussed previously. Carburetor cleaner or Tyme solution contains phenol and methylene chloride, both of which are toxic. The risks associated with the use of methylene chloride, including its potential for causing cancer, have also been discussed previously. Phenol has the potential for causing-cancer, particularly when present with polycyclic aromatic hydrocarbons, which are also present in Tyme solution. It is believed that polycyclic aromatic hydrocarbons account for the increased incidence of skin cancer in workers exposed to cutting oils.

Phenol is also caustic, causing tissue destruction in a manner similar to acids and other strong chemicals. Although the seven percent in Tyme solution is only slightly higher than that used in some topical applications, in medical practice it is applied only to very small areas, usually only to abnormal tissue. This solution should not be permitted to come in contact with the skin, and the vapors should not be inhaled. Skin irritation frequently occurs following contact with phenol.

In repairing automobile radiators the mechanic should be aware that the auto manufacturers in the United States have reduced the tin content of the solder from the normal 50 to 60 percent to a mere 5 percent. As is the case in all such innovations, this has been done solely to increase profit. This change makes the manufacture more difficult and it makes the product develop problems sooner. This explains why you have to replace your radiator core after four to five years. In addition to assuring a repair sooner, it increases the risk of lead exposure during that repair. When these repairs are undertaken, great care should be taken to avoid inhaling the fumes generated. Even when the job is undertaken outdoors the worker usually has his nose close to the project and the smoke, because that's where his eyes are.

When doing brake jobs, the first task after removing the wheel has been to blow the dust out of the wheel and rotor, either with compressed air or with the mouth. This should NEVER be done. This dust contains asbestos particles, which pose a serious risk of cancer or asbestosis (see Asbestosis, Chapter X). Although the manufacturers have removed asbestos from brake pads on current auto production lines, asbestos pads will be rolling down the highways for some time. This dust should be vacuumed, preferably with a central vacuum system vented to the outside. Asbestos fibers pass through conventional vacuum cleaner filters, and a vacuum cleaner should never be used on brakes, then taken inside for use in the home.

III

HAZARDS OF CHILDHOOD AND ADOLESCENCE

Train up a child in the way he should go: and when he is old, he will not depart from it.   — Proverbs 22:6 (KJV)

Accidents are the leading cause of death in children. More children die as a result of accidents than cancer, meningitis, congenital defects and heart disease all combined. More than 4,000 children 6 years and under die each year in the United States as a result of accidents.[1] At age 16 years and up the number increases dramatically, reflecting the expansion of activities into a larger society. Attacks by dogs cause 10 to 20 deaths in the United States each year, mainly in children.[2] There are over 3,000 deaths per year in infants under one year of age from falls, burns, drowning and suffocation. For every death, there are one hundred children seriously injured. Curiosity is the most common cause for most of these accidents and injuries. Young children demand constant attention and supervision. This is difficult to provide among the many other demands of a household, especially if other children are in residence. Accidents occur much more frequently when young children are left with a baby-sitter. They are also more frequent during an illness of the parent, during a pregnancy, or when the parent is occupied by other demands in general.

Given the great number of playgrounds in our society, and the volume of children using them, it is not surprising that about 200,000 children each year suffer injuries on playgrounds serious enough to require medical care. Approximately 17 children die each year from these injuries. About 60 percent of these injuries result from falls to the ground beneath playground equipment, and 75 percent of these result in head injuries. Children 12 years old and under account for 95 percent of these injuries. It has been a routine practice for the past forty years to pave the surfaces where these children fall with asphalt. Hard surfaces are finally being replaced with more forgiving materials such as wood mulch.

Injuries from contact sports range from minor bruises and injuries to more serious fractures and torn ligaments or muscles.

Fractures in joints can result in permanent disabilities, particularly if not properly set and immobilized. Ligamentous tears similarly can result in a diminution or loss of their function if not immobilized adequately and long enough to permit their healing. Surgical re-attachment is required in some cases. Of even greater concern is the more recent studies that have demonstrated evidence of small infarcts in the white matter of the brain in football and soccer players. It has long been known that boxing produces brain damage, sometimes with alarming brain dysfunction. The lesions demonstrated by magnetic resonance imaging (MRI) in these recent studies have also shown a correlation with a subtle cognitive dysfunction.[3] In view of the seriousness of these findings and the popularity of these activities this issue needs to be carefully assessed.

Burns from hot metal surfaces of slides, steps and decks provide many more playground injuries. Less dramatic but no less significant is a splinter that children may acquire from equipment that is constructed from lumber that has been treated with a wood preservative. The most commonly used substance contains arsenic, which causes skin cancer. Simple contact with this material presents a serious toxic hazard for it is well absorbed through the skin. The risk is particularly high during the first year that the lumber is placed in use. Swingsets, seesaws, jungle gyms, and sandboxes are frequently made from treated lumber. Additional contact may be present at home where treated lumber is used to construct porches, decks, steps and flower boxes. Walking barefoot and skin contact on arms, hands and legs causes significant absorption and skin cancer risk. A protective coating such as varnish should be applied to all equipment that is constructed with treated lumber.

A particularly tragic injury that occurs in young children involves wading pools that are common in private as well as public recreational facilities. Young children who sit over the suction drain in these pools have had their rectum pulled out with severe injury and tearing of the intestines. Several cases have required surgery and colostomies, a very tragic event for a person of any age, but particularly so for a child. Design changes to prevent this tragedy are being instituted currently, but older pools will remain in place for some time. Protective devices over the drains and closer supervision of children will remain necessary in the interim.

Although the sale and use of fireworks has been curtailed drastically since I was a young, they still account for many injuries and loss of sight. Almost 10,000 people are treated in emergency medical facilities each year during the Fourth of July celebration. About one-half of these injuries occur in young people under 15 years of age. Over one-half of minor children who are injured by fireworks are under the supervision of adults at the time of injury. Burns are the most frequent injury, many of these from sparklers, which are generally considered by parents' to be safe. Since they don't explode children do not fear them and many burns to the eyes result from getting them too close to the face. This usually happens to children younger than 5 years.

Debris from bottle rockets and more powerful exploding devices inflict injury to the eye ranging from a scratch of the cornea to a complete loss of an eye. Particularly dangerous is the practice of placing any of these explosive devices in bottles. Flying glass provides very dangerous shrapnel. These injuries usually happen to the person lighting the device, but many people suffer permanent eye injuries when they are more than 20 feet away from where the device explodes. Young children should not be permitted to handle even sparklers without very close and constant supervision. There is a serious need to educate adults to the risks from sparklers, and parents need to be much more vigilant in supervision of children than they currently are. When older children discharge even legal fireworks, injuries are going to occur. Danger and injury are inherent in the process. Two thirds of the injuries that require hospitalization result from the use of fireworks that are illegal under federal law.[4] Additional laws will not solve the problem; only parents can.

Blunt trauma may occur as a result of a fall, being struck by a motor vehicle, or by a baseball bat. Air bags in automobiles have inflicted many serious injuries and deaths upon children as discussed in the Introduction. Injuries to children also occur when a rock or similar object is thrown by a power lawnmower. Children should not be permitted outdoors in the yard when this chore is being performed. They certainly should not be permitted anywhere near this equipment when it is being operated. The majority of the lesser accidents do not result in serious injury, but that possibility must always be considered. Certainly, whenever there is drowsiness or a visual change such as blurred vision or double vision, careful examination by a physician is imperative. Similarly, when a blow in the region of the eye is sustained, examination should be made to determine the extent of injury, if any. Blood in the anterior chamber of the eye is common in children following a contusion to the eye or the region surrounding it. This is a serious injury that requires prompt medical attention.

Dislocation of the lens of the eye, abrasion of the cornea, laceration of the eyeball and retinal detachment are other complications of blunt trauma to the eye that require medical attention. These are injuries that cannot be detected at home, and neglect can result in loss of vision. Cold packs can be applied following blunt trauma, but great care must be taken to avoid applying any pressure to the eyeball itself.

Burns of the retina of the eye that result from looking at an eclipse of the sun occur every time we have this solar event, and permanent loss of vision results. There is no safe way to view a solar eclipse directly. An ophthalmologist should be consulted when this injury occurs. Ultraviolet burns of the eye (keratitis) resulting from looking at a welding arc is much more common in adults than in children, but it does happen. It can also happen on the ski slope as a result of the reflection of the sun on the snow, and as a result of a child looking at a sunlamp. Adequate eye protection will prevent it on the ski slope, and proper supervision will avoid the sunlamp accident.

Thousands of children suffer burns in the home each year. Most of these are preventable with closer supervision, but parents have become very lax in this responsibility. In an effort to reduce the number of fires started by children childproof cigarette lighter are now marketed. Curiosity prompts young children to pull hot cooking utensils from the stove, a common source of burns each year. The simple expedient of making certain that the handles are always turned in so that the child cannot reach them would prevent many of these accidents. A cord dangling from a hot curling iron in the bathroom produces 6,400 serious burns in children under 5 years of age each year. These appliances are frequently left unattended while they are plugged in and hot. Burns on the face of children frequently involve the eyelids. The threat here is secondary infections that are common with all burns. The most feared infection, and one that is common, is that of *Pseudomonas*. It is resistant to most antibiotics, and can destroy the eyeball.

Another threat to vision in children is that of a foreign body. These may be simple to remove, or they may penetrate the eye and require surgery. One such injury results from pounding on a metal object with a hammer, for instance. Another serious and common injury is that inflicted by an air gun or BB gun. About 35,000 individuals are injured by these each year, and about 2,000 of these involve the eye. The majority of eye injuries sustained in this manner (over 70 percent) occur in individuals between the ages of five and eighteen years. The loss of vision in this injury is the rule. No one should be permitted to handle these guns until they have a thorough understanding of their safe use. Children should not be permitted to handle them without careful supervision.

Leaving teenagers at home alone, with no supervision, while both parents work is a certain formula for disaster. The assumption that they are old enough to look after themselves is proven false by the statistics from accidents and social misadventures. It is especially foolish to leave a loaded gun "hidden" or supposedly secure in the parents' bedroom. When children happen across these weapons it happens all too often that someone is injured or killed. Every parent who has a gun in the home should store the gun and ammunition separately, under lock and key. This is especially important when parents are going to be away from the home. A secure lock on the bedroom door would be an important step in dealing with this threat. There are many items such as medications, razors and scissors in the parents' bedroom and bathroom that should be securely locked away from children and teenagers. The sewing box can be conveniently locked in this room, thus denying access to the hazards contained therein.

Electric shock is common in young children, resulting from the insertion of metal objects or fingers into electric outlets, or from chewing on lamp cords. The latter results in burns of the mouth in addition to the other threats from electricity, frequently with destruction of tissue around the mouth that requires plastic surgery. Safety caps should be placed in all electric outlets in homes where children are exploring. Protecting them from lamp cords requires vigilance. Children and adolescents also are electrocuted as a result of flying kites, and climbing trees in the proximity of power lines.

Death due to asphyxia, heart irregularities or respiratory arrest can occur within minutes if the child remains in contact with the electricity. In removing the child from the contact with electricity, care must be taken to avoid winding up with two casualties instead of one.

Approximately 20,000 children under the age of 5 years are hospitalized each year for having swallowed a potent toxic substance. Medicines account for about 45 percent of these cases and aspirin and other analgesics are the most common medicines involved. Acetaminophen, considered to be a safe and innocuous medicine, can cause severe damage to the liver when the recommended dose is exceeded. This toxicity is greatly accentuated in the fasting state and by the concomitant consumption of alcohol. Medicines include both prescription and nonprescription drugs, and the latter are increasing in number and availability year by year. In 1985 the American Association of Poison Control Centers reported over 60,000 incidents of unintentional prescription medicine ingestion by children under the age of 5 years. In a review of 2,000 of these cases, the medicine was in a child resistant container in 80 percent of the cases. The medication was in the original container in only 65 percent of the cases. Grandparents' medication accounted for 17 percent of the cases. The chief factors contributing to these poisoning were found to be:
• Not replacing the cap securely
• Not keeping the medication in a container
• Keeping the medication in a container other than the original one
• Availability of medication in the kitchen and bedroom
• Medication being left where it is accessible
• The natural tendency of children to explore, and to put things in their mouth

Deaths resulting from accidental ingestion of these substances have reportedly declined by 70 percent since the enactment of the Poison Prevention Packaging Act in 1970. Even these containers, however, need to be kept out of the reach of children.

In 1983, 110,000 children under the age of five years were treated in emergency rooms for the ingestion of a potent toxin. While accidents are the leading cause of death in children, poisoning is the fourth most common cause of fatality. The peak incidence occurs at age two years, the majority of cases occurring under the age of five. Accidental poisoning is uncommon after the age of five. If poisoning is suspected, and if the poison is unknown, if the child vomits, the vomitus should be saved for analysis. In general, vomiting should not be induced after the ingestion of certain agents such as furniture polish, kerosene and other hydrocarbons. The family physician should be called immediately. If unable to contact the family physician, the hospital emergency room or emergency medical team should be called.

There seems to be little excuse for accidental poisoning of children with medications in view of the use of mandated safety caps. The hazard of aspirin has long been known, and it should never be removed from safety cap containers. It should never be left where children can get their hands on it. The most toxic salicylate is methyl salicylate (oil of wintergreen), commonly used in liniments. Next to aspirin and other salicylates, caustics, lead and hydrocarbons are the most common poisons in children.

Strong alkali substances (caustics) produce more severe chemical burns and greater damage, in general, than do acids. Caustics are seen in drain cleaners, toilet bowl cleaners, oven cleaners, fertilizers (potassium hydroxide, potash), electric dishwasher detergents and Clinitest® tablets for diabetics. The newer liquid dishwasher detergents are much easier for children to swallow and are much more damaging. With the powder, the crystals stick to the lining of the mouth and burn, which discourages further consumption. There is a tendency to swallow much more of the liquid products. Severe burns of the mouth, throat and esophagus result from ingesting caustics, and the esophagus is frequently completely destroyed. Household bleaches, which are 3 to 6 percent sodium hypochlorite, are not corrosive and produce less damage. Rust removing cleaners such as ZUD® and BAR KEEPERS FRIEND® contain oxalic acid and result in damage to the kidneys in addition to burns. (See Chapter I for information on the hazards of kitchen, bathroom and household cleaners.)

Lead-based paint pigments have not been used in interior paints for homes since the sixties. Since 1977, legislation has restricted the lead content of paints used in households to no more than 0.06 percent (600 parts per million). Paints manufactured in the forties for indoor use contained as much as fifty percent lead (500,000 parts per million). This paint remains in 27,000,000 households today. This continues to be a major source of lead intoxication in children each year. In some cases the under layers of paint are scraped off by children. Remodeling of these older homes is currently popular, and children are poisoned by the particles produced by the scraping and sanding of these projects. Lead pigments are still used in paints on some objects, and this presents another source of poisoning. Other sources of lead in cases of lead poisoning in children are:

• Artists paints
• Lead shot, fishing weights, toys, curtain weights
• Storage of acid foods such as fruits and their juices, tomatoes and tomato juice, pickled fruits and vegetables, wine, cider and soft drinks in improperly glazed ceramic utensils (usually imported)
• Burning lead-painted wood in the fireplace
• Casting lead bullets, sinkers or toys at home
• Solder and soldered joints

Iron deficiency anemia may create a craving for dirt or paint. This may at least partially explain the habit among children of eating paint. Lead intoxication in children produces brain damage with decreased intelligence that is permanent, and behavioral disorders. It is most harmful between the ages of one and six years. Periodically, an episode of gasoline sniffing results in lead toxicity among young people, but with the disappearance of lead from fuels this should be a problem of the past. There are hazards other than lead toxicity from this practice, the most serious being brain damage from the multiple toxic substances present and the risk of leukemia.

Hydrocarbons include petroleum distillates such as gasoline, kerosene, paint thinners, furniture polish and some pesticides and weed-killers. As strange as it seems, these continue to be among the most popular substances for children to experiment with and to drink. These substances are very toxic, especially in the lungs, where they are 140 times more toxic than in the stomach. They are frequently aspirated into the lungs when swallowed, and only a few drops in the lung can produce a serious pneumonia. They can also cause destruction of red blood cells and damage to the central nervous system. Furniture polish (mineral seal oil) is particularly lethal. It produces damage to the kidneys and bone marrow in addition to the pneumonitis that it provokes.

The recent popularity of oil candles, which contain a wick

encapsulated in a glass sleeve that children can use as a straw, has added a significant household risk for poisoning from lamp oil. During August 1997 four children under the age of two years were hospitalized in Columbus, Ohio following ingestion of oil from these devices. In 1996 the regional poison control center in Columbus reported 95 cases of lamp oil ingestion. Throughout the United States in 1996 there were 2,879 cases of lamp oil ingestion reported.[5] Parents need to be aware of this serious new hazard in the home and take the necessary precautions.

Another group of hydrocarbons is the halogenated hydrocarbons, which include carbon tetrachloride, trichloroethylene, trichloroethane and ethylene dichloride. These substances are used for general cleaning, including the dry cleaning of clothes, for degreasing and as solvents. They are found in many compounds in the home even if not present in their pure form. They produce severe damage in the liver, kidney and brain.

A list of some of the more common poisons in the home that pose a threat to children includes:
• Nail polish remover (acetone): inhalation is toxic to the brain
• Household ammonia (ammonium hydroxide)
• Ethyl alcohol (beer, liquors, wines)
• Rubbing alcohol (isopropyl alcohol or denatured ethyl alcohol)
• Methyl alcohol (paint solvents, shellac, canned fuel); causes blindness
• Pesticides: virtually all are readily absorbed through the intact skin
• Ant poison (Thallium)
• Rat and roach poisons; various agents, see Chapter XIV
• Glues and cements, such as contact cement
• Cleaning fluids (carbon tetrachloride, trichloroethylene)
• Cosmetics
• Hair removers
• Permanent wave neutralizers (high degree of toxicity)
• Permanent wave lotion
• Cresol antiseptics and creosote compounds
• Moth repellents (naphthalene, para-dichlorobenzene): children's clothing should not be stored in naphthalene, since this substance is absorbed through the skin; it is also very toxic when ingested
• Floor wax (carbon tetrachloride)

- Turpentine (paint thinners)
- Antifreeze (ethylene glycol)
- Bath oil
- Hair dyes
- Hair tonic (alcohol)
- Shaving lotion
- Cologne, toilet water
- Tobacco (ingestion and skin absorption)
- Liniments and balms (methyl salicylate, oil of winter green)
- Nitrates and nitrites in well water (and spinach); produce methemoglobinemia in infants
- Artists paints (lead and cadmium pigments)

Many houseplants are also toxic, and are commonly ingested by children. Those generally held to be toxic are philodendron and dieffenbachia (dumbcane), both of which contain oxalic acid, amaryllis, calla lily and poinsettia. Symptomatic poisoning from the ingestion of plants in children almost always involves the philodendron or dieffenbachia. These are the two toxic exposures to plants most frequently reported to poison control centers in the United States. Castor beans from the castor oil plant are very toxic if chewed, or if the shell is cracked. They contain a potent poison, ricin, which was used by the KGB to assassinate a Hungarian dissident, Georgi Markov, in London in 1978. The ricin was incorporated into a pellet that was fired from a modified umbrella shaft into Markov's thigh.[6] There is no known antidote for ricin. The knowledge of its value as an agent for terrorism and assassination has apparently spread for it has been discovered in the possession of dissidents arrested by police since 1990 both in the United States and Canada. Fava beans have also been responsible for poisoning in children. Outdoor plants that are poisonous include hemlock (respiratory paralysis), rhododendron, yellow jasmine, crocus, foxglove, oleander, sorrel and larkspur. For a more complete listing of poisonous plants see the table at the end of this chapter.

Boric acid was a popular home medicinal agent until about the fifties when a number of poisonings and deaths occurred from it. It remains useful in certain applications best left to professionals. It has no place in the home. A study published in a medical journal in 1977 recommended boric acid for the treatment of fungal vaginal infections.[7] It would be very unwise to follow this recommendation. Fatalities have resulted from mistaking boric acid eye solutions for a mouthwash. Fatalities also resulted from absorption of boric acid from baby powders when a diaper rash was present. It is no longer found in these products. Childhood poisoning is best prevented, rather than treated. This is done by:

• Locking up all household cleaning supplies, medicines, pesticides, auto polishes and supplies, paints and paint supplies. It is not enough to place these on a shelf "out of reach;" children have repeatedly demonstrated that the top shelf is not out of reach

• Not storing cleaning supplies with food

• Leaving medicines and chemicals in original containers

• Not storing household supplies under the sink

• Not leaving medicines or chemicals available when answering the telephone or attending the dryer

• Reading the name on the label prior to administration of any medication

• Not taking medication in front of children; they are great imitators

Unfortunately, many medications have a very narrow safety margin, and even a moderate overdose in children can result in death. Iron tablets, even though they are available without prescription, are a medication, and many children have died as a result of consuming them. During the period of June 1992 to January 1993, five children in the Los Angeles area aged 11 to 18 months died as a result of eating iron supplement tablets. Iron supplements account for 30 percent of all deaths from poisoning by accidental ingestion of medications among children. It is the most common cause of poisoning death in children. During 1991, 5,144 cases of children ingesting iron supplements were reported to poison control centers in the United States. Eleven of these cases were fatal.[8] Iron supplements are very lethal in overdose. Unused supplies should be disposed of by flushing them down the toilet, not placing them in the trash.

The telephone number of the family doctor, hospital emergency room or emergency squad, or all three, should be at the telephone, readily accessible. In any household with children, the family physician should be consulted regarding recommended procedures to follow in the event of an emergency, and what supplies such as ipecac should be kept on hand. In general when a substance such as a pesticide is spilled on the skin, it should be flushed with copious amounts of water, washed well with soap and water and then thoroughly rinsed. Never induce vomiting in the following circumstances.

• If unconscious
• If petroleum distillate has been swallowed
• If a corrosive has been swallowed (lye, drain cleaner)

The family physician should be contacted immediately when a child has suffered a poisoning event. If he cannot be contacted immediately these guidelines may provide assistance while efforts to reach the doctor continue:

• If medicine has been swallowed, give nothing.
• If a household product has been swallowed, give one glass of milk, water if milk is not available.
• Do not give the antidote listed on the label, they are frequently not current.

If these measures seem onerous or unduly cautious, one should visit one of the large children's hospitals to view a child with a severely damaged esophagus, or other serious injury from poisoning. Remember that 20,000 children are hospitalized for such tragedies each year, and they suffer, many of them permanently.

Many children choke as a result of swallowing items that are not poisonous, but which obstruct the airway. These include buttons and small objects from toys, but also coins found in the couch and pieces of puzzles and other games such as checkers. All of these dangers should be searched for and removed for as long as young children are in residence.

The problem of methemoglobinemia produced in infants as a result of nitrates in the drinking water is discussed in Chapter V. Botulism in infants as a result of using honey in the formula is covered in the same chapter. Botulism in infants has also been traced to contamination of food by soil or dust from the vacuum cleaner. Central vacuum systems, which exhaust the dirt to the outside, reduce this risk. Botulism spores exist in the soil everywhere. Other cases of botulism in infants have resulted from breastfeeding because the mother failed to properly cleanse the breast.

SIDS: Sudden Infant Death Syndrome, in which infants are found dead in their cribs with no apparent cause, is a phenomenon that has appeared only since the 1940s. It has become the leading cause of death in infants in the United States. Studies in Great Britain suggested that the deaths might be due to the release of phosphine, arsine and stibine gases that are formed when the fire retardant antimony trioxide in the crib mattresses is degraded by fungus. Wrapping the top and sides of mattresses in polyethylene (not PVC) reduced the deaths by 90 percent in Great Britain.

This solution has not gained acceptance in the United States. In June 1992 the American Academy of Pediatrics recommended that infants be placed in their cribs on their backs or sides rather than on their stomachs. In 1996 the Academy modified its policy to recommend placing infants only on their backs.[9] The supposition has been that infants born after the 1940s were burying their heads in the mattress and suffocating. This is an illogical thesis, but it is still adhered to by some authorities. The repositioning of infants has resulted in some reduction in deaths, albeit not as dramatic as in Great Britain, because the child is breathing less of the toxic gases released. The fact that infants did not suffocate in their cribs for generations, until newer materials such as fire retardants were used, has been ignored entirely in the United States.

An environmental threat of a different nature is rheumatic fever. This disease, which damages the heart valves, has been under control for the past twenty-five years, thanks to vigilance and adequate treatment of streptococcal infections with penicillin. Recently, however, there has been a resurgence, with an increase in the number of cases reported. This renewal was ushered in by an epidemic in Utah in 1985-86. The reasons for this upsurge are not clear.

Rheumatic fever rarely occurs prior to age five years, and a primary episode rarely occurs after age eighteen years. The disease itself is not an infection, but is a hypersensitivity reaction that follows an infection by certain strains of group-A streptococci. It occurs two weeks or more after the infection has cleared. It can be prevented by prompt treatment of any streptococcal throat or tonsil infection for a full ten days. It is essential, however, that the full ten-day course of treatment be completed. Discontinuance of treatment before the full ten days compromises the treatment and risks the affliction of rheumatic fever, with its damage to the heart valves. It also risks the development of resistance to the antibiotic by the streptococcus. Repeated attacks increase the damage to the heart significantly.

Until recently the streptococcus that causes rheumatic fever has been universally sensitive to penicillin. This has been remarkable good fortune for us, and unique in that virtually every other species of bacteria has developed a resistance to penicillin. In recent years some strains of streptococcus have developed a tolerance to penicillin, requiring abnormally high doses. This unfortunate situation has developed because of the penchant of people to discontinue medication once they begin to feel better. The family physician and the pediatrician must fully explain the necessity of continuing treatment for the full ten days, and the risks of failure to comply. Unfortunately there is no simple way of telling when an infection is due to a strain of streptococcus that requires the higher dosage.

Some individuals are carriers of streptococcus, showing no outward evidence of illness. Pets have also been shown to be carriers of this bacterium, and must also be considered as a source when repeated infections occur in a family. The role that the great increase in the number of household pets plays in the increase in the incidence of rheumatic fever has not been fully explored.

Kissing pets has become an extremely common practice in our society, reflecting an abysmal ignorance of disease and hygiene. Whether this is a side effect of or part of the sinister objectives of the campaign to create a docile and compliant populace,[10] the results have been devastating. As Charles J. Sykes states in *Dumbing Down Our Kids*, theories of teachers turned amateur psychologists, such as cooperative learning, Outcome Based Education, and cultivation of self-esteem have largely replaced reading, writing and arithmetic as the goals of education. The result has been the delivery into society of individuals who are not only illiterate and ignorant of science, math, our government's operation and our history, but are lacking in interpersonal and job skills. These individuals are totally unprepared to earn a living for themselves or a family, or to serve their vital civic role in a self-governing society. The alarming increase in the incidence of sociopathic behavior, especially among young people, can be attributed directly to the confused and misguided social and behavioral standards that have been instilled during these vital formative years.

Strangely enough, my mother, with a very limited education, was very aware of the principles of personal hygiene and the risks of disease transmission. She educated her seven children regarding these basics in their very early years. The potentially serious consequence of kissing animals was demonstrated very dramatically in New Jersey in 1990 when an eight-week-old boy was hospitalized with meningitis. The infection resulted from the parents having the family dog lick the face of the infant for the purported purpose of "bonding." *Pasteurella multocida* was cultured from both the dog's mouth and the boy's spinal fluid. This organism frequently colonizes the mouth and respiratory tract of dogs, cats, guinea pigs and birds, and infections with this bacterium are common following a bite or scratch involving pets. Resulting infections may necessitate the amputation of a finger. Many cases of meningitis and infection in the blood of young children result from contact with a pet's saliva as occurred in this case. Bonding with pets develops from the normal association and play and does not require an exchange of saliva.

ASTHMA

About 12 million people in the United States suffer from asthma, and it is the most common chronic illness among children. It is an inflammatory reaction in the lungs that results in spasm of the bronchi and swelling and increased mucus production in the cells lining them. This reaction in the lungs is the same as what occurs in the nose with hay fever victims. The reaction in both cases is triggered. by the inhalation of a foreign protein such as various pollens, molds, dust mite excrement, residue from cockroaches and other insects and animal dander. Household pets such as dogs and cats are common causes of not only asthma, but also other respiratory allergies in children. In cats the offending allergen is in the saliva, and the constant grooming by the cat makes it a particularly troubling source. Studies have demonstrated that the cat allergen can accumulate on furniture and carpeting even where there is no cat present, because it is readily carried on clothing. It has also been shown to be present on very small airborne particles.[11] Horses also provoke these allergies, but fewer people come in contact with these animals. Rabbits have joined dogs and cats as house pets and they are as prone to provoke allergic reactions as are cats.

Desensitization through weekly injections of a precalculated mixture decreases the frequency and severity of attacks, as is the case with hay fever. Those individuals with severe disease must utilize aerosol inhalants of two different types of medication. One, a beta agonist, serves to relax the spasm of the bronchi, while the other is a cortisone analogue that tends to suppress the inflammatory reaction. Many people must use these medications regularly on a continuing basis, and continuous medical supervision to detect any undesirable side effects such as might develop in the eye is essential. As is the case with all medications in all fields, their powers are limited, and avoidance of the offending agent is necessary for control. This may mean removing all carpeting, drapes and upholstered furniture from the bedroom. Encasing the mattress and pillows in an impermeable cover helps to protect against dust mites. All bedding should be selected to be as free of lint as possible. Frequent vacuuming with a central vacuum system that is ducted to the outside is also important. Placing a HEPA filter in the room will additionally help to reduce the dust level (see Chapter VI).

COMMUNICABLE DISEASES

VACCINE PREVENTABLE:

I grew up in a family of seven children during lean times, long before the politicians discovered poverty and its value as a political weapon. We had to do a lot of sharing, and we certainly shared all of the communicable diseases. I can recall our mother suffering from mumps along with the seven children. In spite of her considerable discomfort it didn't interfere with her household duties, which were many.

We had no vaccines in those days. I was introduced to the world of immunizations when I entered the U.S. Navy in 1943. They made up for lost time. When I entered medical practice in 1956 we had DPT (diphtheria, pertussis, tetanus) injections and small pox vaccination in our armamentarium. We started every newborn on this routine at three months and saw to it that they had their DPT booster at 18 months. Parents of that era were very dutiful about seeing to it that their children received this protection. These illnesses were virtually eliminated in the United States. The most serious illness that remained was paralytic poliomyelitis.

During my first year in medical school a good friend died of bulbar polio, leaving behind a wife and two small children. In my junior year at medical school a neighbor child had polio, and I administered gamma globulin injections to my three children. Polio was a very dread disease that we had to contend with every summer. To be delivered from this threat and its burden of fear is a great blessing.

The introduction of the Salk injectable polio vaccine in 1955 sharply reduced the incidence of polio. The licensing of the Sabin live oral polio vaccine in 1961-62, and the widespread public immunization programs that followed, further reduced the incidence. In 1963 over 280 cases of paralytic polio were reported in the U.S. In 1964 the number had dropped to 91. During the period 1978 through 1991 a range of 6 to 9 cases per year were reported. This has been one of the great success stories in medicine, and it was accomplished against a disease that was caused by three different strains of the poliovirus. One cloud over the enthusiasm that accompanied the success of the Salk vaccine arose in 1955 when incomplete inactivation of the live virus during production by Cutter Laboratories resulted in 192 people contracting polio after being immunized with their vaccine. It is also known that some batches of polio vaccines were contaminated with the simian virus 40 (SV40), and this has been associated with a significant increase in brain tumors among those who received the vaccines in the 1950s and 1960s.

More recently vaccines for measles, mumps and rubella have been developed, with a dramatic drop in the incidence of these diseases. In 1964 over 1,800,000 cases of rubella were reported. The vaccine was introduced in 1969 and by 1986 only 551 cases were reported, an all time low. The number of cases of measles (rubeola) declined to 1,497 cases in 1983, but that number doubled every year following that, and 27,786 cases were reported in 1990. These cases were seen mostly in older individuals whose immunity needed a boost. The vaccine has not been recommended for those individuals born before 1956 because virtually everyone experienced natural infection prior to that time. Over 90 percent of people had experienced the disease by the age of 20 years.

The number of cases dropped dramatically the following year, 1991, and has fallen since then to fewer than 500 cases per year. The low point for mumps after that vaccine was introduced was 2,982 cases in 1985. Since that time about 5,000 cases per year had been reported, but that number started to decline after 1990, and since 1995 fewer than a thousand cases per year have been recorded. It is obvious that more diligence in obtaining these available immunizations is needed. In the United States that is the responsibility of parents, however, not the government bureaucrats who have usurped that authority.

There has developed considerable laxity among parents in getting their children immunized in recent years, and the result has been a recurrence of some of these infections. Several studies in different cities and populations have revealed that greatly inadequate percentages of infants and young children are receiving the recommended vaccines. It is true that the cost of these immunizations, which used to be very reasonable, has increased in recent years. This is partly due to the influence of lawsuits and partly the cost of a federal tax, which produces a slush fund for a federal compensation program. This tax adds a cost of $4.56 for each dose of DPT, $4.44 for each dose of MMR (measles, mumps and rubella), and 66 cents for each dose of polio vaccine. Through 1998 the National Vaccine Injury Compensation Program had paid out $925 million in claims for vaccine-caused injuries and deaths.

All of the childhood immunizations are available free of charge or for a nominal fee at health department clinics for low-income populations. A lack of understanding of the importance of this protection is a factor among some parents. A greater effort to correct this is currently being planned. No amount of effort by health officials can solve the problem of those individuals who refuse to be burdened by the responsibilities of parenthood. This attitude has become pathetically widespread in our society, and is the basis for many of our societal problems.

Immunization of a population has the potential to virtually eliminate those diseases for which vaccines have been developed, or at least to suppress them. In order to accomplish this it is necessary to induce immunity in a minimum number of the susceptible population, usually considered to be 80 to 90 percent. This phenomenon is referred to as **herd immunity**. The goal in the United States at present is to achieve a level of 90 percent immunization among the susceptible population. At that level of immunization herd immunity serves to suppress the transmission of the disease. This concept is based upon the principle that when such a large percentage of the population is protected from the disease, the infectious agent is reduced to such a low level that even those who are not immunized are protected.

It is necessary to keep in mind that a small percentage of individuals who are administered vaccines do not develop protective levels of immunity. This percentage varies with the type of vaccine, and the mechanism in the body through which it cultivates immunity, but it may be up to 10 percent. This is a more common problem in adults, and in individuals who have deficient immune systems. When the level of immunity in a community falls below a critical level we see outbreaks of a disease that had been controlled previously, as has happened with rubella, diphtheria and others. During recent years, the level of immunization in many communities has fallen to 60 to 70 percent. As a consequence we have seen a resurgence of some diseases that need not occur. We have even seen epidemics of some diseases such as measles, although that has been due at least partially to expiring immunity in the late teens.

The successful establishment of infant and childhood immunization programs after 1940 virtually eliminated those communicable diseases for which vaccines had been developed. Infants and young children are particularly vulnerable to communicable diseases. Newborns carry into life with them immunity to some of these diseases that is acquired from the mother. This dissipates by about six months, however, and the need for acquired immunity becomes urgent. It is therefore important to begin immunization schedules as soon as they are safe and effective. If given too early immunity does not develop to the fullest extent, so some delay and some compromise is necessary. Maximum protection is not achieved until after multiple doses for most of the vaccines. It is imperative, therefore, that parents return with their children on schedule to complete the immunization series. Overall in the United States only about one half of the children are fully immunized by age two years. This percentage increases dramatically at school age, because of laws requiring immunization for entry into schools.

Rubella is particularly worrisome in view of the serious

effects that it has on the fetus when the disease occurs during the first three months of a pregnancy. Immunity levels for rubella should be measured in all females in the late teen years, prior to pregnancy. Rubella vaccine should be administered to all who have low titers of immunity in the blood. This must be done well before any pregnancy occurs, not only to ensure protection, but because the vaccine cannot be given during pregnancy.

The long established caveat of medical practice, *first do no harm*, must also be adhered to in the application of vaccines. Immunization should be limited to those diseases that the individual is likely to be at risk for, and only with vaccines that are safe and without untoward side effects. In recent years there has been an energetic push to develop new vaccines for every conceivable infectious disease. Over 200 such vaccines were under development in 1999. Some vaccines have serious side effects, including death in some cases. Studies have also suggested that the assault on the immune system of infants results in as much as a five-fold increase in their risk of allergic phenomenon such as asthma.[12]

Monetary considerations have been too dominant a factor in the efforts to market some of these products, overshadowing their adverse reactions. Another disturbing development has been the usurpation of parental authority by government bureaucrats, who have been successful in instituting laws that mandate the administration of immunizations to children, under penalty of law. These bureaucrats have already announced their intention to mandate the immunization of all 12-year-olds with an AIDS vaccine once it is marketed. This is the same perverted mentality that mandated an unneeded hepatitis B vaccine on all newborn infants. Lord Acton's observation that power corrupts has certainly been demonstrated here.

The Centers for Disease Control has established the Advisory Committee on Immunization Practices (ACIP), whose members it appoints. Some of these members have financial links to the vaccine manufacturers, whose interests are primarily in promoting the increased use of vaccines. The ACIP decides what vaccines should be administered to children, and then the CDC endorses this schedule. The American Academy of Pediatrics, which previously made this judgement, decided in 1995 to simply endorse the schedule that was established by federal authorities. These mandates are then endorsed by the states, sometimes with the passage of laws by the legislature, and endorsed by HMOs and other third party payers. This removes parental authority completely and places parents at risk of legal action and prosecution if they fail to follow the mandates. This is fascism pure and simple and it violates the most basic tenents of the Constitution.

One of the most blatant abuses of this fascist power has involved the hepatitis B vaccine. In November 1991 this vaccine was added to the list of routine immunizations to be given to newborn infants. This decision was made by the ACIP, endorsed by the Centers for Disease Control, and supported by the American Academy of Pediatrics. They concluded that they would never be able to get the at risk population (IV drug users, male homosexuals and prostitutes) to become immunized. They concluded that if they immunized the entire population they ultimately would reverse the upward spiral of the disease in our society. There has been some resistance from both parents and physicians to adding this unnecessary immunization to the already long list of childhood immunizations.

It does not seem rational to immunize newborns against a disease that is contracted only through aberrant behavior that is not engaged in by the general public. For the majority of infants born there will be no risk of contracting hepatitis B throughout their lifetime. Additionally there have been a significant number of deaths among newborn infants as a result of the administration of this vaccine. The precise number is not known because these deaths have been ignored or mislabeled as SIDS (sudden infant death syndrome) in an effort by the CDC and the FDA to conceal this information. At least some of these deaths have been deliberately omitted from the FDA's Vaccine Adverse Effects Reporting System. It is also prudent to recall that recently developed technology has revealed that some of the vaccines that have been considered benign have been discovered to be contaminated with undesirable viruses. The contamination by simian viruses of polio vaccines that were administered to millions of children and adults, as mentioned previously, is one example.

Diphtheria immunization is accomplished by the administration of a toxoid, the dose of which is reduced after age 7 years. There is no immunity after natural infection, and vaccine immunity diminishes with time. Toxigenic strains of the causative agent, *Corynebacterium diphtheriae*, have been virtually eliminated in most Western countries. There has been a major eruption of diphtheria in the former Soviet republics recently, however, with over 40,000 cases in Russia alone in 1994. Immigrants from these regions present the potential to reestablish these strains in the U.S.

Pertussis: the vaccine for pertussis is derived from killed bacteria, and is not given after age 7 years due to adverse reactions. A new acellular vaccine is now available and it has a lower incidence of fever and local reaction. There is no immunity after natural infection, and vaccine immunity diminishes with time. Large outbreaks have occurred when vaccination programs have been neglected. (170,000 cases with 42 deaths in the United Kingdom in 1977-1979)

Tetanus: although tetanus is not a communicable disease it's toxoid is one of the three components of the first universal childhood vaccine, and will be discussed in this section. It is very effective and provides immunity for at least 10 years after the initial series. Booster doses should be administered every 10 years, or at the time of tetanus prone injuries. Human tetanus immune globulin should also be administered with high-risk injuries. The mortality rate with tetanus was 90 percent in the 1940s, but this has declined to about 25 percent with appropriate care. Tetanus and wound botulism have become an additional risk for injecting drug abusers as a result of injecting through unclean skin and/or from contamination of the drug being injected such as Mexican black tar heroin.[13] The incidence of this complication of drug abuse has been increasing recently. Neonatal tetanus kills one million infants each year in the developing countries as a result of the custom of dusting the umbilical stump with animal dung, or a powder of dried local clay sold for this purpose. Tetanus spores are ubiquitous in the environment, surviving for years in soil. As with most spores they are difficult to inactivate, requiring boiling for at least four hours or autoclaving for 12 minutes at 250°F. A natural reservoir for tetanus is the intestine of horses and other animals, where they produce no illness.

Hemophilus influenza: there are several species of *H. influenza*, but type b is the most important. Immunization for this strain is now included in the routine schedule for infants. It is discussed further under meningitis below.

Poliomyelitis is an acute infection that destroys motor neurons in the spinal cord and brain stem, resulting in a flaccid paralysis. Prior to the development of a vaccine this was a dread disease that occurred in epidemic form during the summer months, and crippled 20,000 people in the United States each year. Some of those who escaped paralysis with the initial attack developed a progressive paralysis 20 to 30 years later in what has been labeled the post polio syndrome.

Polio is caused by three antigenically different strains of poliovirus, types 1, 2 and 3, and a vaccine for each strain had to be developed. This was accomplished in 1955 with the introduction of the Salk injectable vaccine. The Sabin live attenuated oral vaccine was licensed in 1961-62, and we have been virtually free of this devastating disease in the United States since. The last documented cases of naturally acquired wild strains of polio in the United States were reported in 1979. There is a risk in adults of acquiring paralytic polio from the oral vaccine, however. It is therefore not recommended for adults currently, unless they will be traveling to areas where wild polio persists. Parents have become lax in having their children immunized, however, and the threat of a renewal of this disease is with us. Travel to areas where polio remains endemic also requires a careful assessment of the immunity status of the traveler, especially during the polio season.

Measles (rubeola): this is an acute, highly communicable viral disease characterized by a rash, cough and nasal discharge. Prior to the development of a vaccine over 90 percent of people had experienced the disease by the age of 20 years. The live attenuated vaccine is now part of the routine childhood immunization program, and this had virtually eliminated the cases in the United States. There was a marked increase in the number of cases in 1989-1991 however, primarily due to neglect of immunizations. Some cases resulted from the failure of a single dose to provide protective levels of immunity, and in 1989 a second dose, to be administered prior to entering school, was added to the schedule. Intensified immunization programs have markedly reduced the number of cases in the United States, to 138 cases in 1997.[14,15] Currently imported cases present the greatest threat to plans to eradicate the disease in the U.S. In 1998 a total of 33 cases of measles occurred in one school in Anchorage, Alaska as a result of importation from Japan of a genotype that had not been seen in the United States.[16]

Mumps is a highly contagious viral disease that is spread by droplet from the nasopharynx and through saliva. The virus most commonly causes inflammation in the salivary glands, particularly the parotid, but may also cause orchitis, especially in adults. Overt meningitis occurs in about 15 percent of the cases of mumps, but about one half of patients with mumps demonstrate an increased number of cells in the cerebrospinal fluid (pleocytosis). A live attenuated mumps virus vaccine has been used in the United States since 1967 as part of the MMR vaccine routinely administered at 12-15 months of age. In Canada and Japan a different strain of virus has been used in their vaccine, which has produced a higher incidence of mumps meningitis following administration of the vaccine.

Prior to the development of the vaccine mumps was endemic, with over 90 percent of children developing antibodies by age 15 years. Routine administration of the vaccine has suppressed the disease in the general population, as has been the case with measles. The challenge is to maintain a high level of immunization in children.

Rubella (German measles) is a milder measles, with the rash usually lasting 3 days. Its main risk lies in its proclivity to produce congenital malformations when infection occurs during the first three months of pregnancy. These congenital defects result from a transplacental infection in the fetus that causes malformations involving all three germ cell layers. The malformations occur in 20 to 80 percent of cases where infection occurs in the first four months. Hearing loss has been the most publicized, but mental, heart, eye, and musculoskeletal defects are common. Prior to the development of a vaccine, rubella was also a common childhood disease that "everyone" experienced. A vaccine was marketed in the United States in 1969, and there has been no major epidemic since. The disease is worldwide, and epidemics continue in countries where the vaccine has not been utilized. Lifelong immunity follows a natural infection, as is true with the vaccine.

Varicella (chickenpox) is caused by the varicella-zoster virus, a member of the herpes family, and is the most communicable of all of the childhood diseases. As a result it is experienced by virtually everyone early in his school years. It is for the most part a mild illness with few complications. Complications, including death, can occur however. Perhaps more important is the reactivation of this virus later in life to cause shingles. As with all herpes viruses, after the initial acute infection subsides the virus remains in the nerve ganglia in a latent state for life. Reactivation of the virus later in life, usually after age 50, concomitant with a reduction in the effectiveness of the immune system, gives rise to herpes zoster, or shingles, when the intercostal nerves are involved, or more serious problems when the cranial nerves are involved. The ophthalmic nerve is the most frequently involved of the cranial nerves, and can result in a loss of vision.

Reactivation of the varicella-zoster virus is also common in AIDS and in patients with Hodgkin's disease. Early administration of acyclovir can prevent the spread of the virus along the nerves, and this is especially important where the cranial nerves are involved. Shingles results in a permanent painful neuralgia in some victims that is very difficult to treat. In 1995 a live attenuated vaccine for varicella became available, and this has been added to the schedule of recommended immunizations. It should be administered after 12 months of age, and a booster dose after 4 to 6 years may be recommended in the future. Inclusion of the varicella vaccine in the childhood immunization schedule will help to eliminate the serious problem of herpes zoster.

Variola (smallpox): Inoculation against this deadly disease with material from the lesions of patients who had the disease was practiced as early as 1701 in Constantinople and 1713 in England.[17] The ensuing disease following this technique was less severe than when acquired through inhalation, but it was still readily transmitted to others. It had been noted that individuals who survived smallpox were immune to subsequent infections. Edward Jenner observed that milkmaids who acquired cowpox were similarly immune to smallpox. In 1798 he published the results of his successful immunization of 23 individuals with the cowpox virus who proved to be protected from smallpox. The subsequent development of a further attenuated vaccinia virus led to the inclusion of smallpox in the routine immunization schedule of infants and children. A disease that had been responsible for the deaths of many of the early pioneers and settlers in the United States was thus eradicated.

By the mid 1940s man to man transmission of smallpox had been eliminated in Europe and North America. Routine smallpox vaccination was discontinued in the United States in 1971.[18] Hundreds of cases continued to occur in other countries, however, and a worldwide campaign to eradicate the disease was undertaken. The last naturally occurring case of smallpox occurred in Somalia in 1977, and the disease was officially declared by the World Health Organization to be eradicated on May 8, 1980. It was believed that no natural reservoir for the virus existed at that time.

Other closely related poxviruses remain, however, including cowpox and monkeypox. Monkeypox has been reported in man with increasing frequency recently. About 400 cases were reported in Africa between 1970 and 1990. During the first eight months of 1996, seventy-one cases of human monkeypox, including six deaths, were reported in Zaire.[19] Smallpox vaccination with the vaccinia virus protected against these other poxviruses as well as smallpox, and as the number of people who are not protected increases, so will infections with these alternative poxviruses. Cowpox occurs only in Europe, but monkeypox is endemic in Africa, probably in a squirrel reservoir. In retrospect the conclusion that smallpox had been eliminated from the earth was naive, and the decision to eliminate stores of vaccine unwise. It is obvious that smallpox vaccination should be ongoing in at least some populations in Africa. Additionally, the terrorist attack on the World Trade Center on September 11, 2001 clearly demonstrated the folly of having no stock of vaccine for the American public. Smallpox is spread through the respiratory route, and it would be feasable to expose a large population in a terrorist attack. Protection against smallpox persists for five years following vaccination in most individuals, decreasing gradually. This is variable, and immunity lasts longer in many cases.

As late as 1994 cultures of the smallpox virus were supposed to exist in only two research laboratories in the world, one in the United States and the other in Russia. In 1998, however, U.S. intelligence discovered that Iraq, North Korea and Russia were all storing cultures of smallpox virus for military purposes. Russia had apparently shared its supposedly secure stock. In early 2001 the *Independent* of London reported that the U.S. Government had ordered 40 million doses of smallpox vaccine from a British company, to be delivered to the Centers for Disease Control in Atlanta. The government apparently is convinced that the genie has been released from the bottle. In 2001 a vaccinia virus vaccine (Dryvax®, Wyeth) that does not contain the smallpox virus was licensed in the United States, but none is available for the civilian population.

The current recommendations for immunization of children are listed in a table at the end of this chapter.

OTHER COMMUNICABLE DISEASES

BACTERIAL MENINGITIS

Hemophilus influenza type b (Greek haima=blood, philos=lover) was formerly the most common cause of bacterial meningitis, prior to the development of *Haemophilus b* conjugate vaccines. About 70 percent of the cases of meningitis from this organism in the United States involve children age 2 months to 5 years. The bacterium, which is found only in humans, can also cause other serious infections such as pneumonia, pericarditis, epiglottitis, tracheobronchitis, cellulitis and osteomyelitis. The introduction of the vaccine in the late 1980s made a significant contribution to the elimination of these diseases in children. An increasing number of cases are being seen in adults now, however. It is still a major problem in developing countries, with most cases occurring prior to 6 months of age there. *Hemophilus influenza* is spread by droplet and is acquired by inhalation through the naso-pharynx. About 30 percent of the strains of this organism have become resistant to the treatment of choice, ampicillin, due to their production of beta-lactamase. Current recommendations are that a third generation cephalosporin be given either alone or with ampicillin until sensitivity tests are received. It is further recom-mended that the patient be given rifampin prior to discharge to assure elimination of the organism.

Meningococcal meningitis is caused by *Neisseria meningi-tidis*. Since the introduction of the Haemophilus influenza type b protein-capsular polysaccharide conjugate vaccine as part of the infant immunization schedule it has become the most common form of bacterial meningitis in children in the United States. It is endemic in the United States at present, and carries a fatality rate of about 12 percent even with prompt treatment. Prior to the development of effective treatment the fatality rate exceeded 50 percent. Children under the age of 2 years are much more susceptible to the infection. The infection is seasonal with the highest incidence in February and March. The organism is spread by respiratory, droplet transmission, transmission being facilitated by crowded conditions such as nursery schools, school dormitories and military barracks. Cigarette smoking, upper respiratory infections, poor nutrition and lax hygiene also facilitate the spread of the organism. Nasopharyngeal colonization precedes the spread to the meninges of the brain, and communicability is high during this period. Some individuals are asymptomatic carriers; the meningococcus can be cultured from the nasopharynx of about five percent of the general population. The organisms thus cultured represent a diversity of serogroups and serotypes, many of which are not pathogenic.[20]

Culture of blood or cerebrospinal fluid is positive only in 60 to 80 percent of patients suffering from this form of meningitis, even when cultures are obtained prior to the initiation of antibiotic therapy. A gram stain of the cerebrospinal fluid can provide a rapid diagnosis by demonstrating the gram-negative diplococcus. A petechial or purpuric rash, typical in generalized septicemia, in the presence of signs of meningeal irritation must be considered to be meningococcal meningitis until proven otherwise.

Treatment of systemic meningococcal infection must begin immediately, preferably within 30 minutes of a tentative diagnosis. Death can occur within a matter of hours. Penicillin remains the treatment of choice in the United States, since the strains here do not yet produce β-lactamase (as of 2001). Significant numbers of cases resistant to penicillin have been reported in Spain and Greece. Thus far the organism remains susceptible to the third generation cephalosporins and quinolones also. Chemophrophylaxis of intimate contacts with rifampin is urgent. Epidemics occur world wide, especially in those countries with crowding and poor hygienic conditions.

Streptococcus pneumoniae occasionally causes meningitis in young infants, the elderly and in individuals with compromised immune systems. The fatality rate of this form of meningitis in these high risk individuals remains at 20 to 40 percent, although it has dropped to 5 to 10 percent in the general population with prompt and appropriate antibiotic therapy. Infection with this organism is discussed under pneumonia below.

Staphylococcus aureus meningitis is usually a complication of a neurosurgical procedure following trauma to the skull. Treatment is guided by sensitivity studies as with all staphylococcal infections.

Listeria monocytogenes is the etiological agent in about one percent of the cases of acute bacterial meningitis, primarily in the immunocompromised, such as those with AIDS, cancer, transplant patients, and patients receiving cortisone medications. There is also a higher incidence during pregnancy, in diabetics and in those with cirrhosis of the liver. It accounts for more than 20 percent of the cases of bacterial meningitis among cancer patients. Although the organism is widely distributed in nature, most human infections are foodborne, usually from unpasteurized milk, inadequately cooked hot dogs, meats at delicatessen counters or soft cheeses such as Brie, Queso Blanco, Queso Fresco, Camembert and Roquefort (see Chapter V). Intravenous penicillin G is the treatment, and it must be continued for at least 10 to 14 days after the temperature has returned to normal to assure a cure. The cephalosporins are not effective.

VIRAL MENINGITIS

Viral, or aseptic, meningitis (inflammation of the meninges in the absence of pyogenic infection) is relatively common, and it can be caused by a multitude of viruses from several different groups. In addition to the arboviruses (arthropod borne viruses) that are transmitted by ticks and mosquitoes, over 50 members of the Coxsackie virus, echo virus, and some newer enteroviruses have been found to cause meningitis. The virus of lymphocytic chorio-meningitis is acquired by contact with food or dust that has been contaminated with the excreta of mice. Herpes simplex virus type 2 causes meningitis in association with genital herpes in about 10 percent of the cases of primary infection. Newborns who are exposed to this virus during delivery may suffer encephalitis, which can carry a mortality rate of 60 to 85 percent, and survivors develop normally in only 40 percent of cases, even with antiviral therapy. HIV-1 can involve the meninges in the early stage of infection, as well as other components of the central nervous system. The aseptic meningitis that accompanies the multitude of central nervous system disorders in the later stages of HIV-1 infection is more serious, and is frequently accompanied by other infections, such as *Cryptococcus neoformans*, toxoplasmosis and many viruses other than HIV-1. Aside from HIV-1, the etiological agent in viral meningitis is identified in only about one-half of the cases.

PNEUMONIA

Pneumococcus: Pneumonia caused by *Streptococcus pneumoniae* has been seen in 400,000 to 500,000 people in the United States each year, and is a common cause of death in infants and older individuals. The fatality rate in those populations and in alcoholics and patients with significant disease remains at 20-40 percent, while it has fallen to 5-10 percent among those not so burdened and who are afforded prompt hospitalization and appropriate antibiotic treatment. The organism is commonly found in the upper respiratory tract of healthy people throughout the world, and it is the most common cause of community acquired pneumonia in the United States. The pneumococcus is spread by droplet and through direct oral contact, or indirectly through contact with contaminated articles. Susceptibility to infection is increased with virtually any of the multitude of chronic diseases, especially in the elderly, and with AIDS and alcoholism. Not surprisingly cigarette smoking significantly increases the incidence of invasion of *Streptococcus pneumoniae*, causing pneumonia or meningitis.

The treatment of choice is penicillin, although resistance is being reported more frequently. A polyvalent vaccine consisting of 23 of the known 83 capsular types is available, providing protection against about 90 percent of those strains known to cause infection in the U.S. It should be administered to everyone 65 years of age and older, and to those with chronic diseases such as diabetes. It is not effective in children under 18 to 24 months, and it provokes less protection in the very old. Immunity wanes after about 4 years, and re-immunization should be considered at that interval.

Mycoplasma or primary atypical pneumonia is caused by the bacterium *Mycoplasma pneumoniae*, which is spread both by inhalation of droplets and by direct contact with infected persons or articles soiled by them. It is frequently transmitted to other family members, health care personnel and associates in dormitories and barracks. Doxycycline and erythromycin are effective in treating the acute illness, but do not eliminate the organism from the respiratory tract. Strains resistant to erythromycin have emerged recently.

Pneumocystis pneumonia is caused by *Pneumocystis carinii*, a protozoan parasite. It is seen primarily as an opportunistic infection in AIDS patients, but may also afflict others with impaired immune function. Studies suggest that the majority of the general population have experienced a subclinical infection by the age of 4 years. A normally functioning immune system appears to prevent overt clinical disease.

Chlamydia trachomatis is a common cause of pneumonia in infants aged 3 to 8 weeks, but not in older children or adults. It is a subacute pulmonary infection transmitted to the infant during birth from infections of the uterine cervix. Treatment is erythromycin.

Chlamydia pneumoniae (formerly TWAR, Taiwan acute respiratory strain) causes an acute but mild pulmonary infection that is seen most frequently in young adults. The organism is antigenically distinct from *Chlamydia Psittaci*. It is transmitted by aerosol and by contact with objects contaminated by secretions. Treatment is tetracycline or erythromycin for 10 to 14 days.

Other: virtually any of the viral or bacterial pathogens that colonize the mouth, nose and throat can cause pneumonia. This is also true of the viruses of measles, chickenpox and influenza.

EXANTHEM SUBITUM (Roseola Infantum)
This disease is seen in infants from 6 months to 4 years of age. It resembles measles, with a rash and a fever as high as 105°F. Convulsions may occur whenever a temperature elevation in that range occurs. These symptoms persist for 3 to 5 days but no serious sequelae ensue. Enlargement of the lymph nodes in the neck and behind the ears may also be seen. The incubation period is 5 to 15 days, and the disease is seen mostly commonly in the spring and fall. Although the disease has been recognized and labeled for over forty years, the causative agent, the human herpesvirus type 6 (HHV-6), was not identified until 1992.

ERYTHEMA INFECTIOSUM (Fifth Disease)

This viral infection was recognized as early as 1900 as the fifth disease that produced a rash in children, thus the name. It was not until the 1980s that it was discovered that it was caused by parvovirus B19. It is spread by the respiratory route (cough, sneeze) and most commonly occurs in schools during the winter and spring months. The disease is characterized by a low-grade fever, malaise and a rash that includes a characteristic "slapped-cheek" appearance. It is a mild disease except in those children who have hemolytic disorders such as sickle cell anemia. The virus interferes with the production of red blood cells for 7 to 10 days, and thus can cause serious complications in that group of children. The virus can also present the same complications during pregnancy as are seen with rubella, including spontaneous abortion.

REYE SYNDROME

Reye syndrome was first diagnosed in the United States in 1963, but the cause and the full nature of the disease is still not known. It is seen only in children under the age of 15 years. It usually follows a viral upper respiratory illness, especially influenza, or chickenpox. Most cases occur between the months of December and March. Frequently an association between the administration of salicylates (aspirin) during these viral infections and the subsequent development of the disease has been made. Reye syndrome has clearly occurred on many occasions where salicylates were not used, however. Histologic examination reveals cellular changes in the brain, kidney and liver, with fatty deposits in the latter. These changes suggest that some toxic mechanism is at work.

Reye syndrome begins with sudden and very persistent vomiting accompanied by abnormal sleepiness and confusion. This is followed by a stupor that rapidly progresses to convulsions and coma. Death ensues in about 30 percent of the cases. Early diagnosis is difficult, but at the same time it is very urgent. There is no specific treatment, but measures can be taken to counter the swelling in the brain and the low blood sugar that frequently is found.

Fortunately the number of cases of Reye syndrome that are reported each year has been declining steadily since 1980. During 1987, thirty-six cases were reported; for 1988, twenty cases. This decline most likely reflects success in educating parents not to administer aspirin during viral infections.

There are still many communicable diseases for which we have no immunization available. Many of these can be prevented by common sense precautions such as hand washing and covering the mouth when coughing or sneezing. The foodborne infections, for instance, can be prevented by proper storage and handling of food and by hand washing (see Chapter V). Personal hygiene is one of the most important disciplines that children need to be taught, and it will require some parental effort over a period of years. If it prevents one case of gastroenteritis or parasitic infestation in the family the effort will have been rewarded.

Parental responsibilities extend far beyond conception. Being a parent demands many years of patience and persistence. Parenthood requires loving and caring, and teaching. All that a child learns after his introduction to this world he learns from others. Contrary to the misguided convictions of politicians, bureaucrats and even many educational officials, parents MUST be the prime source of this learning. In addition to the basic principles of personal hygiene and disease transmission, the rules of society, acceptable and unacceptable behavior must be taught. Failure in these responsibilities will of a certainty yield pain and grief for both the child and the parents, as well as for society. We have already witnessed an abundance of social disasters from this neglect, and this is only the beginning. Usurpation of parental authority by miguided totalitarian officials has greatly compounded this problem.

ROTAVIRUS

Rotavirus enteritis is one of the most common and most severe forms of diarrhea in children under 3 years of age. About 90 percent of all infants and children have experienced a rotavirus infection by 3 years of age. Approximately 65,000 children in the United States are hospitalized each year with rotavirus infection. About 100 of these children die as a result of the pronounced dehydration that results from this diarrhea. Rotavirus enteritis accounts for about one third of all hospitalizations for diarrhea in children. More than 3 million children acquire the disease in the U.S. each year without being hospitalized. Almost one million children under the age of five years die worldwide each year from this enteritis.

In the underdeveloped nations lack of sanitary water supplies accounts for most of the infections, especially in infants on formula. Early aggressive use of oral rehydration fluids prevents the more serious sequelae that result in death. The disease is seen primarily in the winter months in the U.S. The virus is transmitted from human to human by the fecal-oral route, frequently by people who change diapers then prepare food without washing their hands. This is yet another disease where cleanliness and hand washing could significantly reduce the risk and the incidence. This should be the basic, primary approach to controlling all communicable diseases. Rotavirus is another disease that is readily spread in day care centers, where diligent hand washing is an urgent necessity.

Two oral vaccines for rotavirus have been developed, and both have been shown to be effective. One is of bovine origin; the other is a combination rhesus-human product. The latter, which was licensed by the FDA on August 31, 1998, contains the four serotypes that most commonly cause disease in man. Immunization requires an oral dose at approximately 2, 4, and 6 months of age. It can be administered concurrently with the DTP, oral polio and hemophilus vaccines. The rhesus origin presents the usual concerns regarding viral vaccines from primates. The tetravalent vaccine has been reported to be about 50 percent effective in preventing rotavirus infections. There has been concern recently, however, about the increasing burden of vaccines administered to children and the possible adverse effect that this might have on their immune system.

CRYPTOSPORIDIOSIS

This is another of the so-called emerging diseases that was not a threat to us before the advent of our modern enlightened society. It is discussed in detail in Chapter V, but it is mentioned here because it has become another threat in day care facilities, demanding careful hygienic measures including hand washing. It presents a high risk of transmission, since only a small inoculum is required to cause infection. It also is difficult to diagnose, requiring special laboratory techniques and skills, as well as a high index of suspicion.

TUBERCULOSIS

Tuberculosis is an infection that most commonly affects the lungs but may invade other organs and tissues. In humans it is caused by a bacterium, *Mycobacterium tuberculosis*, an acid fast, aerobic, non-spore forming bacillus. The disease in cattle and other animals is caused by *Mycobacterium bovis*. All of the Mycobacterium species are resistant to virtually all of the antibiotics that have been developed over the past fifty years. The only reservoir in nature is infected people and for this reason efforts to control tuberculosis have centered on isolation of those with active disease, and the promotion of natural defenses. Prior to World War II every community of any size had tuberculosis sanitariums for the purpose of isolating and treating people with active tuberculosis. Finally in 1945 isoniazid was discovered to be effective against the organism and the prospects for control improved. The period necessary for the isolation of active cases was shortened to a few weeks. Since family members and other contacts could also be given isoniazid prophylactically, the period of isolation could be served at home in most cases. Gradually the disease was brought under control, and the number of new cases started to decline.

Isoniazid is the only drug that is used in the prophylaxis of tuberculosis. This medication must be taken faithfully, for six months in most cases, for 12 months for HIV positive individuals. Daily dosage is ideal, but twice weekly is acceptable for prophylaxis. Supervised administration (DOT, Directly Observed Therapy) for those with active disease is frequently necessary because failure to comply with the schedule risks not only the spread of the disease to others, but the development of resistant strains. Exposure to the disease is much more serious in infants, adolescents and in immunosuppressed individuals. These patients must be treated very aggressively to prevent progression to active disease.

The tubercle bacillus is spread primarily by droplet infection (aerosol), through a cough or sneeze, or even through talking and singing. Infection in the larynx is particularly communicable. The droplet, which is in the range of one to five microns in size, evaporates and leaves the organism suspended in the air for many hours. When another person inhales these organisms they are deposited in the lungs. Materials in the capsule and other components of the bacillus stimulate the defense mechanisms of the body, and the organism is inactivated in about 95 percent of healthy individuals thus infected. This containment results from the body's immune system in general, and specifically the immunity at the cellular level in the lungs. This process takes place over a period of several weeks, however, and during this period the organisms multiply in great numbers and are disseminated to other tissues of the body such as the kidneys and bones. The skin test usually becomes positive 4 to 6 weeks after infection, although it may be delayed for up to 20 weeks. It is of little value in patients with AIDS, since the majority of these victims do not react to the skin test even with active disease.

Even though they might be inactivated after being deposited in the lungs and other tissues, the microorganisms are merely dormant, and present the potential for later activation. Reactivation characteristically occurs during pregnancy, old age, serious illnesses, alcohol abuse, administration of cortisone, and any condition that suppresses the body's immune system. In the past, active tuberculosis in the United States has resulted primarily from such reactivation of a latent infection. Since 1985 not only has the incidence of reactivation of dormant tuberculosis increased, but the number of people progressing directly to active disease from the initial infection has also increased. Worldwide tuberculosis is currently the leading infectious cause of morbidity and mortality. In Africa more than a million people a year are contracting tuberculosis, with 500,000 deaths annually.

Meningitis caused by *M. tuberculosis* can be expected to result in death. Infection in the spine is called Pott's disease and causes destruction of bone there. Infection in the kidney, ureter and bladder can cause obstruction with impediment of urine flow. All of these have been uncommon in the United States, seen mainly in older patients and those with immune deficiency. Infections with *M. bovis* have been rare in the United States due to the universal pasteurization of milk and control of the disease in cattle. It has been found in deer herds in recent years, however, and their explosive population increase and spread to neighborhoods presents a new threat. *M. Bovis* has been a continuing problem in Mexico and in the border regions of the United States because the disease in cattle has not been controlled there and milk products there are not pasteurized.

During the period from 1953 to 1985 the total number of cases of tuberculosis in the United States had steadily declined by about five-percent per year. This success had resulted from the continuation of aggressive surveillance and treatment programs by public health officials, and by the development of isoniazid, and later, other drugs that were effective against the *Mycobacterium tuberculosis* organism. From 1985 to 1992, however, there was a persistent increase in the number of new cases reported each year. In 1990, 25,701 new cases were reported, up 9 percent over 1989, and the largest annual increase since 1953. In 1991 this number increased to 26,283. It has since remained at about 22,000 cases per year. In addition to the increase in the number of new cases of tuberculosis, patients with disease caused by strains of the organism that are resistant to the four drugs that are effective in combating it have been reported with increasing frequency. Both the increase in numbers and the development of resistant strains have been due primarily to the AIDS epidemic.

Both the increase in numbers of the disease and the development of resistant organisms also have been influenced to some extent by the increased numbers of immigrants from areas where resistant organisms are known to exist. An epidemic of unprecedented proportions has developed in Russia, Belarus, Moldova and Ukraine. In 1998 there were over 86,000 new cases of tuberculosis in Russia, and the Russian Red Cross expected that figure to double in 1999. As elsewhere resistant strains are present among these new cases. The general poor health of the population and lack of medicines that has ensued since the breakup of the Soviet Union is responsible for this catastrophe.

Another factor in the United States and elsewhere, which has been increasing in significance, is the growing AIDS population in the U.S. This group provides a fertile ground, not only for the spread of the disease, but also for the development of resistant strains of *M. tuberculosis*. The AIDS epidemic was a major factor in the resurgence of tuberculosis. Not only were AIDS patients much more likely to succumb to active disease upon exposure, but the destruction of their immune system resulted in the activation of latent disease. The increase in the number of young individuals with active disease has resulted in the exposure of increasing numbers of people in the general population. The cultivation of organisms that are resistant to the few anti-tuberculosis medications that we have is a further complicating, serious development.

As the incidence of tuberculosis increases in the adult population we can expect to see a concomitant increase in the disease among children. Because of their increased susceptibility to tuberculosis, the numbers of these exposed children progressing to active disease will be proportionately higher. This will add fuel to the already expanding epidemic. The current recommendation of skin testing for TB at age one and five years will most likely need to be revised to a more frequent schedule. These increased needs will place an added burden on public health programs and budgets.

The incidence of AIDS in adolescents aged 13 to 19 years more than tripled during the period from 1987 to 1991. A primary exposure to the tubercle bacillus in these immunosuppressed individuals is much more likely to progress to active disease, and the progression is much more rapid than has been seen in patients in the past. This progression results from the failure of the cell mediated immunity in the lung, and from the severely impaired immune system of the body in general. The incidence of disseminated tuberculosis and tuberculous meningitis, both of which can be expected to be fatal, is thus much higher in these pediatric AIDS patients. The development of resistant strains that render our medication less effective or useless will have a profound effect on both the morbidity and mortality in this age group. All of these factors will significantly increase the exposure of the general population to tuberculosis, and to resistant tuberculosis.

The lack of reactivity in skin testing among AIDS patients, which is a reflection of the suppression of the immune system, will also complicate the task of screening in this group. Physicians will need to be acutely alert to the early symptoms of the disease, particularly a persistent cough. Because tuberculosis is spread by droplet infection it will be urgent to teach these individuals to cover their mouths when coughing and sneezing. It may be necessary to return to the practice of teaching this and other basic hygiene principles at an early age. Both parents and schools will need to participate in this effort.

The increased incidence of tuberculosis conversion and active disease in the pediatric and adolescent population will also translate into a proportionate increase in the numbers of family members who will need to be placed on prophylactic medication(s) and surveillance. This will probably add to the problem of the development of resistant strains of the tubercle bacillus. Periodic monitoring of liver function through blood tests is essential with all patients placed on these medications. These needs will mandate that the resources devoted to tuberculosis programs, both in monetary terms and in personnel, be increased significantly in the future. The additional question arises of how to deal with the growing population with active disease caused by organisms that are resistant to all of our medications. In essence this returns us to the position that we were in prior to the advent of isoniazid. We may need to once again consider the establishment of facilities for isolation of patients with active disease.

BCG VACCINE

In Africa in regions where HIV infection is widespread among infants and young children, tuberculosis is a common complication. It is a particularly severe disease in this population and a frequent cause of death. Because of the serious problem of communicability of tuberculosis, the World Health Organization has recommended vaccination against TB at birth with BCG vaccine (bacille Calmette-Guérin). This live attenuated vaccine that is derived from *Mycobacterium bovis* has been widely used in Europe and some other parts of the world such as India for many years. It has been the subject of a prolonged disagreement between health officials of these regions and those in the United States.

There has been a wide variation in the effectiveness of the vaccine and in the level of side effects seen with it. These have been some of the arguments against its use. A recent fifteen- year study in India found that BCG vaccination was ineffective in preventing tuberculosis transmission.[21] When it is used it also totally invalidates the tuberculin skin test, and in fact introduces the risk of a local reaction in those who have received the vaccine. Up to the present time the value of the skin test has far outweighed any need for the BCG vaccine in the United States. The AIDS epidemic could conceivably force a re-evaluation of this policy, however.

NUTRITION

Inadequate or improper nutrition is a significant and common, although widely unrecognized, hazard of childhood. Nutritional needs during the first year of life are particularly not understood and thus neglected. It is important to supplement the milk diet with other essential nutrients as soon as feasible, without provoking problems such as food allergies. These essential nutrients are basically the same as those for adults, and are discussed below and in Chapter XV. A feeding schedule for solid foods for infants is included at the end of this chapter.

Growth and development continue through the teen years, and for this to proceed successfully the proper building materials must be available. A robust child does not guarantee a healthy child. Many obese infants and children are significantly malnourished. This can be readily demonstrated by a simple blood count, which will reveal a low hemoglobin level and red blood cell count.

One of the symptoms of iron deficiency anemia in young children is pica, the eating of non-food substances such as plaster, dirt or even poisonous substances. Zinc deficiency can also cause this, but it is much less common than iron deficiency. Pica frequently has been the underlying cause for the lead intoxication that results from children eating paint. Although the use of lead in paints has been restricted since 1977, it remains in many older buildings, often buried under coats of newer paint. When children eat any substance that contains clay (geophagia) it makes the anemia worse because it binds to ingested iron, preventing absorption. Both iron and protein are required to maintain a proper red blood cell and hemoglobin level. The latter is frequently seen in the 11 gram level, which is never satisfactory. A deficiency of iron in children has an adverse effect on mental and physical development and performance, as well as on resistance to disease. Teenage girls in particular are likely to be deficient, and thus benefit from iron supplementation.

All individuals require an adequate quantity of and a proper balance between protein, fat and carbohydrates. Certain vitamins and minerals are required additionally. In children where these basic needs are neglected while maintaining body weight 30 to 40 percent above normal, deficient growth and development will occur, and a higher frequency of illness will be noted. A normal balanced diet will supply these needs in most cases, but vitamin supplementation is frequently advisable, especially during the first year or two of life.

It is difficult for us in our land of plenty to visualize the serious nutritional deficiency states that are every day occurrences in other lands. Vitamin A deficiency, for instance, is the leading cause of permanent blindness in the developing countries. It is easily preventable by dietary supplementation of Vitamin A, which is synthesized and is cheap. Protein, which provides not only essential building materials, but also vital elements of the body's immune, protective and recovery processes, is widely deficient in the third world countries. This can be seen readily in the photographs of infants and young children with potbellies. We should be very grateful that we truly live in the land of plenty where we are spared these tragedies and suffering. Sadly, these blessings are universally taken for granted.

It is not difficult to fulfill the nutritional needs of the body. The protein needs are readily supplied by one half to one third the quantity of meat that most of us consume on a daily basis. The requirements other than protein are normally supplied by a well-balanced diet. Some elements are not always present in the diet in adequate quantities, and these can be provided by supplementation. Vitamin C, for instance, is not abundant in most diets, and it is easily destroyed by cooking and by oxidation from contact with zinc-coated containers or strainers. It is easily and cheaply synthesized, however, and 250 milligrams per day readily supplies our needs. The two vitamins that can cause harm in overdose are A and D. Vitamin D should rarely be taken in supplementation, certainly not in doses exceeding 400 international units daily. Many foods such as bread and milk are universally "enriched" by vitamins A and D, ensuring their presence in our diets in adequate amounts.

Consumption of potato chips, cheese chips, tortillas and any of the multitude of products that are made with the new synthetic fats should be completely avoided (don't ask me how). These products can rob the individual of whatever vitamin A, D, E and K that he does ingest. They bind to these vitamins so that they pass through the intestinal tract without being absorbed. These synthetic fats should never have been approved for marketing, but money not only talks, it barks.

For the child who is allergic to cows milk, calcium, which is essential for proper growth, can be supplemented by oyster shell calcium. Mineral sources of calcium such as dolomite, which also contains magnesium, are contaminated with other minerals that may be harmful. The most significant of these is lead and talc. Animal sources of calcium (bone) carry the risk of containing other harmful substances. This was the case when strontium-90 was found in the bones of animals during atmospheric testing of nuclear weapons. Care must be exercised also with calcium to not overdose and risk damage to the kidneys.

There is overwhelming evidence that the administration of small amounts of fluoride to children from birth and throughout childhood virtually eliminates dental caries. Dental caries is caused by a destruction of the enamel of the teeth by acid that is produced by bacteria in the mouth. This is the most common cause of tooth loss up to about age 45 years. Fluoride alters the enamel of the tooth in such a fashion that it becomes almost impervious to this action. Fluoridation of municipal water supplies is the most efficient means of accomplishing this. Widespread and irrational public objections have prevented this from being done in many communities. In localities where the public water supplies are not fluoridated, vitamins that contain fluoride should be administered to the infant. This should be continued throughout childhood. This simple practice will save the child much discomfort at the dentist and the loss of teeth. It will also save your pocketbook.

It is essential that supplemental fluoride NOT be administered in locations where an adequate fluoride content exists in the water. In addition to public water supplies where fluoride has been added, well water in some localities contains significant levels of fluoride. Your family physician or the local health department can give you this information, and tell you whether or not administration of fluoride is advisable. Excess fluoride will damage the teeth by producing mottling. This has happened in some regions of the United States where the natural fluoride content of the water is too high. Excess fluoride also causes increased bone density with brittleness and even neurological disturbances in high enough doses.

The objections to fluoridation of public water supplies have been based upon its toxicity and claims that it is a poison. These statements apply no more to fluoride than they do to other trace minerals in the diet, such as chromium, selenium, cobalt, nickel, copper and zinc. Iron overdose kills many children every year. Every substance is a poison if taken in overdose. This is true even of water. The point is that every substance taken into the body must be kept within the range dictated by genetics and physiology. Any substance that provides a benefit to health and well being should be supplied to the body within that range. Those of us who did not have the benefit of fluoride, and who suffered the dental consequences, can well be envious of today's generation.

PARASITIC DISEASES

Scabies and head lice have rejoined our society as scourges that are all too common. This emergence reflects the development of a laxity in personal hygiene and cleanliness in our society. That is not to say that you must be "dirty" if you acquire the diseases. A child from the most fastidious of families can bring home head lice from a companion at school. These organisms are easily shared. If the parents of all of the children in the school were likewise fastidious in cleanliness, however, it is unlikely that head lice would be present. Scabies finds a bountiful home on children, and this also is shared, requiring a somewhat closer contact than is the case with head lice. Scabies is frequently transmitted during sexual activities, and this is discussed in Chapter XI. Both scabies and head lice are discussed in Chapter XV.

HYPERACTIVITY

Attention deficit-hyperactivity disorder (ADHD) occurs in about 5 percent of the population in the United States. Higher percentages have been reported in some studies, depending upon the accuracy of diagnosis and criteria used for definition. A genetic component to this disorder that is inherited has been demonstrated. Recent MRI studies have localized the disorder to the dopamine receptors of the brain, which explains why stimulant drugs are effective in ameliorating the symptoms. The administration of either methylphenidate (Ritalin®) or dextroamphetamine (Dexedrine®) produces dramatic improvement with a single dose. Both drugs are equally effective and both without significant side effects at the appropriate dose. Methylphenidate is much more widely prescribed, primarily because it has been more intensely promoted, and because the federal bureaucracy has demonized dextroamphetamine. It is true that some children are on doses that appear to be excessive. The lowest dose that produces relief should be sought. In order to give a rest from the drug, it may also be discontinued during vacation periods from school. Enthusiasm for relief for the parent or teacher should not influence dosage decisions. God created few children who could pass for an angel; they require patience, attention and effort, and above all else, love.

ADOLESCENCE

Accidents are the leading cause of death among adolescents also. In addition, many nonfatal accidents result in hospitalization of young people. In many of these cases, emotional disturbances are a significant underlying factor. This may be suspected where a history of running away from home, depression or truancy is obtained. In many cases, however, truancy is merely a reflection of a low priority for education on the part of the parents. In those families where the parents give a low priority to the children in general, additional problems evolve. Society seems to be far more concerned about these problems than are some parents.

Approximately 15,000 to 18,000 of the accidents in adolescents each year are due to automobiles, and many of these are alcohol related. Alcohol is the substance most frequently abused in this age group. Its use is reported in about three million adolescents each year. In addition to accidents, other risks associated with abuse of alcohol are cirrhosis of the liver and its sequelae, malnutrition and vitamin deficiencies. Increased frequency and severity of infections of all forms, including tuberculosis, may accompany the malnutrition.

In the presence of a family history of alcoholism there may be a genetic predisposition. Alcohol and other substance abuse may be purely recreational, or may be an indication of a deeper psychological disturbance. It may reach a level where it interferes with interpersonal relationships with family, friends and working cohorts, and may interfere with attendance at and performance on the job. With the recent development of widespread substance abuse testing in the workplace these problems are being discovered more frequently and at an earlier stage.

Suicide is the third leading cause of death among individuals between the ages of fifteen to twenty-four years (homicides rank number two). Suicide is the second leading cause of death among college students. The rate of suicide among young people has doubled since 1960. The majority of these people are depressed. Other psychological disorders prompt this drastic action in others. Signs are frequently in evidence when looked for in retrospect. Frequently these individuals have been withdrawn and have isolated themselves from friends and family. An increase in problems at home, at school and at work is often in evidence.

Some events that may precipitate the psychological trauma are loss of a family member or loved one, breaking up with a friend, or divorce or separation of the parents. Difficulty in coping with these traumas is usually apparent. In many cases suicide attempts are unsuccessful at first, a genuine wish to die may not exist. In some cases where the wish to die is not real, the suicide succeeds by accident or unexpectedly. The suicide attempt may reflect a desire to punish a parent or other person for a perceived injustice, or may represent an act of retaliation. It may also represent self-perceived guilt.

OBESITY

Since the 1960s the incidence of obesity in the United States has doubled, and the magnitude of the excess weight in individuals has increased dramatically. The cultivation of this pathology among adolescents is particularly alarming because the number of excess fat cells that are added during this period can never be removed by any means short of surgery. Obesity presents many hazards to health. One of these is represented in the increased incidence of elevated cholesterol and triglyceride levels in teenagers, and the early onset of atherosclerosis. Emotional and self-image problems also accompany obesity in many cases. Of equal importance is the poor nutrition that frequently accompanies this disorder. It is difficult for parents to channel food intake toward the essential nutrients during this period, yet the fact that growth and development continue through these years makes it virtually as urgent as it is in the earlier years.

Parents have much less influence over nutrition during adolescence today, since the combination of increased freedom, cash in the pocket and a fast food or ice cream facility on every corner almost guarantees consumption of these items. These are difficult obstacles to overcome, but neglect of nutrition during these formative years will almost certainly penalize the individual throughout the remainder of life. In addition, gross obesity acquired during these formative years can never be totally reversed. Many of the cases of childhood malnutrition and obesity in our society today are simply the result of parents abdicating the responsibilities that are mandated by parenthood. In December 1996, a 6-year old boy who was admitted to a hospital in New Orleans for a limp was found to have scurvy. His diet for the past 12 months had consisted of cookies, yogurt, milk and biscuits. Administration of vitamin C resolved his symptoms, but the developmental damage could not be undone. This was a case of gross parental neglect.[22]

Several studies, including the 35-year follow-up of the Framingham Heart Study, have demonstrated the tragic consequences of obesity in childhood and adolescence. Another recent very comprehensive study was that of the Harvard Growth Study of 1922 to 1935.[23] After 55 years of follow-up this study revealed that death from all causes, and specifically from coronary heart disease and stroke, was significantly higher in individuals who were overweight in adolescence, regardless of adult weight. A higher incidence of other health problems such as arthritis, especially of the knees, gout, diabetes and hip fractures was also found. The significance of this for the current generation, which has experienced an epidemic of obesity, is ominous.

SLIPPED CAPITAL EPIPHYSIS

This is a disorder of the femur (the bone in the thigh). It is a more serious complication of obesity, at least from an immediate standpoint. The disorder is a separation of the upper portion of the femur at the growth plate of the head. It occurs more commonly in overweight individuals, during adolescence, and no hormonal imbalances have been found to explain its occurrence. It may follow a fall, but most cases present no history of trauma. Onset is insidious and marked by pain and limping. The pain may be referred to the knee, misleading the search for the cause. An x-ray reveals the diagnosis. In about one-third of the cases, the head of the femur is destroyed by necrosis (decay). Medical treatment is urgent, although it frequently does not prevent the unfortunate sequelae. There is a high incidence of premature degeneration and arthritis of the hip joint in overweight adolescents even without this disease.

LEGG-CALVÉ-PERTHES DISEASE

A similarly destructive disease of the hip joint strikes mostly male children between the ages of 5 and 10 years. For unknown reasons the head of the femur undergoes degenerative changes, resulting in deformity in the hip joint. The disease runs a 2 to 3 year course, requiring prolonged bedrest and orthopedic appliances for support. The damaged hip is prone to develop degenerative arthritis later in life.

SCHEDULE FOR SOLID FOODS FOR INFANTS

• Feed same food for several days before adding another
• Start with a small amount, one-half to one spoonful first day, gradually increase.
• Pushing food out is normal, does not indicate dislike. Infants must learn to swallow.
• No egg white before 10 months to avoid allergy. Also avoid wheat and orange juice for same reason.
• The surplus of iron that the infant is born with (assuming good nutrition during pregnancy) becomes depleted by the third month. Dietary sources of iron become important at this time.
• Both breast milk and cow's formula are deficient in iron and thiamine (unless added).
• Start feeding strained foods at about 2 to 3 months. Feed before breast or bottle, once daily at first. Gradually increase feedings to three times daily. Introduce these foods as follows:
FIRST: Precooked infant cereal (oatmeal) enriched with iron. Avoid wheat. Make consistency thin until infant learns to swallow solids.
SECOND: Egg yolk, hard-boiled, mixed with milk. Start with one-half spoonful or less, gradually increase. Good source of iron. May mix with cereal or other foods.
THIRD: Meats, strained.
FOURTH: Vegetables; start with peas first then add green beans. No spinach, beets or rhubarb which contain oxalic acid which will

108

cause diarrhea.

LAST: Fruits (other foods may be rejected if these are fed first).
• As teeth come in (6 to 8 months) give graham crackers and toast to chew on. Do not permit the quantity of these and other foods such as potatoes, noodles and deserts to diminish the intake of the more essential foods listed above.
• During second year of life the rate of growth slows, and thus food intake will diminish accordingly. Do not force quantity of food on infant.

RECOMMENDED IMMUNIZATION SCHEDULE FOR CHILDREN*

IMMUNIZATION	COMMENTS
HBV**	Initial dose of series, newborn
HBV**	Second dose of series, 4 weeks later
DTaP, IPV§, Hib***	At 2 months, as part of routine check
DTaP, IPV§, Hib***	At 4 months, 2 months between OPV
DTaP, HBV, Hib***	At 6 months
Varicella	At 12 months, booster after 4 to 6 years may be advisable
MMR, Hib	Combined vaccine at 12-18 months
DTaP	Third dose at 15-18 months
DTaP	At 4-6 years, prior to starting school
MMR#2	At 4-6 years, prior to starting school
MMR#2 if not given previously	Prior to entrance to middle school
Td	Repeat every 10 years for life

* Current as of January, 2002 (Advisory Committee on Immunization Practices)
§ In October 1998 the ACIP changed its recommendations and replaced the initial two doses of oral polio immunization with IPV, with the goal of reducing the incidence of vaccine-associated paralytic poliomyelitis.[24] It now recommends an all IPV program.
**HBV, hepatitis B vaccine, recombinant. Routine immunization controversial, see text.

***DTaP and Hib now available as a combined vaccine.
DTaP, diphtheria, tetanus, acellular pertussis
OPV, oral polio vaccine
IPV, inactivated poliovirus vaccine
MMR, measles, mumps, rubella
Hib, *Hemophilus influenza* type b, conjugate vaccine
Td, tetanus, adult (half strength) diphtheria.
BCG (Bacille Calmette-Guérin) vaccine for tuberculosis is not recommended for routine use in U.S.
TB skin test should be administered at age 1 and 5 years, and after exposure.

SOME COMMON POISONOUS PLANTS IN THE UNITED STATES

COMMON NAME	POISONOUS PORTION OF PLANT
Azalea§	Andromedotoxin is similar to aconite, depressant to heart and muscles of body (curare-like effect).
Baneberry, red & white (Dolls-eyes)	Berries & roots poisonous.
Bittersweet (Red Nightshade)	Green berries contain solanine. The riper, the less poisonous.
Black nightshade (Deadly Nightshade)	Leaves & berries contain several very toxic glucosides, especially solanine.
Blue cohosh (Papoose Root)	Leaves & blue berries (seeds) are poisonous.
Buttercup	Leaves & flowers cause salivation, peeling of tongue, loss of taste, & abdominal cramping.
Caster beans	Colorful, attract children. Contain ricin, very poisonous, may be fatal.
Celandine (Rock Poppy)	Leaves & seeds. Severe irritation & burning mouth, stomach pain, diarrhea, collapse. Skin irritation.
Dieffenbachia (Dumb Cane)	Oxalic acid. Chewing leaves produces immediate burning in mouth & lips, difficulty swallowing & breathing.
Ergot (from moldy grain, espe cially barley)	Gangrene of fingers & toes.
Fava beans	Serious destruction of red blood cells in susceptible persons.

Foxglove (Digitalis purpura)	Entire plant, but leaves are very poisonous, may cause death. They contain a series of glycosides including ouabain and digitoxin.
Indian Tobacco (Lobelia)	Leaves & seed contains lobeline; vomiting, stomach pain, diarrhea may lead to death. Plant labeled poison by FDA.
Jequirity Beans ("Crab-eyes, Rosary Beads)	Imported from Africa to Florida & Caribbean. Very attractive, very dangerous. Powder from beads is often fatal when inhaled.*
Jimsonweed	All parts contain belladonna alkaloids. Plant labeled a poison by the FDA.
Mistletoe	All parts, but especially the berries contain tyramine.
Monkshood (Aconite)§	Common in gardens. All parts severely toxic. Sometimes mistaken for horseradish.
Moonseed	Berries can be mistaken for wild grapes & have resulted in death.
Morning Glory	Seed contain a mild hallucinogen.
Mountain Laurel§	Leaves & flowers contain a toxin similar to aconite.
Mushrooms, various	All parts. Especially Amanita species which contains excitotoxin.
Oleander§	Leaves, flowers & bark may be fatal. Poisoning has occurred from using as spindle on barbecue grill.
Poison Hemlock (Fool's Parsley)	All parts contain coniine. Looks like Queen Anne's Lace.
Pokeweed	All parts, esp. unripe berries. Abdominal pain, impaired vision, respiratory depression.
Poppies, California	Depressant action on heart & muscles of body.
Poppies, Oriental	Contain opium alkaloids. Narcotic poisoning.
Potatoes	Sprouts, leaves, berries & seeds contain solanine.
Rhododendron (family)§	Foliage & shoots andromedotoxin; symptoms similar to aconite & curare.
Sorrel	Contains oxalic acid, dangerous to children and older people.

Tomatoes	Leaves and stem contain solanine.
Tung Nuts (look like Brazil nuts)	Severe stomach pain with vomiting, profuse diarrhea, shock and respiratory depression.
Water Hemlock (Spotted Cowbane)	Entire plant contains cicutoxin; may result in death in few hours.
White Snakeroot	All parts poisonous; cattle avoid it, get "the trembles" if they eat it. Poison in milk. Other species medicinal.
Wild Cherry (Chokecherry)	Leaves and fruit pits contain hydrocyanic acid.
Yellow Jasmine (Gelsemium)	Weakness, unsteady, unable speak or swallow, pupils dilate, eyelids drop. The alkaloid gelsemine is related to strychnine.
Yew (Ground Hemlock)	All parts of all yews are poisonous; contain a toxic alkaloid, taxine.

* Contains abrin, one of the most toxic substances known.

§ Toxin may be carried to honey by bees.

1. National Safety Council. Accident Facts, 1997 edition.

2. Fleisher GR. The management of bite wounds. *N Engl J Med*. 1999;**340**:138-140.

3. Autti T, Sipila L, Autti H, Salonen O. Brain lesions in players of contact sports. *Lancet* 1997;**349**:1144.

4. CDC. Fireworks-related injuries. *MMWR* 1992;**41**:451-454.

5. CDC. Near fatal ingestion of household lamp oil — Ohio, August 1997. *MMWR* 1998;**47**:880-882.

6. Kalugin, O. The First Directorate. St. Martin's Press. New York, 1994.

7. Sobel JD, Chaim W. Treatment of Torulopsis glabrata vaginitis: Retrospective review of boric acid therapy. *Clin Infect Dis* 1997, April; 24:640-52.

8. CDC. Toddler deaths resulting from ingestion of iron supplements — Los Angeles, 1992–1993. *MMWR* 1993;**42**(6):111-113.

9. American Academy of Pediatrics Task Force on Infant Positioning and SIDS. Positioning and sudden infant death syndrome (SIDS); update. *Pediatrics* 1996;**98**:1216-1218.

112

10. "The aim of totalitarian education has never been to instill convictions but to destroy the capacity to form any." (Hanna Arendt, *Totalitarianism* [New York: Harcourt Brace Jovanovich, 1968], p168. Also see *Dumbing us Down* by John Taylor Gatto, New Society Publishers, 1992, and *Dumbing Down our Kids* by Charles J. Sykes, New York, St. Martin's Griffin, 1995.

11. Siebers R, Weinstein P, Fitzharris P, Crane J. House-dust mite and cat allergens in the Antartica. *Lancet* (353) June 5, 1999, p. 1942.

12. Odent MR, Culpin EE, Kimel T. Pertussis vaccination and asthma: is there a link? *JAMA*, 1994;**272**:591-592.

13. CDC. Tetanus among injecting-drug users — California, 1997. *MMWR* 1998;**47**:149-151.

14. CDC. Summary of Notifiable Diseases, United States, 1997. MMWR 1997;**46**(No. 54):74-75.

15. CDC. Measles Eradication: Recommendations from a Meeting Cosponsored by the World Health Organization, the Pan American Health Organization and the CDC. *MMWR* 1997;**46**:RR-11.

16. CDC. Transmission of measles among a highly vaccinated school population — Anchorage, Alaska, 1998. *MMWR* 1999;**47**:1109-1111.

17. Garrison FW. *An Introduction to the History of Medicine,* ed 4. WB Saunders, Philadelphia, 1961.

18. CDC. Public Health Service recommendations on smallpox vaccination. *MMWR* 1971;**20**:339.

19. Mukinda VBK, Mwema G, Kilundu M et al. Re-emergence of human monkeypox in Zaire in 1996. *Lancet* 1997;**349**:1449-1450.

20. Infectious Diseases and Immunization Committee, American Academy of Pedriatics. Meningococcal Disease Prevention and Control Strategies for Practice-based Physicians. *Pediatrics* **97**:1996, p404.

21. Kumar S. 15-year follow-up shows BCG vaccine is not effective in India. *Lancet* 1999;**354**:1619.

22. Shetty AK, Steele RW, Silas V, Dehne R. A boy with a limp. *Lancet* 1998;**351**:182.

23. Must A, Jacques PF, Dallal GE, Bahema CJ, Dietz WH. Long–term morbidity and mortality of overweight adolescents. *N Engl J Med* 1992;**327**-(19):1350–1355.

24. CDC. Impact of the Sequential IPV/OPV Schedule on Vaccination Coverage Levels — United States, 1997. *MMWR* 1998;**47**:1017-19.

IV

HAZARDS OF REPRODUCTION

— for whatsoever a man soweth, that shall he also reap.

— Gal. 6:7

FAMILY PLANNING

The goal of family planning is to permit a couple to have children at a time of their choosing, and in numbers that they feel comfortable with. A successful program would provide for happier circumstances for a family, both economically and socially. It would also avoid the less than desirable time spacing between children that has been a common problem in the past. We have not had the necessary tools for such a program until about forty years ago. Although we had many programs and plans, we lacked the necessary tools to carry them out successfully. Abstinence was an early solution to the problem, but not surprisingly this system never gained wide acceptance. The rhythm method, based upon calculating when conception was possible and refraining from intercourse during that period, prompted a greater effort but with little more success. Barrier methods such as diaphragms, condoms, and spermicidal foams and jellies gained even greater acceptance and use, but it is doubtful that many couples realized the 70 percent rate of effectiveness that was claimed for them. They were almost guaranteed to fail for both the enthusiastic performers and the repeat offenders. Additionally, the use of diaphragms requires premeditation and advance planning, which frequently are not components of sexual activity.

The first oral contraceptive was introduced in 1958, and it was virtually 100 percent effective in preventing pregnancy. Adverse side effects with these "high dose" pills (10 mg norethynodrel) were significant, however. These included nausea and the general metabolic effects that are also seen during pregnancy. Of greater concern was the increased incidence of cardiovascular events, including thromboembolic phenomena and myocardial infarction. Those women who smoked cigarettes experienced substantially more of these side effects than did those who did not smoke.

Within a short time pills with one half the estrogen content (5 mg) were introduced, and this significantly reduced the incidence of side effects, while making no sacrifices to efficacy. This was followed, by trial and error, by a pill containing 2.5 mg of estrogenic substance, with a further reduction of side effects, and a retention of greater than 98 percent effectiveness in preventing pregnancy. By 1973 we had tablets containing 50 μg (.05 mg) of estrogen. Even lower dose pills with 35 μg of estrogen and 1 mg of progestin are currently available, and these very low dose pills are the mainstay of contraception today. They have a failure rate of about 0.1 percent when taken faithfully. Oral contraception is the most widely used method with approximately 50 million women world wide utilizing it.

These contraceptive pills are not teratogenic and deliver none of the adverse effects on the fetus that had been observed previously with other hormones such as diethylstilbestrol. They also reduce the risk of benign breast disease such as fibroadenoma and fibrocystic disease, both of which are a factor in the subsequent development of breast cancer. Oral contraceptives also reduce the risk of endometrial carcinoma by 50 percent and of ovarian cancer by about 40 percent, depending upon how long the pills are taken. The benefits persist for at least ten years after discontinuing their use. Another benefit is a lighter menses with reduction in the blood loss that is common during menstruation. Amenorrhea is sometimes experienced after cessation of the pill, but this usually resolves within four to eight weeks. Oral contraceptive pills should not be taken by women who are obese, who smoke, who have thrombophlebitis, cardiovascular disease, impaired liver function, varicose veins, or malignancies that are stimulated by estrogen. They also should not be taken at the same time as antacids, which may interfere with their absorption.

Injection of a long-acting progesterone has become a popular alternative to oral pills. This form of contraception carries a success rate similar to the pill when properly administered. It relieves the recipient of the burden of remembering to take a pill, but has to be repeated every 3 months. A large percentage of women experience significant disruptions of the menstrual cycle with this method. A more serious risk is the promotion of osteoporosis due to the reduction in circulating estrogen. This is especially damaging in teenagers, a group especially targeted for this form of contraception, since a women's maximum bone density is normally developed at about age 25 years. Long term injections of progesterone interfere with this and the result is a permanent reduction in bone mass. The same complication results from the use of the implantable capsules. Another side effect of injectable progesterone contraception is weight gain.

The intrauterine device (IUD) was introduced in the United States in 1961, although it had been used in Germany as early as 1929. These have been highly effective in preventing pregnancy, with a failure rate of about 0.7 percent in the first year and two percent over a ten year period with the copper-bearing devices currently available. IUDs became very popular, especially after the introduction of the Cu-7 in 1972. This new smaller device could be inserted into women who had never delivered a baby. In 1973 there were 3.2 million women in the U.S. using IUDs. In 1983, however, the CDC reported that women using the Dalkon Shield experienced a higher incidence of pelvic inflammatory disease that did women using the other designs. In that same year both the CDC and the FDA issued a well-publicized recommendation that women wearing a Dalkon Shield have them removed.

That report unleashed a torrent of damage suits by trial lawyers, not only against the maker of the Dalkon Shield, but the other IUDs as well. As a result liability insurance became unavailable and the manufacturers of the Cu 7 and Tatum-T withdrew their products from the market in 1986 (over 800 lawsuits had been filed).[1] Thereafter no IUDs were available in the United States for several years. They continued to be widely promoted and used elsewhere in the world, however, with over 40 million people in the People's Republic of China alone using them.[2] With an effectiveness of 98 percent and low cost the IUD has been invaluable in less developed countries where excess pregnancies are a particular burden.

With the onslaught of unwarranted lawsuits no domestic manufacturer was willing to risk the cost of litigation. Finally in 1988 one copper wound IUD, the Copper T-380A (or TCu-380), was imported into the U.S. and is currently available as the ParaGard T 380A.® It provides protection against both intrauterine and ectopic pregnancies by preventing the fertilization of ova[3] for up to 10 years. In 1993 the Chinese government began using only copper-wound devices. Although a copper-bearing IUD is the method of choice for contraception in most women, sharing the effectiveness but lacking the side effects of the pill, less than 1 percent of women in the United States using contraception utilized it in 1992.[4] By contrast about 100 million women worldwide use an IUD for contraception.

It has been argued that IUDs increase the risk of infection, and especially pelvic inflammatory disease (PID). PID may result in infertility, which is especially troublesome in women who have not had children. Women who have multiple sexual partners are at higher risk of infections and PID, with or without an IUD. There is no more excuse for an infection that results from insertion of an IUD than there is with any other surgical procedure. Infections generally result from a failure to abide by generally accepted aseptic surgical procedures. Obviously an IUD should not be inserted in the presence of a current infection. The wizards in our fascist federal bureaucracy mandated that physicians must issue the detailed information in the package insert to patients before inserting an IUD (Federal Regulations, 21CFR 310.502). They neglected to include a mandate that physicians follow standard sterile techniques.

It is a sad commentary on our current society that we have such a large number of unplanned pregnancies and unwanted children born. Fifty years ago the unplanned pregnancies were understandable, for we had no effective methods of contraception. In spite of that the unplanned children that were born were not neglected and abused as extensively as is the case today. Especially tragic is the epidemic of young girls becoming pregnant currently. That we have reached a point in the United States where over 11,000 babies are born each year to girls younger than 15 years of age is shocking and deplorable. The social problems engendered by these events are serious enough, but the resultant health consequences are equally serious. Prominent among these to the mother is the high risk of sexually transmitted diseases and their consequences, including HIV and its long, unpleasant journey to death. For the babies there is an increased incidence of prematurity, low birth weight, birth defects, impaired development and mortality.

In addition to the above, over 500,000 babies are born each year to girls who are between the ages of 15 and 19 years. The same social and health consequences apply to both the babies born and to their mothers as is seen in their younger counterparts. Some of these babies are fortunate enough to receive the appropriate rearing, love and guidance, but many other children are unloaded on government social agencies, which cannot substitute for parental and family guidance. The current alarming outbreak of sociopathic behavior by young people gives some indication of the price that we as a society will pay for this carelessness and neglect for years to come.

There is no greater joy on earth than the introduction into the family of a newborn baby. It is a great tragedy, however, to have this joy marred by physical or mental malformations in the infant. Such sorrow is visited upon couples far too often, and in many instances unnecessarily. Some such defects are familial; the result of inherited genetic defects. Many, if not the majority of such malformations, however, are the result of external factors that could be avoided. Cigarette smoking and alcohol and cocaine use during pregnancy account for a very large number of defective, malformed and mentally deficient newborn infants in the United States. This places an enormous burden on society and is a national disgrace.

PRENATAL CARE AND CONGENITAL MALFORMATIONS:

Serious congenital malformations are observed in about 3 percent of the infants born in the United States. However such defects can be found in about 7 percent of infants autopsied. About 500,000 pregnancies terminate each year in spontaneous abortion or in death of the infant due to congenital malformations. Spontaneous abortion prior to twenty-eight weeks occurs in ten to twenty percent of pregnancies diagnosed, and in approximately twenty to twenty-- five percent of conceptions. Approximately one-third of these demonstrate chromosomal abnormalities, and about one-half of the remaining have malformations of one form or another. Some authorities estimate that one half of all conceptions are lost in the first 2 to 3 weeks due to major chromosome abnormalities. This loss passes unnoticed, and thus no accurate data is available.

Thus about sixty-five percent of spontaneous abortions result from imperfect fertilized germ cells. These are, for the most part, zygotes that would result in a significantly abnormal infant. This so-called "wastage" is a phenomenon that is common to all animal species. The process protects against the birth of many severely deformed offspring, but it is not an absolute protection. It seems to work best in those instances where serious defects exist at the time of fertilization, or at least early after implantation. Developmental defects that are cultivated well after development is under way appear to escape this natural protective process in large measure. Spontaneous abortions that are not associated with chromosomal abnormalities usually occur later in pregnancy, at about three months, and are most frequently associated with maternal age of more than 35 years (see infertility below).

Birth malformations date back to the earliest days of mankind. These are evident in recorded art from previous eras before language recorded the events. Aside from inherited genetic influences there were many environmental factors that led to malformation. Many of these remain to the present. Nutritional deficiencies were recognized in the 1930s to be a factor in malformations, with vitamin A deficiency being the first nutritional influence to be identified. From that point to the present the single major advance in the management of pregnancy has been the recognition that adequate vitamin-mineral supplementation from the earliest days of pregnancy continuing to delivery is vital to the development of a normal fetus.

This presupposes good nutrition, for the development of a new organism requires the same growth materials that are needed after birth, namely adequate protein, fat, carbohydrate and essential vitamins and minerals. Additional calcium is needed to supply that needed for the development of the fetal bones and teeth. Sufficient calories to sustain both the mother and infant are needed, but this can usually be accomplished with little more than 1800 to 2100 calories daily. An additional 500 calories are needed during the last half of pregnancy and an additional 1000 during breast-feeding. During the first half of pregnancy 60 grams of protein is sufficient, but during the last half this should be increased to 80 grams; during breast feeding it should be increased to 100 grams. As the fetus enlarges and crowds the stomach it is advisable to divide the days food needs into five or six smaller meals to avoid the heartburn that is common.

The first three months is the period of most rapid development of the fetus, and this period is crucial, not only in providing proper nutrition, but in avoiding drugs known to interfere with the normal development of the fetus. Alcohol and tobacco are the most commonly used drugs that adversely affect fetal development. Generalized malnutrition with inappropriate caloric restriction and protein deficiency in the mother during pregnancy lead to severe growth retardation, thyroid deficiencies and delay in the maturation of the central nervous system in the fetus. These are not reversible with feeding or any level of care after delivery. Deficiency of folic acid, which is common in the general public, may lead to neural tube (spine) defects such as spina bifida, and perhaps to other birth defects that develop in the first month of pregnancy. These can be prevented by routinely taking 400 micrograms of folic acid, which is present in therapeutic strength multivitamins, daily before pregnancy ensues and continuing in prenatal vitamins for the duration of the pregnancy.

About 40 percent of all women in the United States in the childbearing years have low body stores of iron. This usually reflects a dietary deficiency, but seldom a caloric deficiency. It is the custom for people to eat what they like rather than what they need. We have far too many pleasure foods in our society, and the bulk of the population has the surplus funds to buy them. Dietary intake of iron containing foods is more critical in women than in men. Menstruation doubles the daily requirement of iron, and thus compounds the anemia that is so common among women. Pregnancy greatly increases the need for iron because 500 mg. of iron is transferred from the mother's iron stores to the fetus during pregnancy. If sufficient iron is not available to the fetus, deficient development, both physical and mental, ensues. These deficiencies are assigned to the individual for life.

It is essential for iron supplementation to be started at the onset of pregnancy. Tea should not be taken with food sources of iron since the tannates in tea interfere with the absorption of iron. It is very difficult to improve a maternal anemia during pregnancy; it is a battle to just maintain the mother's iron level and to provide the iron needed by the developing fetus. Iron deficiency anemias should ideally be corrected before pregnancy occurs. Good professional prenatal management should be instituted early in pregnancy, not merely after the third month. The first three months are the most critical as far as the development of the fetus is concerned, and this period is frequently neglected. Very often, women wait for two to three months to be certain that a pregnancy exists before scheduling a visit with the physician.

It is also vital that vitamin-mineral supplementation and good nutrition be instituted at the earliest possible time during pregnancy. Neglect of these imperatives, especially during the critical early months of development, can result in developmental defects that can never be corrected. The discussion on nutrition in chapter XV should be reviewed for more detail. The essential blood count, chemistries and other tests need to be done early. Most women are aware of being pregnant as a consequence of the symptoms that they feel, in conjunction with a missed period. The newer pregnancy tests confirm this rapidly and inexpensively.

All too often a couple view the need for professional guidance as involving only the actual delivery of the infant. Pregnancy and the growth of the fetus are viewed as a natural process that will proceed without any assistance or interference. This benign neglect frequently results in children with unnecessary congenital malformations. Aside from abstaining from drugs, adequate nutrition is essential. This can be provided by about 1800 calories daily where excess weight is a problem. These calories must come from essential foods in a proper balance, however, not junk foods. Even in overweight women an extra 500 calories are needed during the last trimester. Nutrition must be attended to early in pregnancy, preferably starting with day one. Ground lost in the early months is very difficult to regain, especially as pregnancy progresses. Birth defects that develop during this period cannot be corrected.

The hemoglobin level always drops about one gram in the last three months due to dilution of the blood by the fetal circulation. This apparent anemia is not harmful if the hemoglobin level has been maintained at a satisfactory level up to that point. If the hemoglobin levels fall to eleven grams or below, however, harm can be done to the developing fetus, and there is a serious risk of complications at delivery.

Overeating and eating junk foods can be just as harmful as undernutrition. These eating habits, in fact, are responsible for the majority of the cases of malnutrition in our society. Total weight gain during pregnancy should ideally be between eighteen and twenty-four pounds, assuming normal weight when pregnancy begins. If this weight gain is realized while adhering to good nutritional guidelines, avoiding foods with no essential nutritional value, it will be adequate. The higher weight gain recommendations that have surfaced recently assume that a significant proportion of the caloric intake during pregnancy will be from "pleasure foods" that are of no nutritional value. Excessive weight gain during pregnancy introduces the risk of toxemia of pregnancy (eclampsia) with its threats to both the mother and the fetus.

Along with good nutrition, exercise takes on added urgency during pregnancy. It provides all of the benefits to health that are seen at any stage in life, but provides added prophylactic value during pregnancy. Proper and adequate exercise facilitates good circulation to both the mother and the fetus. It reduces the risk of phlebitis in the mother that is so common during pregnancy, and keeps the heart and lungs "tuned up." Simple walking meets this need in most cases and is seldom contraindicated in any pregnancy.

The problem of insuring adequate nutrition during the first trimester of pregnancy is often compounded by morning sickness. This is due to the hormonal changes that accompany pregnancy, and can be severe in some women. In addition to the nutritional deficiency that results, unacceptable fluid and electrolyte imbalance can ensue. This disorder was formerly well controlled by Bendectin®, a combination of doxylamine and pyridoxine that was very effective. During the 1970s many lawsuits were filed falsely claiming that Bendectin caused birth defects. As a consequence the manufacturer withdrew the drug from the market in 1982, and it has not been available in the United States since then.

There is no other drug available for the treatment of this serious and troublesome side effect of pregnancy, and hospitalizations for it have doubled since the withdrawal of Bendectin. It has continued to be used in Canada under the name Diclectin®, and studies and experience have demonstrated that it is not responsible for birth defects.[5] Pyridoxine alone, 50 mg taken once or twice daily is helpful in controlling some cases of nausea and vomiting of pregnancy. Injections of pyridoxine may be necessary in the more refractory cases.

Deficiency of vitamin A and folic acid each individually

produce growth retardation, abnormalities and fetal death. A deficiency of folic acid has also been linked recently to the development of neural tube defects such as spina bifida. Neural tube defects, spina bifida and other conditions where there is a failure of the spine to close around the spinal cord and nerves, are serious developmental defects. About 4,000 such infants are born each year in the United States.[6] Some studies have suggested that the routine use of multivitamin supplementation during pregnancy reduces the incidence of these defects. A British study published in 1991 demonstrated that the use of a higher than normal dose of folic acid, taken daily prior to conception and during early pregnancy, reduced the incidence of repeat neural tube defects by 70 percent.

This study group was composed of women who had experienced a previous pregnancy that had yielded a neural tube defect. The chance for a repeat of these defects in subsequent pregnancies is 12 times greater in women with such a previous birth. An additional study suggested that a much smaller dose similarly was protective. Folic acid has been routinely included in prenatal vitamins in a dose of 0.5 mg for many years. The managing physician must be alert to the development of megaloblastic anemia in the mother that sometimes occurs during pregnancy, however. Folic acid masks the symptoms of this complication, and if it is not detected and treated, permanent nerve damage can ensue.

Following a review of at least 8 of these studies in the U.S., Great Britain, Wales, Hungary, Australia and Cuba, the United States Public Health Service recommended in September, 1992 that all women of childbearing age who are capable of becoming pregnant take 0.4 mg (400 μg) of folic acid daily in order to reduce the risk of spina bifida and other neural tube defects.[7] The studies demonstrated that these defects occur during the first month of pregnancy, before most women begin prenatal vitamins and care. It is estimated that following this recommendation would reduce the number of these defects by one half. Many multivitamin preparations have now added folic acid in this amount. Some studies indicate that higher doses might reduce the incidence even more, but higher doses carry a serious risk, and should be used only under a physician's supervision.

In one of the greatest demonstrations of the type of ignorance and incompetence that we have come to expect of elected officials and political bodies, the state of Florida in 1989 enacted a workmen's compensation type of fund to compensate women who give birth to infants with neural tube defects, such as spina bifida. To fund this boondoggle, an annual tax was levied on every physician with a Florida license. The tax ranges from $50 for those who do not manage patients in Florida to $5000 annually for those delivering babies in Florida. It is unlikely that physicians are responsible for any but a small percentage of these pregnancies. It would seem that a direct tax on sex, levied for each time at bat and directly against the participant, would be a more reasonable assignment of responsibility.

This creative approach to extorting more money from productive citizens without raising taxes has been a trend during recent years among politicians at the federal, state and local level. So called "user fees" are seen as cash cows which people cannot complain of paying for, over and over again. Thus you will pay an additional fee (tax) on your fishing or pleasure boat, the dock where you keep it or launch it, a user fee when you fly out of your local airport, a fee to use the highway that you have already paid for during construction, a user fee for the use of the public land that was purchased with your tax dollars, etc. The politicians mistakenly believe that people will not recognize these "fees" for the taxes that they indeed are. Some sources estimate that the sum of these and other hidden taxes equals the total of published "on the book" taxes collected from the public.

This venture into fantasia will do nothing to solve the problem of these tragic defects. It is simply a job creation program for the trial lawyers who were responsible for its passage. The efforts and money should have been expended toward educating women to the simple expedient of adequate nutrition and proper prenatal care, which could reduce these defects by 70 percent.

In 1992 the New York State legislature picked up on this new source of taxation, and studied legislation that would provide a pay-off to parents who have children who are born with cerebral palsy. The proponents of this bill acknowledge that no one is at fault in 95 percent of these cases. In fact that is precisely why the legislation was proposed, since 95 percent of the cases taken to court lose. This is a scheme to award monies in those cases where the courts have ruled that there is no merit in doing so. The

124

funding for these payments will come from special assessments on physicians. This is another in a never-ending stream of money transfer schemes that assume that the funds are plucked from the mythical money tree. The increase in the costs of goods and services, as well as the drag on the economy from these hidden taxes has escaped scrutiny thus far.

The next recognized cause of birth defects was rubella, which produced such an epidemic of birth defects in 1941 that the association between the disease and the defects was finally made. Rubella in the mother during the first trimester (three months) of pregnancy produces a high incidence of defects in the heart and eye, as well as deafness and mental retardation. The incidence of defects when the infection occurs in the first four weeks of pregnancy is as high as 60 percent. The infection in the mother does not have to be pronounced. Subclinical cases of rubella can produce malformations. We now know that other infections, especially viral infections such as cytomegalovirus, similarly can cause defects.

The most notable parasitic infection that produces malformed infants is toxoplasmosis, which may result in blindness and severe mental retardation. This disease is acquired by the pregnant woman from cats (see chapter VII), but no illness is usually apparent in the mother. Infection acquired just before pregnancy may be transmitted to the fetus by the mother. Congenital toxoplasmosis is most severe if acquired early in the first trimester. Although toxoplasmosis is common, as is the case with birth defects that result from malnutrition, there is seldom any association made between the defects and the cause. Diabetes and hypothyroidism in the mother are two metabolic disorders that commonly result in birth defects. Proper medical management can reduce the incidence of congenital defects in both conditions.

A normal, healthy infant requires a normal, healthy ovum and sperm prior to fertilization. Together they form a normal, healthy zygote, barring inherited genetic disorders. The zygote then rapidly develops into a fetus. It is during this period of rapid development that all of the environmental influences take their toll. Few of the agents that adversely influence the developing fetus have any effect on the ovum or sperm. Age does, however, and in women who experience pregnancy after the age of 35 to 40 there is a significantly increased risk of malformations. This is because all of the remaining ova at this time bear the same age as the female. They are less receptive to fertilization and more likely to produce defective zygotes. The most prominent and best documented of these abnormalities is Down's syndrome (trisomy 21), which is much more common in women over the age of 40. Whereas the incidence is one in 1,667 live births in women at age 20, it increases to one in 40 births at the age of 43. (One in 385 at 35 years, one in 175 at age 38 years).

Various other malformations result from late life pregnancies, all less well delineated than Down's syndrome. Hydrocephalus is definitely more common. Various malformations of the central nervous system, such as anencephalus and spina bifida also occur with increased frequency. It should ever be kept in mind that congenital malformations tend to be multiple. When one obvious defect is found, other more obscure problems should be looked for. The risk of breast cancer is also increased significantly in women who have not had children by their early thirties. Estrogen levels in the breast tissue of these women are higher than in women who have had children. Estrogen increases the rate of cell division, which increases the risk of cancer developing. Ramazzini reported in 1700 that there was a very high incidence of breast cancer in celebate nuns, and correctly ascribed it to the absence of pregnancies.

It has always been standard procedure to study the effects of drugs on animals, and particularly on reproduction, before marketing them for human use. There has been an increased interest in the investigation of the influences of drugs and chemicals on the developing fetus during the past thirty years. Much of this interest was spawned by the epidemic of malformed infants in 1961 that resulted from the administration of thalidomide for nausea and vomiting during pregnancy. The most notable defect was incomplete development of the arms and legs, to varying degrees, but defects in the heart, eyes, kidneys and intestines also occurred. These cases were first recognized in Germany where the drug was marketed. No cases occurred in the United States because the drug was never approved or marketed here.

It is of interest to note that these birth defects did not show up in tests on laboratory animals; the rabbit and rat appear to be resistant to these effects of thalidomide. This is another demonstration of the fallacy of the mouse to man obsession (see chapter XIII). A very large body of knowledge regarding teratogenesis has evolved during the past 50 years, even to the point of documenting the time during pregnancy when specific defects are likely to develop with various exposures.

Substances that produce fetal abnormalities are referred to as teratogens. There are 600 therapeutic agents known to produce these defects in laboratory animals, but only 20 that produce them in humans. Some of the latter substances and the associated sequelae are:

• Anti-convulsants, especially phenytoin, trimethadione and para-methadione, are associated with the production of cleft palate, cardiac abnormalities, cranio-facial abnormalities, immature development of nails, fingers and toes, chromosomal aberrations, defects in the internal organs and mental deficiencies Valproic acid is associated with neural tube defects (see above).
• Phenothiazine can produce an abnormal development of the eye (retinopathy).
• Tetracycline taken during the middle to the end of pregnancy produce a permanent staining of the teeth, defective enamel with caries and retarded bone growth; they are suspected of causing congenital cataracts.
• Streptomycin, gentamicin, kanamycin damage hearing and the labyrinth.
• Sulfonamides near delivery can produce severe jaundice.
• Propranolol can produce a slow heart rate and hypoglycemia in the fetus.
• Cortisone in high doses causes abnormalities such as cleft palate.
• I-131, used to treat maternal goiter, destroys the fetal thyroid gland.
• Triiodothyronine, propylthiouracil and methimazole cause goiter in the fetus.
• Salicylates such as aspirin in the latter stage of pregnancy can damage the brain of the fetus (kernicterus).
• Nonsteroidal anti-inflammatory drugs such as ibuprofen in the last three months of pregnancy are known to stimulate closure of the ductus arteriosus; other possible cardiovascular effects are as yet unknown.

• Angiotensin-converting enzyme (ACE) inhibitors for high blood pressure taken in the second and third trimester may cause serious developmental defects, kidney failure and death in the fetus.
• Acetazolamide (Diamox), commonly used for glaucoma and for mountain sickness, is known to cause congenital defects.
• Maternal viral infections such as rubella (German measles) in the first three months; in 1964, 20,000 infants died or were permanently disabled due to intrauterine rubella infections.

During pregnancy the only safe course is to take no drugs, including alcohol and nicotine. Lead is one of the most serious exposures during pregnancy, and it has been common in the past. For sources of lead exposure around the house see chapters III and V. Some of the occupational exposures to lead include auto workers and body shops, service stations, lead battery manufacturing and reprocessing, manufacture and application of inks, paints and pigments, electronics (soldering), and gray iron foundries. One need not be "on the line" to suffer lead toxicity — working in the atmosphere is sufficient. In any of these setting, no eating, drinking or smoking should take place. Lead is carried from the hands to the mouth during all of these activities.

There are many occupational exposures that can produce serious damage to the developing fetus. Virtually all toxic substances, including mercury, readily pass through the placenta to the fetus. These should be reviewed in chapter X to help determine the safety of any given job. Many forms of employment on the other hand can be continued safely virtually throughout pregnancy.

The adverse effects of alcohol consumption during pregnancy on the fetus have been recognized since ancient times but were officially rediscovered by modern medicine in 1973. Low birth weight is the most common and most readily identified consequence. The severity of the malformations appears to be dose related, but any dose over two ounces a day can yield abnormalities. A characteristic set of features in an infant with the fetal alcohol syndrome has been described. These include a small head, a set of typical facial features, an I.Q. significantly below the mean, learning disabilities, poor memories, short attention span and speech disorders. The fetal alcohol syndrome is a major cause of mental retardation. The facial features include small, wide-set eyes, defects of the lids, a short nose and small upper lips. The defects can be pronounced and graphic. A single photograph of one of these tragic cases tells more than a volume of prose. There may be many more hidden defects of the heart, kidney and other internal organs. These have not been catalogued yet.

As with all mutagenic drugs and chemicals, the most pronounced defects that are produced by alcohol intake occur during the first three months of pregnancy. This is the period of most rapid growth, the period when the body and its organs are being formed. This is the period when geno-toxic, mutagenic agents exert their greatest influence. In addition to the risk to the developing fetus, alcohol places an added burden on the maternal liver. Any anesthetic presents some risk, but a liver compromised by alcohol greatly adds to that risk. As with most poisons no safe dose has been established, but two drinks per day have been associated with low birth weight.

Aspartame (Nutrasweet®) and glutamate (MSG and other food additives), both excitotoxins, have been shown to destroy brain cells in the developing fetus. Aspartame is found in virtually all diet soft drinks and deserts, and is consumed in huge quantities by the public. It should NEVER be ingested during pregnancy. Whereas most developmental abnormalities that result from drug and chemical exposure during pregnancy occur during the first three months, the excitotoxins can destroy brain cells at any time, up to the time of delivery. They similarly destroy neurons in the brains of adults, and contribute to degenerative brain diseases such as Parkinson's disease, Huntington's disease, Amyotrophic Lateral Sclerosis and Alzheimer's dementia. (See chapters XII and XV)

Cigarette smoking frequently interferes with conception, presenting a readily curable cause for apparent infertility in some women. Smoking has also been associated with abnormal fetal development, and it appears to be synergistic with alcohol. Infants born to mothers who smoke during pregnancy weigh an average of 170 grams (six ounces) less than do those who are born to non-smoking mothers. This is most likely due to the reduced blood flow to the developing fetus, although direct feto-toxic influences may also play a part. Smoking during pregnancy may result in retarded physical and mental development in the child that persists through-out life. It is also frequently an unrecognized cause of the sudden infant death syndrome during the first year of life.

When nicotine is administered to rabbits the vaso-constricting properties can be immediately and readily observed in the blood vessels in the ears. When this action reduces the amount of blood flowing to the fetus, incomplete and abnormal development of the various organs results. This is identical to the results seen with the use of cocaine during pregnancy. The results of interference with the blood flow to the fetus have been studied extensively in experimental animals by clamping the placental arteries sufficiently to partially restrict the blood flow. An additional effect of cigarette smoke is the direct action of the multitude of chemicals in the smoke, many carcinogenic, all toxic to the fetus.

Infections caused by *Listeria monocytogenes* bacteria as a result of eating certain meats and cheeses have presented us with a new foodborne disease since 1988. Pregnant women are more likely to acquire this infection, and it may lead to miscarriage, stillbirth or meningitis in the newborn infant. The bacterium is acquired most frequently in foods from delicatessens, soft cheeses, undercooked chicken and inadequately heated hot dogs and cold cuts. All of these foods these should be avoided, especially during pregnancy. This problem is discussed in more detail in chapter V.

GUIDE TO A NORMAL, HEALTHY BABY

- See your physician at the first suspicion of pregnancy. Assume that you are pregnant until this appointment can be kept, and follow all of these guidelines.
- Follow your physician's dietary recommendations scrupulously. It is essential to consume an adequate quantity of protein (meat) and other essential nutrients daily, maintaining normal weight gain at the same time. The appropriate prenatal vitamin-mineral supplementation, with folic acid, should be started at the very onset of pregnancy.
- DO NOT smoke during pregnancy. Smoking causes an immediate constriction of the arteries, both in the fetus and in the blood supply from the mother. This is comparable to choking off the air to the fetus, but it deprives him not only of oxygen but of essential nutrients as well. This leads to defects in development of the heart, brain and other vital organs and systems.

- Drink no alcohol during pregnancy. Even small amounts have been shown to cause small birth weight and fetal abnormalities.
- Take no drugs, including over the counter medications without clearing them with your physician first.
- Exercise daily in accordance with your physician's recommendations. Walking every day does no harm except where certain complications exist, and it promotes good circulation, essential to the health of the mother and the infant. The circulation in the legs is always compromised during pregnancy due to the pressure of the enlarged uterus on the veins and lymphatics in the pelvis. Walking helps. Brisk walking also exercises the heart and lungs, important to the health of mother and baby, and in preparation for delivery. Follow your physician's advice for specific exercises to tone up muscles.
- Get adequate sleep, usually 8 to 9 hours each night. You may require more sleep during pregnancy. Get enough to feel rested the next day.
- Nine months of these sacrifices is not too great a price to pay for the reward of a normal, healthy baby. A baby with serious congenital defects and health problems provides not only heartbreak, but also requires sacrifices for the rest of your life.

POSTNATAL CARE:

Shortly following delivery, the infant should be subjected to a complete and thorough physical examination to assess its health status and detect any abnormalities. Circumcision of male infants may be done during this period or subsequently in the office. In the case of infants with no abnormalities or special needs monthly visits are adequate. These visits should include assessment of nutrition, with feeding schedules outlined and adjusted as necessary. Measurement of height and weight should also be done and documented in the permanent record. Any problems that arise should be dealt with at interim visits, not postponed to the regularly scheduled visit.

Equally important during this period is to initiate and carry out the routine immunization schedule, a copy of which is included at the end of chapter III. A measurement of the hemoglobin level should be made at six months and one year to assure that proper nutrition and development are progressing.

INHERITED RISK FACTORS

There is a long list of disorders that are inherited through genetic or chromosomalmechanisms. Some of these are specific to certain races of people such as sickle cell anemia to people of African ancestry, and a longer list that is characteristic of the people of the Mediterranean. Some of the inherited disorders are listed below.

INHERITED DISORDERS

Alpha$_1$- antitrypsin deficiency	Marfan's syndrome
Adrenogenital syndrome	Muscular dystrophy
Adult lactase deficiency	Niemann-Pick's disease
Color blindness	Osteogenesis imperfecta
Cystic fibrosis	Phenylketonuria
Down's syndrome (trisomy 21)	Polycystic kidney disease
Familial hyperlipidemia	Retinoblastoma
Familial Mediterranean fever	Sickle cell anemia
Familial polyposis	Subaortic stenosis
Friedreich's ataxia	Tay-Sach's disease
Gaucher's disease	Thalassemia
Gout	von Recklinghausen's disease
Hemochromatosis	von Willebrand's disease
Hemophilia	Wilm's tumor (kidney)
Huntington's chorea	Wilson's disease
Hurler's syndrome	Xeroderma pigmentosum

In addition to the above disorders, also inherited is a proclivity toward some other diseases that require additional influences (such as cigarette smoking and other chemical exposures) for their development. Some examples are breast and lung cancer, leukemia and lymphoma. Inherited disorders that produce disease when provoked by exposure to environmental stimuli are discussed below. Proposals to genetically screen employees and potential employees for these abnormalities have raised a storm of protest from labor organizations. The goal of such proposals is to avoid placing individuals who are at risk in jobs where exposures to various agents might provoke these disorders. This issue has expanded the already hot debate over permitting women in jobs where they might be exposed to lead (see chapter X).

G6PD (glucose-6-phosphate dehydrogenase)

Deficiency of this enzyme is a genetically transmitted metabolic disorder. It is X-linked (transmitted on the X chromosome), fully expressed in males and homozygous females, and variably expressed in heterozygous females. Ten to fifteen percent of American black males and one to two percent of American black females have this disorder. It is also seen in people from the Mediterranean basin, such as Italians, Greeks, Arabs and Sephardic Jews, but at a lower frequency than that seen in blacks.

Hemolysis of the older red blood cells in the circulation, sometimes with a profound hemolytic anemia, occurs after exposure to certain drugs or other substances that cause oxidation of the hemoglobin and red blood cell membrane. More than forty substances are capable of provoking this response, including aspirin and other preparations containing salicylates, sulfonamides, nitrofurans, phenacetin, naphthalene, chloramphenicol, antimalarial drugs such as primaquine, some forms of vitamin K and fava beans. Since most of these are passed into the maternal milk, breast-feeding of a newborn with G6PD deficiency risks hemolytic reactions.

Hemolytic anemia may also be precipitated in these individuals by acute viral and bacterial infections and by diabetic acidosis. Characteristic Heinz bodies may be seen in a blood smear early, but these are removed by the spleen, and a specific enzyme assay is the best test. Recovery occurs after removal from the offending agent.

SICKLE CELL ANEMIA

This disorder is a chronic hemolytic anemia that occurs almost exclusively in blacks. Homozygous individuals have sickle cell disease (about 0.3 percent of blacks in the United States). Hemoglobin levels in these individuals usually runs about 8 grams compared to a normal of 14 to 15 grams. Heterozygous individuals demonstrate the sickling trait but no anemia (8 to 13 percent of blacks in the United States). The frequency of the inherited gene is greatest in regions with a high prevalence of malaria, such as central Africa. About 30 percent of the population of Nigeria have inherited the trait. The inheritance of this form of hemoglobin provides some protection against one of the forms of malaria (falciparum). The individuals with this gene thus tended to survive onslaughts of malaria more successfully than did those without the disease. This is a graphic example of the principle of the survival of the fittest.

Acute hemolytic episodes, which are variable in their occurrence, may be accompanied by thrombosis, infarction and pain. Episodes of severe abdominal pain with vomiting may mimic an acute abdominal problem such as appendicitis. There is no treatment for this disorder, and many patients die during childhood of pulmonary emboli, renal failure, intercurrent infections or thrombosis of an artery to a vital structure.

ALPHA-1-ANTITRYPSIN DEFICIENCY

Homozygous expression (present in both alleles of the chromosome) of this disorder is rare. About 10 to 15 percent of the population demonstrates a heterozygous deficiency (present on only one of the two alleles), which results in a mild impairment of the ability to inactivate proteolytic enzymes in the lung. Proteolytic enzymes are released in the lung by the alveolar macrophage as a defense against bacteria and other foreign substances. Normally these enzymes are inactivated by alpha-1-antitrypsin before the enzyme damages the lung tissue. Deficiency of this substance permits accumulation of the enzyme with resultant damage to the lung tissue.

Individuals with this deficiency may develop emphysema by middle age, even in the absence of exposure to dust and other substances that might damage the lung. The disease progresses even more rapidly and to a more severe stage in the presence of exposure to dusts and all of the other substances that tend to affect the airways adversely. The emphysema progresses to chronic obstructive lung disease, which is a major cause of disability and death. Chronic obstructive lung disease is second only to heart disease as a cause of death in the United States. It is found in 15 percent of older men and 10 percent of women. The mortality rate from this affliction has been doubling every five years.

Measurement of the level of alpha-1-antitrypsin is easily done by a blood test, and this should be done in any individual with an unusual degree of problem with bronchitis. It should be done early in such cases, and also should be measured in anyone with a family history of bronchitis, emphysema or chronic obstructive lung disease.

MALIGNANT HYPERTHERMIA

This is a genetic, inherited disorder marked by the onset of an acute, life threatening hyperthermia following the administration of any of the commonly used inhalation anesthetics and muscle relaxants. Early and prompt recognition of the disorder is essential when it occurs. Unless aggressive action is taken to correct it, 70 percent of the cases will terminate in death. The disorder can be diagnosed in susceptible individuals, and these tests should be conducted on anyone with a family history of this disease. This inheritance should be discovered before any surgery or obstetrical delivery is needed.

PORPHYRIA

Porphyria is a condition characterized by an excess production or accumulation of porphyrins in the body. Various porphyrins are produced in the natural metabolic cycle that produces heme, the iron carrying pigment in the blood. One type of this disorder is caused by a genetic inherited disorder of metabolism that causes excess porphyrin to be produced when the individual takes certain drugs, such as barbiturates, sulfonamides, phenylbutazone and hexachlorobenzene.

Since the reactions provoked can be serious, and since several commonly encountered agents can precipitate the disorder, identification of individuals at risk should be accomplished before the onset of a crisis. Laboratory measures aid in this identification, but the family history is a starting point. All members of a family with a previous history of porphyria should undergo screening tests. Those who are identified as being at risk should avoid the medications and other environmental exposures that are likely to provoke attacks. The potential for this disorder should be part of the occupational health screen also.

INFERTILITY

Infertility, the inability to become pregnant, or in the case of males to impregnate, has become a more common problem in recent years. The significant increase in the incidence of sexually transmitted diseases has been one of the factors responsible for this trend. Historically gonorrhea has caused sterility because of its proclivity to infect and thus scar the fallopian tubes. Any infection in the pelvis can produce this result, however, and *Chlamydia* infections have been an increasingly frequent culprit in this process (see chapter XI).

There are many causes for infertility, all of which must be investigated. The cause for the inability to get pregnant is about evenly divided between male and female. Both partners must be fully evaluated. A thorough medical history and physical examination of both individuals is the first step. The next step in the male is an analysis of the sperm for both quantity and quality. Ionizing radiation, excess heat and some chemicals can cause a reduction in sperm production. An example of the latter is the soil fumigant, DBCP, which was used in Kern County, California (see chapter V).

Undescended testicles can also produce sterility, and this will be detected during a physical examination. The scarring of a testicle from mumps orchitis should be a problem of the past with a vaccine available now. Unfortunately not everyone avails himself of the vaccine. Chronic abuse of alcohol, marijuana and anabolic steroids can also impair sperm production. The result of chronic abuse of anabolic steroids has become dramatically apparent in recent years. It has produced not only sterility but impotence as well. Use of anabolic steroids is near epidemic proportions among high school and other young athletes. (See also chapter XII).

There are over 100 medications that are commonly listed as having the potential to cause sexual dysfunction in humans.

Impotence, the inability to achieve an erection, and decreased libido (sexual desire) are the most common side effects listed. Less common but more serious is priapism, persistence of a painful erection. Fortunately all of these consequences are relatively uncommon, occurring in a small percentage of the individuals taking the medications. The most likely category of drugs to elicit a significant reaction is the psychotherapeutic agents, especially some antidepressants. Some of the antihypertensive agents in common use 25 years ago presented a fairly high incidence of impotence. The newer drugs, especially the angiotensin-converting enzymes (ACE) inhibitors have not been shown to cause sexual dysfunction.

In women, scarring of the tubes is a common cause of infertility as mentioned above. This can be demonstrated by a tubal patency radiographic test and by laparoscopy. The ovaries can also be visualized during laparoscopy. Aberrations of ovarian function can be suggested by a history of irregularities in menstrual function, but this can also indicate a thyroid deficiency. The occurrence of ovulation can be timed and confirmed by charting the basal body temperature. A perceptible rise in temperature will be noted when ovulation takes place.

Another cause of infertility that is almost unique to the current generation is waiting too long to attempt pregnancy. The incidence of infertility increases dramatically with age. Couples in the 30 to 35 year age group experience about a 30 percent chance of having fertility problems. This risk increases to 50 percent at age 40 and beyond. The reason for this is aging of the ovaries. A woman is born with her full complement of eggs, which enjoy the same age progression as does she. She does not produce additional ones at any time after her birth. As they age they are less receptive to sperm penetration. They are also more likely to be spontaneously aborted if they are fertilized. These are most likely protective mechanisms to prevent birth of defective infants. Spontaneous abortion reflects imperfect zygotes in many cases.

The evolution of the apparent increase in infertility delivered to the environmental extremists another opportunity to perpetrate a fraud upon the public. They conducted "studies" that supposedly demonstrated that sperm counts and the quality of semen in men had been diminished by environmental exposures such as "dioxin-like" compounds and pesticide metabolites such as DDE. Subsequent studies, prompted by these claims, disproved these claims, and showed that sperm counts had not declined during the past 15 to 25 years. It must also be noted that the oral intake of naturally occurring estrogenic compounds in vegetables, fruits and other foods is several thousand times greater than dietary exposures to synthetic compounds such as the organochlorines (DDT, DDE) and PCBs.[8] Additionally, exposures to these chemicals had diminished dramatically during the period that these effects were claimed to have occurred.

The increased incidence of inability of couples to conceive has created a new industry. Although artificial insemination is not new, it does carry some new and serious risks, especially when donor sperm is utilized. The risk of unknown inherited diseases has always been present, and in theory this can be screened for in the donor. Less likely to be uncovered are diseases such as HIV, and hepatitis B and C, all of which can be transmitted through donor semen.

HEPATITIS

In 1991 the Immunization Practices Advisory Committee[9] recommended that testing for hepatitis B be incorporated into the routine laboratory tests done on all pregnant women, and that infants born to women who test positive be given both hepatitis B vaccine and immune globulin within 12 hours of birth. Hepatitis B is spread very efficiently through the placenta from the mother to the infant. Most infants born to mothers who have active disease or who are chronic carriers will acquire the disease. Ninety percent of these infants will become carriers of the virus and about 25 percent of these will die in adulthood of cirrhosis or cancer of the liver.

In November 1991 the Advisory Committee and the Centers for Disease Control recommended that all newborn infants be started on the three-dose immunization regimen for hepatitis B. They reasoned that since they were having little success persuading those with the aberrant behavior that placed them at risk for hepatitis B to be immunized, immunizing every newborn would solve the problem. This recommendation has been slow to gain acceptance by parents and some physicians, since the overwhelming majority of infants born are not at risk of contracting hepatitis B, either at birth or later in life. The recommended routine screening of all pregnant women will identify those infants who are at risk, and thus those who should receive the immunization. The routine administration of hepatitis B vaccine to all newborn infants is irresponsible, and has resulted in tragedy in many cases.

There are currently two vaccines for hepatitis B that provide immunity for those who might be exposed to the disease. One vaccine is derived from whole blood, while a more recently developed bio-engineered recombinant vaccine is cultivated in yeast cells. This latter is as effective and is more palatable to those worried about AIDS transmission.

The incidence of hepatitis B increased by about 37 percent from 1979 to 1989, largely as a result of the great increase in the abuse of IV drugs, and the sharing of needles. Chronic liver disease and cancer of the liver develop in a significant number of individuals who have hepatitis B, and 4,000 to 5,000 of these people die each year. Routine vaccination of individuals at risk could protect them from this disease. Routine screening and vaccination of those newborn babies who are at risk could prevent chronic disease in about 6,000 individuals annually. These are individuals who are destined to die in the mid-twenties if no such preventative action is taken. The characteristics and concerns regarding hepatitis B are discussed in greater detail in chapters XI and XV.

URINARY TRACT INFECTIONS

Urinary tract infections are very common during pregnancy. Any woman who has had a history of cystitis, or the more serious pyelonephritis, is particularly at risk. The increasing mass of pregnancy in the pelvis produces pressure that impedes the normal drainage from the kidneys that is an important natural defense against ascending infections. It becomes more urgent than ever to drink an adequate supply of water daily. Cystitis is a far more common infection in females than in males because of the anatomic position of the urethral opening, and its short length. A good nutritional status is also important, as it is in preventing any infection. Any other needed prophylactic measures, such as acidification of the urine should be outlined by the managing physician, for virtually any medication taken during pregnancy presents a risk to the developing fetus. Any infection in the kidney introduces the risk of chronic infection that can produce permanent damage to that very vital organ.

CRADLE CAP

Cradle cap is a form of seborrheic dermatitis of the scalp that is common in infants up to about six months of age. It then disappears, but may recur at puberty. It is characterized by yellowish oily scales on an eczematous base. Treatment consists of daily applications of a selenium sulfide shampoo, left on for five minutes, then thoroughly rinsed off. Care must be taken to remove the shampoo completely and to not get it on the face or in the eyes. After improvement these treatments may be decreased to once or twice weekly.

NURSING

One of the most important and most neglected elements in breast-feeding is careful cleansing of the breast prior to feeding. In addition to the many microorganisms present on the skin, clothing and bed linen, the spores of *Clostridium tetani* persist in the soil for years, and are present in most of our environment. Neonatal tetanus kills thousands of infants each year in the developing countries (277,400 in 1997) as a result of nonsterile delivery and the custom of dusting the umbilical stump with animal dung, or a powder of dried local clay sold for this purpose. It is rare in the United States, but one case was reported in 1998 in a 9-day-old newborn. A multibacterial infection and tetanus resulted from applying a "Health and Beauty Clay" powder provided by a midwife to the umbilical cord. The infant was hospitalized and required mechanical ventilation for 12 days.[10] Tetanus immune globulin and penicillin was administered, and the infant survived.

Virtually all drugs and chemicals that are taken into the body through any route are carried to the mother's milk and transmitted in it. This includes all forms of mercury with their dire consequences. All of the exposures discussed in chapters V and X should be studiously avoided during pregnancy and nursing. The quantity of a substance that is delivered to an infant through breast milk depends upon a number of variables, such as the concentration of the substance in the milk, the frequency of feedings and the total quantity of milk consumed. The concentration is influenced by such factors as the solubility of the compound, whether it is fat-soluble, the degree to which it binds to protein and the time after dosing. The substance can reach breast milk only after it has been absorbed into the maternal blood. Most medications reach a peak concentration at 1 to 2 hours, then decline. Some are inherently long acting, however, and some are delivered through slow release tablets. Both of the latter will persist in breast milk for a more protracted period.

Breast milk at the beginning of feeding is highest in protein and lowest in fat. Toward the end of feeding this ratio is reversed. One would expect that a drug with protein binding would be delivered at a higher level early in feeding, while a higher level of a fat soluble drug would be delivered late in feeding. No studies have been done to verify this hypothesis, however. The lower pH of breast milk relative to blood also influences the concentration of substances in the milk. Weakly alkaline substances generally have a higher concentration than acidic ones.

In general, most antibiotics, antihistamines, isoniazid, antidepressants, metronidazole (Flagyl®), chlorpromazine and all alkaloids that are taken by the mother are delivered to the infant in a higher concentration than is present in her blood. Barbiturates, sulfonamides, diuretics and penicillin are delivered in the milk at an equal concentration. Nursing is generally not permitted when the mother is taking atropine, oral anticoagulants (coumarin and phenindione), antithyroid drugs, anticancer drugs, laxatives, iodides, mercurials, narcotics, radioactive drugs, bromides (sleeping and nerve medications, most available without prescription), ergotamine (for migraine headaches), tetracyclines and metronidazole (for *Giardia, Trichomonas* and *Gardnerella* vaginitis). These restrictions have been relaxed some recently, and that trend will continue. As medications are taken during pregnancy with no apparent serious consequences, there will be a tendency to categorize them as safe.

Medications for high blood pressure (hypertension) such as the beta-blockers may cause low blood pressure and a slow heart rate in nursing infants. The newer selective agents in lower dose ranges may be safe, however. Calcium channel antagonists generally do not present a problem. Infants are particularly susceptible to anticholinergic drugs such as atropine, belladonna and scopolamine and, tricyclic antidepressants, which have similar properties. High doses of caffeine or theophylline can cause irritability in the infant. Cortisone preparations can suppress growth and seriously interfere with the normal production of growth hormone in the infant. Nicotine also finds its way into the breast milk, but the passive smoking in such a home would be a much greater health risk to the infant.

In premature infants where the physiologic and metabolic systems in the liver and kidney are not fully matured, greater caution is needed. Most of the substances would not only achieve higher levels in the infants blood for a longer period, but damage to these vital organs might result from a direct local action. In infants who are born with a G6PD deficiency, sulfonamides, nalidixic acid, salicylates and any of the other forty some oxidant drugs that might be taken by the mother can precipitate a hemolytic crises in the infant, as mentioned earlier in this chapter.

Antibiotics that have no apparent adverse effect on the infant may alter the normal bacterial flora of the intestine resulting in diarrhea and monilial overgrowth. The infant may also develop a sensitivity to the antibiotic. Cocaine, which persists in the breast milk for up to 24 hours, cannot be used safely at all during nursing. Marijuana persists for an even longer period, being released from fat stores of the mother into the blood stream for up to a week.

In many instances the quantity of substance delivered to the infant through breast milk may have no practical, significant effect. No studies have been done to assure this, however. It would be very difficult to conduct such studies because of moral and ethical considerations. Subtle effects on the infant may not be detected until later in life, and at that time it may not be associated with the responsible agent. These factors and the absence of concrete data largely explain the considerable controversy surrounding the issue of what can be administered to nursing mothers safely. The decision is for the most part a calculated risk.

In preparing formula and in offering water to infants it is important to be certain that the water is nitrate free. Nitrates destroy the ability of the red blood cells to carry oxygen and result in the so-called "blue baby syndrome" which can be fatal. Recent studies have also incriminated nitrates in drinking water as a cause of spontaneous abortion. Nitrates occur naturally in well water in some locations in the U.S., but increasingly they also find their way into wells through contamination. This can result from the septic system or from drainage from animal wastes (see chapters I and V).

If you rely upon a well for your water source it would be wise to check with your local health department, especially if there are large farms, animal feed lots or hog farms in your state. Contamination from these farms can travel underground for miles, and the risk includes exposure to pathogenic microorganisms as well as nitrates.

In the unlikely event that I am blessed with another infant in my household, I will insist upon sterilizing all bottles, nipples and formula. Our society has abandoned this practice and parents have become very lax in their hygienic practices in caring for infants, as they have in their lives in general. Infants are born into this world with a gastrointestinal system that is pretty much devoid of microorganisms. They need to be introduced to the necessary, normal flora gradually, and protected from those that might cause disease. Infants also have not built up the immune system that adults have the benefit of. This is especially true after the first six months when they lose the limited passive immunity acquired in the womb.

INFANT BONDING

The theory that infant bonding must be aggressively cultivated early in life in order to prevent aggressive, antisocial violent behavior later is a hoax that has been perpetrated upon the parents of the United States since about 1972. It was born of some convoluted reasoning and interpretation of some supposedly scientific studies that were in reality a farce. The motivation of most of such crusades by scientists or medical practitioners during the past generation has been to promote a personal social or political agenda, or to enshrine one's name in the pages of history. Not infrequently these efforts succeed.

Bonding between parents and child is a naturally occurring process that evolves out of the love and attention that needs no cultivation among normal people in normal times. This is not to say that serious emotional problems will not arise if a child is abused, neglected, derided or unwanted. These crimes against children are all too common in our society today, and the results are in evidence in abundance. The most frequent failure of parents in our society during the current generation has been to simply let children grow up without teaching them the rules and limits essential to existence in any civilized society. The result has been the cultivation of a very large population of very uncivilized creatures.

Every child, from the day that he crawls out of his crib, needs to have limits established for him. Failure to do so produces a very insecure individual with behavioral abnormalities and a lack of regard for the rights of other members of society. This has been the genesis of the increase in antisocial behavior that has so puzzled and perplexed people. Every society since the beginning of time has recognized that a set of rules of conduct for its members is essential to its survival, and that these must be instilled into the children and adolescents. This issue is addressed several times in the Bible, where mandates are issued. (Prov. 13:24, Prov. 22:6, Prov. 22:15)

Parents have come to expect the schools to correct the aberrant behavior that results from years of parental neglect. This is to expect the impossible. Most of these individuals adjust and enter society, although their behavior is frequently less than ideal. More serious are the individuals who are propagated by adults, or near adults, who do not want children, or the burden imposed by them. These children, in addition to the neglect, are frequently seriously abused, and treated very badly both physically and emotionally. The result is an uncivilized individual who invokes violence upon society. At that point society has an insoluble and expensive problem.

Most parents need no special advice. It is enough to simply do what comes naturally. Love and embrace the child, but do not neglect discipline. Teach the rules, limits and responsibilities that are essential to living in any civilized society. For most of us our parents provided the role model, with only minor modifications needed.

ABORTION

The majority (about 85 percent) of spontaneous abortions occur during the first three months. These are usually followed by a surgical curettage, for if any fragment of tissue is retained in the uterus bleeding will persist. It is important that this be undertaken in the sterile setting of a surgical suite, for infection is a serious threat that can claim the life of the mother. Induced abortions, to terminate an unwanted pregnancy have become very common in the United States, unfortunately. The use of this procedure in lieu of contraception is a serious mistake, and certainly must be condemned in those cases where a women undergoes this procedure three or four times. An induced abortion is not the simple, innocuous procedure, that it is commonly perceived to be.

Even in a surgical setting, with a skilled and experienced surgeon, there are greater risks and possible complications than with a spontaneous abortion. Many of these abortions are not done in appropriate surgical suites, and many are done by physicians who not only are not skilled surgeons, but also are inept in the procedures that they are performing. The horror stories such as the child born with an arm ripped off make the news, but the many other cases of serious bleeding, infections and death are usually ignored or relegated to the obituary pages. The inability to conceive subsequently and carry a child to term is another common complication of this trade.

Young women who elect to abort their first child also increase their risk of developing breast cancer significantly. Several studies have reported this increased risk to be between 50 and 90 percent. There has been a determined effort to obfuscate and reject these findings, both within the medical community and among abortion rights advocates. We are blessed to have very effective and low risk means of contraception that were not available to us fifty years ago.

The current level of abortions performed in the United States (about 1.2 million each year) is a national disgrace. Since the infamous Roe vs. Wade Supreme Court ruling in 1973, there have been more than 38 million babies aborted in the United States. Particularly heinous is the barbaric atrocity that has been labeled partial birth abortion. Although the news media has claimed that this procedure is rarely done, Ron Fitzsimmons admitted in 1997 that he had previously "lied through his teeth" about that number, and estimated that 5,000 were performed annually. There is absolutely no instance where this procedure is needed or justified. Aside from deliberately killing the infant, it introduces a significant additional risk to a delivery, without contributing any benefit. No ethical, moral physician would perform this procedure.

1. Searle Pharmaceutical Group. Searle discontinues IUDs. (Press release) Skokie, Illinois, SPG, January 31, 1986.

2. Population Reports; Intrauterine Devices, B-4, July, 1982.

3. Population Reports; IUDs — an Update. B-6, December 1995.

4. Forrest JD, Fordyce RR. Women's contraceptive attitudes and use in 1992. *Family Planning Perspectives* 25(**4**):175-179. July-August 1993.

5. Koren G, Pastuszak A, Shinya I. Drugs in pregnancy. *N Engl J Med* 1998;**338**:1128-37.

6. CDC. Use of folic acid for prevention of spina bifida and other neural tube defects — 1983-1991. *MMWR* 1991;**40**(30):513-516.

7. CDC. Recommendations for the use of folic acid to reduce the number of cases of spina bifida and other neural tube defects. MMWR 1992;**41**(No.RR–14)

8. Bailey R. ed. *Earth Report 2000*. McGraw-Hill, New York, 2000.

9. CDC. Hepatitis B virus: a comprehensive strategy for eliminating transmission in the United States through universal childhood vaccination: recommendations of the Immunization Practices Advisory Committee. *MMWR* 1991:**40**(No.RR-13):1-13.

10. CDC. Neonatal Tetanus — Montana, 1998. *MMWR* 1998;**47**:928-930.

V

HAZARDS OF FOOD AND WATER

The control man has secured over nature has far outrun his control over himself.   — Ernest Jones

ADDITIVES

At the turn of the century there were no laws governing the adulteration of food by chemicals and preservatives. During the decade of 1870 to 1880 widespread and extensive adulteration of food with many toxic substances became common practice. Additives which were commonly used included boric acid (which is very toxic to the liver), salicylic acid and formaldehyde. While these agents were effective in prolonging the shelf life of food, they lacked similar benefits with regard to the health of humans.

The Food and Drug Act that was passed in 1906 resulted from the efforts of a chemist, Dr. Harvey W. Wiley. Several additions and amendments have been tacked on over the years, but many of these later efforts have been marked by the confusion and inconsistencies typical of legislative bodies. Some of the confusion results from the phraseology, such as a sentence composed of one hundred thirty-five words in the Federal Food, Drug and Cosmetic Act of 1976. Much confusion also results from the scattering of regulations among various sections of the law and among various bureaucracies.

The Environmental Protection Agency, for instance, has waged a relentless campaign to remove lead from our gasoline, house paint and from shotgun shells. One would assume that at least as much concern would have been expressed for the lead that leached into our soup from the soldered seams of the cans. The corrosion that was seen at this seam on the inside of the can was not comforting. The food industry in the United States reportedly discontinued the use of lead containing solder in cans in 1991, at long last. Cans imported from other countries continued to contain lead, however, and some may still. An inspection of canned foods in supermarkets in 1998 suggested that all domestic suppliers were

148

using either extruded or welded cans. This source of lead in foods appears to have been eliminated, at least from U.S. suppliers.

Some companies have been using extruded cans for several years. These cans can be recognized by the absence of a seam along the length of the can and at the bottom. The only seam is where the lid is joined to the body of the can. The bottom of the can is slightly rounded at the bottom margin, and is continuous with the side. More recently many companies have switched to a welded seam in cans, which also eliminates the contamination of the food with lead. Some of these cans are marked as welded, but even when not marked the seam can be identified readily, especially when compared with the soldered seam of the soup can. The welded seam has been ground on the outside of the can and presents an even, ground appearance.

The soldered seam, on the other hand, is an irregular, crimped seam. If you look carefully you can see the small beads of solder. You can also scrape some of the soft solder off with a knife. There has been no excuse for using soldered cans for the past several years, since the technology to eliminate this risk has been available. Lead from soldered seams presents a particularly high risk in highly acid foods such as tomatoes and many soups.

Another source of lead in food comes from improperly glazed dishes, cups and pitchers. The hazard results when the temperature during firing is not high enough (1150° C.) to properly seal the lead in the glaze and the lead in some color pigments. Highly acid foods and beverages then leach some of the lead out of the glaze. Tomato containing foods and orange and other fruit juices are particularly active in this respect. Decals on the inside of cocktail glasses have also been a source of lead contamination of drinks.

Most of the incriminated lead containing dinnerware has been imported. The Food and Drug Administration issued twelve recalls of imported dinnerware between 1982 and 1994. These materials came from Italy, Spain, the Netherlands, Hungary, Mexico, Taiwan and Thailand. One recall by the FDA was in July of 1987, and involved an expensive line of dinnerware from Palermo, Italy. The FDA invoked more stringent standards in 1971, but domestic dinnerware manufactured prior to that continues to be a source of lead poisoning. Even dinnerware and coffee mugs that are properly fired and safe at purchase can be rendered hazardous by washing in the dishwasher. Strong cleaners in automatic dishwasher detergents erode the glaze, releasing the lead in the pigments beneath.

In the summer of 1987 lead poisoning in six adults and one child, all relatives in a family in New York, was reported to the Centers for Disease Control. The source of the lead was a home-made beverage that was stored in a ceramic bean jug that had been brought back from Mexico. Numerous cases of lead poisoning traced to imported ceramic ware have been reported. These cases are especially serious when they involve children since they can result in permanent brain damage. In 1988 the Food and Drug Administration signed an agreement with the People's Republic of China designed to safeguard against unsafe ceramic ware being imported from that source. Japan had already instituted such safety precautions. Items that are brought back by individuals from vacations or business trips are not monitored and continue to be a risk.

Mexico is the most common source of unsafe ceramic ware because much of these products are made in small operations rather than factories. They also are frequently not imported in large shipments that can be monitored, but are brought back by tourists or by residents of the United States visiting relatives in Mexico. Any suspect ceramic ware can be tested for lead by most local laboratories. A qualitative test is simple and inexpensive. If you have difficulty in finding a laboratory that will do this test for you, contact the local health department for assistance.

Lead crystal decanters do not need to be tested. They always contain lead and should never be used for storage of wine, liquor or any other substance intended for consumption. European glass contains 20 to 25 percent lead, while crystal made in America contains from 30 to 50 percent. The American crystal is thus much heavier. The addition of lead to glass permits deeper ornamental cuts. Toxic levels of lead will leach out of these containers, and consumption of even smaller quantities of lead should always be avoided wherever possible. These items should be used as orna-mental displays only.

Questions about the safety of the colored inks found on bread wrappers have also been raised. Most colored inks in any applica-tion, including newspapers and advertising flyers, contain lead and cadmium pigments, both very toxic. The lead and cadmium pigments on bread wrappers do not contaminate the bread, for they do not penetrate the plastic wrapper. There is a risk if the bags are reused to store food, or if the bag is abused to the point that some of the pigments might flake off. These plastic bags should not be re-used for food storage, or any other use in the home. Safe plastic storage bags are abundant and inexpensive.

The greater danger from these bread wrappers, as well as other printed materials, is in recycling paper products that contain toxic pigments such as lead and cadmium. It is extremely unwise to use such recycled material in paper plates and other applications where it comes in contact with food. These products should be carefully avoided by reading the label. Using recycled materials in the production of paper plates has become very popular, however, because of the current mania for recycling with no consideration for its consequences.

An unusual source of lead poisoning in what some might label as food results from consumption of "moonshine" whiskey. It is common practice to use automobile radiators in the illicit distillation of alcohol in this industry. Unfortunately the lead content in the radiators produced in the auto industry has been greatly increased in recent years, to the point that it now constitutes 95 percent of the solder, rather than the conventional 50 percent. This fact greatly increases the yield of lead when producing whiskey with this equipment. Using any equipment made with even conventional solder will result in lead contaminated alcohol, since lead is leached out of the soldered joints of the still. This has been a problem for many years.

During the summer of 1991 the Alabama Department of Public Health identified nine persons who had markedly elevated blood lead levels, one as high as 259 μg/dL (any level over 10 is cause for concern). All had been treated for alcohol related illnesses, but also had symptoms of lead poisoning. All had consumed moonshine, and tests from these stills yielded extremely high lead levels (7400 μg/L and 9700 μg/L).[1] Alabama authorities destroyed 94 stills in 1991. This problem is perennial and present in several different states. It was detected in these cases by virtue of reporting requirements for elevated blood lead levels, and a vigilant and competent state health department.

Even low levels of lead present a serious threat to children. Lead produces mental retardation in infants and infertility in women. Any quantity of lead that is consumed by a pregnant woman presents a threat of brain damage to the developing fetus. It affects the brain less dramatically in the adult, but may result in personality changes. Lead also produces serious damage to the kidneys. The decline in the fertility and vitality of the ancient Romans has been attributed to the lead in their pewter dishes and drinking utensils. As late as 1960 pewter was defined as an alloy of variable composition, frequently 80 percent tin and 20 percent lead. Contemporary pewter should have no lead, being composed of tin, copper and antimony. No pewter utensil should be used for food or drink, however, unless it has been tested and found to be free of lead. It has been discovered recently that harmful effects to the various organs of the body can occur at lead levels below what has been considered acceptable in the past. This will require some reassessment of test results and may result in new standards.

Federal authorities expressed considerable concern during the nineties over the discovery that lead had been found to be leached out of soldered plumbing joints into water supplies. This had occurred in areas where the acidity of the water is unusually high, such as in the Northeast. Water with a low mineral content will also leach lead to a greater degree; this is not a problem in most homes. After about ten years the solder in the joints becomes coated with minerals from the water and lead is much less likely to find its way into the water supply. The lead consumed from this source was much less than that which was consumed from foods.

Extremist groups that make their fortune by exaggerating risks and alarming the public filed lawsuits to force faucet manufacturers to remove the small amount of lead in faucets. Brass often contains a small amount of lead to facilitate fabrication and produce a superior product. Any lead leached out by the water would be minute, and would be detectable only on the first draw in the morning. As in most cases of such legal extortion, however, the manufacturers have agreed to discontinue the use of lead in faucet manufacture. Lead free faucets can be identified from a label stating that they comply with the NSF-61 industry standard. If you are concerned about the lead content of the household drinking water it can be measured readily.

The Environmental Protection Agency recommends that individual households with either public or private (well) water supplies should have a lead content of less than 15 parts per billion in "first draw" water. First draw water is the first water from the tap after sitting over night. A flushed specimen is drawn after flushing the lines for one to two minutes, and the maximum acceptable lead level in this specimen is 5 parts per billion. If a lead content higher than 5 ppb is found after flushing the line, the first source to suspect is the service pipe between the water main and the residence.

Lead pipes were commonly used for water supply lines to houses built before 1930, and many of these remain in use. The local authorities can advise you as to whether or not this problem exists in your area. Bear in mind that this line is the responsibility of the homeowner, and replacement will be at his expense. The federal authorities have not mandated any correction of this problem. If any question exists regarding the threat of lead leaching out of your plumbing from a source other than lead lines, do not use hot water for cooking and drinking. As an added precaution, run the cold water for a short period each morning to flush out the lines as a simple precautionary measure. Where lead lines are in place, water for cooking and drinking should come from another source.

Federal agencies have mandated that ordinary solder be replaced with so called tin solder, or lead-free solder, in the plumbing of all new construction. The solder that was widely available and used up to the present was a mixture of tin and lead, usually in a 50-50 proportion. A eutectic mixture of tin and lead (the mixture which melts at the lowest temperature) is 63 percent tin and 37 percent lead. This proportion flows best, provides the strongest joint and seals most efficiently. Any significant deviation from this formula results in more difficult soldering and the potential for poor results, as many of us discovered during and after World War II when tin was in short supply.

Solders introduced to meet the new federal demand are composed either of 95 percent tin and 5 percent antimony, or a mixture of zinc, silver and antimony in the tin base. They cost about twice as much as the conventional solder. It remains to be seen how satisfactory and durable the new solder will be (see soldering in Chapter II).

Cadmium is another metal that presents serious toxic effects when it finds its way into the food supply. These effects became painfully obvious after the epidemic of "Itai-Itai-byo," ouch-ouch disease, in Japan during and after World War II. With the increased industrial activity the smelting plants produced heavy pollution of rivers and streams with copper, zinc and cadmium. This resulted in contamination of the rice crops, which take up cadmium more readily than lead and the other metals. Shellfish such as mussels, scallops and oysters also accumulate cadmium in significant concentrations from the water. Large numbers of postmenopausal women emerged with excruciating back pain. The cause was unknown for a long time, until autopsies demonstrated high concentrations of lead, copper and cadmium in all of the internal organs. The cadmium produced a pronounced decline in the internal architecture and integrity of the bones, accounting for the pain in the vertebra (spine).

When cadmium is ingested it is deposited in all of the internal organs, but very serious damage results in the kidneys. The renal tubules are severely damaged, with many profound metabolic consequences in the body, one of which is the osteoporosis and osteomalacia demonstrated in Itai-Itai. There is also evidence that cadmium contributes to the development of prostate cancer. Shellfish represent the major source of dietary cadmium from contaminated waters. Drinking water from these contaminated bodies similarly presents a threat, a condition that exists in some regions in Japan. Long term use of fertilizer results in increased levels of cadmium being taken up in crops, especially grain. Even more hazardous is the use of fertilizer derived from commercial sludge, which contains high levels of not only cadmium, but also other toxic minerals. These should not be used in commercial farming.

Over 2500 substances are added to food to render it more tasty, more creamy, smoother, or to give it a more appealing color. Many of these substances are not harmful (ascorbic acid, calcium gluconate, lecithin, carnauba wax), but some are known to carry a risk, and others are yet to be categorized. Coloring agents are used for the sole purpose of rendering the product more pleasing to the eye; they serve no other purpose. With the exception of caramel, all of the widely used food-coloring agents are synthetic substances, so called coal tar dyes for the most part.

Butter yellow, which was found to be highly toxic and to cause cancer in the liver and urinary bladder, was removed from the market place in 1919, after years of acceptance and use. In 1938 "Cadmium red" (cadmium sulfoselenide) was banned from use as a dye in lipstick after it caused sore throats. In 1960 FD&C orange Number 1 and Number 2 were removed from the market for their toxicity to internal organs, and red Number 1 for causing liver cancer. Yellow Numbers 1, 2, 3 and 4 all were removed as a result of intestinal lesions and heart damage in humans. Red Number 4 and citrus red Number 2 were markedly restricted in what they could be used for. FD&C violet Number 1 was banned in 1973.

Ironically the FDA banned the use of red Number 2 (amaranth) in 1976 as a result of great pressure from the news media and the Congress. This pressure was generated as a result of misinformation and a botched experiment. This event was to prove to be the forerunner of the Alar fiasco. Red Number 40, a substance about which we know much less to this day, was substituted. Extensive retesting of all currently approved food colors has been underway. This is an effort by the FDA to establish the safety of all approved colors, and to eliminate provisional approval status.

By 1973 allergists were reporting a growing number of hypersensitivity reactions among patients, especially asthmatics, resulting from food dyes such as red Number 3 and yellow Number 5 (tartrazine). Similar reactions to preservatives such as sodium benzoate were also recorded. More recently sulfites (sodium sulfite, sodium and potassium bisulfite, sodium metabisulfite) have been identified as having caused severe reactions, including life-threatening reactions, in many asthmatics and sensitive individuals. The sulfites were widely used in salads and wine and on fresh fruits and shellfish to maintain freshness. Approximately 11,000 drugs contain sulfites as preservatives.

The Food and Drug Administration banned the use of sulfites in fresh fruits and vegetables effective in August 1986. This restriction applies to salad bars also. Sulfites may still be present in many foods served in restaurants, such as seafood, sauces, soups, coleslaw and sauerkraut. Individuals who are sensitive to sulfites must exercise the same precautions as those who are allergic to seafood. Sulfites are much more pervasive than seafood, however. As of January 1, 1987 all packaged foods containing 10 parts per million or more of sulfites were required to be so labeled.

Sodium nitrate and sodium nitrite have been widely used as preservatives for a long time. They have been very effective in preventing the production of botulism toxin in foods such as sausage and lunchmeats. These additives are also being phased out because of concern over their role in the production of nitrosamines in the stomach. Nitrosamines are among the most dangerous cancer-causing agents yet discovered. Most of our knowledge about them has been collected only since about 1960. They have the distinction of being one of the few substances that have caused cancer in every species of animal studied. In the past it has been very difficult to produce cancer of the stomach in experimental animals. This cancer can be readily induced in the stomach of the rhesus monkey with nitrosamines, however.

Several different nitrosamine compounds have been identified, and they each seem to be organ specific. One causes liver cancer, another lung cancer, and another cancer of the urinary bladder. In addition to being formed by chemical action in the stomach, they are produced when cooking meats, especially in grilling. Nitrosamines are likely to be present when meat is charred regardless of the cooking method. More recently (2001) they have become suspect in the production of colon and breast cancer. Several different nitrosamines are found in tobacco. There is a strong suspicion that the nitrosamines in tobacco play a role in the production of cancer, especially cancer of the mouth caused by smokeless tobacco. Potassium nitrate (saltpeter) also recently has been discontinued as a food additive.

Monosodium glutamate (MSG) is a common food additive, and is used in the preparation of some Chinese foods. It is seen chiefly in meats and meat dishes and it has become well known for the "Chinese Restaurant Syndrome" that it precipitates in some people. This consists of a burning sensation throughout the body, headache and chest pain. It appears to be dose related and varies considerably among individuals. It is not an allergic reaction.

Preservatives are added to virtually every food and beverage that are marketed. Without these the shelf life of most products would be about 24 hours or less. We would like to use preservatives that prohibit the growth of all other forms life, but still permit us to thrive and stay healthy. Such utopian agents cannot be produced, simply because all of life depends upon some similar and basic biologic systems. As with pesticides, compromises are necessary. Some of the most commonly used preservatives at present are ascorbic acid (vitamin C), which is a natural antioxidant, calcium propionate, propyl paraben and sodium bisulfite. Ordinarily several are used so that a lower dose of each suffices. Brominated vegetable oil was widely used in soft drinks to prevent deterioration of flavor until about 1981. Concern over its potential to cause cancer prompted its discontinuance. Brominated compounds in general are suspect in the production of cancer.

Several non-intentional additives find their way into our food indirectly. One of the most common, and one of great concern, is antibiotics. Cattle are frequently administered antibiotics to treat various illnesses. Both beef cattle and poultry are raised on feed that almost always contains antibiotics. Commercial growers have learned that better production of meat is thus achieved, and fewer episodes of illness in the animal encountered. The problem is that these antibiotics are retained and are present in the meat when it is consumed. This can be a problem for those individuals who are allergic to them. Of even greater concern is the problem of resistant strains of bacteria that are a threat to humans emerging as a result of this common practice. We cannot develop new antibiotics fast enough to keep ahead of the emerging resistant strains. The cultivation of resistant strains in growing our beef leaves us defenseless when these strains cause disease in humans.

Other substances are also commonly fed to cattle, pigs and poultry to stimulate greater growth. One of the best known is estrogen, which increases growth in poultry. This has been discontinued after the extensive publicity about the cancer risks of this practice. Other growth promoting substances continue to be used, however, with no assurance of their safety. All of these substances undergo enzymatic transformation in the animal that may render them even more hazardous to humans upon consumption.

Some additional potentially harmful non-intentional additives include animal and insect feces and parts, microorganisms (bacteria, fungi), parasitic organisms, toxic metals and their compounds, glass and toxic chemicals such as solvents.

Decaffeinated coffee was a source of undesirable food additives in our diet for a long time. For many years trichloroethylene was used for removing the caffeine, until someone observed that this was also the substance used in dry cleaning our clothes. It had also been universally used in industry for degreasing metal parts until concern over liver toxicity prompted the substitution of trichloroethane, a substance with no less risk. Methylene chloride (dichloromethane) was then substituted to remove caffeine from coffee. While it has some less toxicity in the liver, recent revelations of its cancer-causing potential have raised fresh concerns. The only safe process for decaffeinating coffee currently known is the so called "water process." This process has been widely used in Europe, and has now been adopted in the U.S.

Aflatoxins, which are the most potent cancer-causing agents known, are produced by a fungus, *Aspergillus flavus*. The fungus grows only when storage conditions are less than ideal. Aflatoxins have been found frequently in peanuts that are not stored properly, and have thus shown up in peanut butter for a long time. Under poor storage conditions that permit mold to grow, aflatoxins are produced in rice, wheat and corn as well as peanuts. They can also be found in tobacco and snuff, again as a result of mold growth. The discovery of aflatoxins in grain and in milk samples in eight states in the Midwest and in Texas in 1988 caused alarm because they had not previously surfaced in this food source. The contaminated corn had been fed to dairy cattle and, as with most substances, the aflatoxins were passed on to the milk. This was an unexpected source of aflatoxins and many states had no means of testing for them or any regulations controlling their entry into the food chain. The risk from corn and other grains as well as milk had been largely overlooked prior to 1988.

The most common source of aflatoxins in the United States has been moldy peanuts and consequently peanut butter. The production of aflatoxins on peanuts by *Aspergillus* can be prevented by proper storage. The Federal Government inspects peanuts and peanut butter for mold and aflatoxins. The amount of money that a grower is paid in price supports is governed in part by the presence or absence of mold. These Government studies had found that certain manufacturers of peanut butter consistently had no or low levels of aflatoxins. This information has never been released to the public, however.

Peanuts (groundnuts) are a dietary staple in large populations in Africa. The high incidence of liver cancer, and its occurrence in young populations (age 20 to 30 years) there is thought to be associated with aflatoxin intake. A positive correlation between aflatoxins in food and the development of liver cancer has been established in Uganda, Swaziland, Thailand, Kenya, Mozambique and China. In the southeast United States where a high intake of aflatoxins in the diet has been noted, a higher than normal incidence of liver cancers has been observed also.

The US Food and Drug Administration has imposed limits on the permissible level of aflatoxins in peanut butter since 1965. In 1969 it set a limit of 20 parts per billion for both peanuts and peanut butter. The US Department of Agriculture has set the same limit on grain fed to dairy cattle.[2] In 1978 a study by a national laboratory found aflatoxin in 67 of 76 samples of peanut butter in the United States. The situation has improved since that time, at least partially due to the publicity. In 1994 a repeat study by the same national laboratory found only very low levels (1 part per billion or less) in samples of peanut butter from the three major companies. By contrast over one-half of the samples from store brands and lessor name brands yielded high levels. The highest levels were found in fresh-ground samples.[3] Even the low levels found present a risk, especially if consumed frequently. With proper storage and handling of peanuts this risk can be eliminated.

PESTICIDE RESIDUE

All fruits and vegetables grown commercially are subjected to repeated applications of pesticides. This greatly increases the yield (and thus reduces our cost) and enhances the quality of the food. Strict regulations exist governing what products may be used on food and how close to harvesting time they may be applied. These regulations are not always adhered to, as witnessed by the poisoning of over one thousand people when aldicarb (Temik) was illegally applied to melons in California (see Pesticides, Chapter XIV). Some residual pesticide is likely to remain on any fruit or vegetable.

Concern has been expressed over the possibility of some quantity of pesticide being incorporated into the fruit itself. Such residue levels are controlled under Section 408 of the Food, Drug and Cosmetic Act. Most of the fruit that reaches our tables is not inspected nor pesticide levels measured, and it is only prudent to wash thoroughly all such products before consumption. Washing does not remove pesticides or other chemicals that are absorbed or incorporated into the fruit or vegetable, however. It is of some comfort to note that in the few instances where these foods have been tested, pesticide residues have been few and of low concentration. Ames has estimated that the intake of natural pesticides is ten thousand times greater than the intake of synthetic pesticides (see Chapter XIII).[4]

FOOD POISONING

Food poisoning can be caused either by consuming a toxin that has been produced in a food or by an infection resulting from consuming food or water that has been contaminated by pathogenic microorganisms. Many thousands of cases are reported in the United States each year and many thousand more are suffered or treated and not reported. The number of such cases has increased dramatically during the past decade. This may be due partly to the increase in the practice of eating away from home, and partly to the increase in travel. Too many people die from such diseases, and many people who are afflicted wonder if they are going to expire because of the severity of the symptoms and the suffering.

Virtually every case of food poisoning could have been prevented very simply by adequate cooking and by proper storage and handling of food. The latter includes the simple measures of hand washing and the wearing of latex or vinyl disposable gloves by food handlers. We have become very complacent in the United States because of the extremely high level of sanitation and refrigeration that we have achieved.

The practice of permitting meat products, particularly an item as bulky as a turkey, to cool slowly at room temperature prior to refrigeration provides the opportunity for organisms such as *Salmonella* to reproduce. Under the same conditions *Clostridia* bacteria produce spores which are very difficult to destroy. Destruction of these spores requires a temperature of 248° F. for thirty minutes, and this can be accomplished only in a pressure cooker. Foods that are canned without the destruction of these bacteria and their spores present the potential for the production of botulism toxin. *Staphylococcus* organisms under these circumstances produce a potent toxin in the food, on the spot. Brief rewarming does not destroy this toxin and eating the food results in a severe illness two to four hours later.

Contrary to what we have been led to believe, all such foods should be placed in the refrigerator or freezer and cooled as rapidly as possible, as soon as possible. Permitting foods to sit at temperatures below 170° F. may permit bacteria to multiply and/or produce a toxin. This activity may take place down to a temperature of 40° F., so refrigerator temperatures must be kept below that level. The lower below that level that the temperature is maintained at, the longer that milk and other perishable products will be preserved. The temperature in the freezer must be 0° F. or below. There is no way to be assured that adequate temperatures have been maintained without an accurate thermometer. Every homeowner should keep a thermometer in both the refrigerator and the freezer.

Meats are the most critical foods with regard to refrigeration both because of the presence of harmful bacteria that may multiply and because of the tendency for this food to deteriorate at temperatures above 0° F. Fresh meat should be kept in the refrigerator no longer than two to three days before use. Ground meat should be used within twenty-four hours. It should be kept in mind that ground meat is a particularly good growth media for bacteria. It should be handled as little as possible. Use of disposable gloves in handling ground meat minimizes bacterial contamination. Meat left sitting at 45° F. or above may be unfit for consumption after as little as two to three hours.

Even at temperatures below 0° F. meat cannot be kept indefinitely. Flavor will deteriorate before spoilage occurs at these low temperatures. Adherence to the following table assures retention of flavor and absence of microbial growth if the freezer temperature is kept at 0° F. or below:

most beef (except ground)	6–12 months
poultry, including turkey	6 months
ground meat, minimal handling	3–4 months

pork	3–6 months
ham	2 months
lamb and veal	6–8 months
fish	6–8 months
shrimp	3 months
vegetables	8–12 months

After meat is removed from the freezer, it should not be left sitting at room temperature to thaw. If the size is reasonable, it can be thawed in the microwave oven prior to cooking. A large item such as a turkey should be thawed in the refrigerator over a period of twenty-four to forty-eight hours. In cooking, it is especially imperative after thawing frozen meats to be certain that the center of the meat reaches an adequate temperature for a sufficient period of time to assure destruction of disease-causing organisms such as *Salmonella*. The center of the meat must reach a temperature of at least 170° F. in order to accomplish this. A thermometer in the center of the meat is the only way to assure this.

Brief rewarming of foods is not sufficient to destroy all of the toxins that are produced by the bacteria in these foods. Some toxins are not destroyed by boiling (212° F.) for one hour. The toxin that is produced by *Staphylococcus* bacteria can withstand this temperature for 20 minutes without losing its toxicity, and it is not inactivated by normal canning methods. The toxin of botulism, on the other hand, is destroyed by heating to 212° F. for 20 minutes. Keep in mind that this temperature is achieved by boiling only at sea level. Elevations of 700 to 800 feet, commonly seen in most of the Midwestern states, do not make a significant difference. If you are backpacking in the Rockies at an elevation of 9,000 feet, however, water boils at 190° F. No higher temperature can be achieved except with a pressure cooker. A longer time will be required, therefore, in order to accomplish the same destruction of toxins or spores.

When more than one person who ate from a common source, or who ate the same food, become ill at about the same time, we can be reasonably certain that we are dealing with food poisoning. For instance when 57 percent of the 343 passengers on board a jetliner became ill, the illness was traced to a toxin produced in the food by a contaminating *Staphylococcus*. The source of the

Staphylococcus was an infection on the finger of one of the food handlers who prepared the food.

The World Health Organization has published "Ten Golden Rules for Safe Food Preparation" which, if followed, would eliminate most of the suffering in the millions of people worldwide who fall victim to food-borne diseases.

1. Choose food processed for safety.
2. Cook food thoroughly.
3. Eat cooked food immediately.
4. Store cooked food carefully.
5. Reheat cooked foods thoroughly.
6. Avoid contact between raw foods and cooked foods.
7. Wash hands repeatedly.
8. Keep all kitchen surfaces meticulously clean.
9. Protect foods from insects, rodents and other animals.
10. Use pure water.

Wooden cutting boards are a common source of contamination for many disease-causing organisms such as *Salmonella*. These cannot be sanitized satisfactorily, and plastic or Corningware™ boards should be used to cut and process all meats. Certainly vegetables and other foods that are not to be cooked should never be processed on a wood cutting board that has been contaminated by any meat.

One of the most significant steps that could be taken to improve the safety of food and reduce foodborne infections is the sterilization of food by irradiation with gamma rays or electron beams at the processing plant. This procedure eradicates all of the common disease producing organisms including salmonella, shigella, listeria and E. Coli. It also eliminates disease from the botulism bacillus, fungus, protozoa (*Cyclospora, Cryptosporidium*, etc), tapeworms and insects. It would increase the shelf life of meats from three days to two weeks. It can produce milk that can be kept on the shelf without refrigeration for long periods. Fruits can be disinfected to retard spoilage, permit shipping ripe fruit to market and to prevent importation of pests such as the Mediterranean fruit fly. Irradiation of imported foods would prevent outbreaks such as the Cyclospora from raspberries and Hepatitis A from strawberries, discussed below.

The U.S. Army began using irradiation for field rations by 1950, and NASA has been using it for the space program. The process leaves no residual radiation in the food and does not alter the taste or texture. The fact that efforts to develop a test to identify foods that have been irradiated have been unsuccessful attests to the safety of the procedure.[5] Over twenty other countries have been using irradiation for four decades. It has been used in the United States to sterilize tampons, contact lens cleaning solutions and adhesive bandages.

An irrational ruling by the Food and Drug Administration in 1958 that radiation must be considered an additive to food stifled its use in consumer food supplies in the US. The FDA finally agreed to permit its use for disinfection of spices, and it belatedly approved its use for pork in 1986 and poultry in 1990. In December 1997 approval was finally given for the irradiation of red meat. This action was in response to a petition that had been filed by a New Jersey medical sterilization company in 1994. Outbreaks of E. Coli O157:H7 can be prevented by routine use of this process, and companies that fail to adopt it will be at a significant risk of litigation. Irradiation is the logical replacement for methyl bromide which has been used as a fumigant for grain, and which the Environmental Protection Agency plans to ban in its battle against the fictional ozone depletion.

Irradiation of all tea imported should be mandated. Until this routine is instituted the popular practice of brewing "sun tea" should be abandoned. In August 1995 the Cincinnati Health Department discovered that all samples of loose tea and tea bags that they examined contained bacteria. Samples of ice tea in restaurants revealed high levels of coliform and other bacteria. Tea is grown in regions where human excrement is still used as fertilizer. These areas are noted for poor sanitation and high levels of gastrointestinal infections and parasites. This is why tourist precautions are issued for these regions. Brewing tea from these areas without using boiling water is tantamount to a visit there. Even with boiling water some risk remains. Irradiation would eliminate this health risk.

STAPHYLOCOCCUS

This is the most common food **POISONING** seen in the United States. The illness is caused by a toxin that is produced in food by

Staphylococcal organisms, usually when the food sits at room temperature. Refrigeration markedly reduces the production of this toxin. The toxin is heat stable and it is not destroyed by heating at 212° F. for 20 minutes. It is not uncommon for an outbreak of food poisoning to occur as a result of contamination of food by pus from an infected wound or pustule on the hands of a food preparer.

Common foods involved in staphylococcal food poisoning are potato salad, cream pastries, meat dishes, especially ham, turkey and chicken, or any dish containing meat or egg products. These foods **SHOULD NOT** be left sitting at room temperature for any length of time. Ham is the most common food reported in staphylococcal food poisoning. Precooked ham has a high salt content which inhibits the growth of other organisms that might compete with *Staphylococcus*, while providing an ideal growth medium for the *Staphylococcus*. Food handlers should wear disposable latex or vinyl gloves when preparing foods for the general public. This includes catering for any occasion and when preparing food for lunch counters, vending machines and the airlines.

Since staphylococcal food poisoning is caused by ingestion of a toxin that has already been produced, the onset of illness is much more rapid. Symptoms normally occur about two to six hours after eating the contaminated food. Characteristically, three quarters of all of the people who eat the tainted food will experience symptoms. These include intense vomiting, lasting up to twenty-four hours. Antibiotics are of no value, since this is not an infection. Intravenous fluid and electrolyte therapy is required in severe cases, usually in about one-fourth of the victims. The organism is usually not recovered in the stool. The suspected food should be examined by health authorities who have the expertise and technology to detect the presence of toxins.

Examination of food for bacteria or toxins should always be conducted when a foodborne illness is suspected. This is particularly important when several individuals who have eaten the same food become ill. In an outbreak at a country club in 1986 where over 800 people were served, one-third of them developed staphylococcal food poisoning. About one-third of those who became ill required emergency medical treatment. *Staphylococcus* was found in the nasal passages of two of the food handlers and in the stool of two. *Staphylococcus* was found in the turkey, which had been allowed to cool at room temperature for three hours. The Centers for Disease Control reported that the most likely source of the contamination of the food in this example was hands. The fingers that prepare food are often contaminated from the nose and/or the stool. Proper hand washing and the wearing of gloves for food preparation would have prevented the illness in these people.

SALMONELLA (other than typhoid)

This species of bacteria is responsible for the most common food-borne INFECTIONS in the United States. About 50,000 cases are reported to the Centers for Disease Control each year, a number which, as stated above, has been increasing. Many cases go unreported. The majority of cases result from the consumption of foods of animal origin, especially eggs and poultry. This is the case partially because *Salmonella* commonly contaminates these foods in their natural form or in processing, and partially because these foods are good culture media for *Salmonella* when inoculated by the hands of a carrier. Potato salad again is a common source of infection. Raw milk is also a potential source of *Salmonella* infection. Unpasteurized milk carries many health risks, but it remains popular in isolated regions of the United States.

Salmonella organisms are found in virtually every animal species, and are found in all of the animals in the food chain of humans. There are over 2200 serotypes of *Salmonella* bacteria, but not all types cause infections in humans. Twelve specific serotypes have consistently been responsible for over 80 percent of reported cases of *Salmonella* infections in humans. There has been a significant increase in the incidence of some previously uncommon types, however. In California, for instance, a large and continuing outbreak of infections caused by *Salmonella newport* was traced to infections in dairy cattle that were used to make ground beef.

There has been much publicity recently over the "discovery" that a large percentage (40 percent or higher) of chicken and turkeys are contaminated with *Salmonella* organisms. This is partially due to feeding habits of these birds, which includes ingestion of each other's excrement. Rupture of the intestines or other careless handling techniques during processing spreads the organisms to the meat. This is a fact that has been well known for the past forty years. It should be assumed that all meat from poultry contains *Salmonella*, and appropriate precautions should be taken.

Since eggs are delivered through a common alimentary port, their shells are also commonly contaminated with *Salmonella*. It is of interest that eggs contain a natural coating that inhibits the penetration of the egg by bacteria. This coating is readily removed by washing or by excess handling, permitting penetration of the shell by the *Salmonella*. The organism then multiplies within the egg, particularly when stored at warm temperatures.

Outbreaks of infection from foods prepared from eggs, such as ice cream, omelets and scrambled eggs, have been reported with increased frequency. Investigation indicates that some of these outbreaks occur because the *Salmonella* has invaded the egg. Failure to maintain cold storage during shipment permits the organism to multiply in the egg. Thorough cooking as well as proper handling can prevent these cases of food poisoning. Products such as eggnog should be pasteurized, and any food to which eggs are added, including custards and pumpkin, should be cooked to at least 160° F. Consumption of any product that incorporates raw eggs carries a distinct risk of serious and unpleasant illness.

Outbreaks of *Salmonella* food poisoning involving as many as one hundred people have also resulted from consuming unshelled steamed shrimp in a restaurant. The simple expedient of having food handlers wear disposable plastic gloves while preparing such foods could prevent much suffering. Frequent hand washing, especially after handling poultry products, including eggs, would also prevent inoculating other foods with this organism. Faucet and refrigerator handles and counter tops that have been contaminated by poultry products should be thoroughly cleansed before handling other food products or utensils.

Poultry products must be kept properly refrigerated at all times. If a large mass of meat such as a turkey is placed in the refrigerator when it is hot, the center can remain warm enough for twenty-four hours to permit *Salmonella* to multiply. In one elementary school 350 children and staff became ill with Salmonella food poisoning after eating turkey salad. The Centers for Disease Control reported that the turkey had been de-boned then stored in the refrigerator overnight in an eight-inch deep pan. The temperature inside any mass of meat this large can stay warm enough to allow bacterial growth. In order to assure that the center of the meat will be chilled promptly, turkey and ham should not exceed four inches in depth when placed in the refrigerator warm. The temperature in the refrigerator should be at or below 38° F., and a thermometer should be kept in the refrigerator to monitor this.

A source of *Salmonella* infections that is neglected because it is not of animal origin is cantaloupe and other melons. Since they are grown on the ground the rinds are easily contaminated by *Salmonella* from the dirt or from animal excreta. If they are then cut without first washing the surface, the *Salmonella* are distributed to the fruit where they multiply. The bacterial growth is particularly significant where the melons are used in salads that sit at room temperature for any period. During June and July 1991 over 400 confirmed cases of *Salmonella* infections from 23 states and Canada resulted from salads containing melons that originated in the Rio Grande region of Texas or in Mexico.[6]

Commercial growers customarily wash the melons in a chlorine solution to prevent this problem. Small growers who pack the melons in the field as they are picked do not take this precaution. Melons that are grown in Mexico have been implicated in *Salmonella* foodborne infections repeatedly. It is wise to wash the surface of all melons before cutting into them, and to use only a clean, sanitary knife. These same precautions apply to all fruits and vegetables that are grown in or on the ground. They also apply to all such food products that are grown in foreign countries, where irrigation with wastewater may be carried out. Gamma radiation of melons as well as all poultry and meats would result in a marked reduction in the more than 50,000 cases of *Salmonella* infections reported each year. Some of these come from unexpected sources. In 1995 two hundred forty-two people in 17 states contracted salmonella infections from contaminated alfalfa sprouts. In the previous year, 600 people in 41 states contracted salmonella infections from contaminated ice cream.

Salmonella organisms reproduce in the intestinal tract of humans, establishing an infection that results in the gradual onset of fever and diarrhea about ten to thirty-six hours after the food has been eaten. Stool cultures will demonstrate the organism. Most antibiotics prolong the course of the disease and increase the risk of recurrence. Resistance has developed to most of the commonly used

168

antibiotics. A more recent group of antibiotics (fluoroquinolones) are effective against *Salmonella* as well as many of the other organisms that cause diarrhea in man. If past experience is any indication, this breakthrough may not benefit us long, since the development of resistance usually occurs. This is one of many diseases that are better and more easily prevented than treated.

CAMPYLOBACTER JEJUNI

Diarrhea resulting from intestinal infections caused by *Campylobacter* species is currenmtly one of the most common foodborne illnesses in the United States, with about 2 million cases each year. It can result from contaminated food or water (see under WATER, below), and only a small dose is required to produce illness (500 organisms, the quantity in one drop of raw chicken juice).[7] Like *Salmonella*, it can be transmitted from most wild and domestic animals. The first outbreak of campylobacter diarrhea in humans reported by the CDC occured in Bennington, Vermont during June 1978, and resulted from inadequate treatment of the public water supply.[8] Infections from food frequently result from drinking unpasteurized milk or dairy products from cattle that are carriers of the organism.

INFECTIONS TRANSMITTED BY NON-PASTEURIZED MILK[*]

Brucellosis (undulant fever)
E. coli, certain strains (gastroenteritis)
Helicobacter (gastroenteritis)
Listeria (encephalitis, septicemia)
Mycobacterium bovis (extra-pulmonary tuberculosis)
Salmonella (gastroenteritis)
Streptococcus (respiratory, scarlet fever)

---

[*]Including all products made from raw milk such as ice cream, cheeses, custards etc. The infections resulting from these organisms are discussed in detail in Chapter V.

Poultry, which may be chronically infected, is also a common source. Other foods can be contaminated from cutting boards or counter tops that were previously used for cutting up poultry. Wooden cutting boards should not be used for meat in general. Plastic and Corningware™ boards can be more thoroughly cleansed. Any food can be contaminated with *Campylobacter* by hands after changing the diaper of an infected infant, or from a sick puppy or kitten. The bacterium can be excreted in the stool for as long as six weeks after an infection.

LISTERIA

Infections caused by *Listeria monocytogenes* bacteria as a result of eating meat had not been reported prior to 1988. A case that resulted from eating frankfurters that contained the organism was reported to the Centers for Disease Control in December of that year. During a follow up surveillance by the CDC, 301 additional cases of listeriosis acquired from food were identified through the end of 1990 in four states selected for the study. One third of the cases occurred in pregnant women or their newborns. The remainder occurred mainly in individuals who had diseases that cause some immune suppression (cancer, cortisone use, kidney disease or diabetes), or in AIDS patients. This confirms previous reports that listeriosis mainly afflicts newborn infants, individuals past forty and those whose immune system has been compromised by diseases such as cirrhosis, lymphomas, other cancers and AIDS. Patients with ulcerative colitis are also vulnerable to infections by *Listeria*.

Although listeriosis is not a large risk for healthy individuals, 23 percent of those who do contract the infection die. This is an unusually high death rate for foodborne illnesses. Recent studies have revealed that *Listeria monocytogenes* is also a common cause of meningitis in adults. When acquired during pregnancy it may lead to miscarriage, stillbirths or serious infections such as meningitis in the newborn. Advice on foods to avoid should be given routinely to pregnant women as part of the early nutritional counseling.

Foods most frequently associated with the cases in studies conducted by the Centers for Disease Control include soft cheeses (Mexican-style such as Queso Blanco and Queso Fresco, Brie, Camembert, and blue-veined such as Roquefort), other foods from store delicatessen counters and undercooked chicken. No cases resulting from ingestion of cottage cheese have been reported. Eating hot dogs without reheating them has been identified as another foodborne source of illness. All leftover foods or ready to eat foods such as hot dogs and cold cuts should be heated until steaming before eating. Foods sold at delicatessen counters should be avoided.[9] Irradiation of these at risk foods would eliminate the many infections caused by them. Between August 1998 and January 6, 1999 at least 50 persons in 11 states became ill from a rare strain of Listeria in contaminated hot dogs and deli meats.[10] During the year 2000 twenty-nine persons from ten different states had illnesses caused by a strain of *Listeria monocytogenes* that they had acquired from eating processed turkey meat that had been contaminated in the plant in Texas.[11] A peculiar feature of infection with Listeria is that illness may not begin until 2-8 weeks after consuming the contaminated food.

At any cafeteria or other food counter where raw food is served in proximity to cooked food, cross contamination is a very real risk, and these foods should be avoided. Such setups have resulted in thousands of cases of various types of food poisonings. Unpasteurized milk and foods made from it also can transmit *Listeria* also. In July 1994 after drinking milk at a picnic in Illinois, 58 people became ill with a febrile gastroenteritis caused by *Listeria*.[12] Although the milk had been pasteurized it had been recontaminated during processing. The storage temperature in refrigerators should be maintained in a safe range as described previously. A thermometer should be in place to monitor this. Permitting the temperature in a refrigerator to range above 38° F. is inviting foodborne infections. Following the World Health Organization's *Ten Golden Rules* listed previously will aid in avoiding listeriosis as well as other foodborne illnesses.[13,14]

CLOSTRIDIUM PERFRINGENS

This is a bacterium that is widely distributed in feces, soil, air and water. It is the third most common cause of food poisoning in the United States. Outbreaks generally result from eating cooked beef, poultry or other meat, or meat products, that have been partially cooked, but not long enough to kill all of the organisms. The meat is then allowed to cool at room temperature during which time the organisms multiply and produce a powerful enterotoxin. The meat is then refrigerated. Upon rewarming, the organisms and their toxin are not destroyed. These organisms also produce additional toxin in the intestinal tract after being ingested. Diarrhea with marked abdominal cramping and pain are experienced after a relatively short period, six to twelve hours. Several large outbreaks have occurred from corned beef served at St. Patrick's Day celebrations.[15] This is another unpleasant illness that illustrates the risks of allowing cooked meats to cool slowly at room temperature prior to refrigeration. The bacteria in such meats multiply and come back to haunt us.

SHIGELLA

Shigella is another group of bacteria that produce an infection in the intestine of humans resulting in diarrhea, often bloody. It has been labeled bacillary dysentery, as contrasted with that caused by other organisms such as amoeba. An abrupt onset of severe abdominal cramping with pronounced straining is common. Since this is an infection in the body, headache, fever, chills and aching are normally experienced. These symptoms are seen twenty-four to seventy-two hours after ingestion of the organisms. Antibiotics are helpful, but resistance to most of these has developed. The newer class of antibiotics mentioned previously (fluoro-quinolones) have proven effective against *Shigella* in laboratory tests, and have been approved for infectious diarrhea recently. Unfortunately, drugs that relieve the cramps prolong the clinical course of the disease.

Approximately 24,000 cases of *Shigella* infection are reported to the Centers for Disease Control each year. About 15 percent of the cases of diarrhea acquired by travelers in Mexico are caused by these organisms. Of fifteen cases of *Shigella* infection among visitors to Cancun, Mexico during an eight-month period in 1988, eight were found to be resistant to the antibiotics commonly used for this disease. The practice of taking these medications prophylactically when traveling contributes to the development of resistance, and thus renders them less useful. For this reason most medical authorities now advise against this practice, recommending greater attention to avoidance of food and drink known to present a risk of acquiring these organisms, and to personal hygiene such as hand washing. Specific antibiotic treatment should be reserved for proven infections. Stool culture in these infections will reveal the causative agent and also determine what medications are effective.

AMEBIASIS

Entamoeba histolytica is a protozoan that produces diarrheal disease in over 5,000 individuals in the United States each year. It is spread from feces to mouth through poor sanitary practices (lack of hand washing), and by contamination of food and water. Fruits and vegetables, including salads, are commonly contaminated by carriers. The infection, known as amoebic dysentery, may be mild or may be marked by a pronounced diarrhea, cramping and flatulence. Abscesses in the liver and infection in the gallbladder are not uncommon. A subacute appendicitis may result, in which case surgery should be deferred until treatment has been instituted and the infection subsides. Stool examination may require special techniques, which can be applied by any competent licensed laboratory. Treatment is available, but antibiotics are ineffective

BOTULISM

Perhaps the best known of all of the food poisonings, botulism results from a very potent toxin produced by the bacterium *Clostridium botulinum*. This organism is present throughout our environment, especially in the soil and anything that comes in contact with it. Poisoning in adults results from consuming food in which the toxin has been produced after packaging, usually in a sealed container or in frozen fish. When the spores of *C. botulinum* germinate they produce the most potent neurotoxin known. It causes a paralysis of muscles throughout the body, beginning with those in the head and neck, spreading to the extremities and the muscles of respiration. The toxin is readily destroyed by cooking the food for thirty minutes at 176° F., or by boiling for ten minutes. Regardless of this, any food exhibiting evidence of spoilage should not be consumed. Any canned food that appears to be swollen from the internal production of gas should be discarded. Contaminated foods may appear and taste normal. Needless to say, any suspected food should **NOT** be taste tested. This is the most potent poison known to mankind. You must also take precautions to avoid contaminating your hands with any suspected food, particularly if any cuts or abrasions are present.

In contrast to the toxin produced by the *Clostridium* organisms, their spores, which are widespread in nature, can survive boiling for several hours. These spores can produce toxin even under refrigeration, and this has been seen in frozen fish many times. The spores are destroyed in a pressure canner after thirty minutes at fifteen pounds of pressure, or after twenty minutes at twenty pounds of pressure (278° F). This is the only system that should be utilized in home canning, particularly of low acid foods such as fruits, vegetables, meats, fish, peppers, eggplant and mushrooms. Home canned foods account for most of the cases of botulism in the United States, since there is minimal chance that the spores will survive commercial canning processes.

The number of cases of botulism that result from eating in restaurants has been increasing however (forty two percent of reported cases between 1976 and 1984). These cases frequently result from home canned low acid foods such as peppers and mushrooms that have been acquired by the restaurant from an individual. Restaurant patrons have suffered botulism poisoning from commercially prepared eggplant and from garlic, however, both of which were canned in oil. Covering a food with oil produces the anaerobic (absence of oxygen) conditions that permits *Clostridium botulinum* to produce the toxin. In one case onions that were covered with grease and permitted to stand overnight resulted in a large outbreak of botulism in Illinois in 1983.[16] It is never safe to allow any food to sit for any period of time at room temperature. This is especially true of roasted vegetables prepared in oil.

Illness and even deaths have resulted in recent years from type E botulism as a result of eating ribyetz or kapchunka, which is ungutted whole whitefish. Smoked freshwater fish such as gelfite has also been associated with type E botulism. Another product that has caused this form of botulism is moloha, a non-eviscerated, salt cured fish. The botulism organism is known to survive in the gut of these fish, and the consumption of smoked or salted uncooked fish carries this risk. The fish tastes and smells normal.

Of the 123 cases of botulism reported in 1984, 99 cases occurred in infants. This occurs most frequently among infants two to three months old. Unlike the adult cases, those in infants result from the production of toxin in the stomach of the child by the organism after it is swallowed. This occurs by virtue of the fact that the immature digestive system is unable to inhibit the activity of the organism. Honey used in preparing formula has been responsible for numerous cases, and this should never be fed to a child of less than one year of age. Botulism spores are prevalent in soil and throughout the environment, so it is no surprise that bees would collect them along with nectar. Wild honey may also contain various plant toxins, depending upon where the bees collect nectar. Poisoning has occurred where bees have collected nectar from mountain laurel, rhododendron, azaleas and oleander. Experienced beekeepers make certain that these plants are not within the range of their bees. All forms of bees require a source of water to make honey, and if this source is contaminated, these contaminants will find their way into the honey. Commercial growers are also careful to provide a safe source of water for their bees.

Other sources of botulism identified have been contamination of food by soil or vacuum cleaner dust. Installation of a central vacuum system that exhausts all of the dust to the outside will serve to minimize this as well as the many other risks from dust that is recirculated through conventional vacuum cleaners. Careful cleaning of the breast should always precede breast- feeding of infants in order to eliminate the risk of this disease as well as others.

Botulism carries a high mortality rate if not properly treated. Hospitalization is essential, and reduces mortality to below ten percent. Vomiting and neurological symptoms such as blurred or double vision, dry mouth and sagging of the eyelids appear twelve to thirty-six hours after ingesting the contaminated food. Weakness of the muscles of the arms and legs then sets in. Diarrhea is rare with this disease because of the paralytic effect of the toxin on the nerves that mediate the intestinal activity. The toxin is a potent poison to the nervous system and paralysis of respiration is life threatening.

CHOLERA

Cholera is an acute bacterial infection caused by *Vibrio cholerae* that establishes itself in the jejunum (smallintestine). There it produces a toxin that results in a profuse watery diarrhea that leads to severe and rapidly progressive dehydration. Death can result in a matter of hours unless aggressive treatment is undertaken. The fatality rate is less than one percent when adequate treatment is rendered. Treatment is directed not at eradicating the organism, but at replacement of the fluid and electrolytes that have been lost in copious amounts. If the patient is in shock this must be done expeditiously by the intravenous route. This may require the administration of 10 liters or more of electrolyte solution each day until the patient is stabilized. If the case is less urgent the replacement can be accomplished by administering adequate amounts of oral rehydration fluids. This should be started as soon as possible after the onset of diarrhea and continued as long as the diarrhea persists. A delay of 6 to 8 hours may result in shock that requires hospitalization. *Vibrio cholerae* is one of several organisms that have a propensity to produce an acute infection in the gallbladder that requires surgical removal.

Over 70 subtypes of *Vibrio cholerae* exist, but two produce the most severe illness. The world base of operations for the disease is the Ganges delta in India. During the 19th century it spread from there throughout the world in several pandemics. Since 1817 there have been seven world pandemics. The last of these to reach the United States was in 1911 when the sixth pandemic entered New York and Massachusetts. It has remained endemic in most of the regions of the world where sanitation systems and public health laws are lacking. The majority of cases in these countries result from human fecal contamination of water supplies. It is then spread among family members by contamination of food and water, either by hands or flies.

Attention to cleanliness and hand washing are imperative in cholera infections as with other infectious diseases. Fly control is equally important in areas where they are present, since they can carry the organism to food and water. Large epidemics occur periodically in those regions where cholera is endemic, occasionally being carried to other countries. In 1988 thirty countries reported over 44,000 cases. Cases are brought into the United States sporadically by travelers. This was the only source of cases of cholera in the Western Hemisphere between 1911 and 1973. During August 1991 three cases of cholera in Maryland resulted from the use of frozen coconut milk imported from Thailand.

Since 1973, 91 cases of cholera have occurred from eating raw or undercooked shellfish taken from the Gulf of Mexico and coastal waters. In 1978 several cases occurred in Louisiana, apparently from consumption of inadequately cooked shellfish. In 1981 an outbreak occurred among 16 workers on an oilrig off the

Texas coast. Most cases of cholera that occur on offshore oilrigs result from contaminated drinking water. Sporadic cases continued to be reported almost every year. Eight cases associated with the consumption of raw oysters taken from the Gulf of Mexico occurred in 1988.

Most of the cases reported in Louisiana in recent years have been traced to crabs taken from lake and estuary waters. All of the aforementioned cases were caused by a strain of *Vibrio cholerae* different than that causing the current epidemic in South America. On July 2, 1991, however, that strain was identified in oysters and oyster eating fish in Mobile Bay. This strain was found subsequently in oysters in Mobile Bay, and again in June 1992. The introduction of this strain of *Vibrio cholerae* into the Gulf Coast waters, probably through the ballast of ships from South America, presents a very real risk of the spread of this epidemic to the United States.[17] A reservoir of Cholera is now established in the Gulf of Mexico in the waters of Texas and Louisiana.

Epidemic cholera surfaced in Peru in January 1991 after an absence from South America throughout the entire 1900's. It subsequently spread to Ecuador, Columbia, Chile, Brazil, Mexico and Guatemala. As of August 12, 1991, 15 persons had returned to the United States from the epidemic areas with cholera. In one case a New York man returned from Ecuador bringing with him crabmeat that he had purchased on the dock. After his return he shared the crabmeat in a salad, without cooking, with family and friends. Three of these individuals were subsequently treated for cholera.

By the end of 1991 an additional 11 cases of cholera were reported in the United States, for a total of 26 cases. Eleven of these cases were related to crabs brought back in suitcases. Crabs are a common source of cholera. *Vibrio cholera* can survive in crabs that are boiled for up to 8 minutes. The common propensity to eat seafood with only minimal or no cooking has resulted in many cases of foodborne infections.

During 1992, 102 cases of cholera were reported in the United States, more than in any previous year since surveillance began in 1961. All but one of these cases was contracted outside of the United States during travel. Cases were reported from 12 states. Seventy-five cases occurred among 356 passengers who had been served contaminated seafood salad on an airline flight from Argentina to Los Angeles in February 1992. One person died. Travel by international airline flights presents many opportunities to share in diseases not customarily seen in the United States.

By the end of 1992, 731,312 cases of cholera from 21 countries in South and Central America had been reported to the World Health Organization. Deaths resulting from this epidemic totaled 6,323.[18,19,20,21,22,23] One of the most recent countries to be invaded by the epidemic is Mexico, where 2690 cases were reported in 1991. In 1994 over 300,00 cases were reported in 66 countries. The disease has also spread to the countries adjacent to the Caribbean, threatening those islands next.

Cholera will persist in some of these regions for years, mandating careful precautions for travel to affected areas. This requires constant awareness of the risk and rigid adherence to the standard health recommendations for travel. Do not eat any uncooked food, including fruit and vegetables. It is a little known fact in our country that in Peru and many other countries throughout the world raw wastewater, including human excrement, is used to irrigate crops. In 1991 after the outbreak of the cholera epidemic in Peru, officials in Trujillo discovered clandestine taps into sewage lines that were being used to irrigate crops such as cabbage, lettuce, carrots and watermelon.[24] These practices automatically contaminate crops with disease-causing organisms that have been discharged into the sewage system. This is especially true of surface crops such as lettuce and cabbage.

With an epidemic of the magnitude that has hit South America this source of spread of the disease is as readily apparent as the lack of chlorination of public water supplies. The latter is also common in many countries throughout the world as a result of lack of funds to purchase equipment and chlorine. In the absence of an epidemic to call attention to the problem, the many other diseases that are transmitted by the irrigation of crops with wastewater are ignored.

Cold seafood and salads are especially risky for the transmission of cholera. Ceviche, the Latin American version of sushi, has been responsible for some of the cases of cholera in the current epidemic. Ceviche should be avoided like the plague that it is, and all fish and shellfish should be thoroughly cooked. Even then they may be contaminated after cooking by raw seafood placed next to them. The hands of food handlers can also contaminate food. Food and drink from street vendors should never be consumed. Ice should never be used in food or drink. The only water used for drinking, brushing teeth, douching, an enema or any other internal application should be bottled water known to be safe. Carbonated bottled water and carbonated soft drinks are usually safe if no ice is used. Public drinking fountains, even in airports should be avoided. The last drink before the flight home is all that it took for many.

Cholera organisms can be eradicated from the intestine if they are susceptible to one of the antibiotics known to be effective against that specific strain. Immunizations were required for many years for travel into regions where the disease is endemic. These injections provide little immunity, and the protection that it does confer is short lived. The side effects are significant. Cholera immunization is no longer recommended, but may be required by some authorities outside of the United States. Two new oral vaccines are available in some countries, but are not available in the United States as of 2001. Native populations in lands where cholera is endemic acquire antibodies to the disease by early adulthood. Individuals from these regions who display no apparent illness can introduce cholera to regions free of it.

Noting this, efforts have been under way to develop an oral vaccine. One such oral vaccine was tested in 1992 in more than 3,000 people, and it provided a high level of immunity with minimal side effects.[25] Recent studies however have demonstrated that an oral vaccine that is effective against one strain of cholera does not protect against another strain.[26] Two strains currently account for most of the cases worldwide, but one of the other many strains could emerge at any time. Continued efforts would be needed to keep any vaccine current. The program at Wyeth Laboratories to develop an oral vaccine has been discontinued.[27] In the meantime, in traveling to areas with cholera the only protection is constant vigilance and scrupulous attention to hygiene and to food and drink. It is very difficult to remain constantly focused on this threat when visiting other countries, but the consequences of neglect are very unpleasant.

VIBRIO PARAHEMOLYTICUS

This is a vibrio species separate from *Vibrio Cholerae* that also causes a bacterial diarrhea. It also is acquired from eating seafood, particularly saltwater fish, shrimp and crab. The practice of eating these foods with only brief cooking increases the risk. Frequently outbreaks have occurred as a result of contamination of cooked shellfish in a kitchen by shellfish that has not yet been cooked. Contamination of foods by using seawater for rinsing has also transmitted the disease. Several outbreaks have occurred on cruise ships. An inspection of cruise ships in early 1989 revealed that one-half failed to meet acceptable sanitary and food handling standards. Cruise ships are not subject to the inspection and regulation by local health departments that apply to restaurants, and have thus delivered a higher incidence of food-borne illnesses. The incidence of this disease is much higher in Japan due to the common practice of eating uncooked seafood.

The disease is ushered in by acute diarrhea and moderately severe abdominal cramping, about 6 to 48 hours, most commonly 12 hours, after eating the infected food. Vomiting is seen in approximately one third of the victims. The organism grows both in the seafood and in the human gut and produces a toxin in both sites. No deaths have occurred in the United States as a result of this infection.

VIBRIO VULNIFICUS

This is a less common *Vibrio* bacterium that is also acquired from consuming raw or undercooked shellfish, producing not only a gastrointestinal infection but also serious infections throughout the body by spreading through the bloodstream. Death occurs in a high percentage of victims (up to 35 percent) and early treatment is imperative. Both this and *V. parahemolyticus* can be treated with doxycycline or ciprofloxacin. Those most at risk are individuals who abuse alcohol, who suffer from an impaired immune system (cancer, AIDS), diabetes and the elderly. Several deaths have resulted from cuts or abrasions while handling crabs and other shellfish. In other cases infection has resulted in the amputation of fingers or limbs. Exposing any open wound to contaminated waters risks serious infection. Thick gloves will help protect from injury, but contaminated water can still soak through the gloves and infect through an abrasion of the skin.

Vibrio vulnificus infections in humans was first reported in the U.S. in 1979[27], and surveillance since then had been limited to four states along the Gulf Coast. It is common in the bodies of water that empty into the gulf, where oysters and other shellfish are contaminated. Infection had most frequently followed consumption of raw oysters. Retrospective studies in 1995 in North Carolina, however, revealed that serious infections and deaths from the organism had occurred there at least as far back as 1992. These cases escaped attention because there has been no national surveillance for infections caused by *Vibrio vulnificus*. The problem is more common than previously believed, and is a risk even in those coastal rivers and streams that have not suffered increased contamination in recent years. This additional risk has added to the woes of the residents near the Neuse and Pamlico Rivers in North Carolina where *Pfiesteria* has been discovered to be causing serious neurologic disorders in recent years.

PARALYTIC SHELLFISH POISONING (RED TIDE)

During the months of May to October conditions are favorable for the reproduction of certain dinoflagellates that are part of the marine phytoplankton in the Pacific and New England coastal waters of the United States. When these organisms reproduce in great numbers they turn the water a reddish color as they remain suspended near the surface, thus the name "red tide." They produce a very potent nerve toxin, saxitoxin, which is an alkaloid that does not readily break down when heated. It interferes with the transmission of nerve impulses to muscles, and thus results in weakness or paralysis in these muscles. When bivalve mollusks such as clams, oysters, scallops and mussels feed on them, these shellfish accumulate and concentrate the nerve toxin.

When humans consume the contaminated shellfish they may experience numbness of the face, arms and legs in addition to muscular weakness, diarrhea, nausea and vomiting. These symptoms may begin in as brief an interval as thirty minutes. In severe cases of this "paralytic shellfish poisoning" paralysis, respiratory arrest and death may occur. These latter sequelae are more common in the Pacific Northwest and New England coastal waters than in the Gulf Coast. State health departments in New England, California and Alaska routinely collect shellfish from their waters and test them for the toxin. When levels of the toxin exceed a preset limit a quarantine against harvesting shellfish is placed in effect and their sale is prohibited. Gathering shellfish during these periods of quarantine is likely to result in great suffering or worse. Not all toxic shellfish originate from "red tide" areas, and not all such reddish areas contain toxic dinoflagellates. It is essential for residents of these areas to heed the posted warnings of health authorities, regardless of personal observations.

In an incident in June 1990, six fishermen in a boat in the Georges Bank area off the Nantucket coast developed the severe symptoms of paralytic shellfish poisoning after eating blue mussels that they had harvested in deep water. They had boiled these for 90 minutes before consuming them. The area had been previously identified to be contaminated with the toxin through deep-sea sampling by the health department.

The neurotoxins that cause paralytic shellfish poisoning (saxitoxin and related compounds) are among the most potent toxins known. Cooking or steaming the shellfish does not destroy them. They are water-soluble and thus can be concentrated in the broth by the evaporation of water during cooking.

SCOMBROID FISH POISONING

This poisoning results from eating improperly handled dark meated fish including tuna, albacore, bonito, bluefish, mackerel and mahi-mahi. When these fish are not refrigerated or placed on ice immediately and continuously after being caught, bacteria in the fish convert the amino acid histidine to histamine. Since histamine taken by mouth is metabolized in the intestine it is normally not toxic even in large doses. Other elements produced by the bacteria in the fish thus are necessary to produce the toxicity. Researchers have postulated that other toxins are produced that either inhibit the metabolism of the histamine, or otherwise enhance its absorption. These elements have not been identified as yet.

In any event, cooking does not destroy the toxins. The only means of preventing the disease is by prompt and continuous icing or refrigeration of all dark meated fish. No change in appearance, smell or taste can be relied upon. The history of the handling of imported fish of this class cannot be readily obtained, thus consumption carries an obvious risk. One must rely upon the integrity of the supplier. Investigation of four cases of scombroid poisoning that resulted from eating tuna salad in a restaurant in 1998 revealed that the tuna had been caught on lines that were up to 60 miles long, with up to 3000 hooks. Retrieval of the fish could take up to 12 to 24 hours, and the tuna could remain in the warm water for up to 20 hours. These are conditions favorable to the production of histamine in the fish.[28]

The onset of illness occurs from one to several hours after consumption of the fish. Symptoms include nausea, abdominal cramping, diarrhea, sweating, redness of the face and burning of the mouth and throat. More severe allergic like symptoms typical of excessive histamine levels may occur. Prompt medical attention is urgent.

CIGUATERA FISH POISONING

This affliction is separate and distinct from scombroid poisoning. It has caused illness in large numbers of diners in restaurants in Florida, Puerto Rico, Cuba and the Virgin Islands. In July 1997 eight people became ill after eating grouper that was served in a restaurant in Chapel Hill, North Carolina, once again reminding us that illness can be imported into regions where it is not expected. Ciguatera poisoning had been reported previously in Alabama from amberjack that had been shipped from Key West, Florida.[29] The poisoning results from a toxin, or more likely a mixture of toxins, produced by a single-celled plantlike protozoa similar to the one that produces the red tides. This dinoflagellate and its toxin, however, do not float near the surface and cannot be observed. As the fish feed on algae attached to coral, they consume the dinoflagellate. These fish are then consumed by larger fish such as barracuda and yellowfin grouper, resulting in a high concentration of the toxin in these species. As with scombroid poisoning, this toxin also is not destroyed by cooking.

In excess of 400 different species of fish have been reported to cause Ciguatera poisoning, including barracudas, groupers, jacks, parrotfish, sea basses, snappers, surgeonfish, wrasses and eels. Many of these are common sources of food for humans. The toxin occurs only in warm waters and only in certain regions. These regions cannot be predicted, however, and it cannot be safely ascertained where any given fish have been feeding. This is particularly true of the high-risk barracuda, yellowfin grouper and hogfish. It is unsafe to eat any of the native fish caught in the waters around the Virgin Islands. Virtually every resident who has done so has experienced this disease. Some aggressive restaurant owners in Florida have been known to sell barracuda as red snapper, which presents the potential for a very unpleasant surprise besides the price.

Symptoms include abdominal cramping, nausea, vomiting and diarrhea that may persist for from eight to eighteen hours. Headache, face pain and muscle pain are also experienced. Numbness and tingling may persist for months. There is no specific treatment available.

PUFFER FISH

Most of the members of this group of fishes contain an extremely potent neurotoxin, tetrodotoxin, which is concentrated mainly in the ovaries and liver. Lessor amounts may also be present in the intestines and skin. A similar poison has been found in salamanders, newts and frogs. Consumption can result in death from respiratory paralysis, with a rapid onset of symptoms, within 30 minutes. With proper handling and cooking the risk of poisoning can be reduced. Fugu, a genus of Japanese puffer fish, and a delicacy in Japan, results in about 250 cases of poisoning each year. Previously 80 percent of those who developed symptoms died, but this has been reduced to about 40 percent through special training of cooks and licensing of Fugu restaurants. Cases of Fugu poisoning are reported also in Thailand and other Asian countries.

VIRUSES

When we consider infectious diseases we invariably think of bacteria or perhaps fungi. These are both easy for us to visualize and understand. We can recover the respective microorganisms from infections fairly easily; we can grow them in the laboratory, place them under a microscope and actually see what they look like. We can further classify those that look alike by the types of media that they grow on, or their characteristic reactions to various substrates. Viruses are much more elusive. They cannot be grown in the average microbiology laboratory; some cannot be grown with any known technique. They cannot be seen under the light microscope, although most can be imaged with an electron microscope. Most viruses range from 0.01 to 0.02 micron in diameter compared to 0.3 to 0.5 micron for bacteria. Most require indirect physical and chemical techniques for classification.

Whereas bacteria have a cell wall, a nucleus and some intracellular substances much as the cells in our body do, the viruses are totally different. They do not have a cell wall, and can reproduce and cause disease only by entering and parasitizing living cells. The viral particle consists of a nucleic acid core (RNA or DNA) with an outer cover of protein. These features help to justify classifying viruses as living entities, and render them susceptible to some degree to chemotherapeutic agents and heat. The fact that viruses stimulate the production of antibodies in the host (as do bacteria) aids in diagnosing diseases produced by them.

Retroviruses were first discovered in the early 1900's as filterable agents that produced tumors in chickens that could be transmitted to other chickens. In the 1950's a retrovirus that caused leukemia in mice was isolated. The first human retrovirus to be isolated was the human T-cell lymphotrophic virus, HTLV-1, in 1979. Four pathogenic human retroviruses have been identified at present, and these are divided into two separate groups. The human T lymphotrophic virus, HTLV-I is responsible for adult T-cell leukemia/lymphoma. HTLV-2 is closely related to HTLV-1, but has not been linked to any specific disease as yet. Several closely related retroviruses that cause cancer in primates have been identified, as well as the FeLV in cats that produces both T-cell leukemia and an immunodeficiency disease very similar to AIDS in humans.

The central core of retroviruses contains two identical copies of the single stranded viral RNA reproductive message, which is unusual among viruses. Retroviruses also contain an enzyme, the DNA polymerase called reverse transcriptase, that causes the transcription (conversion) of the RNA in the cytoplasm of the virus to the double stranded DNA form. This DNA then migrates from the cytoplasm to the nucleus and integrates with the DNA of the cell of the host (human). This form is known as the provirus and it remains for the life of the cell. In this capacity it dictates the structure of cells produced by the infected cell. The original genetic code of the human cell is thus permanently altered. This change persists for the life of the individual, and there is currently no means to correct this alteration, or to eradicate the virus from the body. The retroviruses that infect humans have an affinity for lymphocytes, especially T4 lymphocytes.

More difficult to classify is a group of agents that have never been visualized by any means. Some scientists, who believe that they are unique proteins that are capable of replicating by some as yet unknown mechanism, have labeled them prions. They are also unique in that they do not stimulate any detectable immune response in the host. They are responsible for slow, degenerative diseases of the brain such as Creutzfeldt-Jakob disease and kuru. The latter was seen exclusively in natives of New Guinea as a result of a ritualistic rite that involved eating the brains of dead relatives. The practice has been virtually abandoned and the disease is now seldom seen. Scrapie in sheep is a similar disease that is also caused by a prion.

Although these agents cannot be visualized they can be transmitted to other animals, with a reproduction of the disease. Creutzfeldt-Jakob disease has been acquired by pathologists as a result of performing autopsies and more recently in patients as a result of organ and tissue transplants from donor banks. Onset of Creutzfeldt-Jakob disease has been noted in patients less than two years after receiving dura mater from cadavers in surgical procedures.[30,31] It has also been transmitted from known victims of the disease to two uninfected individuals through brain electrodes. During the 1960s thousands of children who suffered severe growth deficiencies received injections of human growth hormone that had been extracted from the pituitary glands of human cadavers. Decades later many of these individuals are dead or dying of Creutzfeldt-Jakob disease (125 as of 2000), and the count continues. Since 1985 human growth hormone has been produced synthetically through recombinant DNA techniques, eliminating the risk of disease transmission.

The Creutzfeldt-Jakob prion is particularly resistant to inactivation by heat, irradiation, chemicals (formalin) and all of the usual disinfecting techniques. It can be inactivated in a steam autoclave or pressure cooker by heating to 270° F. for one hour.

Every other disease-causing organism that we have identified is destroyed after 20 minutes in an autoclave at 270° F. Surgical instruments that are used on patients with Creutzfeldt-Jakob disease are discarded rather than sterilized and re-used.

VIRUSES IN FOOD AND WATER

Diarrhea resulting from viral enteritis is attributable to two categories of viruses, for the most part. The rotaviruses include a group of agents that causes disease worldwide, mainly in infants and young children. This affliction frequently attacks adults, however, especially family members of younger children who have the disease. It is also seen in older people and in immunodeficient individuals (such as in AIDS patients). This disease, which occurs mainly during the winter months in the United States, is the chief cause of diarrhea that results in severe dehydration and hospitalization in children. It can be fatal in young children if adequate fluids and electrolytes are not administered (see Chapter III). Administration of oral rehydration solutions, such as the World Health Organizations solution, is usually adequate in all but the severely ill. There is no specific treatment for the virus.

The rotavirus replicates only in the small intestine, where it causes significant damage to the lining by destroying the cells there. This results in impairment of the normal absorption of nutrients, which accounts for the diarrhea and dehydration. Large numbers of the virus are shed in the stool, and the disease is readily spread from hands to mouth by virtue of this. Adequate hand washing after visiting the bathroom or changing diapers could prevent virtually all of these cases. The failure of this most basic personal hygiene measure accounts for the spread of this virus as a food-borne disease. Contamination of drinking water by improper handling or treatment of sewage is another common source of infection.

NORWALK AGENT

This is the other category of viruses causing diarrheal disease, and this includes a variety of related viruses, most of which have not been fully defined. The Snow Mountain agent and the Marin agent are two examples of viruses in this group that have been recognized to cause disease. These agents are about one-half the size of the rotaviruses, and they cannot be grown in cell culture or in laboratory animals. They are also shed in the stool but in much smaller quantities than is the rotavirus. As a consequence, our knowledge of this group is extremely limited and incomplete.

In contrast to the rotaviruses, the Norwalk agent causes diarrheal disease all year long, not seasonally. There is serological evidence of a previous infection in 60 to 70 percent of adults world-wide. The Norwalk agent accounts for about one-third of all of the epidemics of acute gastroenteritis in the United States. Many of these have been related to food items such as oysters, salads and ice in beverages. Outbreaks on cruise ships, in nursing homes, summer camps and schools have been traced to contamination of the water supply. Spread of this disease is also by fecal contamination of water or of food by improperly washed hands. In November 1993 seventy people in Louisiana developed an acute gastroenteritis after eating raw oysters. Investigation revealed that the oysters had become contaminated by infected harvesters, who routinely dumped their sewage overboard into the oyster beds.[32]

The Norwalk agent group causes a less serious illness in infants than does the rotavirus group. Malabsorption also occurs in this disease, but it is less severe. This virus also replicates only in the small intestine (jejunum), but no one has been able to demonstrate the precise cells where this takes place. The vomiting and diarrhea begin approximately twenty-four to seventy-two hours after consumption of the contaminated food or water. This persists for about twenty-four to forty-eight hours. There is no specific treatment, no test to demonstrate the disease, and no immunity following infection. For this latter reason, a vaccine is unlikely.

In the fall of 1987, following a college football game in Pennsylvania, 158 students were treated at the health center for nausea, vomiting, diarrhea, fever, chills, headache and muscle aches. Fifty-five members of the football team later developed the same complaints after exposure to ice from the same source. These symptoms began about thirty-six hours after the game. A virus of the Norwalk group was identified as the cause of illness. Two days later an outbreak of acute diarrheal disease struck a group of 750 people attending a fund-raising event in Delaware.

In both outbreaks the disease was traced to drinks that contained contaminated ice that had been purchased from the same manufacturer in Pennsylvania. The source of water for the manufacturer of this ice was wells that had been flooded two weeks previously by a stream following heavy rains. Several residents along the stream who draw their water from wells also developed the disease. The ice had been sold in Pennsylvania, Delaware and New Jersey. A total of 5,000 people became ill as a result of this distribution of ice. Disinfection of the wells ended the outbreak.[33]

ESCHERICHIA COLI

E. coli is a bacterium that is universally found in the intestinal tract of humans. Because of this fact, and the fact that it is easily cultured and identified, it is frequently tested for to identify fecal contamination of water. There are numerous strains of *E. Coli* and those normally inhabiting the human intestine do not cause disease unless introduced to other parts of the body. Some strains, however, produce toxins that cause serious disease. One such group is labeled enterotoxigenic *E. coli*, and it is the most common cause of travelers' diarrhea, accounting for between 50 and 75 percent of the cases. It has been considered to be rarely acquired in the United States, although outbreaks among newborns in nurseries in the US have occurred, with disastrous results. This pathogenic strain produces a toxin that results in diarrhea and vomiting about twenty-four to seventy-two hours after eating. Agents to relieve the abdominal cramping are useful. Little is known or understood about the production of toxins by some strains of this common intestinal organism in humans, and why the problem is rampant in some countries.

A rare strain of *E. coli* was first reported as a cause of severe bloody diarrhea in the United States during a multistate epidemic in 1982. That epidemic was traced to contaminated hamburgers. The bacterium responsible is a specific serotype that has been labeled O157:H7. It has been seen in a growing number of cases of diarrhea since the initial episode. It was responsible for four deaths among 243 persons identified with this illness during an outbreak of waterborne disease in 1990. Fecal contamination of the public water supply during repairs was the source of the organism. Failure to properly chlorinate the water following repairs exposed large numbers of the population.[34]

About 73,500 cases of illness, 2000 hospitalizations and 60 deaths occur in the United States each year as the result of *E. coli*

O157:H7 infections.[35] From November 15, 1992 through February 28, 1993 over 500 confirmed cases of bloody diarrhea, with four deaths, caused by this organism resulted from eating incompletely cooked hamburgers from a fast food restaurant chain in four western states, Washington, Idaho, California and Nevada. A single source of the contaminated ground beef could not be identified. Five slaughterhouses in the United States and one in Canada were identified as potential sources. The meat had come from farms in six western states.[36,37] During the spring and fall of 2000 outbreaks of *E. coli* O157:H7 infections among school children in Pennsylvania and Washington resulted in 56 illnesses and 19 hospitalizations. The illnesses resulted from visits to farms where the children had direct contact with farm animals.[38]

E. coli O157:H7 is found in the intestines of healthy cattle, and contaminates the meat during slaughter. Most of the outbreaks have resulted from eating undercooked beef. Drinking unpasteurized milk has also transmitted the organism, however. The udder of cows is frequently contaminated with excrement, and cleansing prior to milking is not always complete. Virtually all of the pathogenic organisms normally found in milk are inactivated by both the holding and flash methods of pasteurization. In 1990 an outbreak at an agricultural show, with at least 70 people infected, resulted from eating roast beef.[39] Cooking beef until the internal temperature reads at least 160° F. as recorded by an accurate thermometer kills this organism. Irradiation of the meat at the packing plant would eliminate the risk of *E. Coli* from that source.

In the fall of 1991 an outbreak of diarrhea caused by *E. coli* O157:H7 resulted from the consumption of apple cider. The apples had not been washed or cleansed and no preservative had been added to the cider. Twenty-three persons in Massachusetts were identified as having contracted the infection from cider. Four children developed hemolytic uremic syndrome, the serious kidney complication of this infection. In retrospect, it is believed that previous outbreaks of diarrhea from cider were caused by this strain of *E. coli*. It can survive in apple cider for 20 days at 46° F. Contamination of the apples with cow manure was the source of the organism.[40] It is common practice to use apples picked up from the ground for cider.

In October 1996 an outbreak of *E. coli* O157:H7 from apple cider occurred in Connecticut even though the apples had been washed.[41] Even with washing, *E. coli* has been found surviving in the core of apples. During the same month 66 people became ill from the same bacteria after drinking commercially prepared canned apple juice. One of these individuals died. In New York during this same period an outbreak of cryptosporidiosis resulted from drinking apple cider. This outbreak resulted from washing the apples with water from a 45 foot deep well that was contaminated from a dairy farm across the road. Such shallow wells are always at risk of contamination, especially when a concentration of cows or other animals is in close proximity. These cases have resulted in a call for the pasteurization of all apple cider and juice, a measure that would greatly complicate this large, important market. Clearly a new risk has been introduced into these popular products, however. Denying access to the orchards by cows, and discontinuing the practice of applying cow manure to orchards are simple measures that can be taken readily without any new laws or significant investment.

In July 1997 more than 100 cases of *E. Coli* O157:H7 infection that resulted from eating contaminated alfalfa sprouts were reported in Michigan and Virginia.[42] Although *Salmonella* infections have been reported from alfalfa sprouts, these are the first cases of *E. Coli* from this source. The source of the contaminated sprouts was traced to the Western United States, including seven farms along the Snake River near Boise, Idaho.[43] The precise mechanism by which the contamination occurred is not known, but it most likely involved animal wastes, especially cattle. Irrigation with contaminated water is one possible mechanism. There is no known acceptable method of decontaminating seeds used for sprouting, other than perhaps irradiation.

In addition to a severe bloody diarrhea, *E. coli* O157:H7 produces two very potent toxins, verotoxins 1 and 2, which often cause acute kidney failure requiring dialysis. The toxins also produce bleeding disorders, and deaths have occurred in most of the outbreaks. In addition to the production of these toxins, this strain of *E. coli* differs from the common strains that we have dealt with in the past in that it is very infectious, requiring only a very small dose for infection. This feature is responsible for the ease with which it is transmitted between persons in nursing facilities and day care centers. It also has a longer incubation period; infection usually ensues between 3 and 7 days after ingestion, whereas symptoms begin within 24 to 72 hours with other strains of *E. coli*. There is no effective antimicrobial or chemotherapeutic regimen for this organism. The serious sequelae of infection with this organism make it imperative to avoid it, but it is gradually spreading and becoming more prevalent.

Besides the presence of the organism in cattle and thus beef, it is also commonly spread from person to person through the fecal-oral route; in other words improper hand washing. It has been spread among family members in this fashion, as well as among patients in long term care/nursing home facilities. This was the mechanism of transmission during an outbreak among children in nine day care facilities in Minnesota in 1988 and 1989.[44] Fecal-oral transmission of disease is common in day care centers, and children with diarrhea should not be permitted to attend regardless of the suspected cause. Routine hand washing by children and staff in these facilities upon first arriving, after toilet and before eating is urgent. Where diapers are handled disposable gloves should be worn. *E. coli* O157:H7 has been overlooked in many outbreaks of diarrhea because it requires special culture techniques that laboratories have not been set up to do routinely. It also may require repeat cultures because it may be found intermittently, especially in the recovery phase. It may be shed in the stool for up to 30 days after recovery, even in the absence of symptoms.

CYCLOSPORA

Outbreaks of a prolonged diarrheal illness associated with what was initially called cyanobacterium (blue-green algae)-like bodies appeared in the literature as early as 1988. This illness was first noted among foreign travelers to Nepal, but an outbreak of diarrheal illness among the house staff of a Chicago hospital was reported in 1991[45]. This was the first reported outbreak from this new organism in the United States[46]. It had been noted as a pathogen in AIDS patients as early as 1987, but prior to 1996 only two outbreaks besides the one in the Chicago hospital had been reported in the United States. In May and June of 1996 infections with what has now been labeled *Cyclospora cayetanensis* were reported from 20 states and in Ontario, Canada. A total of 1465 cases were reported, but as with all such food borne outbreaks many cases were not reported[47,48] During the first half of 1997 an additional 510 cases were reported from events such as wedding receptions and banquets, and an additional 224 cases from a cruise ship that departed from Florida.[49,50] Whereas previous outbreaks had been associated with drinking or swimming in contaminated water, these recent cases were attributed to the consumption of berries, especially raspberries, that had been imported into the United States from Guatemala.[51,52]

Diarrhea from *Cyclospora* usually results from fecal contamination of food or water. The use of human excrement or sewage waste on crops would account for such disease transmission, but this practice is not common in the United States. The use of sewage wastewater is common in many of the areas of the world where food crops are grown, however. The contamination of the berries could also have resulted from using contaminated well water for pesticide applications. After the 1996 outbreak Guatemala took steps to improve water quality and sanitary conditions on the farms where berries are raised.

The continuation of the problem into 1997, with 1450 cases from fresh raspberries and mesclun lettuce (a mixture of varieties) reported in the first half of the year, indicated that not all of the farms were successful in these efforts. In addition during June and July 1997 at least 25 episodes of cyclosporiasis, involving 185 persons, were reported in the Virginia–Washington D.C.–Baltimore area. These cases resulted from eating imported fresh basil that was not from Guatemala, but the source of the contamination has not been determined.[53] During the spring of 1998 importation of fresh raspberries from Guatemala into the United States was not permitted. Canada imposed no such restriction, however, and during May 1998 thirteen additional outbreaks involving 192 people were reported there.[54] These were again traced to berries imported from Guatemala. These additional outbreaks demonstrated that the control measures instituted by the authorities there had not been adhered to by all of the growers.

Importation of fruit, vegetables and spices into the US is becoming more and more common, introducing a health risk that we have not faced in the past. A large outbreak of hepatitis A in

March 1997 caused by contaminated strawberries imported from Mexico (see Chapter XV) demonstrated this risk graphically. These reports reinforce the importance of thorough washing of all fruit, but that does not guarantee the elimination of the risk of any microorganism from berries. All lettuce and salad components should be thoroughly washed, two to three times, even though they may be labeled as washed. Even if it has not been contaminated in the field, it may be inoculated with E. Coli or other disease-causing organisms during handling and transport, or by customers handling it in the store. The safest source of salads in this new era is the prepackaged ones by large manufacturers such as Dole or Fresh Express. They utilize a cleansing process designed to kill bacteria, and certify on the package that it has been washed and is ready to eat. Packages that do not carry this certification carry a greater risk.

Outbreaks of Cyclosporiasis typically occur during the warmer months since the oocysts must sporulate after being shed in feces before they become infective. This takes several days to weeks in a warm environment. The watery diarrhea is accompanied by nausea, loss of appetite and abdominal cramping. In the healthy individual this may persist for 1 to 4 weeks. In immunocompromised patients (AIDS) it may persist for months. Persistent cases have also occurred in travelers to Asia, South and Central America and Mexico. As with most protozoan infections there is no specific drug to eliminate the organism.

TRAVELERS' DIARRHEA

Virtually all cases of travelers' diarrhea are caused by the consumption of food or water, including ice, contaminated by feces. Hands are frequently the transportation agents. Obviously all of these cases could be prevented. Hand washing would eliminate much of the problem, particularly in the case of those waiters who serve your soup with their thumb in the bowl. Especially risky foods are raw fruits (particularly berries) and vegetables and raw or inadequately cooked meat and seafood, especially shellfish. Hepatitis and cholera are a serious risk from the latter. Lettuce, spinach and salads in general should not be consumed when traveling outside of the United States. Hands easily contaminate these and, as stated above, wastewater (sewage) is used for irrigation of crops in many regions of the world. Additionally, human excrement is still used as fertilizer for crops in agricultural areas of China, such as around Xian and Guilin. This explains in large measure why hepatitis A is endemic throughout China.

Fruits that are cut up also can be expected to be contaminated by hands, and should not be consumed. Milk and dairy products (cheese), deserts and ice in beverages, should be avoided when traveling to areas of risk. Foods that are served steaming hot are safer than those served cold. Avoid buffet food that is served at room temperature. Food from street vendors has been responsible for many outbreaks of foodborne disease, and it should **ALWAYS** be avoided.

Sealed carbonated bottled beverages are generally considered safe. Coca-Cola and Pepsi products are widely available throughout China and Eastern Europe. Bottled purified or spring water is available in sealed containers in most areas, and this should be the sole source of water for consumption, face washing, brushing of teeth and for enemas and douches. For the latter two procedures, commercial packaged preparations carried from home are much safer. Do not use any bottled water that does not have an intact seal. Do not rinse the toothbrush under the faucet, rather carry a supply of 3 to 4 ounce plastic cups in your luggage and use bottled water.

In some areas, Hong Kong for instance, some hotels have their own purification systems. These hotels will have a placard in the bathroom guaranteeing the safety of their tap water. In regions where the water that comes out of the faucet is not safe to drink, such as in Poland and China, sealed bottled water is widely available in hotels, stores and street stands. Safe bottled spring water is sold throughout China at the many souvenir and street stands at the Great Wall, Forbidden City, Ming Tombs and in Beijing, Shanghai, Xian and Guilin in general.

As discussed above, enterotoxigenic *Escherichia coli* account for somewhere between 50 and 75 percent of the cases of travelers' diarrhea. *Shigella* organisms account for approximately fifteen percent of the cases from Mexico. Various viruses, amoeba and *Giardia* together are responsible for fewer than 10 percent of cases. Recently *Campylobacter* has been reported as an important cause of travelers' diarrhea. Most cases of simple travelers' diarrhea can be resolved in a reasonable period of time without serious conse-quences. Amebiasis, shigellosis, salmonellosis and hepatitis are far more serious illnesses, however. The prevention of these diseases assigns great urgency to strict adherence to frequent hand washing and the other hygienic measures outlined above.

Much advice has been dispensed about what drugs the traveler should take with him to deal with this vexing and common problem. It has been common practice for physicians to prescribe trimethoprim/sulfamethoxazole (Bactrim® or Septra®) or doxycycline (Vibramycin®) for their patients to take prophylactically when traveling outside of the United States. Unfortunately, antibiotics worsen some types of diarrheal diseases. This practice has also led to the bacteria developing a resistance to these drugs, so that they become useless when the treatment of infection is needed. Such is currently the case with doxycycline in some parts of the world such as in Thailand and Honduras. Resistance to trimethoprim/sulfa-methoxazole has also become common in many areas. Another problem with such prophylactic use is the development of sensitivi-ties to the drugs by the traveler. This has been a particular problem with sulfa preparations. The most common reaction is skin rash, but nausea may also develop. Doxycycline (Vibramycin®) produces a photosensitivity that makes the traveler much more susceptible to sunburn.

The consensus among medical experts is that antibiotics should not be taken prophylactically when traveling; rather they should be reserved to treat any infection that might occur. This was the recommendation of the National Institute of Health Consensus Conference on Travelers' Diarrhea in 1985, and it has gained general approval in the medical world since. Drugs to relieve the painful cramping also may worsen some infections by delaying clearing of the organism, thus permitting uninhibited reproduction and infection.

One drug that should **NOT** be taken without close supervi-sion by a competent physician is iodochlorhydroxyquin. This drug is sold without a prescription outside of the United States under the name of Clioquinol®, Vioform® and Entero-Vioform®. It is effective for amebic dysentery, but has the potential for loss of vision and other nervous system damage through the destruction of the lining of the nerves, including the optic nerve. From 1955 to

1970, 10,000 cases of this serious toxic side effect of the drug were reported in Japan, and the sale of it was banned. This is a classic case of the cure being worse than the disease.

A relatively new group of antibiotics, the fluoroquinolones, have proven to be effective against all of the organisms that commonly cause travelers' diarrhea. They are are effective against *Salmonella, Shigella, Aeromonas, Yersinia, Vibrio, Escherichia coli,* and *Campylobacter.*[55] These agents will provide a much welcome addition to a long-time plague to travelers. Some of these have been approved recently for infectious diarrhea, and should prove to be effective in many cases of travelers' diarrhea that do not respond to the conventional agents. They should be reserved for proven cases of infections where they will work, however. Otherwise they will become as useless as some of the previously effective agents have. They cannot be given to children because of their proclivity to damage developing cartilage in joints.

Pepto-Bismol in a dose of two tablespoonfuls (or two tablets) four times daily gives relief in travelers' diarrhea and does not interfere with recovery from any of the diseases. Taken prophylactically during periods of exposure it may prevent diarrhea. It should not be taken at the same time as any other medications, however, since it may interfere with their absorption. In recent studies it has been shown to be more effective than antibiotics in eliminating *Helicobacter* infections. Several studies and clinical trials of this subject are currently underway.

In any case of prolonged vomiting or diarrhea, replacement of fluids and electrolytes (sodium, chloride and potassium) is essential. This may be done by mouth if vomiting does not preclude this approach. Premixed chemicals for making these solutions are sold in drugstores, or they may be mixed much more economically by following the World Health Organization formula. This latter formula has saved thousands of lives in developing nations. After a cholera stricken passenger became severely dehydrated during a flight in July 1992 the Centers for Disease Control recommended that all airlines serving cholera infected regions stock these replacement solutions,

In any instance where vomiting or diarrhea persist for longer than twenty-four hours, or in the event of a high fever or bloody stool, medical attention should be sought. This is a difficult problem when outside of the United States. Directories of physicians outside of the United States are available from travel agencies and health authorities. The traveler also can seek assistance at the US consulate, during working hours. This cannot be relied upon over weekends. Local health departments have personnel who have current information on travel conditions throughout the world. It is advisable to consult with these authorities, either directly or through your physician, regarding conditions at your travel destination. They can advise you as to what immunizations and other prophylactic measures are recommended. Make these contacts at least three months prior to departure in order to allow adequate time to complete all necessary prophylactic measures.

The enormous growth of the restaurant and fast food industry in the United States over the past two decades is abundantly in evidence as you drive through the streets of your hometown. This growth stems in large measure from the affluence that has been achieved by the middle-class and workingclass of our society. Many families who never ate in a restaurant a generation ago now eat out on a regular basis. A considerable proportion of this increased expenditure at food establishments is contributed by teenagers, who also enjoy a level of wealth unimaginable a generation ago.

That we do not suffer the level of food related diseases experienced by some other societies is a testimonial to the public health laws and endeavors of the state and local governments. These have evolved over the past fifty years to the present commendable levels. In spite of this, many thousands of food-borne illnesses are reported each year. A study of the many outbreaks clearly illustrates the need for greater efforts in public education regarding these risks, and how to avoid them. The low level of knowledge among United States citizens of communicable diseases and how to prevent them by simple hygiene measures is a national embarrassment. Such education should be instilled at home, but certainly this subject deserves attention in the public schools equal to that assigned to "sensitivity training," sex education, the application of condoms, and the hazards of AIDS.

Even the most intense public educational effort will fail, however, if a strong sense of responsibility is not instilled at home. No level of effort by the school system or the government can compensate for the shortcomings of parenthood that neglects its obligations. As a representative from the Centers for Disease Control recently remarked, "How do you arrest people for not washing their hands?" It should not be necessary to even pose the question.

SUSHI and CEVICHE

Sushi is a Japanese dish that has become very popular in the United States recently. It consists of thin strips of raw fish wrapped around cold, cooked rice. The principle risk in the case of fish that is fresh and not contaminated with disease-causing microorganisms is parasites such as *Anisakis* and similar larval nematodes. Fresh, uncontaminated fish is the exception in the United States, however.

Ceviche is a dish that is popular in South America, and it has played a signal role in the spread of the epidemic of Cholera that began in Peru in January 1991. It is made from raw fish or shellfish marinated in spicy sauces and lime juice, and served cold. It has received little attention prior to the current epidemic, so the number of other foodborne infections caused by it is not tabulated.

Unlike the seafood illnesses produced by heat stable toxins, all of the parasitic infestations from fish can be prevented readily by adequate cooking. This is not the customary practice, however.

ANISAKIASIS

ANISAKIASIS is a parasitic infestation caused by the ingestion of a small white worm, *Anisakis marina*, one millimeter in diameter and 1.5 to 2.5 centimeters in length. It is found in haddock, mackerel, cod, pike, herring, anchovy, sardine, bonito, salmon, squid, tuna, Alaskan pollack and Pacific red snapper. It occurs only in fish that share waters with dolphins, whales, seals, porpoises and other large sea mammals. It is common in Japan and some parts of Europe, but it has been reported with increasing frequency in the United States with the rising popularity of Sushi.

A. marina lives in the intestine of the fish, and theoretically if the fish is iced down immediately after harvest, the worm stays there. If the fish is not cooled adequately and kept cold the worm migrates into the muscle of the fish. After ingestion by humans the worms burrow into the lining of the stomach and small intestine where they produce tumor-like granulomas. They may penetrate the intestinal wall and invade other organs. The typical case produces fever, vomiting and abdominal pain and tenderness. Peritonitis and intestinal obstruction can occur, and anaphylaxis has been reported[56]. Diagnosis is difficult unless the worm is seen in vomitus, since no test exists to detect it. The admonition to examine the sushi visually to manually remove the worms, then chew well to destroy the remaining parasites is appropriate if one is adventuresome. Otherwise, cooking is advisable. Consumption of uncooked seafood carries a significant risk of contracting this and a number of other diseases. No treatment is available to eradicate the worm, as is true of many parasites.

DIPHYLLOBOTHRIUM LATUM

The fish tapeworm is acquired by eating inadequately cooked freshwater fish. Salmon also has been incriminated in the Northwest. The organism is present in fish in the United States in Florida, the Great Lakes region and along the Pacific Coast. The increased contamination of bodies of water by sewage has increased the incidence of the disease. The recent popularity of sushi has also resulted in an increase in the number of cases reported. Symptoms are mild in most cases, consisting of mild abdominal discomfort. The infestation can be treated with praziquantel although some unpleasant side effects may be experienced.

TRICHINOSIS

Earlier in this Chapter we discussed the importance of cooking meat adequately, reaching a high enough temperature in the center of the meat for a sufficient length of time to kill the microorganisms that are always present. This is certainly no less urgent in the case of parasites, some of which can cause irreparable damage to health and even death. *Trichinella spiralis* produces such a disease. This parasitic disease is acquired by eating inadequately cooked meat, virtually always pork, that contains encysted larvae of the roundworm, *Trichinella spiralis*. A few cases have been reported in recent years from walrus meat, bear meat and wild boar.

The pig or bear usually becomes infected from eating raw garbage, although eating infected rats is also a source. The rats feed on raw pork scraps thus helping to maintain the cycle of infection (see also Chapter VII). The risk of this parasite has been greatly reduced by laws that require commercial farmers to cook all garbage and scraps fed to pigs. An increase in the incidence of the disease in the northeastern states recently has resulted from noncommercial farmers feeding raw garbage to pigs.

Prevention of trichinosis is accomplished very simply by adequate cooking of meat. Particular care must be exercised when cooking pork in a microwave oven, for the core of the meat may remain cool even though the surface is quite hot. An adequate internal temperature (170° F.), as measured with an accurate thermometer, must be reached to assure inactivation of the larva. There is no means of eradicating the larva from the human body. All garbage fed to pigs must be cooked. This simple measure has markedly reduced the incidence of this disease in the United States.

TAPEWORM

Taenia saginata is a tapeworm acquired from eating inadequately cooked beef. Public health and sanitation measures have helped to reduce the incidence of this parasite in cattle. The risk of acquiring *Taenia saginata* has thus diminished accordingly. Adequate cooking of all meat will prevent acquisition of *Taenia* from beef where it does exist.

Taenia solium is a parasite that is acquired from eating inadequately cooked pork. It is a more sinister disease than the beef tapeworm in that the eggs passed in the stool of humans with this tapeworm are infective to the host of the worm and to other humans. When those eggs are swallowed, either by direct contact or contaminated food and vegetables, the eggs hatch. They then migrate through the wall of the intestine and are carried by the lymphatics and blood stream to other organs of the body, notably the eye, heart and brain. This involvement carries serious consequences such as seizures and death. The eggs have been found on the skin and clothing and in the dirt under the fingernails of people who have the tapeworm.

The pork tapeworm, and the very serious neurocysticercosis, has been very uncommon in the United States because of the extensive sewage and water systems in place. The laws requiring that foods fed to commercially raised hogs are cooked has been a major contribution to this accomplishment. Recently an increasing number of cases of neurocysticercosis have been reported in household or other contacts of immigrants from Mexico, Latin America, Asia and Africa, regions where cysticercosis is widely endemic. It also has become more frequent in cities that are in proximity to Mexico, notably Los Angeles, San Diego, San Antonio and Tuscon, Arizona. There is no medication to eliminate the parasite from the human brain or other organs.[57]

In one recent case a man acquired neurocysticercosis from farm workers who had immigrated from countries where it is endemic. In another case a 16-month old girl was diagnosed with the disease after she suffered seizures. She acquired the disease from her father who had immigrated from the Cape Verde Islands where the disease is also endemic. He was demonstrated to be carrying the eggs. Another girl in South Carolina was also diagnosed with the disease after she suffered seizures. She acquired the eggs from neighbors who had immigrated from Mexico. Between 1988 and 1990, ten cases of locally acquired neurocysticercosis were reported in Los Angeles. Reporting of this disease is not required, so the actual incidence is unknown. It is obviously increasing.

Trichinosis, Taenia saginata and *Taenia solium* are discussed in more detail in Chapter VII, along with other zoonoses.

WATER

In 1900 typhoid epidemics were a common place annual occurrence in virtually every city in the United States. Cholera epidemics imported from Asia repeatedly struck both the United States and England. These two water borne diseases accounted for many deaths and much suffering. These epidemics resulted from the contamination of food and drinking water by the excrement of infected individuals. The incidence and severity of such epidemics became more intense as the population density increased following industrialization of the United States. A few perceptive individuals of the time deduced that contaminated hands from handling the sick or their bed clothing transmitted the disease to otherwise healthy individuals.

This was graphically demonstrated by John Snow in the now classic case of the Broad Street pump in London. John Snow, from New York, had graduated from the London Medical School in 1844. He theorized that cholera was waterborne, and transmitted thereby.

During a major epidemic of cholera in London in 1854 he advised the authorities that the spread of the disease would cease if they would remove the handle of the pump. They heeded his advice and the cholera epidemic promptly subsided.[58] During this same year the chlorine treatment of sewage in London was authorized. Chlorine remains the most effective agent that we have to kill bacteria in water to this day. Its universal use in public water supplies is the principal reason that we have had safe drinking water supplies throughout the United States for almost one hundred years. It has saved countless thousands of lives, and prevented millions of people from suffering illnesses that are common in other areas of the world.

By 1870 several states in the United States had established boards of health to deal with sanitation and the control of filth. These efforts resulted in a pronounced decrease in the incidence of typhoid, cholera and dysentery by the early 1900's. Today every major city, county and state have well organized and effective health departments. The result is a level of sanitation and safety of food and drinking water that is unmatched in the world. The public water supply in virtually every city in the United States is remarkably safe and free of disease-causing organisms. A visit to many large cities in Europe, Russia and Asia where no one dares drink the water that comes from the tap instills a deep appreciation for this fact. This has been accomplished by the construction of sophisticated treatment plants, at great cost to the taxpayers. These are maintained by professionals (again paid by the taxpayers) who are educated and kept current in the science of these systems. We have taken all of this for granted at the very time that a few people are working to extend some of these practices to the many regions of the world where thousands of people die annually because of their absence.

The safety and integrity of these systems is being threatened currently by environmental extremists such as Greenpeace who are waging a campaign to force the discontinuation of chlorination of these water supplies. Their claim is that the chlorinated drinking water that we have been consuming for the past century causes cancer. It does not. As Dr. Bruce Ames at the University of California at Berkeley points out, if there is any cancer risk at all from chlorinated water it is one-thirtieth that of one serving of peanut butter. The great risk to us is from the peanut brains who have successfully promoted this garbage propaganda. Abandonment of our chlorinated water systems would be insanity, tantamount to returning to the dark ages. No other system, neither ozone nor ultraviolet light, can be substituted.

In 1994 the Environmental Protection Agency issued a proposal to decrease the use of chlorine to treat public water supplies. It had speculated that up to 700 cases of cancer occur each year in the United States as a result of chlorine treatment of water. It had been successful in convincing the Peruvian government to take this action,[59] and the result was the current cholera pandemic that has killed ten thousand people in South and Central America and Mexico, and caused cholera in more than a million more. The EPA is determined to inflict a similar catastrophe upon the United States. This is another example of ignorant and irrational individuals with the power of the federal bureaucracy and its purse inflicting great pain and suffering upon us, and demanding that we pay for it. It is a repeat of the Freon fiasco, except that it will result in millions of cases of illness and thousands of deaths in a short time frame. The EPA is one of the most serious threats that the American people face, not only to our health but also to our freedom and economy as well.

The safety of these public water supplies is also coming under threat by irresponsible and dishonest politicians and bureaucrats at the local level. In early July 1996 the Washington, D.C. officials warned residents that bacterial levels of the public water supply were so high that elderly and those with weakened immune systems faced health hazards unless they boiled their water prior to consumption. This disgraceful situation resulted from gross mismanagement and corruption by the city government. It was unprecedented in modern American public health history, but may surface in other cities where similar mismanagement might exist.

When earthquakes, floods or power outages strike, the water delivered from the tap must be considered unsafe until certified by responsible authorities. Under these circumstances boiling is advised for all water used for human consumption, including brushing of teeth, douches and enemas. Some authorities recommend boiling for as brief a period as 3 minutes. This harks back to the early 1900s when typhoid was the chief pathogen transmitted in drinking water. To inactivate the newly emerged contaminants in water today such as *Giardia, Cryptosporidium, Cyclospora* and *Amoeba* requires closer to 20 minutes. It should be kept in mind that the spores of *Clostridium botulinum* can withstand boiling for one hour, and can survive a dry heat temperature of 212° F. for a period of 3 to 5 hours. Water for consumption does not have to be sterile, but it must be remembered that with some of these organisms such as *Cyclospora* and *Cryptosporidium* it takes only a small number of surviving organism to cause disease.

We cannot continue to be complacent, however, for once again population density and industrial development are threatening our environment and food and water supply. With the growing move to rural areas more and more people are relying upon wells and septic systems. Approximately one-half of the households in North America are served by these systems. The installation of these facilities is supervised and controlled by the local health departments. With increasing frequency the underground aquifers from which wells draw their water are discovered to be contaminated by chemical and industrial waste, however. Seepage from landfills has accounted for some of this contamination. Some of it has resulted from improper storage and disposal of substances by industry. In some areas the aquifers are even contaminated by local septic systems. The full extent of contamination from landfills and industrial sources is yet to be established.

Such seepage more readily contaminates the aquifers in some geologic strata than in others. Sand and limestone in some areas permit seepage of wastes from dumps and septic systems into the underground water supplies. Some wells in these areas are grossly contaminated and unsafe. Many older homes have septic systems on small lots, and wells that are forty to sixty feet deep on the same lot. Wells in such circumstances are very likely to be unsafe. The finding of nitrates in the well water, a simple test, will usually confirm contamination either by the septic system, or by seepage from animal feed lots or hog farms.

Dumping of industrial wastes into streams and other bodies of water is another source of contamination of our water, and this practice threatens even municipal water supplies. The standard treatment techniques of filtration, aeration and chlorination do not remove toxic chemicals. They also are not always effective against some viruses and the cysts of *Giardia* and *Amoeba*. The great increase in the recreational use of bodies of water from which municipalities draw their water, coupled with the increased incidence of diseases caused by organisms such as *Giardia* and *Cryptosporidia*, add to the urgency of this problem.

GIARDIA LAMBLIA

Giardia is a protozoan that establishes itself in the small intestine of humans and other animals where it persists and reproduces. In excess of 26,000 cases of acute diarrheal disease caused by this organism are reported in the United States each year. This represents only a fraction of the people actually infected with *Giardia*. Formerly it occurred mainly in the developing countries, where wells are consistently and chronically contaminated. It is now the most common cause of outbreaks of water-borne diarrheal disease in the United States. Previously it occurred most commonly in the Rocky Mountain States and more frequently in visitors there. Drinking from mountain streams that are assumed to be pristine, but in reality are contaminated by excrement from beavers and perhaps other animals, accounts for many of these cases. Outbreaks are still common in mountain communities that derive their water supply from streams and rivers and fail to provide adequate filtration.

The concentrations of chlorine customarily used in municipal treatment plants do not kill the cysts of *Giardia*. Proper filtration is essential. Since the organism is a protozoan, its relatively large size makes it feasible to remove it by filtration. Pockets of communities have emerged elsewhere in the United States where wells have become contaminated with this organism, most likely by animals. More recently, concurrent with the increased incidence of this disease in humans in the United States, contamination of bodies of water with *Giardia* by human excrement has become common. During 1999 a study of formed stool specimens that had been deposited in recreational waters such as swimming pools yielded *Giardia* in 4.4 percent. During 1989-1998 approximately 10,000 cases of diarrheal illness resulted from exposure to these recreational waters that had been adequately treated.[60]

Among 26 outbreaks of waterborne disease from drinking water reported by 16 states during 1989 and 1990, *Giardia* was the causative agent for seven. No organism was identified in 14 of the episodes. All of the outbreaks of giardiasis resulted from consumption of unfiltered surface water or surface contaminated groundwater. Four of the seven outbreaks of *Giardia* resulted from drinking water from community water systems. *Giardia* has become the most frequently recovered parasite in human stool specimens, occurring in over 7 percent of those examined.[61] This incidence has almost doubled during the past decade, perhaps due to immigration from South America and Southeast Asia during that period.

Giardia forms cysts in the small intestine of man and other animals. The cysts are then passed in the stool, thereby infecting others when food or water is contaminated. These cysts may survive in water for months and are not destroyed by the customary means of chlorination. Boiling the water for a sufficient time effectively destroys the cysts. It must be remembered, however, that at higher elevations this will require a much longer time than at the lower levels, as is true of cooking. Since they are fairly large (on the order of ten microns) filters sold for backpacking remove them. Cases of *Giardia* induced diarrhea have resulted in individuals who used these filters, however, possibly due to faulty handling of the filter or contamination of the filtered water.

Giardia can also be acquired by eating food that has been contaminated by a carrier who has neglected hand washing. Individuals who have previously had a gastrectomy, or who are on acid inhibiting medication for an ulcer are at a particularly high risk of contracting the disease upon exposure to the *Giardia* cysts. The normal acid level in the stomach provides some protection against this and some other diseases. This organism is shed in the feces of pets, which may be an additional source of infection in the home and among children playing on the ground or in sandboxes (see Hazards of Pets, Chapter VII).

Outbreaks of giardiasis have also occurred in day care centers and nurseries. Careful hand washing after handling diapers and the use of disposable gloves is effective in preventing transmission in these circumstances. These practices also help guard against the acquisition and transmission of hepatitis, which is also a significant risk in day care centers.

The water supply in St. Petersburg, Russia is heavily contaminated with *Giardia*, and over fifty percent of visitors to that city have suffered the disease. The tap water in that city is not only infested with Giardia, but also is contaminated with heavy metals that give a greenish tint to the bath water. These conditions persist to the present.[62] The incubation period for Giardia is ten to twenty days, so the onset of symptoms frequently occurs after one returns home, fortunately. This onset is marked by a profound watery diarrhea, with as many as forty to fifty stools per day. Bloating, abdominal pain and cramping that may be severe accompany the diarrhea. These symptoms may persist for weeks or even months if untreated. Effective treatment is available.

Diagnosis of *Giardia* is difficult. Cysts are found in the stool in less than one-half of the victims. Repeated laboratory examination at intervals of five to seven days for several weeks may be required to demonstrate the organism. After the acute phase, however, the cysts are seen infrequently. Duodenal aspiration or biopsy will usually help to establish the diagnosis. This is an unpleasant procedure, however, and is not as readily accomplished as a stool examination. A nylon string that can be swallowed, then retrieved, is now marketed as a diagnostic tool for recovering *Giardia* from the duodenum.

CAMPYLOBACTER JEJUNI

Prior to 1972 this organism was not associated with intestinal infections, but by 1979 it had become second only to *Giardia* as a cause of water-borne diarrheal disease in the United States. It is found in milk that is contaminated by cattle that are carriers of the organism and in contaminated water. This is yet another disease acquired by drinking raw milk. Since 1983 several instances of *Campylobacter* illness among school children visiting dairies and consuming raw milk products have been reported in California, Michigan, Minnesota, Pennsylvania, Vermont, and British Columbia. About 60 percent of people drinking contaminated raw milk or dairy products will succumb to diarrhea. *Campylobacter jejuni*, as well as other *Campylobacter* species, is present in the intestine of domestic and wild animals and poultry. Excrement from these sources contaminates streams and water supplies also.

Like *Giardia*, many cases of *Campylobacter* diarrhea have resulted from drinking water from mountain streams. Contamination of food by excrement from pets in the home is a frequent source of *Campylobacter* infection. Puppies and kittens are a common source, particularly when they are sick. Infections have been seen frequently in slaughterhouse workers who are in contact with the intestines of animals. The diarrhea, which begins an unusually long 2 to 6 days after exposure, may be pronounced. It is accompanied by a fever, and bloody stools may be present, especially in children. Also like *Giardia, Campylobacter* is seldom cultured from the stool during an infection because a special media and atmosphere are required to grow this organism. No blood test is available to identify it, so unless the local labs are equipped to do this culture, the diagnosis depends primarily upon the symptoms.

HELICOBACTER PYLORI

Several additional species of *Campylobacter* have been identified in humans, causing a variety of infections, including systemic infections. All that have been identified seem to come from animals, but exact sources and the course of the disease have not been mapped out as yet. One of these has attracted much interest for its role in the production of gastritis and duodenal ulcer. Previously termed *Campylobacter pylori,* it was renamed *Helicobacter pylori* in October, 1989, based upon the observation that the flagella was sheathed, uncharacteristic of *Campylobacter* species. The organism reproduces in the human small intestine.

Up until 1983 gastritis and ulcers of the stomach and duodenum were considered to be the result of excess acid produced by stress or aspirin intake and foods that increased acid production, such as coffee. In that year, however, the presence of *H. Pylori* was discovered to be associated with gastritis and peptic ulcers.[63] Since that initial report numerous studies have confirmed that at least 90 percent of the cases of peptic ulcer are caused by infection with this organism. Initially diagnosis required the passage of a scope into the stomach but several tests have been developed, most recently a breath test, that have rendered this invasive and onerous procedure unnecessary.

Initially studies indicated that bismuth preparations were more effective than antibiotics in eradicating *Helicobacter pylori* in ulcer patients. Ulcer healing and relief of symptoms in gastritis were noted when the organism was eradicated, but recolonization and return of symptoms followed discontinuance of the treatment. More recent studies have demonstrated that a combination of bismuth, metronidazole and tetracycline can eradicate the organism in more than 90 percent of patients, and prevent recurrence of ulcers. This regimen must be adhered to rigidly for 14 days, however. Reinfection continues to be a problem because the organism is readily reintroduced from the oral secretions of an infected person, either by direct contact or by contaminated food and utensils. This is another argument for not sharing these items. *Helicobacter pylori* is the most common human infection worldwide.

TYPHOID

Only about 400 cases of typhoid fever are reported each year in the United States currently, thanks to the public health measures described previously. About one-half of these cases are acquired outside of the U. S. It continues to kill many people worldwide, however. This occurs chiefly in underdeveloped countries and in nations where water and sanitary systems are of inferior quality or non existent. The only source of *Salmonella typhi*, the causative organism, is human beings. It is theoretically possible, therefore, to eliminate it. We have accomplished this with smallpox, but never with the infectious diseases that require simple modification of the health and hygiene habits of people. The same observations apply to the sexually transmitted diseases.

The typhoid organism is dispensed in large numbers in the feces of infected people. Infection of others occurs only by fecal contamination of water supplies or of food, either by flies or by contaminated hands. The latter could be prevented if hands were washed appropriately with soap and warm water, and if latex or vinyl disposable gloves were worn at all times when preparing and handling food for public consumption. Both of these should be standard practice for all food handlers.

Typhoid fever, which has killed thousands of troops during wars, and tens of thousands of civilians throughout history, is a systemic infection spreading through the blood stream to every organ in the body. It has a particular predilection for the gallbladder and multiplies there in great numbers. It may remain there permanently in the carrier state. Antibiotic therapy cures most cases, but the response is not as rapid and dramatic as with most bacterial infections. Every effort should be made to eradicate the organism, especially in chronic carriers because of the risk of transmission to others. Immunization is available for travelers to areas where a risk exists, but its protection is not absolute. Even with immunization typhoid can still be contracted if a heavy exposure occurs.

CRYPTOSPORIDIOSIS

Cryptosporidiosis, which has long been associated with diseases in animals, was first recognized in humans in 1976. In 1981 severe enteritis in 47 AIDS patients was identified as being caused by *Cryptosporidium*. Since then it has been seen with increasing frequency as a cause of severe, resistant diarrhea in AIDS patients, and has now been transmitted to the general population. *Cryptosporidium* is a protozoan that infects the intestinal tract in most animals, and now many humans. It sheds small cysts in the stool, which may remain infective for up to six months. Because of their small size these cysts are successfully removed from water supplies only by special filtration techniques and careful maintenance thereof. No chemical is effective against the cysts, but boiling the water does inactivate them. No effective treatment is available, but the disease is normally self-limiting in healthy individuals. Water supplies may be contaminated by human waste or by cattle or other animals. Calves with diarrheal disease particularly require careful handling to avoid acquiring this infection from them.

Cryptosporidium has also caused gastroenteritis in individuals with intact immune systems more recently, sometimes in epidemic form. In 1987 approximately 13,000 residents of a Georgia community experienced a cryptosporidiosis gastroenteritis as a result of contamination of their community water supply. This occurred in spite of the fact that the water was processed in a treatment plant that met all of the standards. The cysts from the organism most likely passed through filters during servicing of the equipment. The source of the contamination of the water supply was never found.

In another outbreak in the summer of 1988, at least 44 persons suffered acute gastroenteritis caused by *Cryptosporidium* that contaminated a school swimming pool when one person accidentally defecated in the pool. Chlorination met required levels, but this does not inactivate *cryptosporidium*. A more extensive outbreak occurred in Delaware County, Ohio in July 2000 when 700 clinical cases of cryptosporidiosis that resulted from a contaminated swimming pool were identified.[64] The spores of this organism are even more resistant to chlorine than Giardia. A concentration 640 times greater than that required for Giardia is needed to inactivate *cryptosporidium*. This process of hyper-chlorination must be maintained for 18 hours, and the pool must be closed during this time.

Swimming pools are easily recontaminated from individuals passing *cryptosporidium* cysts after this onerous and expensive - process has been completed. It is impossible to maintain a high enough chlorine concentration to protect against contamination. *Cryptosporidium* unfortunately possesses a high infectivity potential; infection requires only a small dose, as contrasted to some other infections, notably *Salmonella*.

The only practical alternative for controlling *cryptosporidium* is by fine filtration using diatomaceous earth (**AVOID INHALING THE DUST**) rather than the sand filtration that is customarily used in swimming pools. The cysts of this organism are small, in the order of 4-6 microns. This deficiency in filtration was responsible for the diarrhea transmitted in the school pool mentioned above. There is no protection possible for swimming in bodies of water such as lakes, streams and ponds.

In 1993 an outbreak of cryptosporidiosis in Milwaukee, Wisconsin caused acute enteritis in over 400,00 persons, 4,400 of whom were hospitalized. This episode resulted from contamination of the public water supply, initially thought to be from animal waste. Further tests revealed the cause to be a new strain, and humans to be the source. Investigation disclosed that the intake for the water treatment facility was two miles downstream from the sewage disposal pipe in Lake Michigan. The discharge of sewage into Lake Michigan was discontinued and the intake pipe for the water treatment facility was extended further out into the lake. The city spent 80 million dollars on construction of an ozone treatment plant, which they believe will inactivate *cryptosporidium*.

NITRATES

Nitrates, which are found naturally in well water in some areas, are a hazard chiefly to infants under three months of age. The nitrates, when transformed to nitrites in the stomach by bacterial activity, convert hemoglobin to methemoglobin (oxidation of ferrous hemoglobin to ferric hemoglobin), which has a much reduced capacity to carry oxygen. The result is oxygen starvation of the tissues in the body. Thousands of cases of methemoglobinemia have been reported, and about eight percent of the infants afflicted with this "blue baby" syndrome die. It has been claimed that agricultural run off of fertilizers can deposit these substances into drinking water supplies in some areas. A far greater source of such contamination, however, is the inadequate treatment of sewage by municipalities. The nitrates that are present in well water in some localities are the result of natural deposits in the underground aquifers.

More serious is when nitrates in well water result from fecal contamination of the water supply from septic tanks. The presence of nitrates in these circumstances results from contamination with fecal bacteria, an indication of the potential presence of disease-causing organisms. This problem is widespread throughout the United States. In many cases septic tanks are placed in close proximity to shallow wells, frequently wells that are only 40 to 60 feet in depth. Contamination is much less likely to occur where wells are 200 to 400 feet in depth, unless abandoned wells permit surface water to contaminate the deep aquifers. In some regions, however, such as southwestern Virginia and much of Florida, underlying porous limestone rock formations permit septic tank effluent to percolate rapidly through to the underground aquifers. There is no means to remedy this contamination of the water supplies.

Another source of nitrates in well water is contamination from animal wastes. Wells as far as 2 miles from a hog confinement facility in Indiana were found to have excessive nitrate levels that were associated with spontaneous abortions in women.[65] In those regions with sandy or porous geologic strata this effluent can reach the underground aquifers, contaminating even deep wells with nitrates and dangerous microorganisms. This is a newly identified source of nitrate levels in drinking water and urgently needs further study. Such studies are particularly needed in regions such as North Carolina where effluent from commercial hog farms has seriously polluted the Neuse and Pamlico Rivers. The increased levels of nitrates in these rivers and the coastal waters have resulted in a pronounced increase in the growth of algae. One of these, a dinoflagellate called *Pfiesteria piscicida*, has caused serious brain damage in humans. This problem has more recently been discovered in Virginia and Maryland as well.

Your local health department can inform you as to whether or not nitrates are a problem in your area. They can also assist in determining the source of the nitrates if they are present. If the source proves to be contamination from a septic tank, this is a serious matter that should be corrected. Under these circumstances the well water should not be used except for cooking where the bacteria will be destroyed. The use of bottled water in preparing formula is mandatory in those regions where nitrates are present in drinking water in significant amounts, regardless of the source. Some areas where nitrates are known to be present naturally in well water include southern California, Illinois and other scattered areas throughout the US. The integrity of the source of bottled water should be determined, for purchasing water in a sealed container is no guarantee of its purity. No public agency currently enforces purity and safety standards for bottled water. History teaches us that this product is therefore not always of the highest purity. If any doubt exists, even bottled water should be boiled before using it to mix formula for infants.

DBCP

Dibromochloropropane has similarly contaminated wells in southern California's Kern County. This chemical was used extensively to control rootworms in commercial agriculture until it was discovered in 1978 that it caused sterility among male workers in the fields. This sterility is caused by a direct toxic effect on the germ cells and is accompanied by a reduction in the number of Sertoli cells in the testicle. This reduction is sometimes profound and the sterility has been permanent in some workers, both in agriculture and in the manufacture of this chemical.

More recently it has been observed that there is a tenfold increase in the incidence of childhood cancer and leukemia in areas where this chemical is found. These toxic and carcinogenic risks were noted by researchers, who warned of its dangers long before it was widely used in agriculture. Brominated compounds in general should always be viewed with suspicion. Ethylene dibromide, which is also used as a fumigant, and TRIS, which was widely used as a flame retardant on children's pajamas, both share these toxic and carcinogenic risks with DBCP. Since testing began in 1979, forty percent of the wells in the San Joaquin Valley of California have been found to be contaminated with DBCP as a result of its previous application in agriculture.

TRIHALOMETHANES (THM)

Trihalomethanes is a group of chemicals that includes chloroform and trichloroethylene, and these compounds have also been found to be contaminating public drinking water supplies. These substances are formed in municipal water supplies by chemical action between the chlorine used to treat the water, and organic matter occurring naturally in the water as a result of the decay of plant and animal material. While experimental studies suggest that trihalomethanes cause cancer in laboratory animals, there is no evidence that this is the case in humans.[66] The move by the EPA to ban the chlorination of drinking water is based upon the fallacious extrapolation of data from mouse to man that has been discredited long ago. Thalidomide demonstrated no teratogenic effect in several species of animals prior to its marketing. On the other hand many substances that are toxic in animals present no risk to humans, because, unlike the animals, we are protected by many enzyme defenses that inactivate most of the toxic substances that we ingest. The overwhelming majority of these are from natural sources, not man made.[67]

MERCURY

The greatest source of mercury in our environment is the natural release from the earth's crust, including rivers, lakes and the ocean as well as land areas. Because of this it is impossible to accurately determine what portion of mercury measured in the environment is the result of man-made releases, and what is from natural sources. Large quantities of mercury are extracted from the mined ore cinnabar. Its industrial and commercial uses are many, although most of these have been curtailed significantly. The once common use of mercury compounds to inhibit bacterial and mold growth in paint and on seeds, as a topical antiseptic and to treat diapers has been discontinued. One of the largest sources of industrial release of mercury has been chloralkali plants, and this has been reduced 99 percent in recent years. The use of mercury in the paper pulp industry also has been reduced dramatically. The fact that mercury readily vaporizes and created illness in miners and others was recognized and described in the fifteenth century (see Chapter X). Inhaled mercury vapors are readily absorbed in the lungs. Mercury that is left open or spilled onto carpeting in dental offices thus creates a hazard that was not well appreciated in our generation until relatively recently.

Both metallic mercury and its various compounds have been the cause of many tragedies when discarded into rivers, streams and lakes. It has been common practice to dump inorganic mercury waste products into these bodies of water because it was felt that these compounds were stable and nontoxic. The inorganic forms of mercury are absorbed from the intestinal tract in humans only in very small amounts, and thus pose little threat in themselves. The inorganic compounds that are dumped into bodies of water are bioaccumulated by plankton and algae present in the silt of rivers, streams and lakes, as well as by fish.

Previously it was believed that all organic mercurial compounds were man-made. Studies have demonstrated as long ago as the mid 1960's that microorganisms in contaminated bodies of water convert the inorganic mercury compounds to methyl and di-methyl mercury, which are organic mercury compounds. These deadly mercurial compounds are concentrated in the plankton and shellfish and other smaller sea life, which are in turn consumed by the fish. The organic mercury compounds become further concen-trated in each form of sea life as they pass up the food chain, with man as the ultimate victim. These findings pose serious questions that will require further careful assessment. They have added to the concern about the risks of consuming fish taken from bodies of water that contain other chemicals that accumulate in the fish, such as PCBs.

One of these organic compounds, methyl mercury, is particu-larly toxic, as was tragically demonstrated at Minamata Bay in Japan in 1953. In that year 202 men, women and children who lived in villages surrounding the bay became severely ill. Fifty-two people died. The mercury had poisoned some infants before their birth. The people developed severe nervous system disorders that included inability to walk, deafness and visual defects. Similar uncoordinated walking was noted in cats in the towns. The epidemic of poisoning was recognized as being due to mercury after autopsy of those who died revealed the destruction of brain cells that was typical of mercury poisoning. The destruction of cells in the cerebellum of the brain explained the uncoordinated walking of the victims.

The source of the mercury was traced to the fish in the bay. Fish was a staple of the diet of the people in these villages, and was consumed as often as 3 times daily. A facility of the Chisso Corporation that is situated on the bay was manufacturing acetaldehyde and vinyl chloride. Mercury was used as a catalyst in the production of acetaldehyde and a waste sludge containing the mercury was discharged into the streams that emptied into Minamata bay for a long time. The aquatic plant life converted the elemental mercury to organic mercury, including methyl mercury. The fish and the shellfish in the bay acquired the mercury from both the plant life and from the water. In 1974 the Japanese government placed a net 1.2 miles in length across the Bay to prevent the contaminated fish from escaping to the open sea. In July 1997 the Bay was officially declared free of mercury and the net was removed.

Another episode of mercury poisoning from a similar plant occurred later in 1964 at Niigata on Honshu Island. Between 1964 and 1974 a total of 520 residents of the Niigata region were identified as having mercury poisoning. Following this incident the government identified the source of the poisoning, after intensive investigation, and moved to prevent further environmental contamination from mercury.

Several episodes of poisoning of people by these organic mercury compounds have resulted from eating seed grain treated with the chemical, and from eating birds that had eaten seed grain. The largest recorded epidemic occurred in Iraq in the winter of 1971–72, resulting in the admission of 6,530 victims to hospitals, and 459 deaths. Eating bread containing wheat that had been imported as seed grain, coated with methyl mercury as a fungicide, was responsible for this disaster. This was not the first such poisoning in Iraq, where similar poisonings had occurred in 1956 and 1960. Other incidents of mercury poisoning involving fewer people occurred in Guatemala, Pakistan and Guiana during this same period.

The mercury compounds used in agriculture, which include phenylmercuric salts used as fungicides and herbicides, are also washed into lakes and streams, where they are taken up by the resident fish. Recommendations for restricting the consumption of fish taken from these bodies of water, which include the Great Lakes, have been published. Lake St. Clair and Western Lake Erie were heavily polluted with mercury from chlor-alkali plants treating wood pulp in the past. This source of pollution has been discontinued and the water quality had improved greatly.

In 1970 a family in New Mexico suffered a severe tragedy at the hands of mercury treated seed grain. The seed grain was fed to hogs, in spite of the fact that it was colored with a pink dye, and a clear poison warning label was on the package. When the family ate the meat from one of the hogs, four children suffered severe nerve damage. One child was born blind and retarded. Another became blind, was unable to speak, and suffered the typical uncoordinated walking. Subsequently the US Department of Agriculture banned the use of methyl mercury as a seed preservative.

In retrospect none of these tragedies need to have happened. Virtually everyone in our society, except for the scientists in their respective fields, is blissfully ignorant of the dangers inherent in mercury and other very toxic substances. This represents an educational failure, a serious deficiency. An increased emphasis on these dangers, and on the sciences in general, in our educational system would help. These topics certainly deserve equal time in our schools to that devoted to teaching the art of condom application. The media could play a significant role also if it were more responsible, and less obsessed with proselytizing socialism.

In order to keep these facts in their proper perspective we must keep in mind that the major source of mercury in our environment is the natural degassing of the earth's crust, including land masses, lakes, rivers and oceans. The volume contributed from this source has been estimated to exceed 100,000 tons per year. Clearing of forests increases the amount of this degassing. With the exception of the clearing of land, we cannot influence nature to deliver up less mercury. All of the efforts of government and the environmental extremists will have no influence on this.

PCB (polychlorinated biphenyls)

PCBs have also been found in hazardous quantities in fish in the Great Lakes. They have been found in particularly high concentrations in fish that have been taken from the Hudson River and Lake Ontario, as well as several other rivers and streams throughout the United States. These substances serve as fire retardants and are widely used in industry in electrical transformers and capacitors. They also are used in the manufacture of paper and waxes, in many plastic products such as telephones, and a multitude of other items. They are extremely persistent in the environment, enduring even longer than the pesticides that have evoked such great concern. The toxic ramifications of the PCBs in man and animal include suppression of the immune system, adverse effects on liver enzymes and tumor production. The fact that they are stored and accumulated in the body fat depots is of particular concern.

SEWAGE

Residential septic systems were discussed in Chapter I. They are the rule in rural homes, in contrast to the widespread use of outdoor privies as late as the 1940's. These private systems are effective and safe when design standards are adhered to and if proper maintenance is not neglected. It is ironic that the major threat to public health today comes from municipal sewage systems. Many municipalities foolishly constructed combined storm and sanitary sewer systems years ago, and this has come back to haunt them. During periods of heavy rain, the sewage treatment plants are inundated, and raw sewage pours directly into the rivers, streams and oceans. These cities now face the necessity of digging up streets and neighborhoods, at enormous expense, to install systems that should have been put in place 50 to 75 years ago.

A few cities in the United States had the foresight to install dual, separate systems initially. Even some of these cities of foresight suffer pollution of their water supplies when communities upstream deliberately dump raw sewage into the rivers. This has occurred frequently in recent years purely as a result of greed when housing developments were permitted to be constructed without concomitant sewage treatment facilities. These acts of misfeasance by public officials invariably go unpunished. *La plus ca change, la plus ces't la même chose.*

Even more disgraceful is the practice of dumping raw sewage directly into the ocean, as many cities along the eastern seaboard have been doing for the past fifty years. This practice has contaminated all of the shellfish from these regions with the hepatitis A virus, introducing a major public health threat. In a vain effort to mitigate the hazards presented by this shortsightedness, sewage pipes have been extended ever further seaward, to no avail. Bathing in these waters carries a significant risk, but eating shellfish from them entails an even greater one. These sad facts may help to explain why hepatitis A, which in the past occurred as an epidemic approximately every seven to eight years, is now with us year round, every year.

Sodium in drinking water supplies should be of concern to anyone who has high blood pressure, or a significant family history of high blood pressure. It is known that a high salt intake early in life has an adverse effect on blood pressure later in life. It was only after years of effort that salt was finally removed from baby foods (it was put there for the benefit of the mother's taste, not the infant's). Many municipal water supplies are relatively high in sodium content. The highest concentration, however, is in drinking supplies drawn through a water softener. This water should never be used for drinking or for cooking where a restricted salt diet is desired. Anyone with hypertension, kidney or heart disease, or with a family history of hypertension, should be on a restricted salt diet. A separate tap that bypasses the water softener should be installed at the sink whenever a water softener is installed.

1. CDC. Elevated blood lead levels associated with illicitly distilled alcohol — Alabama, 1990– 1991. *MMWR* 1992;**41**:294-295.

2. U.S. Department of Agriculture website, May, 2001.

3. *Consumer Reports.* Aflatoxin in peanut butter. September 1990:591.

4. Ames BN and Gold LS. Environmental pollution and cancer, KR Foster, DE Bernstein and PW Huber eds., in Phantom Risk; Scientific inference and the law. Cambridge, Mass: MIT Press, 1993.

5. *Food Technology* 1994;48-5.

6. CDC. Multistate outbreak of Salmonella poona infections — United States and Canada, 1991. *MMWR* 1991;**40**(no.32)549- 551.

7. Tauxe RV. Epidemiology of *Campylobacter JEJUNI* infections in the United States and other industrial nations. In: Nachamkin I, Blaser MJ, Tompkins L, eds. *Campylobacter jejuni*: current status and future trends. Washington, DC: *American Society of Microbiology* 1992:9-19.

8. *Environmental Health Letter*, July 1, 1978;**17**(13):6-7.

9. CDC. Update: foodborne listeriosis — United States, 1988–1990. *MMWR* 1992;**41**(15):251-258.

10. CDC. Update: Multistate outbreak of Listeriosis — United States, 1998-1999. *MMWR* 1999;**47**:1117-18.

11. CDC. Multistate outbreak of Losteriosis — United States, 2000. *MMWR* 2000;**49**:1129-30.

12. Dalton CB, Austin CC, Sobel J. et al. An outbreak of gastroenteritis and fever due to *Listeria Monocytogenes* in milk. *N Eng J Med* 1997;**336**:100-105.

13. Schuchat A, et al: The role of foods in sporadic listeriosis: 1. Case-Control Study of Dietary Risk Factors. *JAMA* 1992;**267**:2041-2045, .

14. Pinner RW, et al: The role of foods in sporadic listeriosis: 2. Microbiologic and epidemiologic investigation. *JAMA* 1992;**267**:2046-2050.

15. CDC. Clostridium PERFRINGENS Gastroenteritis Associated with Corned Beef Served at St. Patrick's Day Meals — Ohio and Virginia, 1993. *MMWR* 1994;**43**:137-144.

16. CDC. Type B botulism associated with roasted eggplant in oil — Italy, 1993. *MMWR* 1995;**44**:33-36.

17. CDC. Isolation of Vibrio cholerae O1 from oysters — Mobile Bay, 1991–1992. *MMWR* 1993;**42**(5):91–93.

18. CDC. Cholera — New York, 1991. *MMWR* 1991;**40**:516-518.

19. CDC. Update:Cholera — Western Hemisphere, and recommendations for treatment of cholera. *MMWR* 1991;**40**:562-565.

20. CDC. Cholera associated with an international airline flight, 1992. *MMWR* 1992;**41**:134-135.

21. CDC. Cholera associated with international travel, 1992. *MMWR* 1992;**41**-(36):664–667.

22. CDC. Update: Cholera — Western Hemisphere, 1992. *MMWR* 1992;**41**(36)-:667– 668.

23. CDC. Update:Cholera — Western Hemisphere, 1992. *MMWR* 1993;**42**:89–91.

24. Swerdlow DL, Mintz ED, Rodriguez M, et al. Waterborne transmission of epidemic cholera in Trujillo, Peru:lessons for a continent at risk. *Lancet* 1992;**340**:28-32.

25. Suharyono, Simanjuntak C, Witham N, et al. Safety and immunogenicity of single–dose live oral cholera vaccine CVD 103–HgR in 5–9 year-old Indonesian children. *Lancet* 1992;**340**: 689—94.

26. Coster TS, Killeen KP, Waldor MK et al. Safety, Immunogenicity and efficacy of live attenuated *Vibrio cholerae* O139 vaccine prototype. *Lancet* 1995;**345**:949-952.

27. Personal communication with Wyeth Laboratories, January 18, 2002.

28. Blake PA, Merson MH, Weaver RE, et. al. Disease caused by a marine vibrio: clinical characteristics and epidemiology. *N Engl J Med* 1979;**300**:1-4.

29. CDC. Scombroid fish poisoning — Pennsylvania, 1998. *MMWR* 2000;**49**:398-400.

30. CDC. Ciguatera Fish Poisoning — Florida, 1991. *MMWR* 1993;**42**:417-418.

31. CDC. Rapidly progressive dementia in a patient who received a cadaveric dura mater graft. *MMWR* 1987;**36**:49-55.

32. CDC. Update: Creutzfeld-Jacob disease in a patient receiving a cadaveric dura mater graft. *MMWR* 1987;**36**:324-325.

33. Kohn MA, Farley TA, Ando T et.al. An outbreak of Norwalk Virus gastroenteritis associated with eating raw oysters. *JAMA* 1995;**273**:466-71.

34. CDC. Outbreak of viral gastroenteritis — Pennsylvania and Delaware. *MMWR* 1987;**36**(43):709–711.

35. Swerdlow DL, Woodruff BA, Brady RC. et al. A waterborne outbreak in Missouri of *Escherichia coli* 0157:H7 associated with bloody diarrhea and death. *Ann Int Med* 1992;**117**:812–819.

36. Mead PS, Slutsker L, Dietz V, et al. Food-related illness and death in the United States. *Emerg Infect Dis* 1999;**5**:607-25.

37. CDC. Preliminary report: foodborne outbreak of *Escherichia coli* O157:H7 infections from hamburger — Western United States, 1993. *MMWR* 1993;**42**(4):-85–86.

38. CDC. Update:multistate outbreak of *Escherichia coli* O157:H7 infections from hamburgers — western United States, 1992–1993. *MMWR* 1993;**42**(14):258-263.

39. CDC. Outbreaks of Escherichia coli O157:H7 infections among children associated with farm visits — Pennsylvania and Washington, 2000. *MMWR* 2001;**50**:293-297.

40. CDC. Foodborne outbreak of gastroenteritis caused by *Escherichia coli* 0157:H7 — North Dakota, 1990. *MMWR* 1991;**40**(16)265–267.

41. Besser RE, Lett SM, Weber JT, et al. An outbreak of diarrhea and hemolytic uremic syndrome from *Escherichia coli* 0157:H7 in fresh-pressed apple cider. *JAMA* 1993;**269**:2217–2220.

42. CDC. Outbreaks of *Escherichia coli* O157:H7 Infection and Cryptosporidiosis Associated with Drinking Unpasteurized Apple Cider — Connecticut and New York, October 1996. *MMWR* 1997;**46**:4-8.

43. CDC. Outbreaks of Escherichia coli O157:H7 Infection Associated with Eating Alfalfa Sprouts—Michigan and Virginia, June–July 1997. *MMWR* 1997;**46**:741-744.

44. Personal conversation with Doug Park, Michigan Department of Agriculture.

45. Belongia EA, Osterholm MT, Soler JT et al. Transmission of *Escherichia coli* 0157:H7 infection in Minnesota child day-care facilities. *JAMA* 1993;**269**:883–888.

46. Hoge CW, Shlim DR, Rajah R, et al. Epidemiology of diarrhoeal illness associated with coccidian-like organism among travellers and foreign residents in Nepal. *Lancet* 1993;**341**:1175-79.

47. Huang P, Weber JT, Sosin DM et al. The first reported outbreak of diarrheal illness associated with *Cyclospora* in the United States. *Ann Intern Med* 1995;**123(6)**:409-14.

48. CDC. Update:outbreaks of *Cyclospora cayetanensis* infection — United States and Canada, 1996. *MMWR* 1996;**45**:611-12.

49. Herwaldt BL, Ackers ML. An outbreak in 1996 of cyclosporiasis associated with imported raspberries. *N Engl J Med* 1997;**336**:1548-56.

50. CDC. Update:Outbreaks of Cyclosporiasis M United States, 1997. *MMWR* 1997;**46**:461-462.

51. CDC. Update:Outbreaks of Cyclosporiasis — United States and Canada, 1997. *MMWR* 1997;**46**:521-523.

52. CDC. Outbreaks of *Cyclospora cayetanensis* Infection — United States, 1996. *MMWR* 1996;**45**:549-551.

53. CDC. Update:Outbreaks of *Cyclospora cayetanensis* Infection — United States and Canada, 1996. *MMWR* 1996;**45**:611-612.

54. CDC. Outbreak of Cyclosporiasis — Northern Virginia–Washingon, D.C.–Baltimore, Maryland Metropolitan Area, 1997. *MMWR* 1997;**46**:689-691.

55. CDC. Outbreak of Cyclosporiasis — Ontario, Canada, May, 1998. *MMWR* 1998;**47**:806-809.

56. The Medical Letter. Enoxacin — a new fluoroquinolone. *The Medical Letter* 1992;**34**:103–105. (November 13, 1992)

57. Alonso A, Daschner A, Moreno-Ancillo A. Anaphylaxis with *Anisakis simplex* in the Gastric Mucosa. *N Engl J Med* 1997;**337**:350-351.

58. CDC. Locally acquired neurocysticercosis — North Carolina, Massachusetts, and South Carolina, 1989– 1991. *MMWR* 1992;**41**:1-4.

59. Snow, John. "The Broad Street Pump." In B. Roueche, *Curiosities of Medicine* (1963). Boston, Little Brown.

60. Anderson C. Cholera epidemic traced to risk miscalculation. *Nature* 1991;**354**:255.

61. CDC. Prevalence of Parasites in Fecal Material from Chlorinated Swimming Pools — United States, 1999. *MMWR* 2001;**50**:410-412.

62. CDC. Waterborne-disease outbreaks, 1989-1990. *MMWR* 1990;**40**(SS-3).

63. Brookhiser R. I stuck around St. Petersburg. *Forbes-FYI*, Spring 1998.

64. Marshall B, Warren JR. Unidentified curved bacilli on gastric epithelium in active chronic gastritis. *Lancet* 1983;**1**:1273-1275.

65. CDC. Protracted Outbreak of Cryptosporidiosis Associated With Swimming Pool Use — Ohio and Nebraska, 2000. MMWR 2001;50:406-410.

66. CDC. Spontaneous abortions possibly related to ingestion of nitrate-contaminated well water — LaGrange County, Indiana, 1991-1994. *MMWR* 1996;**45**:569-571.

67. U.S. Department of Health and Human Services, Public Health Service, National Toxicology Program. *Report on Carcinogens*, Ninth Edition, 2000.

68. Ames BN, Gold, LS. The Causes and Prevention of Cancer: The Role of Environment. In *The True State of the Planet*. R. Bailey ed. New York: Free Press, 1995..

ERRATUM: Endnote number 27 for page 180 should be number 28. Every subsequent note should be one number higher.

VI

HAZARDS OF THE AIR THAT WE BREATHE

Science begets knowledge; opinion, ignorance

— Hippocrates

As has been the case on the job (see Chapter X), air quality at home has become an increasing source of symptoms and complaints. In the extreme, a number of families have been forced to evacuate their homes as a result of excessive levels of formaldehyde that caused respiratory complaints. The formaldehyde came from urea foam insulation that was blown into the walls. Similar complaints have come from residents of mobile homes. High levels of formaldehyde in these units were traced to not only urea foam insulation, but to the plywood and particleboard components as well.

All of these complaints have increased in recent years because residences have been sealed more tightly to make them energy efficient. Improvements in insulation materials and techniques have facilitated these efforts and have contributed to the problem. This has resulted in a reduction in the amount of outside air that is circulated through the home. Many substances that have previously produced no symptoms are now increased in concentration to levels that produce discomfort.

Formaldehyde levels that are greatly above the limit of one part per million set by the American Conference of Governmental Industrial Hygienists have been measured in new homes. New materials used in home construction have contributed to the problem. The increased use of particle board, plywood and adhesives adds to the level of formaldehyde and organic solvents in the air. The escape of these gases into the air is not detected by conventional measuring instruments and techniques.

Some of the organic solvents contributed from building materials include 1,1,1-trichloroethane, toluene, styrene, xylene and benzene. The latter has been associated with the development of leukemia and is closely controlled in industrial and laboratory use. The level of these and other gases has been found to be particularly high in mobile homes. This is due to both the greater quantities of materials containing them being used, and to the relatively smaller air volume. These levels in new units gradually subside over a period of six to twelve months.

Carbon monoxide, which kills many people in their homes and apartments every winter, reaches higher levels in a tight home. Most people who are exposed to elevated levels do survive, but they suffer vague symptoms such as headache that are frequently not attributed to this potentially lethal gas. Lower levels of carbon monoxide that do not produce symptoms have been suspected of contributing to arteriosclerotic heart disease and angina. These diseases have been noted to occur at a higher than normal rate in cigarette smokers. The level of carboxyhemoglobin (from carbon monoxide) in cigarette smokers is five to fifteen times normal values.

Some carbon monoxide is produced in homes from gas cooking stoves. Potentially lethal levels can result from using space heaters, even supposedly safe kerosene heaters. Most serious exposures result from defective or obstructed chimneys, flues or furnaces. A number of deaths have occurred as a result of cooking indoors with charcoal. Charcoal should never be used for cooking or heating in any enclosed space. This is particularly true in homes, mobile homes and recreational vehicles.

Hazardous levels of carbon monoxide build up during a variety of indoor sports events such as ice hockey games and tractor pulls. Both ice edgers and ice resurfacing machines produce carbon monoxide in arenas during games. The levels for these events can reach or exceed hazardous levels unless concerted efforts to provide adequate ventilation are made. The hazard is much greater during events such as tractor pulls and other indoor vehicle contests. Carbon monoxide levels of more than 70 parts per million have been measured at the beginning of these events. The carbon monoxide is produced by the idling of engines in the building. Levels well over 400 ppm have been recorded before the event was over.[1,2] A level of 10 ppm is high enough to adversely affect health. Several cases of serious carbon monoxide poisoning have occurred among farmers while using gasoline powered washers to clean the interior of buildings. One death resulted from this activity in 1993.[3]

Carbon monoxide is colorless and tasteless and its presence is never suspected until symptoms are well advanced. Early symptoms are subtle and do not arouse suspicion of air contamination. Headache is the first symptom noted, followed by weakness, shortness of breath, confusion and visual disturbances. In individuals with heart disease, angina is aggravated, as is shortness of breath in people with emphysema. Irregularities of the heartbeat may be precipitated. Harm to the fetus in pregnant women will not be evident until after delivery, and carbon monoxide usually will not be associated with these abnormalities when they are noted.

Nitrogen oxides are also produced by gas stoves and by kerosene space heaters. These gases are not only respiratory irritants but also have been incriminated in the production of cancer. Gas stoves and all space heaters should be vented to the outside. An overhead hood vented to the outside is sufficient for the kitchen gas range if the blower is on during cooking.

Cigarette smoke is the most hazardous indoor air pollution problem that many people face. It is the cause of virtually all bronchial carcinoma, the only type of cancer that is on the increase. The only cancer epidemic in the United States today is lung cancer. Cigarette smoking causes 80,000 deaths from lung cancer each year in the U.S. Only about 10 percent of the people with lung cancer live for five years after the diagnosis is made. Only about 15 percent of all cases of lung cancer in the United States are due to occupational exposures. The remainder are due to cigarette smoking.

Statistics from the National Cancer Institute show that people who smoke one to nine cigarettes per day have over four times the death rate from lung cancer that is seen in nonsmokers. For those who smoke ten to nineteen cigarettes per day, the rate climbs to about eight times as high. For those who smoke twenty to thirty-nine per day it is about thirteen times, and over forty per day the rate is about seventeen times as high. Fifty times the quantity of tobacco is smoked today as was the case in the early 1900s.

More than four thousand chemical substances have been identified in tobacco smoke, several of which are known carcinogens. The mean particle size of cigarette smoke is 0.2 to 0.5 micron, which assures access to the deepest reaches of the lungs. The most potent cancer-causing agent in cigarette smoke is benzopyrene. It is also present in coal tar, in wood smoke and in many other instances of combustion. Benzopyrene is used in the laboratory to produce cancers in animals for research purposes.

Polonium, a breakdown product of radon, is another serious cancer producing substance in cigarettes. Some of the polonium in tobacco originates from the soil where it is grown. Some of it comes from the decay of radioactive lead in the phosphate fertilizer used to grow tobacco. Nitrosamines are also present in tobacco, and their cancer-causing propensity was discussed in Chapter V.

Some of the other pollutants in cigarette smoke are irritants and are responsible for the bronchitis and productive cough that is so characteristic of smokers. Acrolein and acetaldehyde, common components of smog, are two such irritants. They produce irritation of the eyes, nose, throat and lungs. Hydrogen cyanide and nitrogen oxides are other irritants. The cadmium in cigarette smoke is worse than an irritant. It is a potent cause of emphysema, a disease seen commonly in silver solderers and welders who inhale the fume. Cadmium undoubtedly plays a significant role in the production of the chronic lung disease and emphysema that is so common in cigarette smokers.

The carbon monoxide in cigarette smoke has been widely studied. It plays a significant role in the production of arteriosclerotic heart disease. Carbon monoxide attaches to hemoglobin in the blood, producing carboxyhemoglobin. This form of hemoglobin is incapable of carrying oxygen. The desirable level is zero, but levels up to one percent are commonly found in nonsmokers. The level of carboxyhemoglobin in moderate cigarette smokers (one pack per day) is about 5 percent, and it ranges up to 15 percent in heavy smokers. In clinical practice it is not uncommon to see levels of 8 to 10 percent among smokers.

In those who already have a compromised circulation to the heart due to arteriosclerosis, this reduction in the oxygen carrying capacity of the blood further deprives the heart muscle of oxygen. These individuals have more severe angina than nonsmokers do. Repeated studies of large groups of people in several cultures throughout the world have all shown that males who smoke cigarettes have a 70 percent higher death rate than nonsmokers do. This mortality is primarily due to coronary heart disease. It is most pronounced in the 45 to 55 year age group. Adverse effects on the nervous system are also caused by these elevations of carboxyhemo-globin over time.

The adverse effect of nonsmokers inhaling the cigarette smoke from smokers has been the subject of several recent studies. In the workplace this exposure has produced irritation of the eyes, nose and throat with coughing and sneezing. The presence of smokers in a room increases the level of particulates that are inhaled into the lungs by three to twelve times. The presence of a smoker in the home increases the level of these respirable particulates to two to three times the normal level. The "passive smokers" in these settings demonstrate a carboxyhemoglobin level of over 2 percent. This level is detrimental to health, invoking risks such as coronary heart disease. In one study after two hours in a room with a smoker, the carboxyhemoglobin level in the blood of a nonsmoker was increased from the baseline level of 1 percent to 2.7 percent .

Decreased pulmonary function and small airway disease have been measured in passive smokers with chronic exposure. Similar findings have been documented in children whose parents smoke. Sixty percent of the children in the United States today are exposed to cigarette smoke in their homes. These children suffer respiratory illnesses at a rate 10 to 20 percent higher than do children who live in homes free of such pollution. The lung damage in these children persists throughout their life.

Efforts to associate second hand smoke with lung cancer have not been supported by the majority of studies. In 1993 the EPA, following the same fraudulent pattern that it set in the Alar fiasco (see chapter XIII), issued a statement claiming that inhaling passive cigarette smoke causes 3,000 deaths each year in the United States. When 10 of the 11 studies that the EPA relied upon failed to support their claim they ignored them and used the one that did. This was precisely the pattern of deliberate, false propaganda that was followed with Alar. In 1998 the World Health Organization released the results of its 10 year study covering 21 countries that showed no connection between passive cigarette smoke and cancer.

Dust in the home includes fungus (mold) spores, animal dander, pollens, dust mites and bacteria, all of which many people are allergic to. Even if the cat or dog is not in the house, enough of the dander is blown or tracked in to cause grief. Tree pollens plague many people even during the winter months as a result of wood-burning stoves and fireplaces. Desensitization affords some relief, but this requires an injection every seven to fourteen days.

Adequate filtration of the air by an efficient filter on the central heating/air conditioning unit helps, but does not solve the problem completely. All of these filters have limitations in the materials that they will remove from the air, based upon particle size. A significant quantity of particles adhere to drapes, furniture and other fixtures, and thus are not removed by filters. They can be dislodged subsequently to circulate or be inhaled. The particles of cigarette smoke range up to about one micrometer in diameter. Pollen particles range from 10 to 100 microns. Dust particles range from 0.5 to 50 microns in diameter. By comparison, the water particles of fog range from 5 to 50 microns.

One unique type of furnace filter, Space Guard, claims to remove 65 percent of the particles of cigarette smoke and virtually 100 percent of pollen and dust particles. This represents a significant improvement over the simple fiberglass filters commonly attached to furnaces. A high efficiency (HEPA) room filter will clear a 12 by 14-foot room of all cigarette smoke in about three hours. These units can remove up to 70 percent of the particulate circulating in a room. One such filter that is readily available to the consumer now is the Honeywell Enviracaire. It is advertised to remove 99.97 percent of the circulating particulate at the 0.3 micron size in a room. It effectively removes circulating pollens, mold spores, animal hair and dander, dust mite allergens, bacteria, viruses and tobacco smoke. It produces no ozone during operation. The Model 13503 at 359 CFM provides 15 changes of air each hour in a 12 by 14-foot room. Keep in mind that these filters remove only the circulating particulates, not those that are imbedded in the carpet or adhered to the draperies and furniture.

Addition of one of these HEPA filter, especially in the bedroom, makes a significant contribution to cleaning up the air. The cost of these units is around $200, but they can be moved readily from room to room. Some filters and humidifiers may serve as a source of microorganism and spore propagation. This is less of a problem with a HEPA filter, but the filter element needs to be replaced periodically. Humidifiers and any unit where water stands must be cleaned and disinfected with household bleach to destroy bacteria and fungus that tend to collect and multiply there. Many people are allergic to these organisms and may suffer cough, wheezing, stuffy nose and eye complaints. Permanent damage, especially to the lungs, can result from prolonged exposure to these microorganisms.

One common organism that causes allergies and is especially troublesome to asthmatics is dust mites. These have not been given much attention until recently, primarily because they cannot be seen and are difficult to study. They are one of the chief culprits in "house dust" causing allergic reactions. Recently the ACAREX Test Kit has been marketed in the United States, which aids in the detection of mites when they are present. When dust mites are present, a powder containing benzyl benzoate can be sprinkled on the carpet of the bedroom (or other rooms where they are found) and allowed to penetrate into the carpet. One such product currently available is AllerCare. A thorough vacuuming then removes the mites and their excreta, both of which cause allergic reactions. This treatment for dust mites has been shown to relieve asthma for as long as 7 to 12 months. Anyone who suffers from asthma, bronchitis, eczema, rhinitis or any other respiratory allergy problem should investigate dust mites in the home as a cause.

The collection of dust can readily be seen on furniture and woodwork, but accumulation in carpeting is hidden from view. Both sources must be cleaned regularly. Furniture polishes are effective for the hard surfaces, but an efficient vacuum cleaner is required for carpeting. This should be a central vacuum system that discharges the exhaust air to the outside. Conventional vacuum cleaners, the type in virtually every home, merely raise the dust from floor level to nose level. Their filters permit significant quantities of the dust particles of the most harmful size to pass through. Installation of a central vacuum system is not a difficult do-it-yourself project, and is highly recommended for every home.

During the winter months central heating systems produce a very dry atmosphere. This is irritating to the respiratory membranes and it increases the incidence of cough and respiratory infections. This dryness can and should be remedied by humidification of the air. The most efficient means of doing this is by use of a humidifier on the furnace. These units frequently provide less than the optimal level of humidity, however, usually due to improper setting or poor maintenance. The elements within these humidifiers that transfer the moisture to the air become caked with minerals and lose their efficiency unless serviced regularly. Bacterial and fungus growth also needs to be cleaned out of humidifiers regularly to avoid dissemination throughout the house. This can be accomplished readily by using household bleach.

The area where humidification is most needed is the bedroom. This is particularly important for young children. An ultrasonic humidifier in the bedroom is very effective in providing the needed humidification during the night. The ultrasonic units also are quiet enough to permit sleep. The simple measure of adding humidity to the air in the bedroom frequently solves a troublesome cough in people with bronchitis, and thus permits sleep. One problem that does arise with the use of ultrasonic humidifiers is that they deposit a light film of minerals on the furniture. This can be avoided by using distilled water, but this requires sizeable quantities, perhaps a gallon or more each night. Most of the ultrasonic units now sold have a replaceable cartridge that removes the minerals from the water if distilled water is not readily available.

Humidification of the air in the home should not be overdone. This is most likely with the use of a portable unit, and in the bathroom. Dust mites require a relative humidity of over fifty percent to feed and reproduce. Keeping the humidity below that level will help to control a major source of allergens in homes. A relative humidity above about 70 percent encourages the growth of mold, especially on windows and in bathrooms. This growth can also take place inside walls, where it is hidden from view. This has been demonstrated during investigations of complaints of illness in buildings, such as a courthouse in Florida.[4,5]

Humidification should be limited to about 55 percent. The spores that are released into the air from the growth of mold are disseminated throughout the house. Such growth should be cleaned and treated regularly with a solution of household bleach, which is very effective in killing both bacteria and mold (see Chapter XV). Permitting stagnant water to stand in any location in the house encourages the growth of bacteria and mold.

One of the most serious and most insidious hazards from humidifiers and other sources of stagnant water is *Legionella* pneumonia. This serious and often fatal disease was first recognized in 1976 after several persons who were attending the American Legion convention in Philadelphia succumbed to it. Several other outbreaks have occurred since. The organism had previously escaped recognition because it is not demonstrated by the typical Gram stain and requires special culture media for growth. It can be visualized on slides prepared from culture on special media when basic fuchsin is substituted for safranin as a counterstain.

The organisms grow slowly, and prefer a warm environment. Much like tetanus spores they are ubiquitous in soil and in bodies of water such as lakes, rivers and streams. Infection is most common in men over age 55 years, the debilitated and in the immunocompromised. Individuals suffering from chronic bronchitis, emphysema and diabetes, and smokers and patients on steroids are particularly at risk.

Infection frequently results from aspiration of or inhalation of aerosolized standing water from air conditioning towers, humidifiers and even showerheads. In 1996 patients in two hospitals, one in Arizona and one in Ohio, acquired Legionnaires Disease through persistent contamination of the hospital hot water system, either from the shower or through nebulizers.[6] As many as 6,000 patients acquire Legionnaires' disease each year in the United States, with a death rate of 40 percent. Much of the cause for this relates to the unfortunate obsession with low temperature water heaters. The bacteria cannot thrive in temperatures above 140 degrees F. This was found to be a factor in a case in an Ohio hospital in May, 2001.

Survival requires an early diagnosis, which frequently is not forthcoming, and aggressive treatment with the appropriate antibiotic(s). This disease adds urgency to the need for regular cleaning of humidifiers. Chlorine (household bleach) in adequate concentration is effective in killing the bacterium. In plumbing systems hyperchlorination is required, but the organism can survive even this treatment in dead spots or areas of low flow.

In addition to dust and dust mites, mold spores, dander, pollen and bacteria all cause sensitivity reactions and a cough. Hydrocarbons and particulates from smoking, formaldehyde from urea foam in furniture and adhesives in plywood and particleboard, and detergent residue from improper carpet cleaning also add to the irritation of the eyes, nose, throat and lungs. Far more sophisticated

air cleaning equipment than exists in the average home would be required to control all of these hazards to health. Some of the many hazardous chemicals that have been identified in the home are:
- Tetrachloroethylene: from dry-cleaned clothes
- Methylene chloride: paint thinners and strippers
- Ammonia: from cleaning agents and oven cleaners
- Chlorine: from cleaning agents, laundry bleach, automatic dishwasher detergent and toilet bowel cleaners
- Hair spray: methylene chloride and other irritants
- Para-dichlorobenzene: moth crystals and air freshener (a cancer risk)
- Trichloroethane: aerosol sprays and solvents
- Formaldehyde: furniture stuffing, particleboard and plywood (counter tops)
- Benzo-*a*-pyrene, a potent cancer producer: tobacco smoke and wood burning stoves
- Insecticides
- Fingernail polish
- Cosmetics

All painting projects in the home should be deferred until the weather is warm enough to permit the doors and windows to be opened. Paints cause a build up of vapors and chemicals in the room air that is irritating to the respiratory tract, and potentially toxic to the liver, kidney and nervous system. Since the series of acute mercury poisonings from interior paint in Michigan in 1989, this hazard should no longer be present. Furniture refinishing similarly should not be done indoors without adequate ventilation. This is not a project for a closed basement workshop. There is a danger of explosion if flammable solvents are used. If nonflammable solvents are used, such as methylene chloride, inhalation of the vapors is hazardous to the liver, kidney and nervous system (brain), and presents a risk of cancer development.

A study at the National Aeronautics and Space Administration demonstrated that some common plants, when grown in the home, help to remove some of the chemicals that cause irritation. Philodendron, chrysanthemum, spider plant and aloe vera break down some toxins, such as formaldehyde, in the process of photosynthesis. It is yet to be determined how many plants are required for a given room, and the full extent of substances that these plants are able to devour.

AIR POLLUTION

There has been an intense and acrimonious debate over air pollution during the past two decades. Much of the propaganda delivered to the general public would have you believe that air pollution and the hazards associated with it are of recent origin. In reality, nothing could be further from the truth. Virtually every home in the United States, as with all of the industrialized world, was heated by coal up until the early 1940s. The emissions from the chimneys of these homes were very obvious after a night of new fallen snow. If you had the misfortune to live anywhere near a factory, the soot from the coal that was burned there darkened the atmosphere even more. Coal-burning locomotives during that era also delivered considerable soot and sulfur dioxide to the air in virtually every city. The outdoor air in the majority of these cities and neighborhoods is much freer of pollution today than it was as recently as the thirties and forties.

Writers documented the pollution of the air by the burning of coal as long ago as the fourth century A.D. The burning of coal by industry and in the home was banned in London in the fourteenth century as a result of the pollution of the air. London has experienced many serious air pollution episodes, by virtue of its propensity for periods of prolonged fog. Most of the components of air pollution become attached to or become a part of the water particles of fog. During a two-week period in December 1952, in excess of 3,000 deaths resulted from such an episode in London. The sulfur dioxide level during this fog was raised to nine times the level measured just before this period. Replacement of the limestone figurines on Victoria tower of the Houses of Parliament in 1948 was necessitated by corrosion from sulfur dioxide in the air.

One of the earliest well-documented mass poisonings as a result of air pollution occurred in the Meuse Valley in Belgium in 1930. Many people became ill but the exact number is not recorded. More than sixty people died. The Meuse Valley shares some topographical and climatic characteristics with those of the Los Angeles basin. Both valleys are surrounded by hills that restrict the movement of air that might serve to cleanse the area. Both have a concentration of industry and motor vehicles that deliver a heavy burden of pollutants to the local atmosphere.[7]

Another thoroughly documented disaster occurred in 1948 at Donora, Pennsylvania, south of Pittsburgh on the Monongahela River. About 6,000 people were made ill and 20 of them died. Although sulfur dioxide was considered to be one of the chief culprits in this episode, over a dozen other toxic chemicals were identified. These originated in various steel mills, chemical plants, a glass works, a powerplant and a railroad. The Pittsburgh area was cleared of much of this smog after natural gas replaced coal and fuel oil in these industries.[8]

Smog is a term that was coined to describe the brownish haze in the Los Angeles area that burns the eyes and throat. The term is a contraction of the two words smoke and fog. Accumulations of pollutants such as sulfur dioxide have historically been associated with the occurrence of protracted periods of fog, for the reason mentioned above. In recent years communities such as Los Angeles and Denver have demonstrated that smog can be cultivated without having fog as a matrix. Smog consists of carbon monoxide, particulates such as soot and dust, ozone, hydrocarbons and oxides of nitrogen (NOx).

Photochemical reactions produce many of the more noxious constituents of smog. These reactions often are produced by the ultraviolet radiation from the sun. This requires a stagnant atmosphere and the reaction is accelerated by increased temperatures. The input materials for these photochemical reactions are oxides of nitrogen, hydrocarbons, water vapor and carbon monoxide. The Los Angeles basin provides all of these elements in abundance. It has gained a reputation as the smog capital of the United States. Other cities vying for this honor are New York City, Houston and Chicago, for all share unacceptable levels of ozone. Even Denver, the mile high city, has grown in population to the point that it suffers from smog. About 100 cities in the U.S. currently violate the 1970 Clean Air Act. Population growth is the underlying cause for most of this problem.

Automobiles have monopolized the attention of the politicians and the extremists as the source of the hydrocarbons, oxides of nitrogen and carbon monoxide that go into the production of smog. This is largely because the automobile is visible everywhere, and has no political clout. Equally to blame, however, are diesel trucks and buses (including smoke-belching city busses), diesel locomotives, farm tractors, industry in its entirety and jet aircraft. Even charcoal lighter fluid and the process of grilling on backyard barbecue grills contribute hydrocarbons to the air. Recent proposals for cleaning up the air include banning the sale of charcoal lighter fluid and the use of grills at home.

These same extremists also propose to ban the use of gasoline powered lawn mowers. Substituting electric mowers would not eliminate any of the aggregate air pollution, since the powerplant would have to increase production. It may mean that we would have to return to the hand-powered mower to comply with these far out suggestions. New automobiles today emit 95 percent less hydrocarbons and carbon monoxide and 75 percent less nitrogen oxides than they did in the 1970s. This has been accomplished at a cost to you of over one thousand dollars for each vehicle ($1500 per auto for catalytic converter). This is not enough for the bureaucrats and environmental extremists, however, and they have further plans for your pocketbook.

The plans of the bureaucrats frequently backfire. Aside from the added costs to the taxpayers, new problems are often created. In the Clean Air Act Amendment of 1990, Congress mandated the use of so called "oxygenated" fuels (either ethanol or MTBE), supposedly to reduce carbon monoxide levels in the great outdoors. In response to this mandate, the oil companies began adding 15 percent methyl tertiary butyl ether (MTBE) to gasoline. It had been used previously in a 2 to 3 percent ratio to boost octane, after lead was banned. The EPA predicted that the addition would raise the cost of gasoline by 3 to 5 cents per gallon. The true cost of the addition was 14 cents per gallon.

In addition to the increased cost, complaints of headache and nausea from people refueling vehicles with the new gasoline in Alaska, Colorado, Montana and New Jersey caused concern among health officials. Studies revealed MTBE in the blood of those who suffered the symptoms. The true threat to health has not been determined as yet, but it would appear that carbon monoxide in open country presented much less of a hazard. Another unanticipated disadvantage of the oxygenated fuels is that they have a much shorter storage life. This not only adds to the cost, but also increases the likelihood that tractors, lawn mowers and other devices left sitting with fuel in their tanks will gum up the carburetor and fuel system.

All automobiles built since the late 1980s have oxygen sensors that adjust the fuel/air ratio automatically. Thus there was nothing to be gained by oxygenated fuels, no reduction in emissions, no benefit, only harm. The new regulations imposed by Congress and the EPA were politically motivated to benefit the producers of ethanol, especially Archer Daniels Midland. The EPA itself had stated previously that 1990 model cars run 96 percent cleaner than their 1970 counterparts as a result of the Clean Air Act of 1970 and the 1977 amendments.

The latest gift from the Environmental Protection Agency arrived in late 1993. New limits on the sulfur content of diesel fuel not only increased the price of the fuel, but also resulted in the destruction of diesel injector pumps. These diesel injector pumps, an integral part of every diesel engine in automobiles, trucks, tractors and many industrial engines, rely upon the inherent lubricating properties of normal diesel fuel. Meeting the new EPA regulations seriously compromised the lubricating properties of diesel fuel. The sulfur content of Number 2 diesel fuel marketed by the major oil companies has been below 0.1 percent since at least 1978. Studies have shown that the sulfur content in most diesel fuel throughout the United States has not been above 0.3 percent. Mercedes Benz has recommended for decades that the sulfur content of diesel fuel be kept below 0.5 percent to minimize corrosion in the engine.

In other words there has been no problem with the sulfur content of the high quality diesel fuel and no need for additional bureaucratic regulations. If any control were needed, elimination of the inferior fuel being sold would have been sufficient. Additionally, the specter of acid rain, the reason given for these restrictions, has been disproved as a threat to the environment long ago. The EPA continues to fight windmills, however.

The irritant substances that are produced by photochemical reactions are aldehydes, nitrates and ozone. The latter has enjoyed the greatest level of attention and measurement. It is generally considered to be the most important constituent of smog in the production of respiratory irritation and subsequent death. Copy machines, negative ion generators, electronic air filters, electric motors and lightening all contribute ozone to the air. It is ironic that we are plagued by such a surplus of ozone in our immediate environment at the same time that the environmental extremists are creating such hysteria about a mythical dissipation of the ozone layer in the atmosphere.

Common symptoms produced by smog are burning of the eyes and throat, cough and heaviness in the chest. People with allergies, asthma and bronchitis are particularly susceptible to the irritant effects of smog. Fatalities during severe episodes invariable include victims who suffer from these maladies.

Nitrogen dioxide is reddish brown in color and this accounts for the color of smog. Several other oxides of nitrogen are produced along with the dioxide. For this reason you will see the term NOx to refer to all of these substances. These other nitrogen oxides are colorless. Oxides of nitrogen are produced in many industrial processes such as electric welding, except where an inert gas such as argon is used. Gas welding and cutting torches also produce nitrogen dioxide, as does any acid dipping operation such as metal plating. Even gas cooking stoves and furnaces contribute this substance to the air. Many deaths have occurred from pulmonary edema caused by this gas when it was formed in freshly filled silos. A layer of brownish gas often can be seen in these circumstances. Over 100 deaths were caused by nitrogen dioxide at the Cleveland Clinic in 1929 when fire ignited cellulose based X-ray film.

Sulfur dioxide is an equally lethal component of smog, when it is present in sufficient concentrations. The deaths that occurred in the air pollution disasters described previously were ascribed largely to sulfur dioxide. It was produced by the burning of coal during a period when coal was the only source of cooking and heating in the home and of energy in industry. The main source of sulfur dioxide in ambient air today is the burning of fossil fuels and specific processes in industry, such as smelting of ores. Fossil fuels include not only coal, but gasoline, diesel fuel and home heating oil.

The quantity of sulfur dioxide in vehicle emissions is directly related to the sulfur content of the fuel and to the design of the engine. The amount of sulfur in automotive fuels is generally held below about 0.3 percent out of consideration for its harmful effect on engines. At this level its contribution to pollution is negligible, especially in well-designed engines. Those vehicles that are poorly maintained and those that burn inferior fuel contribute significantly more sulfur dioxide to the atmosphere. These vehicles are frequently identified by the cloud of black smoke that surrounds them. The Environmental Protection Agency has mandated that the remaining sulfur content of even current low levels in automobile fuels be eliminated. This has added at least 5 to 10 cents per gallon to the cost of diesel fuel, without yielding any further benefit. It has also resulted in the unnecessary destruction of diesel injector pumps as discussed previously.

The damage to coniferous trees that was blamed on sulfur dioxide from smokestacks was subsequently found to be caused instead by insects and disease. Enormous sums of money were spent to placate the environmentalists, and this investment was found to have been unwarranted. In order to mitigate the claimed damage to trees from powerplants the height of the stacks was increased to over 800 feet. The discharge from these stacks into the atmosphere is generally three times the height of the stack, so the noxious chemicals are delivered to the air at an altitude of about 2,500 feet. One such chimney in Switzerland was built on a mountain so that the top of the stack was 1,800 feet above the town. The emissions from that stack would enter the atmosphere at an altitude above 5,000 feet.

This neatly solved the local pollution problem, and delivered it to the neighbors. Nuclear powerplants would have eliminated all of the pollution problems associated with power generation. The installation of nuclear powerplants was stopped dead in its tracks, however, by the extremists, politicians and special interest groups, and by bungling contractors. France generates 75 percent of its power needs by using nuclearpower plants. Several other countries are well ahead of the United States in this new technology. The solution to the sulfur dioxide problem from the Environmental Protection Agency was to mandate expensive scrubbers on the smokestacks of everypower plant in the U.S. in the 1980s. This expenditure was required even where no sulfur dioxide was produced. This law costs the consumer over $4 billion every year. The fix actually increased carbon dioxide emissions.

The quantity of all of the most significant air pollutants had actually declined before these huge sums of money were drained from the economy. Sulfur dioxide emissions have declined 25 percent since 1970, carbon monoxide emissions have fallen 41 percent, and smoke, soot and dust are down 59 percent.[9] No cost benefit formula is ever applied to the laws and rules that strive to eradicate every perceived hazard. In many instances nature produces a far greater level of these substances than is acceptable to the bureaucrats. Ninety percent of the volatile organic compounds in air come from trees. This is what produces the haze in the Smokey Mountains, not campfires as the environmental extremists would have you believe.

All of the proposals to resolve the problem of air pollution and smog will prove to be very costly. The burden of this cost will rest upon the consumer and the taxpayer, as is always the case. Many of the proposals are ludicrous, but this is the kind of thinking that goes into most legislation. The eruption of Mount Pinatubo in the Philippines in June 1991 sent nineteen million tons of sulfur into the atmosphere where it was transformed into sulfur dioxide. This had far more effect on the ozone hole than all of man's activities did. The resultant haze from that natural pollution blocked sunlight until the mid-1990s, and resulted in cooler weather. A similar eruption of Mount Tambora in Indonesia in 1816 resulted in that year being recorded as the year without summer, with an unseasonably cold summer recorded in the United States with snow in some areas. A single major volcanic eruption can produce a greater effect on the earth's weather than all of man's industrial activities have over the past one hundred years.

The basic cause of most air pollution today is the massive increase in population, and the propensity for people to settle in areas that the American Indians judged unfit to occupy. There is no simple, quick, easy solution to the problem. It is a problem that should be approached with intelligence and careful study by experts in the various sciences. This is not the manner in which most problems are solved in the United States today, however.

RADON
Concern has been mounting during the past decade over the discovery that homes in certain regions of the United States harbor high levels of radon gas. Levels as high as those that have been shown to cause lung cancer in uranium miners have been found in

many homes. Homes in Montgomery County, Pennsylvania were among the first discovered to have this problem. The problem was discovered in December 1984 when a worker at the Limerick Nuclear Power Plant in Pennsylvania triggered the radiation detectors as he was going INTO the power station in. He and his family lived in one of the homes in this area. When the home was tested radon levels a thousand times higher than the four picocuries that the EPA has established as a threshold level were found. (National Geographic April 1989)

It is known that the geologic formation identified as the Reading Prong, which extends from eastern Pennsylvania through northern New Jersey and south central New York, contains deposits of uranium in the granite. Homes built over these deposits are at a higher risk of having radon gas accumulate, but there is a considerable variation in the concentration among homes in a given region. Even homes built side by side may vary greatly in the concentration of radon gas in the internal air due to construction techniques and the development of cracks in the foundation. Radon gas also enters homes through sump pumps, and sealed covers are now available for these units.

About 70 percent of the homes evaluated in Maine had significant concentrations of radon gas. Similar concentrations were found in homes in Texas (Houston) and Illinois. The Environmental Protection Agency estimates from their surveys that at least seven percent of the homes nationwide exceed its guidelines for maximum exposure, which is four picocuries per liter of air. They contend that houses that exceed this level can be found in almost every state. Some people claim that even the level of four picocuries is not a desirable level, and that it carries an increased risk of lung cancer, especially among smokers. Other experts, such as Dr. Norman C. Rasmussen, a nuclear engineer at the Massachusetts Institute of Technology, contends that "There is a lot of evidence that low radiation doses not only do not cause harm but may in fact do some good. After all, humankind evolved in a world of natural low level radiation."[10]

Radon is a gas that evolves as a naturally occurring breakdown product of thorium and uranium ore. It is much like carbon monoxide in that it cannot be detected by the human senses, since it is colorless, odorless and tasteless. We have known since about

1950 that it causes lung cancer in miners, and that miners who smoke are at a particularly high risk. In 1950 the U.S. Public Health Service conducted a survey among uranium miners in Colorado. They found an increased incidence of lung cancer among the miners, due to the radon and other radioactive breakdown products of radon. The incidence rate of lung cancer was four times the expected rate. No increased rate for other types of cancer was found in this study.

This same observation regarding lung cancer had been made as far back as 1875 among miners of pitchblende in the Bohemian Mountains. It was from this pitchblende that Madame Curie isolated radium and polonium in her laboratory in Paris. Later analysis demonstrated that during the period 1875 to 1939 lung cancers were responsible for 43 percent of all of the deaths among these miners.

The latency period for the development of lung cancer among uranium miners is approximately twenty years. Data suggests that at least ten years of exposure in the mines is required for lung cancer to develop at a later date. A study conducted in Sweden concluded that women who were exposed to high levels of radon at home had double the risk of lung cancer. It is estimated that radon gas in the home is responsible for 5,000 to 15,000 cases of lung cancer deaths each year in the United States.

As in the case of asbestos exposure, the risk of lung cancer among cigarette smokers is not merely additive; it is increased as a multiple. In other words one plus one does not equal two. With asbestos exposure, for instance, cigarette smoking increases the risk of cancer approximately ten fold over the risk of simple exposure to asbestos. Many individuals who develop lung cancer would not do so if they had been exposed only to asbestos, and not to cigarette smoke additionally. The same statement can be made regarding radon.

The risk of lung cancer results primarily from breakdown products of radon gas, chiefly polonium. When these particles are inhaled into the lungs they are deposited there and they produce radiation damage to the nucleus of the cells, which can result in cancer. We do not have enough data or experience to predict accurately how frequently this will occur in exposed individuals. We do have data for the increased risk of lung cancer in uranium miners. Their exposure levels are ten times as high as that seen in most of the homes that were evaluated, however. One worrisome fact is the great amount of time that is spent in the home compared with that on the job.

Radon gas seeps into the home from the earth beneath and can accumulate to a dangerous level. This seepage can be minimized by appropriate construction techniques. It also has found its way into homes as a result of building materials when radon-producing ore was used as aggregate for concrete. Phosphate slag, which emits radon gas as well as other radioactive particles such as polonium, was used in the concrete foundation of homes in southwestern Idaho from 1962 to 1977.

Mining of phosphate rock has long been a major industry in Florida. Thousands of homes in that state have been built over the tailings of these mining operations, on reclaimed land. High levels of radon gas have been measured in these homes. Several thousand houses were also built over uranium tailings from mining activities in Grand Junction, Colorado. Other states where a high probability of radon gas exists, besides Pennsylvania, New Jersey and New York are Idaho, Maine, New Hampshire, North Carolina, Wisconsin, Massachusetts, Connecticut, California and Wyoming.

The presence of radon gas can be detected with appropriate measuring devices. Many laboratories and organizations throughout the United States offer radon test kits for under $35. These test kits primarily use activated charcoal filters. The charcoal filter is left in place, usually in the basement, for several weeks. A minimum period is required for an accurate reading, and this time depends upon the type of measuring device. The basement and the house must be kept closed during the measuring period, and winter is the best time to conduct these assessments. The filter is then sent to the laboratory for an estimation of the radon level. If the screening device indicates that a significant radon level exists, a more definitive measurement can then be made at a cost of $50 to $75. State and local health departments can help in locating reliable laboratories that offer this service. As might be expected, some unqualified, unscrupulous individuals are attempting to make money from this latest scare.

Screening for radon in the home is certainly advisable in areas where the potential for accumulation exists. Health officials in many states have undertaken studies to determine exactly where this risk occurs, but these have been completed in only a few areas. Your health department should be able to advise you whether of not your house is sitting over likely strata. The only solution to the problem in a home constructed over such a hazard is special ventilation systems and a heat exchanger that together conserve up to 80 percent of the heated or cooled indoor air. The cost for these is $1,000 to $2,000.

Plugging all cracks in basements, foundations and floors and around all pipes helps to reduce radon infusion and should be the first step. An airtight cover for sump pumps should be installed at the same time. Ventilation systems can then be considered if levels still measure high. In new construction many measures such as a polyvinyl barrier underneath the ground floor and a subslab ventilation system reduce radon intrusion. Radon mitigation techniques should be a part of the planning of all new homes in areas where a risk exists.

1. CDC. Carbon monoxide levels in indoor tractor-pull events—Manitoba, Canada. *MMWR* 1990;**39**:743-745.

2. CDC. Carbon monoxide levels during indoor sporting events — Cincinnati, 1992-1993. *MMWR* 1994;**43**:21-23.

3. CDC. Unintentional carbon monoxide poisoning from indoor use of pressure washers — Iowa, January 1992–January 1993. *MMWR* 1993;**42**:777-785.

4. Clayton Environmental Consultants. Controlling Microbial Contamination to Prevent Building-Related Illness and Remediation Costs. **15**(2), July 1993.

5. Clayton Environmental Consultants. Microbial Contamination in Buildings: Precautions During Remediation Activities. **15**(3), October 1993.

6. CDC. Sustained transmission of nosocomial Legionnaires Disease — Arizona and Ohio. *MMWR* 1997;**46**:416-421.

7. Nemery B, Hoet PHM, Nemmar A. The Meuse Valley fog of 1930: an air pollution disaster. *Lancet* 2001;**357**:704-708.

8. Amdur MO. Air pollutants. In: Amdur MO, Doull J, Klaassen CD, eds. Casarett & Doull's toxicology; The basic science of poisons. New York: Pergamon, 1991;854-871.

9. Environmental Quality: 21st Annual Report of the Council on Environmental Quality. U.S. Government Printing Office, Washington, D.C., 1991. 311.

10. *National Geographic*, April 1989, p.411.

VII

HAZARDS OF PETS AND OTHER ANIMALS

A physician cannot make a diagnosis unless he first thinks of the disease.   — Osler

Zoonoses: Diseases transmitted from animals to humans

TOXOPLASMOSIS

This is one of the most serious of all of the zoonoses by virtue of its impact on the unborn child. Infection in the mother during pregnancy may result in spontaneous abortion, stillbirth or premature birth. Infection is transmitted through the placenta to the infant in about one-third of the cases where active infection is present in the mother. The mother may have no outward evidence of the disease; symptoms are noticeable in only about 10 to 20 percent of these cases. The diagnosis is never made in 80 to 90 percent of toxoplasmosis infections. Blood tests (serological, antibody tests) will reveal active disease after it has been present for a time, but these are seldom considered in the absence of symptoms. Blindness and severe mental retardation in the newborn may result, and since the cause of these misfortunes is obscure, this infection is usually not related to it then.

Inflammation of the retina and the choroid of the eye leading to loss of vision is most often the result of toxoplasmosis acquired from the mother through the placenta prior to birth. Thirty-five percent of the cases of such inflammation and visual loss in children and young adults are acquired in this fashion. Frequently the disease appears later in life as a delayed reaction to congenitally acquired toxoplasmosis. Strabismus (cross-eyed) may be an early sign of this affliction. Approximately one fourth of young adults test positive for toxoplasmosis.

Toxoplasmosis is caused by *Toxoplasma gondii*, a protozoan parasite that can survive and multiply only within living cells. After the cysts are ingested the active forms of the organism (trophozoites) are released in the gastrointestinal tract. From here they travel through the blood and lymphatics to virtually any tissue or organ in the body where they invade the cells and multiply therein. They are especially common in the brain, heart and skeletal muscle. In most healthy individuals the body's immune system eventually controls the infection and the organism forms cysts within the cells. In this respect the disease resembles tuberculosis. Each cyst contains thousands of the active forms (trophozoites) which may lie dormant within the cells for years.

At some point in life, perhaps when the defense mechanisms of the body are compromised, the cyst may rupture, releasing the trophozoites which initiate active disease. These active forms cannot survive or multiply outside of the host cell, and thus cannot be cultured in the laboratory by customary means. They can be demonstrated by injecting infected body tissue into the peritoneum of a mouse. After a period of proliferation within the cells of the human host, the trophozoites rupture the cell wall and are dispersed through the blood and lymphatics to infect other cells, where the process is repeated.

Occasionally the body's defense mechanisms are not successful in controlling the infection and inflammation of the brain, heart and lungs occur which may be fatal. Inflammation in the eye threatens vision. This outcome is particularly likely in individuals whose immune systems are compromised by diseases such as leukemia, Hodgkin's disease, AIDS or by medications such as those that are given to organ transplant patients and cortisone.

The cat and other felines such as mountain lions are the only animals in which this disease can reproduce, and they are the only animals that transmit it directly to humans. Toxoplasmosis cannot be transmitted directly from one human to another except through the placenta to the unborn child. The oocysts are passed in the feces of the cat, and these are then transmitted to humans through food, hands or inhalation of dust from a litter box. Children frequently acquire the oocysts from playing in a sandbox where cats have deposited feces. The oocysts may also be transmitted to food by insects such as flies and cockroaches.

Toxoplasmosis can be acquired by eating improperly cooked beef or pork (another good reason to assure proper cooking of all meat). The oocysts from cat feces are much more infective, however. One large outbreak in British Columbia in 1995 resulted from contamination of the public water supply by cats and cougars.[1]

The disease also can be transmitted through blood transfusion; the organisms survive for 50 days in refrigerated blood. Toxoplasmosis is present worldwide except on a few islands in the Pacific where no cats exist.

Symptoms, when they are present, are vague and may mimic mononucleosis. These symptoms may persist or recur for months. When inflammation of the heart or brain occurs it carries a significant morbidity and even death. In one case a realtor who cleaned out an old farmhouse developed a severe myocarditis (inflammation of the heart muscle) two weeks later and died as a result of toxoplasmosis. Currently approximately one in every one thousand newborn infants is congenitally infected. This is eighteen times the incidence of phenylketonuria and four times the incidence of muscular dystrophy, but thus far this disease has failed to attract the attention of the fundraisers and the politicians.

There is no successful treatment to eradicate the organisms once they have entered the body. A combination of pyrimethamine and sulfadiazine is effective against the active forms (trophozoites) of Toxoplasma gondii, but this regimen is completely ineffective against the cysts in the tissues. Potentially serious side effects exist when this therapy is used. While we have effective and safe antibacterial agents to treat some bacterial infections, in general we have had far less success in developing comparable agents for protozoan and other parasitic infections. No therapy is available for the treatment of the cysts in the tissues and they persist, to erupt into active infection at a later date.

Having cats in the home presents a significant health threat. Where cats are kept indoors extreme care should be taken in handling litter boxes, and dust levels should be controlled scrupulously. Cats and litter boxes should never exist indoors during pregnancy. Where cats exist outdoors, hands should be washed carefully after gardening. Cats should be denied access to sandboxes by covers, and children should be indoctrinated in the art of hand washing. Inhalation of dust carrying the cysts is much more difficult to avoid. Recalling the extent of the spread of pinworm ova by dust in the household, it is easy to appreciate the difficulty of controlling this disease. In the case of pinworms, this means of transmission is so efficient that eighty percent of the members of the household become infested when one child brings it home. The obscure nature of toxoplasmosis infection is unfortunate in that it is recognized so infrequently.

CAT SCRATCH DISEASE

Ninety percent of the 20,000 some cases of this disease that occur annually in the United States follow a scratch by a cat or intimate contact with a cat. It is usually a self-limiting disease with none of the serious consequences of toxoplasmosis. However, in 1994 five children in Florida were hospitalized with encephalitis that was discovered to be caused by *Bartonella* (formerly *Rachalimaea*) *henselae*, the causative agent of cat scratch disease.[2] Although all five children recovered, these were serious illnesses characterized by seizures and coma. The disease had been contracted by handling stray kittens; no bite or scratch could be identified. In view of the inability to identify the causative organism in cat scratch disease until recently, it is impossible to say how many such cases have gone undiagnosed in the past. More recently endocarditis, bacillary angiomatosis and infections of the eye and central nervous system have been attributed to the cat-scratch disease organism.[3]

Positive classification of *Bartonella henselae* was elusive, due to the difficulty in culturing it. Studies in 1995 isolated two closely related bacteria, *Afipia felis* and *B. henselae*, from lymph nodes of patients suffering from cat scratch disease.[4] Identification of these organisms was made possible by new DNA testing techniques utilizing the polymerase chain reaction (PCR) test described in Chapter XI. It is now generally accepted that *B. henselae* is the causative agent of cat scratch disease.

In most cases a small erythematous papule that resembles an insect bite is noticed within 3 to 10 days after the scratch. This papule fails to appear in as many as 40 percent of individuals, however. Enlargement of the regional lymph nodes draining the site of the scratch develops within 2 weeks. Microscopically these nodes are similar in appearance to those seen in tularemia, brucellosis and mycobacterial (TB) infections. The enlarged nodes may be quite painful, and surgical drainage is required to relieve this pain in about 10 to 20 percent of the cases. Fever and malaise are usually mild but may persist for two to three weeks. Although several antibiotics are currently used, the optimal treatment regime has not been determined.

A skin test has been used in the past, but since this is derived by aspiration of lymph nodes from individuals with the disease, it carries the risk of transmission of the various types of hepatitis, AIDS and other viral diseases, and has been discontinued. An immunofluorescent antibody test is 95 percent accurate, but currently this is available in few clinical laboratories. A PCR test can identify the organisms, but is not generally available yet.

Heat applied to the enlarged lymph nodes provides some pain relief. There has been no consistent improvement with any antibiotic, possibly because of the defective cell wall that is characteristic in Bartonella. Most cases are self-limiting, but when encephalitis ensues antibiotic therapy becomes more urgent. Ciprofloxicin is currently recommended, although doxycyline has enjoyed some success in eliminating the organism from cats. Cats acquire these organisms from the soil and carry them in their mouths and claws for long periods of time, usually without any symptoms of disease.

LEISHMANIASIS

This protozoan infection is not transmitted in the United States, but is common in Central and South America, as well as Africa and the Mediterranean countries, India, Russia and China. Approximately 12 million people who live in those regions have leishmaniasis. The disease is transmitted to man by female sandflies, which are quite small, 1.5 to 2.5 mm. in length. There are over 600 species of phlebotomine sandflies (Old World sandflies). The female sandfly acquires the protozoan parasites by feeding on rodents that harbor them in their blood. The parasites undergo cyclical changes in the gut of the sandfly before becoming infective.

One or more blood meals is necessary for the development of each batch of eggs by the sandfly, thus assuring transmission of the protozoan to another host and continuation of the cycle. This process is very similar to that in the mosquito in the transmission of some viral and protozoan infections. Eradication of colonies of gerbils near villages by using picrotoxin has helped to control the disease in some areas, but domestic dogs may also be a source.

Visceral leishmaniasis or kala-azar is also labeled Dumdum Fever. The protozoan parasite is deposited in the skin by the bite of a sandfly, where it may produce a small hard nodule (granuloma). The organisms then invade the bloodstream, and settle in the liver, spleen, bone marrow and lymph nodes, where they reproduce. They produce fever, an enlarged spleen and liver, emaciation and suppression of the production of all forms of blood cells (red blood cells and white blood cells). These symptoms generally do not appear for 3 months.

Visceral leishmaniasis was seen in members of the U.S. armed forces who had been sent to the Persian Gulf in 1991, but was not recognized until after they had returned home. Through December 1991 seven male members of the armed forces were diagnosed at Walter Reed Army Hospital as having the disease. The parasite was cultured from bone marrow aspirates in all seven. The fatality rate is 90 percent in untreated individuals, 10 percent with treatment. Bacterial secondary infections are common.

The diagnosis of leishmaniasis is made by biopsy of lymph nodes or by bone marrow aspiration where the parasite can be demonstrated. Needle biopsy of the spleen or the liver also would show the organisms but this procedure is not recommended due to the risk of hemorrhage. Skin lesions if present may also be biopsied. A blood (agglutination) test has been developed recently and is positive early. Drugs are available for treatment, but as with all parasite infections they are toxic. Antimony compounds, which must be administered intravenously, have been the classical treatment. A very recent study has demonstrated that allopurinol, which is taken orally and which has been used in gout for many years, is equally effective in the South American cutaneous forms of the disease. It is also much less expensive.[5]

In the cutaneous (skin) form of leishmaniasis the protozoan is again deposited in the skin. With this form it usually does not spread to internal organs. It produces a granulomatous lesion that may become quite large, 1 cm or more. Frequently multiple such lesions are seen on the face, nose, ears, (where they cause considerable destruction) and other areas that are not covered by clothing, such as the hands, arms and legs. The disease also may involve the eyes. The lesions bear a remarkable resemblance to leprosy. They usually ulcerate in the center, and are infectious, with spread of the disease to one's self and to others. The organisms also may be transmitted to dogs in this manner. A number of different species exist in both the Old World (Europe, Africa and Asia) and New World (the Americas). Through December 1991 the cutaneous form of leishmaniasis had been diagnosed in 16 military personnel who had served in Operation Desert Storm.

Spontaneous healing is common in the Old World disease, but not in the lesions of the New World variety. The protozoan is harbored in burrowing rodents, such as gerbils. It also has become well established in domestic dogs, accounting for the widespread extent of the disease even in large cities. The disease is widespread in Brazil, Venezuela and the Dominican Republic. Residents of these regions do not develop cell-mediated immunity. Direct injection of medication into the skin lesions is effective in controlling them.

Some control of the disease has been noted in areas where extensive spraying for mosquito control has been undertaken to prevent other infections such as malaria and dengue fever. These results have been dramatic sometimes. There is no prophylactic medication to prevent the disease. The use of insect repellents and fine netting while sleeping are the only preventative measures that a traveler can take.

SANDFLY FEVER
The troops deployed to the Arabian Peninsula during the Gulf war in 1991 also experienced sandfly fever (3-day fever). Sandfly fever is caused by a virus that also is transmitted by female phlebotomine sandflies. As is the case with leishmaniasis, the sandflies acquire the infectious agent (virus) from rodents, specifically gerbils in the Arabian Peninsula. The virus can also be transmitted directly from humans to humans by the sandfly, however. Recent evidence suggests that the sandfly itself transmits the virus from one generation to the next through its eggs, and thus serves as a reservoir as well as a vector. This sandfly is common in urban settings and is small enough to be able to penetrate ordinary screening. Very fine mosquito netting, 25 to 30 mesh (holes per inch), is required to prevent access by the sandfly. Insect repellents are also effective in protecting people from the fly. Insecticides should be used to eradicate the sandfly in dwellings, sheds and at dumps where it feeds and propagates. Although DDT

is still used in some regions, other newer insecticides are probably preferable, albeit more expensive.

Sandflies usually feed at night, and unless the individual develops a sensitivity reaction to the bite, there is no awareness of having been attacked. Onset of the disease occurs 3 to 5 days after the bite, with fever of 100 to 105°F, headache, aching in muscles and joints, neck stiffness, photophobia with pain upon motion of the eyes and vomiting. A pronounced congestion with redness of the face and neck give the appearance of sunstroke. Although the symptoms appear severe, the disease is self-limiting, lasting for 3 days in most victims. Severe fatigue may persist for weeks, and the symptoms may recur 2 to 10 weeks later. Meningitis may also accompany the disease. No fatalities from sandfly fever have ever been recorded although many thousands of people have been victims of the disease.

Personnel stationed in the Gulf region were also exposed to both epidemic (classic, European, louse-borne) typhus and murine (endemic, rat-flea-borne) typhus fever. Q fever is endemic in western Saudi Arabia, so this risk was also present. Brucellosis from raw milk was another risk in Saudi Arabia.

RINGWORM

Ringworm gets its name from its appearance, not its causative agent. It is a fungus infection of the skin, caused by a variety of different species. It is frequently transmitted to humans from dogs and cats. The infection is seen more frequently in children because of their close contact with animals. The disease may not be readily apparent on the pet. Successful treatment requires attention to the pet as well as to the human, otherwise recurrent infections will be noted. Ringworm, as with bacterial infections, may also be transmitted to the pet from humans.

The diagnosis should be established by a physician through scrapings from the afflicted area placed under the microscope or by culture or both. Cure is accomplished by the application of one of the very effective antifungal creams such as Monistat-Derm,® Micatin® or Tinactin®. These may be combined with sulfur, and sometimes salicylic acid, to increase effectiveness. It is a misconception that these infections cannot be cured. Treatment must be persistent, adequate and continued for several weeks. Failure is usually the result of reinfection from the animal or failure to pursue treatment diligently and long enough. Failure to treat the animal will almost certainly result in reinfection of the child.

BACTERIAL INFECTIONS

Several infections caused by bacteria may be transmitted either from humans to pets or vice versa, as has been seen with impetigo. Dogs and cats have been identified as the reservoir of recurrent streptococcal throat infections in children. It may not be mere coincidence that the upsurge in the number of cases of rheumatic fever in recent years has paralleled the explosion in the dog and cat population. The practice of kissing animals greatly increases the chances of children acquiring streptococcal infections and other diseases from animals. Some parasitic infections can also be acquired in this fashion and they are much more difficult to cure than are bacterial infections.

The case of the infant who was hospitalized with meningitis that was caused by *Pasteurella multicida* as a result of the parents deliberately having the pet dog lick his face is discussed in Chapter III. Many cases of meningitis and infection in the blood of young children result from contact with the pet saliva as occurred in this case. In another case a healthy 31 year old man developed Ludwig's angina, a serious life threatening infection of the jaw and floor of the mouth, after being licked in the face by a friend's dog.[6] The practice of permitting dogs to lick the face, which has become very common in our poorly educated society, is extremely unwise.

The *Salmonella* species of bacteria is the most common cause of food poisoning in the United States, and *Salmonella typhimurium* is the second most common strain, behind *S. enteritidis*. *Salmonella typhimurium* frequently infects cats when they eat raw food scraps (cattle, sheep, pigs and poultry all harbor the organism) or rodents. Once infected the cat sheds the organism from its mouth and in its feces for at least 2 to 3 months. The infection is then transmitted to humans either from their feces, their fur (from grooming) or from contaminated claws (burying feces). This infection has become more serious recently because this bacterium has become resistant to most of the antibiotics that were formerly effective against it. During 1999 *S. typhimurium* infections in individuals that were acquired from cats were reported to health departments in three different states. In each case the organisms were resistant to all of the antibiotics that have been used in the past.[7]

CREEPING ERUPTION

This parasitic disease results from hookworm (Ancylostoma braziliense) infestation in the dog or cat. The ova in the feces of the dog or cat are deposited in the soil where they hatch. The larvae then penetrate the skin when humans sit or lie on the ground. The migration of the larvae in the skin produces a winding, erratic trail as well as marked itching. The larvae do not reproduce in humans, and thus they produce no disease in man other than the burrowing in the skin. This can go on for several weeks or months, however. In the case of a single or few larvae, freezing the area that contains the larvae will solve the problem. If multiple larvae are present giving ivermectin by mouth will eliminate them. On rare occasions an intestinal infection is seen in humans.

ROUNDWORMS

Toxocara are common intestinal infestations of both dogs and cats. Here again the ova in the feces are deposited in the soil. Sandboxes are a particularly popular site for this sport among cats. After humans swallow the ova they hatch in the intestine, penetrate the intestinal wall and spread to any portion of the body. They especially invade the liver, lung, eye and nervous system (brain). They may live for many months, producing hemorrhage, scarring and sensitization as they migrate. Children up to about 5 years of age are more prone to acquire this infestation due to their undisciplined sanitary habits and frequent close contact with pets. Fatalities that have occurred usually have resulted from involvement of the heart or brain. Difficulty with vision, development of crossed eyes and pain in the eye heralds involvement in that organ. A simple blood count will reveal a marked increase in the percentage of eosinophils (greater than 60, normal is up to 4). There is no effective treatment.

Ascaris lumbricoides is another roundworm with a cycle similar to toxocara. This worm, however, is passed from one human to another, again in the feces. It may be acquired from raw vegetables that have been contaminated with human feces. Young children who have not entirely mastered the discipline of the toilet may also deposit the eggs in their feces in the sandbox or the soil. These eggs can survive for long periods in this setting, up to six years, even surviving winters. Other children playing in the sandbox or soil, pick up the eggs on their fingers, especially under the nails, and then deposit them in their mouths, as children are prone to do.

After they are swallowed, the eggs hatch and the larva migrate through the wall of the small intestine. They are then carried through the lymphatics and bloodstream to the lungs. There the larvae travel up the bronchi to the throat where they are swallowed. They grow into mature worms in the small intestine where they feed and discharge eggs.

In heavy infestations obstruction of the intestine can occur, especially in children. Not infrequently an adult worm is passed in the stool and occasionally one is seen in vomitus. The adult worms are large (15 to 30 cm. in length) and resemble an earthworm, from which they get their name. In the intestine they impair absorption of food and other nutrients, and may cause malnutrition. In their migration the larvae can wind up in the bile or pancreatic ducts and cause obstruction. More serious is when they migrate to the brain, carrying the bacteria from the intestine and causing an abscess. Such an infection is very serious and death can ensue.

Although ascariasis is primarily a disease of warmer climates, eggs deposited in northern states by visitors can survive even through winter. It is therefore not uncommon to see this infestation in northern states. About 2 million Americans have acquired ascariasis; 25% of the world's population have it. Few deaths result in the United States, but about 20,000 people die each year of ascariasis outside of the U.S. Medication is available that is effective in eradicating the worms from the intestine, but it is not effective against worms lodged or encysted elsewhere. Re-infestation may also occur from ingestion of eggs deposited previously by the treated individual, or from eggs passed by other family members who have not been treated.

LEPTOSPIROSIS

This is the most widespread zoonosis in the world, and has been reported in every region of the United States. It is caused by a spirochete, the same type of bacterium that causes syphilis, yaws and Lyme disease. It can be carried by virtually every animal species, including the rat, dog, cat, fox, raccoon, skunk, cow and pig, and is shed in the urine. It is by this mechanism that it contaminates streams and farm ponds. The animals may have no sign of disease and yet may shed the organism in the urine for years.

Swimming in contaminated bodies of water or riding motorcycles through contaminated pools of water has accounted for a significant number of cases. It may be acquired through skin abrasions or through the conjunctiva of the eye during these activities. Most cases are acquired by ingestion of food or water contaminated by urine from the cat, dog, mouse, rat, cow or pig. An outbreak of severe disease occurred in Baltimore, Maryland in 1996 among three individuals who had been exposed to rat urine in alleys.[8] This is another of the many hazards that the homeless population faces. During that same year at least nine members of an expedition that engaged in white water rafting in Costa Rica suffered an infection with leptospirosis. In 1995 an epidemic in Nicaragua that was associated with pulmonary hemorrhage involved 2,000 persons. Both of these latter two outbreaks occurred after heavy flooding.[9]

The severity of the disease varies considerably, depending on the serotype of the leptospira and on the age of the victim. Fatalities may occur in one half of individuals past the age of fifty years. The organism can affect virtually any organ in the body, including the liver, the kidneys and the meninges (lining) of the brain. Jaundice indicates a more serious inflammation of the liver and thus a more serious illness. Death can result from failure of either the liver or kidneys. Recovery may take months in untreated survivors.

The most important single prophylactic measure is to avoid swimming in ponds, particularly those shared with cattle or pigs. It is also wise to avoid areas with significant rat populations, an increasing problem in some cities. Precautions are especially urgent during pregnancy.

SCHISTOSOMIASIS

Schistosoma in humans are blood flukes (parasites) that may cause bleeding and inflammation in the urinary bladder, diarrhea when they invade the intestines and cirrhosis of the liver. They are acquired as a result of swimming, wading or bathing in waters that have been contaminated by the feces or urine of an infected individual. The eggs so deposited are processed by fresh water snails, the intermediate host, where they develop into free swimming cercaria. These then penetrate the skin of humans and are carried to the liver where they mature. The adult worms then migrate to the veins of the urinary bladder or intestine.

Three different species of schistosoma account for most of the disease, and are found in most of the warm climates of the world. These include Africa, the Middle East, South America, South China, Indochina, the Philippines, Thailand, Laos, and Puerto Rico. Successful treatment is difficult, and there is none for the liver fibrosis and other complications.

Schistosoma that infest various migratory birds are responsible for swimmers itch, cercaria dermatitis. This is caused by the penetration of the skin by larval forms of these blood flukes (schistosoma). Humans acquire the disease by wading or swimming in bodies of water that are frequented by ducks, geese and some shore birds. Snails are also required in the same body of water to serve as intermediate hosts to complete the cycle for the birds. Man is an end host, and the cercariae from birds never invade other organs of man after penetration of the skin, and do not mature in humans. In the United States the Great Lakes and some of the coastal waters of California are the most common source of this affliction. The disease is self-limiting, but sensitization can result from repeated exposures, in which case the itching can be intense.

TULAREMIA

Also called rabbit fever or deer fly fever, this is a bacterial infection caused by *Francisella (Pasteurella) tularensis*. It is most commonly acquired by humans while handling rabbits, usually in the process of dressing them. Disposable gloves should always be worn when performing this operation, and the hands should be washed carefully afterwards. The organism can penetrate intact skin. Special precautions should be taken in any circumstance where the rabbit appears ill. Infections have occurred in humans when sick rabbits were assumed to have been poisoned by pesticides. Infection has been acquired similarly by inhalation from poking or stepping on a dead animal. The organism is highly infectious and is easily contracted by airborne aerosols. This is one of a handful of agents that have been cultivated for germ warfare. Rabbits are made ill by and die from this disease.

Indirect transmission from rabbits to humans has resulted from the bite of a pet animal as well as by the bite of the deer fly, tick or even mosquito. Use of an effective insect repellent will discourage insect bites and wearing a hat as well will tend to discourage the deer fly (see insect repellents in Chapter VIII). Cases resulting from insect bites are seen more frequently in the spring and summer, whereas cases resulting from contact with rabbits are seen more frequently during the hunting season. Squirrels, deer and other mammals also serve as a reservoir for the organism and thus can transmit the disease.

Pneumonia is a serious form of this disease. Mortality is low if adequately treated for a sufficient length of time. This disease usually confers lifelong immunity. Only 214 cases were reported in 1987, 152 cases in 1990, 193 cases in 1991, down from the peak of 2,291 cases reported in 1939. Education of the hunting public has had much to do with this decline. Gloves should always be worn when handling any animal.

SALMONELLA INFECTIONS (Intestinal)

Several species of *Salmonella* cause gastrointestinal infections in humans, resulting in diarrhea, abdominal cramping and fever (see also Chapter V). Baby chicks, ducks and turtles transmit these organisms. Virtually all birds and reptiles, including iguana, carry *Salmonella*. Iguanas are the latest pet discovery, and their mark has already been felt. In 1998 a healthy 5-month-old boy in Wisconsin died suddenly at home from Salmonella septicemia contracted from a pet iguana in the home. Additional cases of serious *Salmonella* infections acquired from pet iguanas in the home had been reported in 1996 and 1997.[10] Reptiles, including iguanas, are totally inappropriate as pets, and have no place in the home.

Parakeets can transmit salmonella as well as the *Chlamydia psittaci* organism of psittacosis. Pet turtles produced approximately 14 percent of the estimated two million cases per year of salmonella infection in the early 1970s. A ban on pet turtles went into effect in 1975 and cases reported as a result of handling them became rare. Outbreaks continue to occur in other countries where such a ban does not exist. Sporadic cases continue to be reported in the United States also.

In June 1986, a two-year-old and his four-year-old brother developed an acute salmonella infection with fever, abdominal pain and bloody diarrhea after their mother had purchased a turtle that had been sold illegally at a local pet store in Ohio. Turtles carry a very high rate of salmonella contamination. Infections have been spread to humans through handling of the turtles and by emptying the turtle's water into the sink, where dishes were contaminated. No method of controlling this organism in the turtle has been devised, and these reptiles also have no place in the home.

During the spring of 1991 sixteen cases of salmonella infection in Connecticut, Maryland and Pennsylvania were traced to pet ducklings that were kept in the home.[11] Fourteen cases were reported in Ohio during this same period.[12] It is unlikely that any state escaped this annual Easter tradition of buying pet chicks and ducks for children. The animals frequently do not survive the experience. The "Bambi syndrome" gets much more reinforcement through television and Hollywood than does public health and hygiene education.

The symptoms of salmonella infection included fever, nausea, vomiting, abdominal cramping and bloody diarrhea. In some homes the ducklings were allowed to run free, in one home it lived in the bathtub where the children bathed. Young ducklings and chicks frequently contaminate bedding, clothing and food bowls, as well as the hands of children, with salmonella. One mother of an infected 3-month-old infant that she was breast-feeding admitted that she did not wash her hands after handling the ducklings. We might expect this behavior from children, but adults should know better. Many do not. Some states have passed legislation prohibiting or discouraging the sale of baby chicks and ducklings as pets. Ohio has such a law. The laws are easy to circumvent, however, and people readily do so. Baby chicks and ducklings are not appropriate household pets.

Salmonella infections acquired from cats, the most common pet in American households, was discussed previously under bacterial infections.

PSITTACOSIS

Psittacosis is an infection in the lungs of birds that is caused by a bacterium, *Chlamydia psittaci*. Most cases evolve from parrots or parakeets, but it can be contracted from pigeons or even chickens. It causes a pneumonitis (inflammation in the lungs) in humans. The incidence has fluctuated considerably since 1930 (170 cases, 33 deaths) in concert with the variation in control measures. Routine quarantine and treatment of imported birds has reduced the incidence of the disease in the general public, but the incidence among poultry raisers and processors has been increasing. In 1986, 224 cases were reported to the Centers for Disease Control. The number of cases reported has remained at about 100 per year since.

Smuggling of parrots from South America into the United States has reached almost epidemic proportions recently. The birds bring a price of as much as $10,000 in the U.S. It is suspected that many cases of psittacosis are simply treated and not reported. Such practice is encouraged by the fact that the disease is readily treatable with antibiotics. Transmission is accomplished by the inhalation of dust contaminated by the excrement, feathers or nasal secretions of an infected bird. Symptoms in humans resemble other pneumonias, and may be moderate to severe. Heart involvement occurs on occasion. Treatment should be instituted early in the course of the disease to improve chances of recovery.

Studies published in the British Medical Journal reported that people who kept birds for one to five years doubled their chances of developing lung cancer. Those who kept birds for ten years or longer tripled their risk. The cancer may be the result of the inhalation of dust from feathers and other sources, from fungi in the bottom of the cage, from an unidentified virus, or a combination of these.[13,14,15]

HISTOPLASMOSIS

Histoplasmosis is a fungal disease of the lungs caused by *Histoplasma capsulatum*, that resembles tuberculosis in many ways. It is acquired by inhaling dust contaminated by the droppings of pigeons, starlings, bats and chickens. The organism survives best in moist soil, which may account for its distribution. It has been found chiefly in the Ohio and Mississippi River valleys, in a broader range than was previously believed. It is found extending into lower to central Michigan, for instance, including the Ann Arbor area.

Histoplasmosis infections in groups of individuals have occurred among children playing under a tree on a school yard in which starlings roosted, while exploring caves where bats resided, after bulldozing of infected areas and after cleaning of dirt-floored chicken coops. It also has been contracted while harvesting firewood from a tree where infected birds roosted.

Most cases involve the lung, and as with tuberculosis, nodules are seen in the lungs on chest X-ray. The disease may spread to the liver and other parts of the body. Death or severe disability can result, but this is uncommon. An infection in the fundus of the eye, which presents a distinctive appearance upon examination, results in a loss of vision to varying degrees. Individuals who wear glasses normally have an eye exam every one to two years, and this should reveal any involvement. Individuals who have any of the exposures listed above should have a skin test to reveal any past or present infection. Individuals with a positive skin test, and indeed anyone with a significant exposure should have a careful eye exam. Almost all of the chronic progressive lung cases occur in cigarette smokers. Treatment is available for the progressive or disseminated cases, but the drugs are very toxic.

ANTHRAX

Anthrax is caused by *Bacillus anthracis*, a bacterium that is transmitted from animals to humans. It has been rare in the United States, as a result of constant surveillance and control measures such as vaccination of cattle and culling of infected herds. No cases were reported in the U.S. from 1992 to August 2000, when a case of cutaneous anthrax resulted from handling cattle that had died of the disease during a widespread epizootic in North Dakota.[16] Anthrax is endemic in many countries such as Turkey, where an average of 355 cases per year are reported. In China between 1990 and 1994 a total of 9,799 cases were reported, with 380 fatalities.[17]

Anthrax can be acquired from infected cattle, goats, sheep and horses. Most of the cases that do occur in the United States result from handling imported wool, hair, hides or bone meal for fertilizer. Woolsorter's disease is the inhalation form of this disease and it is highly fatal, most individuals dying within twenty-four hours in spite of treatment. No case of this had been reported in the U.S. since 1976 until October, 2000 when anthrax spores were deliberately delivered through the mail in Florida in an act of bio-terrorism, resulting in a fatality.[18,19] Several subsequent cases of inhalation anthrax with deaths, and cases of cutaneous anthrax in Florida and New York resulted from mailed anthrax spores. Q fever, discussed later in this chapter, is acquired in the same manner as inhalation anthrax.

The anthrax bacterium is one of several agents that have been used in developing germ warfare material. It was used in aerosolized form as a spray against the Chinese population when Japan invaded China in the 1930s.[20] It is a very effective and cheap means of eliminating large numbers of people. The spores of *B anthracis* are very difficult to eradicate from the environment, requiring intensive application of large amounts of 40 percent formaldehyde (formalin).[21] Every country that is interested in terrorism or conquest of people has long produced and stockpiled this agent. This includes not only the major powers, but also countries such as Iraq and Iran. This exposure was anticipated and prepared for in the Persian Gulf war, but exposure did not material-ize. We do know now that our troops there did suffer harmful biochemical exposures.

BRUCELLOSIS
Also known as undulant fever, this bacterial infection is caused by several species of brucella, and is transmitted from a wide variety of domestic animals, such as cattle, swine, goats and sheep. Human infection is most commonly acquired from consuming un-pasteurized milk and dairy products, a very risky practice. It can be acquired through abrasions of the skin when handling animals, however, and outbreaks have occurred among workers at meat processing plants. There is a greater incidence among dairy farmers and cattle breeders. This disease may be seen almost anywhere in the body, commonly in bone (osteomyelitis), the spleen, lung, genitourinary tract and heart.

Endocarditis (inflammation of the heart) is the most common cause of death. Treatment is difficult and success limited. About 150 to 200 cases are reported annually in the U.S., but again many cases go unreported. A vaccine for cattle is available, and where it has been used it has reduced the incidence of the disease significantly. The disease has been eradicated in some countries through strenuous control programs.

RABIES

Rabies is a viral disease of the central nervous system (brain and spinal cord) that affects all mammals. It is transmitted in the saliva of an infected animal, usually through a bite. It may be acquired also through a skin abrasion or by inhaling the virus in droplets. Four cases have resulted from corneal transplant operations where the donor had apparently died of undiagnosed rabies. The required immunization of dogs has greatly reduced the risk from domestic animals in the United States. Although about 7800 cases of rabies in animals is reported each year in the United States, the incidence of laboratory confirmed cases of rabies in dogs dropped from 6,949 cases in 1947 to 128 cases in 1988, and has remained at about that level since.

No such success has been achieved in cats, and the number of cases of rabies reported in cats each year now exceeds that reported in dogs. Today, cats represent the greatest danger among domesticated animals for the transmission of this deadly disease. The number of cases of rabies reported in wild animals had been about 4,500 per year through the 1980s, but that number has almost doubled from 1990 (4881) to the current level of about 8,000 (7853 in 1997). This increase has been largely due to the spread of rabies among raccoons in the northeastern United States. In 1995 of the 7,881 cases of rabies in wild animals reported to the CDC, about one-half were in raccoons.[22] Raccoons from the southeastern region of the U.S., where rabies has been established for years, were transported to the Mid-Atlantic States in the mid 1970s to replace hunting stock.

The first cases of rabies in raccoons in this region appeared in West Virginia in 1977. The disease then spread to Virginia in 1978, Maryland in 1981, Pennsylvania in 1982, Delaware in 1987, New Jersey in 1989, New York in 1990 and Connecticut in 1991.[23] Rabies is now firmly established in the raccoon population along the entire eastern seaboard from Florida to Connecticut. The first case in Ohio was reported in May 1996, 3 miles from the Pennsylvania border. Further expansion is inevitable, not only in Ohio but also throughout the Midwest. The large population of raccoons and their propensity to live in densely populated neighborhoods is a matter of some concern. Efforts are currently underway to develop techniques for delivering a newly developed oral rabies vaccine to wildlife populations such as raccoons.

In 1985, the National Association of State Public Health Veterinarians recommended laws requiring the vaccination of all cats. This recommendation has been reinforced periodically since that time, to no avail. Cat owners who ignore this responsibility risk the loss of their pet, but their neighbors risk a horrible death for their child. The risk of rabies transmission by cats has increased greatly in those regions now affected by the epidemic among raccoons. Continued removal of all stray dogs and cats is essential in controlling this dread and virtually 100 percent fatal disease. Although there are over one million animal bites in the United States each year, rabies in humans in this country is rare, with three reported deaths in 1984 and 1991, one death in each of 1989 and 1990, and four deaths in 1997.[24]

Many cases continue to occur outside of the United States. Fatalities probably are in excess of one thousand per year. In India 700,000 people are treated for rabies virus exposure every year. Worldwide more than one million people receive rabies vaccine annually.[25] This imposes an enormous financial burden on many countries that can ill afford it. The disease poses a serious threat when traveling to areas such as Africa, where rabies is common among wild dogs.

The primary reservoir in animals in the United States is the skunk, raccoon, bat and fox, in order of decreasing frequency. Rabid bats have been reported in every state except for Alaska and Hawaii and have caused at least 33 cases of rabies in humans in the United States through 2000.[26] Some deaths from rabies acquired from bats have occurred without any history of a bite. In some cases the only history was that of a bat being in the same room with the victim.[27] The bite or claw wound from a bat is so small that it frequently cannot be seen without magnification.[28] In every case where a bat is found in the same room with a person, post-exposure prophylaxis should be administered unless the bat is examined and found to be free of the rabies virus.[29]

The raccoon is a more recent addition to our risk, and is especially important since it increasingly is joining us in our neighborhoods. This makes it more imperative than ever to make certain that the rabies immunization of all pet dogs and cats is kept current. When traveling with these pets a current rabies vaccination certificate should be taken along.

The ideal procedure following a bite by any animal is the confinement and observation of that animal for ten days. If any illness or abnormal behavior develops in that period of time the brain of the animal should be examined by the health department for evidence of rabies. If the animal is alive and well after ten days, the odds are that it does not have rabies. Confining a wild animal, especially one exhibiting abnormal behavior, is very difficult and not without danger. Under these circumstances killing the animal and preserving the head is the next best course. The animal should be handled carefully with disposable vinyl or latex gloves. The hands should be washed carefully and thoroughly with soap and hot water when the task has been completed. It must be remembered also that rabies can be contracted by inhaling the virus.

In the event of an unprovoked bite by any wild animal, or by any animal exhibiting abnormal behavior, the head of the animal should be preserved (in a plastic bag in a freezer) and the local health department should be called immediately for instructions. Disposable vinyl or latex gloves should be worn while handling any such animals. A vaccine derived from human diploid cell, developed in 1987,[30] replaced the only vaccine available in the United States at that time. It requires five injections, in contrast to the fourteen daily injections previously required, and it provokes fewer reactions. It is highly effective if administered early and if rabies immune serum or globulin is given concomitantly.

In 1985 an additional vaccine that is derived from cells from rhesus monkeys was also approved.[31] A new rabies vaccine for both pre-exposure and post exposure prophylaxis in humans was approved in 1997. As with the original vaccine, it is derived from chick embryo, but purification techniques appear to have diminished the incidence of sensitization that caused reactions in the original rabies vaccine.[32] Rabies, once acquired, is 100 percent fatal. Prevention is the only hope.

Every animal bite should be treated immediately by a physician. Infections from these bites commonly include pasteurella species, but may also include many other orgnaisms not usually considered. Appropriate prophylaxis requires a combination of antibiotics rather than a single agent.[33] In the case of a rabid animal, proper treatment of the wound is an important and integral part of the prophylaxis. Decisions regarding treatment after a bite are complex and require careful professional judgement. A high index of suspicion is necessary to avoid tragedy.

In March 1995 a 4-year-old girl in Washington died of rabies 25 days after a bat had been found in her bedroom.[34] There had been no evidence that the child had been bitten and the bat was buried. Subsequent examination of the bat confirmed that it was the source of the rabies. The diagnosis was delayed until 2 days before the death in this case, during which time some 72 people were exposed and required prophylactic treatment. Rabies prophylaxis is now recommended after exposure to bats in a confined space such as a bedroom, even when there does not appear to have been a bite. There are no second chances with this disease, as it is 100 percent fatal if it is not successfully prevented.

Pre-exposure prophylaxis for rabies is available to individuals with a high degree of risk, such as veterinarians and laboratory workers. It is more complex than other immunizations such as tetanus, however, and it requires the measuring of antibody titers. This protection is not recommended routinely for travelers to areas where rabies is endemic. If someone is attending to business in the remote areas of Africa where no medical facility will be available without many days of travel, prophylactic immunization is probably advisable. Here again this requires experienced professional judgment.

TRICHINOSIS

This parasitic disease is acquired by eating inadequately cooked meat, virtually always pork, that contains encysted larvae of the roundworm, *Trichinella spiralis*. It is acquired most commonly from ready to eat pork sausage. A few cases have been reported in recent years from eating bear meat and wild boar. The pig usually becomes infected from eating raw garbage, although eating infected rats may be a source. The rats feed on raw pork scraps thus helping to maintain the cycle of infection. Laws requiring that garbage fed to pigs be cooked has markedly reduced the incidence of trichinosis in the United States. There has been an increase in the number of cases reported in the Northeastern states in recent years, primarily as a result of noncommercial farmers who are feeding raw garbage to pigs. Thichinosis is rare in France where swine are fed vegetable roots.

Once ingested, the encysted larvae are released in the stomach or duodenum by the digestive process. Diarrhea, abdominal pain and nausea may be experienced at this time, one to two days after ingestion. The larvae mature and mate. The female then burrows into the wall of the intestine where she discharges minute larvae. These are then carried throughout the body by the circulation. They invade and encyst in various muscles, including those of the diaphragm, tongue, eye, arms and legs. This invasion results in severe muscle aching. They may persist in this location in this form for five to ten years. When the larvae invade the brain symptoms of meningitis or encephalitis may appear, in which case the mortality may reach 10 percent. If inflammation of the heart muscle (myocarditis) ensues, the mortality may reach 20 percent.

A blood count will generally reveal 15 to 50 percent of eosinophils, compared to a normal of up to 4 percent. There is no means of eradicating the larvae from the body. Thiabendazole has been used against the parasites in the intestine, and mebendazole against those in the muscles, both with limited success. There is no cure for the inflammatory response evoked by the encysted parasites in the various organs.

Prevention is accomplished very simply by adequate cooking of meat. Particular care must be exercised when cooking pork in a microwave oven. An adequate internal temperature (170 degrees Fahrenheit), as measured with an accurate thermometer, must be reached to assure inactivation of the larva. All garbage fed to pigs must be cooked. This simple measure has already markedly reduced the incidence of this disease in the United States.

TAPEWORM

Taenia saginata, the beef tapeworm is widespread through out the world. The infective immature worm is present in the muscles of cattle. When the meat is eaten uncooked or inadequately cooked, the worm develops into an adult worm in the small intestine, where it may remain for as long as 30 years. The eggs passed in the feces of humans are not infective to other humans, but they are to cattle. When cattle consume the eggs in feed or water that has been contaminated by human waste the cycle is completed.

Symptoms in humans are usually minimal, with mild stomach discomfort, nausea and bloating. Weight loss and diarrhea may occur. The encased eggs are passed daily in the stool and sometimes can be seen on bedding or underclothing. This type of tapeworm cannot be diagnosed from these eggs; the "head" must be retrieved and examined for classification.

In a rare exception to parasitic infestations, a highly effective and relatively nontoxic drug is available for treatment. Recheck of the stool should be made at about 3 months to assure eradication of all of the parasites. Prevention lies in adequate cooking of all beef, which readily destroys the pathogen. Preventing contamination of cattle feeding stations by human feces helps to control that portion of the cycle of this parasite, and thus subsequent infection of humans.

Taenia solium, the pork tapeworm similarly is acquired by eating inadequately cooked meat ("measly pork"). The ingested egg or proglottid matures to an adult worm in the small intestine, where it attaches and may persist for 30 years or more. Unlike *Taenia saginata* where the eggs are infective only to cattle, the eggs of *Taenia solium* passed in human feces can reinfect the host or another person immediately. This may be accomplished by direct contact with feces or through contaminated food or water. Eggs have been found under the fingernails and on the skin and clothing of people who have a pork tapeworm. It may also occur through vomitus from an infected person. The eggs passed in human feces or vomitus can remain viable in the environment for months.

When these eggs are ingested by either man or pigs, the larva penetrate the wall of the intestine. They are transmitted through the lymphatics or blood stream to various organs and tissues of the body, frequently the eye, heart and brain, where they form cysts. The disease when these larval forms penetrate the intestine and invade other organs of the body is called cysticercosis. This disease is not acquired by eating infected pork; it is acquired only from eggs passed by a human who has the tapeworm. It is a far more serious disease than the tapeworm in the small intestine. Involvement in the brain can cause seizures, hydrocephalus or psychiatric disorders, and carries a relatively high fatality rate.

The same drug that is used for *Taenia saginata* (niclosamide) is also effective for removing adult *Taenia solium* from the intestine. This drug releases viable eggs in the intestine, however, that can then penetrate the intestinal wall and migrate throughout the body. This is not a threat with *Taenia saginata* because the eggs are infective only for cattle, not man. Some authorities administer a cathartic after drug therapy to speed up passage of the infective eggs from the body. Other drugs are effective at killing encysted organisms in the various organs, and this can present serious side effects, especially in the brain. These drugs should not be used when the eye has encysted organisms; these must be removed surgically.

Taenia solium is uncommon in the United States due to public health and sanitary standards, and proper handling of meat supplies. Infected pigs have been found in Colorado and New Mexico, however. It is common throughout most of the rest of the world, and is widely endemic in Latin America, Africa and Asia. It is commonly seen in immigrants to the United States, and increasing numbers of cases have been seen in the cities of California, Texas and Arizona that have immigrant populations. These people present a serious risk for the development of cysticercosis in people in the same household, or people who eat food handled by them. Cysticercosis is a serious disease.

Neurocysticercosis, invasion of the brain by the larval forms of the pork tapeworm, has been seen with increasing frequency in contacts and household members of immigrants from Asia, Africa and Latin America.[35] A California schoolteacher who ate a pork taco from a steet stand while in Mexico became ill for three weeks, then began to have seizures. She underwent brain surgery to remove a tapeworm larva.[36] This is a disease with serious consequences, that once more emphasizes the importance of hand washing after defecating and before eating and food handling. Unfortunately many foodhandlers, both at home and in restaurants, have little or no understanding of these risks.

Just as important is the proper handling and disposal of human wastes. Animals should never be permitted access to human waste. This disease, as well as others, is widely reinforced in countries where human waste is used for irrigation and fertilization. The true incidence of this problem in the United States is unknown because reporting it is not required. All immigrants from regions where it is endemic should be screened for the disease (a blood test is available) and treated, especially if they handle food for others.

DOG TAPEWORM

Dipylidium caninum infests the dog and cat, and may be suspected when the pet is observed dragging his bottom across the floor. The eggs deposited on the carpet in this manner are ingested by fleas, where they develop into infective larvae. These infective forms are then acquired by humans when they accidentally swallow the fleas. This may be done through food contaminated with the fleas, or by children crawling on the floor.

Once in the human intestine, the eggs hatch and set up housekeeping. This happens more frequently in children than in adults, and is usually not associated with any symptoms. The infestation is noted when motile proglottids (tapeworm segments) that are passed in the stool are seen around the anus or on the stool. Treatment for humans is available. Periodic de-worming of the pets and controlling fleas is the most effective means of preventing the disease. Humans on occasion may also be afflicted with the rat tapeworm in a similar manner by ingesting rat fleas. This also occurs more frequently in children.

MOSQUITOS

Throughout the history of mankind mosquitos have delivered more death and disease than any other insect. Diseases transmitted by mosquitos have killed more of the earth's human inhabitants than the combined total of all of the wars in history. In the United States we have been blessed to be spared most of these diseases and plagues. Some are being visited upon us now, however, and the list will grow. The increase in world travel by U.S. citizens accounts for the introduction of some of these diseases, immigration for some and international commerce for some. The latter is the mechanism by which the new mosquito strain, *Aedes albopictus*, was introduced into the U.S.

In the United States mosquitos are responsible for the transmission of the four types of encephalitis, California, eastern equine, western equine and St. Louis, all discussed below. In other parts of the world they have been the means of transmission of malaria. We seldom think of malaria as a disease that is likely to be encountered in the United States. Most of our citizens who have contracted this disease have done so in military service overseas or through foreign travel. Mosquito vectors capable of transmitting malaria do exist in California and Florida, however. During the summer of 1952 the California Department of Health recorded 35 cases of malaria localized in an area northeast of Sacramento.

These were the first cases of malaria contracted in the United States since 1945. Investigation revealed that 27 of the cases occurred in girls ages 9-19 who had been camping at Lake Vera under the sponsorship of the Campfire Girls. Lake Vera is a 15-acre artificial lake in the Sierra Nevada mountains northeast of Sacramento. It is blessed with an abundant mosquito population. Five additional cases of malaria were seen in staff members and a volunteer. Two permanent residents of the area also fell victim to the disease.

Additional investigation turned up a recently discharged marine who had returned from Korea in November 1951. He had suffered his first attack of malaria in April 1952 and was hospitalized at that time. He then spent the Fourth-of-July weekend (1952) at Lake Vera, and suffered a relapse of malaria while he was there. The four days that he spent at the camp was more than sufficient to inoculate the mosquito population. Twenty-six additional cases occurred during the following spring and summer, 1953. Intensive spraying of the area with DDT eradicated the mosquito reservoir of malaria.[37]

The next recorded episode of mosquito transmission of malaria in California occurred during the summer of 1986, when 26 cases were reported among migrant workers in a town on the coast of California, north of San Diego. Malaria was introduced into the mosquito population by an infected worker, and subsequently transmitted to other susceptible workers over a 3-month period.[38] Conditions in other states are also conducive to transmission of malaria by this mechanism when individuals carrying the parasite in their blood are in the area. This frequently is the case when migrant workers from Mexico or South America are employed.

There were no subsequent cases of malaria transmission in the United States until 1990, when one case was reported in Florida and one in California. Foreign travel, blood transfusions and IV drug abuse were ruled out as the source of infection in both individuals. Both cases apparently resulted from the bite of an Anopheles species of mosquito that had recently fed on an infected migrant worker nearby. That was the first such case in Florida since 1948. Transmission of malaria through this mechanism occurs periodically in California, as illustrated by the cases reported above.

Two cases of locally acquired malaria were identified in New Jersey in 1991. These cases were most likely transmitted from a recent immigrant from Honduras. Anopheline mosquitos capable of transmitting malaria are resident in that area. In 1995 a man in southeastern Michigan acquired malaria after sleeping outdoors at a campground. Anopheline mosquitos were recovered from the area of the camp.[39] The acquisition of malaria in these northern regions should alert us to a risk that we have not faced here since 1972. It has become more urgent than ever that we prevent attacks by mosquitos as outlined below.

The female Anopheles mosquito acquires the malaria protozoan parasite when it takes a blood meal from an infected host. The male form fertilizes the female form in the gut of the mosquito, producing zygotes. These progress to infective forms which migrate to the mosquito salivary gland from which they are injected into the next human victim that the mosquito feeds upon.

A similar active cycle in the mosquito is customarily associated with the other diseases that this arthropod transmits to man. Transmission of viruses such as those of encephalitis, yellow fever and dengue fever follow a similar pattern. The mosquito ingests the virus when feeding on an infected host. The virus invades the tissues of the mosquito after penetrating the wall of the gut or passing through it. The virus multiplies in these tissues, which include the salivary glands.

The mosquito must ingest a minimal quantity of the virus before such a multiplication process can take place, and this quantity varies for each viral disease. This is an important factor in the transmission of these diseases to man. These viruses persist in the mosquito throughout its life span, and thus survive in mosquitos that hibernate over the winter. A single *Culex tarsalis* mosquito may transmit Western equine encephalitis for up to 8 months. Culex-borne arboviruses can be similarly carried through the winter, but even without this feature the arrival of migrating birds to a given area can initiate a cycle of disease. Unlike *Aedes albopictus*, the majority of mosquitoes, including the Culex species (there are 800 known) attack their hosts at night. While most species require a blood meal to produce eggs, some culex species, such as *C. pipiens*, can lay one batch of eggs without having acquired blood.

Besides viral and protozoan diseases, mosquitos also transmit the white thread-like worm that causes filariasis. After the microfilaria is acquired from an infected host by the feeding mosquito, it bores through the intestinal wall of the mosquito and reproduces. The infective larvae then migrate to the proboscis of the mosquito where they are injected into humans. This parasitic disease is endemic in the warm moist regions of the world, including Africa, Asia, the Pacific Islands, Haiti and parts of South America. It is not transmitted to humans in the U.S. but residents traveling to those regions are at risk.

Another affliction transmitted by mosquitos to travelers to Mexico and Central and South America is myiasis by the human botfly. The adult female fly attaches her eggs to mosquitos. The eggs are then deposited on the skin of humans when the mosquito feeds. The larva in the egg then rapidly penetrates the skin in 5-10 minutes. It continues to develop there for six to twelve weeks, feeding on the tissue fluids. The larvae must be removed surgically, taking care not to leave any remnants.

In addition to the very efficient transmission of the diseases described above, the mouthparts of mosquitos that are contaminated by viruses as the result of feeding on infected hosts may serve to mechanically transmit those viruses to a noninfected human. It has been demonstrated in Africa that *Aedes aegyptii* can transmit the chikungunya virus (fever, rash and polyarthritis) in such a fashion for up to 8 hours after feeding.[40] This fact has an ominous implication for the current AIDS epidemic, although this means of transmission is difficult to document even when it occurs. Very few studies have been undertaken to attempt to clarify this risk.

Several cases of **dengue fever** (pronounced deng'e) have been transmitted by *Aedes aegyptii* in the Rio Grande valley of Texas (Brownsville) since 1980. This disease, which can cause hemorrhage and death, has had a sudden resurgence during the past 30 years, for unknown reasons. The abandonment of mosquito control measures, both in the United States and in South America, is the most likely explanation. Epidemics occurred periodically in the U.S. up to the 1940s, when effective pesticides such as DDT became available. DDT was incorporated into organized, effective mosquito control programs by public officials throughout the U.S. These programs in the southeastern U.S. interrupted the cycle of transmission of dengue, and it was not seen in the U.S. for the next thirty years.

These effective control programs have been virtually abandoned since the late 1970s as a result of the widespread hysteria regarding pesticides. The program to eradicate *Aedes aegyptii* in the United States was officially terminated in 1970. The result has been a pronounced increase in the population of the two Aedes species of mosquito. They are now the dominant mosquitos in the southeast. The introduction of *Aedes albopictus*, discussed below, has added another very effective vector of dengue, not only in the southeast, but also throughout most of the United States.

In an effort to eliminate yellow fever, which is also spread by *Aedes aegyptii*, the Pan American Health Organization established a control program that eradicated *Aedes aegyptii* from most of the South and Central American countries in the 1950s and 1960s. During that period dengue occurred only in some of the Caribbean islands, and only sporadically there. Following the lead of the United States, the control program in South and Central America was also abandoned. The result was a similar expansion of the *Aedes* mosquito population in South America. In 1979 dengue was limited to the northern coastal countries, Columbia, Venezuela and Guyana, and to Cuba. Ten years later dengue had spread to Mexico and all of Central America, and it had spread to most of the Caribbean countries. It would require a massive and costly program now to bring this disease under control. It would have been much more economical to maintain the mosquito control programs, not to mention the suffering and deaths among the victims.

Several large outbreaks of dengue fever have occurred in the Caribbean in recent years. An outbreak in Cuba in 1981 involved 350,000 people who were infected with the virus, and resulted in 158 deaths. In early 1988 during an epidemic of dengue fever in Ecuador, 420,000 people were infected. This epidemic resulted from a resurgence of the *Aedes aegyptii* mosquito population. Ecuador had been declared free of this mosquito in 1958 after a ten-year eradication program to control yellow fever. Spraying with malathion has been resumed since the epidemic. The Pan American Health Organization has reported similar episodes of dengue fever in Brazil, Bolivia and Paraguay in recent years. About 100,000 cases a year occur in the Far East. There is neither a vaccine nor treatment for dengue fever, other than supportive therapy. Effective control of mosquitos is essential in preventing the disease.

The introduction of the Asian tiger mosquito, *Aedes albopictus*, into Houston, Texas in 1985[41] has raised the specter of far more widespread outbreaks, not only of dengue fever, but also of other viral diseases not yet seen in the United States. This new breed of mosquito is known to transmit dengue and will also transmit the LaCrosse virus, which will increase the incidence of encephalitis. In 1990 ten strains of a new virus belonging to a group previously seen only in Africa were recovered from *Aedes albopictus* mosquitos in Potosi, Missouri.[42] This find confirms the fears that new diseases will be introduced and become established in areas of the United States that were previously free of "tropical" diseases. We will be spared filariasis, a devastating mosquito-borne disease of Africa, Asia, South America and the Pacific Islands. *Aedes albopictus* is refractory to infection by the various microfilariae of those regions.

Aedes albopictus, which is native to Japan and China, was brought into Houston through a shipment of used tires from Asia and has since spread well beyond Texas. By 1988 it had been reported in 113 counties in 17 states, including Indiana, Illinois, Ohio, Maryland, Delaware, North Carolina, Tennessee, Kentucky and most of the southern states. In 1986 it had become established in one county in Florida. By 1991 it had spread to 61 of the 67 counties in that state. The *Aedes* species can be readily differentiated from the *Anopheles* by the appearance of the eggs, larva and the adult.

The *Aedes albopictus* population in Florida was also discovered to be harboring the virus for eastern equine encephalitis in 1991. This was the first time this virus had been found in this mosquito species in the United States. The virus is maintained in a cycle between several species of mosquitos and birds. The heavy rains in the spring in Florida in 1991 resulted in an increase in the incidence of eastern equine encephalitis. The fatality rate from this form of encephalitis may exceed 50 percent in humans.

Aedes albopictus has been found to be infected with the eastern equine encephalitis virus in Houston, Texas also. Eastern equine encephalitis has been the most uncommon of the various forms of mosquito-borne encephalitis, but there is no doubt that with this added vector it will become more common. There will be seen an increased incidence of the disease in the areas where it has been recorded, and it will be seen as well in the other areas where *A. albopictus* has become established. This species of mosquito was also discovered to have been introduced into Africa for the first time in 1991. As had been the case in the United States and Brazil, the mosquito larvae were transported into the country in used tire casings from Asia. It was associated with an epidemic of yellow fever in Nigeria, and will undoubtedly increase the incidence of that disease in Africa.

Aedes albopictus is a much more aggressive feeder than the other mosquitos that we have had to deal with. It also feeds on humans throughout the daylight hours, unlike some other species. Individuals unfortunate enough to be in its habitat will suffer significantly more bites and rhus an increased incidence of disease. It has already displaced the local species in some areas in the south, and continues to do so elsewhere. It also has demonstrated some resistance to the pesticides customarily used against mosquitos, such as malathion, temephos and bendiocarb. Its hibernation habits make it adaptable to survive winters as far north as about the Fortieth Parallel (40° latitude), the latitude of Columbus, Ohio, Champaign, Illinois and north of St. Louis.

Aedes albopictus transmits viruses to its offspring through the eggs, which survive freezing. This assures the survival and transmission of diseases that would not ordinarily survive the winter season. The only mosquito in the United States previously that was capable of transmitting dengue fever, *Aedes aegyptii*, cannot survive the winter months in the northern states. This fact explained why indigenous cases of Dengue had been reported only in the southernmost regions of the United States, such as the Rio Grande valley of Texas. In the future a mosquito bite in any of the areas where it has become established may well present a risk of dengue fever transmission.

The only effective natural measure to control mosquito populations is to deny them a breeding pool. Such efforts have been very effective in California but they will prove more elusive in other parts of the country. Many areas of the United States have swamps and marshes all year long that provide excellent breeding sites for mosquitos. Some species breed in small pools of water in tree wells, discarded cans and other containers, and even in the gutters on houses. Organized, methodical programs of application of effective pesticides on a regular and continuing basis will be required to control this new disease vector. That will not occur until after we have seen a number of new, frightening diseases, and a large number of deaths.

Developing new pesticides to replace those that insects become resistant to presents the same problem that we have with antibiotics and bacteria. Unfortunately the current irrational prejudice against pesticides has placed a virtually impenetrable wall between the research laboratory and the marketplace. These new diseases, once introduced, will never be eradicated from the United States. We will have to live with them, and attempt to control them by whatever means remain at our disposal after the hysterical rampages of extremists. The past history of mosquito borne epidemics in the United States, such as the outbreak of yellow fever in 1793 in Philadelphia that killed thousands, is completely ignored.

Old tires are a favorite breeding ground for *Aedes albopictus*. Effective January 1, 1988, the Centers for Disease Control required that all tire casings imported from Asia be certified as clean, dry and free from insects. Fumigation is required as an added precaution, and examination of tire casings since then indicates that these efforts have been successful. These measures all come too late to save us from these new diseases that have already become established, however.

It will become ever more urgent to take every precaution to avoid attacks from mosquitos during recreational activities. Fortunately we have a very effective repellent in diethyl-meta-toluamide (DEET). It is the only effective agent, but it is widely marketed by several different manufacturers. The products with the higher concentrations, 25 to 50 percent, have the longest duration of action. These higher concentrations also present a greater risk of sensitization and toxic effects, however. In order to minimize these risks, it is best to avoid any unnecessary skin contact, applying the repellent to clothing instead, wherever possible. A new formulation of 35 percent DEET combined with a polymer should be effective in prolonging the period of protection.

None of the electronic devices are effective against mosquitos. The zappers that destroy larger insects permit mosquitos to pass through without making contact with the electrodes. These devices have also been shown to aerosolize the viruses from the surface and internal organs of flies, and disseminate them up to six feet away. This presents an obvious risk of inhaling disease causing organisms. When camping, netting on tents is essential. To control a tent full of insects that gain entry as a result of repeated passage by children, spraying the tent with a pyrethroid aerosol thirty minutes before bedtime is effective. Exit the tent after spraying to avoid inhaling the aerosol.

ENCEPHALITIS

Four types of encephalitis transmitted to humans by the bite of certain species of mosquitos occur in various regions of the country. Western equine is seen throughout the United States and carries a mortality rate of only about 3 percent. Only 1 to 2 cases per year have been reported in the past decade. Eastern equine is seen along the eastern seaboard and in western Michigan in recent years. It carries a mortality rate in humans as high as 50 percent. Outbreaks in horses precede human cases in both of these types of encephalitis.

In Florida in 1991 a record number of cases of encephalitis in horses was reported, 70 cases through June. The epizootic spread to the entire southeastern seaboard and into Ohio and Michigan where it also caused deaths among horses. During the 1991 season, eleven cases of Eastern equine encephalitis in humans were reported; five from Florida, two from Georgia, two from Michigan, and one each from Louisiana and South Carolina. Two deaths occurred in Florida. The virus was also found in *Aedes albopictus* mosquitos in Florida for the first time since their invasion of the United States.[43]

St. Louis encephalitis is the most common type of epidemic viral encephalitis in the United States and has occurred throughout the country. It is most commonly seen in the central U.S. and in Florida. Occurrences are sporadic and unpredictable. A total of 247 cases in humans were reported in 1990 and 78 cases in 1991. These were the largest numbers since the epidemic of 1975 when 1,957 cases were reported. Since 1991 about 15 to 20 cases per year were reported through 1996. Many cases are mild and inapparent, but fatalities may reach 7 percent in full-blown cases. The California group, which includes the LaCrosse virus, has been widely distributed throughout the U.S., and is the most common form of encephalitis. Reported cases range from 40 to 75 per year, chiefly in Illinois, Indiana, Iowa, Minnesota, North Carolina, Ohio, West Virginia and Wisconsin. *Aedes albopictus* is known to be capable of transmitting this form of encephalitis also.

Mental retardation, seizure disorder and speech and behavioral problems may persist after recovery from any of these diseases, the pattern varying somewhat according to the type. Encephalitis occurs during the period from spring to fall, when mosquitos are active. Approximately 100–200 cases per year of these mosquito born encephalitides are reported in the United States, but periodically an epidemic is seen. A total of 2,254 cases of all four types of encephalitis were reported in the United States for 1975.[44] This was the last large epidemic to date through 2000. Outbreaks can be predicted by placing sentinel chickens in areas known to be candidates for the disease. Periodic monitoring of the chickens for signs of the disease forewarns that it is in the area.

Control of mosquitos is highly effective in controlling the incidence of these diseases, as has been demonstrated in California. In that state, the elimination of pools of water in agricultural irrigation systems and the planting of larva eating fish, such as Gambusia, in bodies of water where mosquitos breed have produced significant successes. Outbreaks of St. Louis encephalitis (SLE) are frequently associated with standing water in drainage ditches and in containers such as flowerpots, birdbaths and discarded containers. This was the finding in Pine Bluff, Arkansas in the summer of 1991 when 25 cases of SLE were reported from July through August. The simple measure of removing these breeding sites for mosquitos would yield great benefits by reducing the incidence of this serious disease.

TICKS

Ticks belong to the same family as mites (acarina) and are the larger cousin of the clan. Two different groups of these arthropods transmit a variety of diseases to humans. Those that have a hard shell (ixodid ticks) transmit viral encephalitis, tularemia, Colorado tick fever, Q fever, Rocky Mountain spotted fever, babesiosis, ehrlichiosis and Lyme disease in the United States. Twelve different families of hard-shelled ticks exist in Africa, Europe and North, South and Central America. The ticks with a soft-shell (argasid ticks) transmit the various species of borrelia spirochetes which cause relapsing fever. Soft shelled ticks are widespread throughout parts of Africa, India and South America, where they commonly attacks humans in camps and huts that are universally infested.

Tick exposure is seasonal, primarily from late April through September, with June and July as the peak period. They can be encountered on the golf course and in some back yards as well as during picnics and hikes. When involved in any of these activities in tick country a daily inspection of the body for ticks is important, keeping in mind that some nymphal stages are the size of a pinhead. Some specific ticks are geographic in distribution, although the range of some of these seems to be expanding. Ixodes scapularis (dammini), the black legged or deer tick, has been located in the northeast (Massachusetts to Maryland) and in the upper Midwest to Wisconsin and Minnesota. Lyme disease has been reported in northern California and in Oregon more recently, however. The western blacklegged tick, Ixodes pacificus, is found in Washington, Oregon, California, Arizona, Nevada and Utah, and is the vector of Lyme disease there. A history of travel in these areas is as important as residence in diagnosing a potential illness.

Specific illnesses are associated with certain ticks, and some ticks transmit no known disease at all. Ixodes scapularis (dammini), the deer tick, carries the Lyme spirochete, the protozoan parasite of babesiosis, and the bacterium of ehrlichiosis. The reservoir for

Lyme disease includes deer and small mammals. Dermacentor varabilis, the dog tick and Dermacentor andersoni, the wood tick both are the reservoir in nature for Rocky Mountain Spotted Fever, a rickettsial disease, which is seen in every state except Vermont and Hawaii. It carries a 25 percent mortality if not treated promptly. Both of these ticks and the lone star tick also transmit tularemia from rabbits and other animals. Dermacentor andersoni, the wood tick, also transmits the virus of Colorado Tick fever from ground squirrels and chipmunks in the mountainous regions above 5,000 feet elevation in the western United States and Canada. The ticks as well as the mammals serve as a reservoir for the virus. Ticks are the reservoir for and/or transmission agent for many serious viral diseases outside of the United States.

Ticks have become resistant to DDT in some areas, but the synthetic pyrethroids and other pesticides such as malathion are still effective. Soft-shelled ticks usually lay about 1000 eggs each, while hard-shelled ticks may lay up to 5000. Some ticks can survive for up to two years without feeding. This characteristic helps to guarantee an abundant population year after year.

In the battle to control tick populations a unique product that utilizes a similar principal as the ground squirrel dusting in California has been marketed under the name of Damminix. It is a biodegradable tube stuffed with cotton that has been treated with a pesticide. These baited tubes are strategically placed in fields in areas where a disease such as Lyme disease is a threat. The field mice then carry the cotton to and incorporate it into their nests, thus killing the *Ixodes scapularis* (formerly called dammini) tick nymphs that feed on the mice. This promises to break the transmission cycle for Lyme disease in those areas where the mouse is the chief host. Techniques for protecting against and removal of ticks from the skin are discussed in Chapter VIII.

RELAPSING FEVER

Relapsing fever is an infectious disease caused by several different species of *Borrelia* spirochetes that are transmitted from ground squirrels or other small rodents to man through the bite of a soft-shelled tick (genus Ornithodoros). It may be transmitted from humans to humans by the human body louse also, as was demonstrated once again in 1991 in refugee camps in Ethiopia. Relapsing fever is endemic in the western mountain states where individual infected ticks may live for decades. This tick has a particularly long life span. It is a nocturnal biter, and feeds on inhabitants of mountain cabins while they sleep. The tick is a slow feeder, and cannot extract much blood except from a sleeping host. It is thus that visitors to this popular resort area are infected. Cases occur mainly in the spring and summer. Untreated the mortality rate ranges from 30 to 70 percent. With antibiotics the mortality rate is reduced to less than 1 percent.

During the summer of 1990, 19 persons who had stayed in cabins at the Grand Canyon North Rim were identified as victims of relapsing fever. These cases were identified by contacting representatives of more than 10,000 visitors from nine states, Canada and Germany. Inspection of the cabins revealed rodent nests above the ceilings and below the floors of the cabins. Ticks that harbor the spirochete of relapsing fever are known to infest such nests. The cabins were sprayed with acaricides and measures taken to prevent nesting by rodents in the future.

This was the first outbreak in this park since 1973 when 62 cases were recognized.[45] That outbreak was associated with an epizootic of plague that resulted in a marked reduction in the rodent population. The ticks then were forced to turn to human visitors as a substitute meal ticket. Visitors who contract the disease usually do not become ill until after their return home, where relapsing fever is frequently not considered in the diagnosis.

LYME DISEASE

Lyme disease (borreliosis) is another spirochetal disease, caused by *Borrelia burgdorferi*, that is transmitted to humans by ticks. The tick vector is of the hard variety (*Ixodes scapularis* in the eastern U.S., *Ixodes pacificus* in the western U.S.) and in the nymph stage is tiny, being only one to two millimeters in length, about the size of a pinhead. This presents a significant problem when inspecting the body for ticks, for it may give the appearance of a pigmented mole or other skin lesion and can be overlooked easily. The nymph stage is the one that most frequently transmits the spirochete to humans, and they feed primarily in late spring and early summer. The adult ticks are parasites of deer, but they have normally acquired the spirochete from mice when they feed on them during their larval stage. *Ixodes scapularis* also transmits ehrlichiosis and human granulocytic babesiosis (see below).

Lyme disease was first detected in 1977, but by 1985 it had become the most frequently reported tick-borne illness in the United States. It is currently the most common vector-borne illness in the United States. In 1980 when 226 cases were reported from eleven states it was limited chiefly to the northeastern United States and Wisconsin and Minnesota. Since that time it has spread to an increasing number of states each year, with a marked increase in the total number of cases reported. In 1984 a significant number of cases were reported from each of the six regions of the United States, with a total of 1,498 cases reported from twenty states. In 1987, 2,368 cases were reported. By 1988 Lyme disease had been reported in 32 states and on every continent except Antarctica. In 1990, 7,943 cases were reported, and in 1991 approximately 9,344.[46]

Lyme disease became a nationally reportable disease in 1991, which improved the accuracy of statistics. In 1992 cases were reported from 48 states, in Canada and many countries in Europe, with a total of 9,908 cases reported in the United States that year. A total of 11,700 cases were reported to the CDC from 44 states in 1995, and in 1996 a total of 16,455 cases were reported from 43 states. In 1999 the CDC reported 16,273 cases, more than double the number reported for 1990.[47]

Ixodes scapularis has been discovered also on well kept lawns of suburban homes, not limited to brushy and wooded areas as previously believed. Periodic application of pesticides to these lawns will help to control the tick population. Removal of leaf litter, brush and woodpiles, and clearing of trees to admit more sunlight will also reduce the deer, rodent, and tick habitat

One reason for the significant increase in Lyme disease is the explosion in the deer population in wide areas of the United States, and their movement into populated areas where they thrive. This problem is especially acute in residential communities serving the major cities of the Northeast, where the human population suffers a severe case of the Bambi syndrome. Residents in some areas are adamantly opposed to culling the deer, the only solution that has proven successful in such circumstances. It is ironic that in the region where the Lyme disease outbreak started, the increase in the deer population has resulted in some residents suffering the disease two or three times. This is a serious illness that should be avoided at all cost. The hundreds of collisions with automobiles that have evolved are also costly in monetary terms.

The mouse and the deer serve as the reservoir for *B. burgdorferi*. The bacteria are transmitted to the tick when it feeds on the animals, and then from tick to man. They are transmitted from the tick to humans slowly, requiring that the tick remain attached for 24 to 48 hours. If the body is inspected carefully daily and all ticks removed, infection is unlikely to occur. Infection with this organism following a tick bite can be suspected when the classical lesion, "erythema chronica migrans," appears. This is a circular area of erythema (redness) surrounding the bite, with some clearing in the center. The erythema is caused by the spread of the spirochete into the tissues. The lesion generally appears two or three days after a bite and is quite large, ranging from 8 to 50 cm. in diameter. Itching accompanies the lesion as with any insect bite, but the area of erythema is also painful under pressure. This lesion is present in about 75 percent of individuals with early Lyme disease.

Early symptoms of Lyme disease include fever, headache, muscle and joint aching and fatigue. These symptoms reflect the dissemination of the spirochete throughout the body. Multiple erythematous skin lesions may appear, presumably as a result of the dissemination of the *Borrelia burgdorferi* spirochete. At this stage the disease may resemble flu or meningitis. Lyme disease is not often considered in the diagnosis unless the erythema chronica migrans is noted. The onset of these symptoms may be anywhere from a few days to a month after the tick bite. The tick bite is seldom noticed because of the smallness of the tick. Many cases go undiagnosed and unreported.

In about 10 percent of victims infection in the heart causes inflammation (myocarditis and pericarditis) and abnormalities in the heart beat. In an additional 10 to 20 percent of individuals inflammation of the brain and nerves produces symptoms of encephalitis or pain and weakness in the arms and legs. Bell's palsy (paralysis of facial muscles) is a common complication of Lyme borreliosis, and results when the seventh cranial nerve is involved. Infection in joints with resultant pain is seen in about one-half of infected individuals. This early phase of Lyme disease can last for several weeks.

Proper administration of appropriate antibiotics in this early stage generally cures the disease and prevents the development of the serious late sequelae. However, more than one-half of individuals infected with Lyme borreliosis do not seek medical attention until well past this stage. If it is not diagnosed early, it can progress to a chronic stage where the diagnosis is even more obscure. The chronic stage persists for a long period, with no relief. In addition to the serious heart involvement, chronic arthritis and nerve disorders are the prominent features of the chronic disease. Among the nervous system problems of chronic Lyme disease are Bell's Palsy, palsy of other central and peripheral nerves, meningitis and encephalitis.

Even with adequate treatment some people develop the above complications in Lyme disease. Whereas antibiotic therapy is curative in the early phase, it does not seem to resolve the chronic cases. For this reason some abnormality in the immune system is suspected to be responsible for the prolonged and persistent symptoms.

Unlike most other bacterial infections, the organism cannot be cultured from the blood or organs affected. It can be identified in skin biopsies taken from the erythema migrans in about 80 percent of patients prior to antibiotic administration. No laboratory test is available to detect the disease in its early stages. Diagnosis can be made only from the clinical evidence in the victim. The ELISA test currently available is of no value prior to the fourth to sixth week. It delivers many false results, and is of limited value. Newer tests, especially a PCR test for the viral DNA, are being developed (1999) in an effort to arrive at an earlier diagnosis. A characteristic of all of the current tests is that they remain positive even after a cure has been apparently accomplished.

Lyme disease shares many characteristics with other diseases caused by spirochetes, such as syphilis (see Chapter XI). It is far better not to get the disease at all. Tight clothing with pants legs tucked into boot tops or socks and insect repellent (DEET) applied prior to exposure are essential when walking in infested areas. The insect repellent must be reapplied at appropriate intervals (see insect repellents in Chapter VIII). Recent studies by the U.S. Air Force and others has found that spraying the clothing with permethrin (Permanone Tick Repellent") in addition to using insect repellent greatly increases the protection against ticks. Permethrin kills ticks on contact.

When inspecting for ticks the size (one millimeter, two millimeters engorged) must be kept in mind; they are difficult to see. Wearing light colored clothing makes it much easier to detect them. Clothing and the body surface should be inspected carefully about every 1-2 hours in the field and before entering the home.

Two vaccines for Lyme disease have been developed, one of which has been approved and marketed in 1999. The cost for the three doses is about $100, and the duration of protection is unknown. While there may be some justification for the use of this vaccine in occupations with frequent exposure, it is far preferable to rely upon the prophylactic measures described previously. There has been concern about the proliferation of vaccines for various diseases, and their potential impact upon the immune system. This concern is especially high in the case of infants and young children where an endless array of new vaccines for conditions to which the child is infrequently if ever exposed are being mandated by fascist federal and state officials. The involvement of commercial interests in these decisions is also suspect.

BABESIOSIS

This parasite is transmitted to humans by the same tick involved in Lyme disease. The nymph stage of the tick transmits several different species of a protozoan parasite, *Babesia*, from a variety of animals. The parasite invades and destroys red blood cells, much as occurs in malaria, and with a similar anemia produced. Some cases have been misdiagnosed as malaria. It was first reported in the U.S. in 1968, and again like Lyme disease, the incidence is increasing. More than 450 cases have been reported, mostly in New England, especially in the offshore islands. It has been reported also in California, Washington, Maryland, Virginia, Georgia, Wisconsin and Minnesota. There is no treatment to eradicate the parasite, although quinine plus clindamycin have been used experimentally. This disease presents a particular risk to people who have had their spleen removed. The same precautions regarding ticks that are described above should be observed to prevent babesiosis.

TICK PARALYSIS

Tick paralysis is caused by a neurotoxin that is secreted in the saliva by certain hard ticks while they feed on animals. Dogs, cattle and sheep are affected as well as man. The toxin acts on the cells of the spinal cord to produce a weakness beginning in the legs. This progresses to a paralysis twenty-four to forty-eight hours later, and gradually spreads up the body to involve the trunk, arms, neck, tongue and central nerve centers. Death may ensue if removal of the tick (or ticks) is not accomplished. Tick paralysis is frequently mistaken for polio or one of the other paralytic diseases. The small size of the tick requires very careful scrutiny, including all of the hair and skin fold areas. Removal of the intact tick results in a rapid recovery.

Tick paralysis occurs most commonly in the Northwestern United States and in western Canada, where the wood tick, *Dermacentor andersoni*, is the culprit. The disease has also been reported in the southeastern and Gulf states where the dog tick and a deer tick have been incriminated. People who live in or visit these areas should always take the simple tick precautions of tucking pants legs into boots or socks, and of applying insect repellent, diethyl-meta-toluamide (DEET) to the clothing and to the exposed skin. Also spraying the clothing with the new Permanone Tick Repellent™ mentioned above gives added protection. Since the tick in this stage is about the size of a pinhead, it requires very careful scrutiny for detection. Prevention is far preferable.

EHRLICHIOSIS

Ehrlichiosis is a new, serious disease transmitted to humans by ticks. It was first reported in the United States in 1986. Many of the early cases were misdiagnosed as Rocky Mountain spotted fever. Eighty percent of the victims did not have a rash, and tests for Rocky Mountain spotted fever were negative. Tests for *Ehrlichia canis*, an infection of dogs, proved to be positive in humans with this new disease. It was thus assumed that this was the same disease, transmitted from dogs to man by ticks. Further study isolated the causative organism as a new species of *Ehrlichia*, closely related to *E. canis*. It was named *E. Chaffeensis* after the army base (Ft. Chaffee, Arkansas) where the disease was recognized in an army recruit in 1991. By 1996 more than 400 cases in humans had been reported from 20 different states, mostly in the southeast and southwest.[48] Although it is known that the organism is transmitted to man by tick bites, the natural reservoir of this new disease is not known. It is important to protect dogs from ticks when traveling in these regions.

Ehrlichia chaffeensis, a member of the rickettsia family, parasitizes granulocytic leukocytes. The disease ranges from mild to severe, even fatal and is characterized by fever, headache, nausea and confusion in the more severe cases. The liver enzymes are usually elevated. Early diagnosis and treatment is essential. A blood test to establish the diagnosis is available from the Centers for Disease Control. Prior to 1986 the only known disease in humans caused by *Ehrlichia* was sennetsu fever, caused by *Ehrlichia sennetsu*, first described in 1954 and seen only in western Japan. The reservoir for sennetsu fever is also unknown, as is the means of transmission. It appears to be associated with visits to rivers or swampy areas near the rivers, making insect transmission suspect.

Early diagnosis and treatment is essential; it has proven to be responsive to the tetracyclines if they are administered early enough. A blood test to establish the diagnosis is available from the Centers for Disease Control. Newer PCR tests (polymerase chain reaction) capable of differentiating the different species of Ehrlichia were developed in 1990-91.[49,50,51,52] This newly discovered disease provides an added incentive for travelers to these regions to exercise precautions against ticks.

ROCKY MOUNTAIN SPOTTED FEVER
Not only do ticks transmit Rocky Mountain spotted fever, but they also serve as the natural reservoir for this rickettsial disease. The female tick transmits the rickettsia to subsequent generations of ticks through the eggs that it lays. Thus although the ticks live off of the blood of small animals such as ground squirrels and other rodents, these animals are not necessary for the maintenance and transmission of the disease. The adult ticks can survive for two years without feeding, a very unique and unfortunate characteristic

for a disease transmitting arthropod. Rocky Mountain spotted fever is discussed in more detail in Chapter VIII.

FLEAS

Various species of fleas attack birds, rats, mice, squirrels, and virtually every wild animal, as well as livestock and domestic pets. All of these species will attack humans, given the opportunity. The fleas of wild rodents (squirrels, ground squirrels, chipmunks and rats) are a serious concern in Oregon, California, Arizona, New Mexico, Utah, Nevada and Colorado because they carry the plague bacteria (*Yersinia pestis*). These fleas can transmit plague to humans when they feed on them.

Careful attention should be given to clothing and to the application of insect repellent (DEET) when involved in recreational or farming activities in these geographic areas. Applying permethrin to the clothing adds significantly to the protection. The residential areas of Los Angeles have extended into the hills where ground squirrels abound. This presents a particular risk to everyone living in that area. An innovative program by the health department in California to control the fleas on these creatures by dusting them through feeding devices has helped to control this disease.

The fleas that most frequently attack humans are the dog and cat fleas. The fleas of wild rodents also will feed on domestic pets and humans, however, if given the opportunity. The fleas of ground and rock squirrels are particularly aggressive. Fleas do not establish housekeeping on humans, rather they feed (through bloodsucking) and depart. Their saliva produces raised, reddened areas that may itch intensely. These are most commonly seen on the lower legs, which are within reach of this prodigious jumper.

If you enter an infested house after the pet has been away for a while, you may readily see these creatures leaping to the attack. Secondary infection of the skin from scratching is occasionally seen. The itching is best controlled by the application of a topical steroid cream such as hydrocortisone. This should not be applied to the face, but fleabites are not customarily seen in that location. In South America and in Africa, fleas burrow underneath the skin and cause abscesses to form.

Successful eradication of fleas may be a long-term project. It requires treating the pet, the house, the yard and the kennel. The yard, even when fenced, is commonly reinfested by nocturnal visits of other animals. The pet should be bathed and then dusted regularly with Sevin® (carbaryl). This may also be sprayed on the yard. Fleas in some areas have developed a resistance to some insecticides, which may require substitution of another pesticide if reduction in population is not seen. Malathion may be sprayed on the yard as well as dusted in the kennel, but not in the home.

Chlorpyrifos (Dursban®) also is effective against fleas, and it may be sprayed outdoors. It should not be used indoors on carpets even though it is prescribed for this use by some. It has been marketed recently with a polymer to prolong the release of the pesticide, for use on dogs only. How much safer this renders the chlorpyrifos remains to be seen. DDT is very effective and safe even for the animal but it is no longer available in the U.S.

All rat runs should also be dusted. If you have inherited a population of ground squirrels, you can use the California technique of dusting these animals using tubes lined on both ends with a fabric containing malathion or sevin dust, and bait in the center. When flea eggs hatch, the larva spin a cocoon that may protect it from pesticides. Repeated applications will pick off the survivors after they hatch. It may well be necessary to continue this battle all summer long. Some years are worse than others are.

Eradicating these creatures from the house may be more difficult. They thrive in carpets, as long as they have someone to feed on. Fleas live much of their life cycle off of the pet, in bedding, rugs and crevices. The use of an aerosol spray containing pyrethroids (permethrin, resmethrin, tetramethrin) combined with piperonyl butoxide, designed for household use, should produce extinction of those fleas contacted within a half-hour. The house should be vacated during this period. Thorough vacuuming should then be undertaken to remove as many eggs as possible. The eggs hatch in three days when conditions are favorable, but they may remain dormant in the carpet, dust or the animal nest for months.

The stimulus that prompts hatching of flea eggs is the presence of a suitable host heralded by warmth and vibration. Retreatment may be required to kill the fleas that hatch from the surviving eggs. If this treatment fails, if it is apparent that there is no reduction in the flea population of the living room, a problem exists. Resistance to the insecticide used may have been developed.

While Sevin® and malathion have a low order of toxicity, they are not recommended for general household use. Chlorpyrifos is commonly sold for the control of fleas on pets, and is even prescribed by some as a spray for carpeting. This product is a member of the organophosphate family of pesticides, and is too toxic to be sprayed on the carpeting in the house. It is significantly more toxic than Sevin® or malathion. As mentioned above, it recently has been marketed with a polymer that prolongs its action when applied to dogs. In households where young children are crawling on the floor, all chemicals should be avoided. (See Chapter XIV for more on pesticides.)

MURINE TYPHUS (endemic, rat-flea-borne typhus)

Murine typhus is a rickettsial disease transmitted to humans by the rat flea. This disease infects virtually all rats and mice at some point in their life. Although it does not kill the rodent, the *Rickettsia typhi* organism remains with them for a long time. The rat flea acquires the organism from this source when feeding on infected rodents. It is the nature of all fleas to feed on any available warm host in an emergency, and outbreaks of murine typhus in humans have been reported after campaigns to poison rats. The source of the bubonic plague (Black Death) in the fourteenth century was suspected as a result of the observation that outbreaks were frequently associated with the appearance of dead rats.

Murine typhus has been reported in virtually every state, being much more common in shipping ports, near granaries and food storage areas. It is prevalent in the southeastern United States and along the Gulf Coast. Currently about 60 cases are reported annually, down from the 2,000 to 5,000 cases annually in the 1940s. This dramatic reduction in incidence has resulted from aggressive programs designed to deny rats access to food in storage and in granaries, and by dusting burrows and runs with pesticides to kill the fleas.

This form of typhus, although it is manifested by an acute, pronounced illness, carries a low mortality rate. Deaths occur primarily among the elderly and those with other debilitating illnesses. Shaking chills, headache, temperature of 102 to 103° F. along with malaise and prostration suggestive of influenza character ize the illness. It can be treated with antibiotics, best results being achieved by instituting therapy early.

EPIDEMIC TYPHUS

Epidemic typhus (also called classic, European and louse-borne) is a much more severe form of typhus caused by *Rickettsia prowazekii*. It is transmitted to non infected humans by the body louse after they feed on an infected individual. As such it is not commonly a zoonoses, although it can be transmitted from flying squirrels by their fleas. Fifteen cases from this source were reported in 1980 and 1981. It was prevalent in England and Europe throughout the sixteenth and seventeenth centuries, due to poor hygienic conditions. All of Europe was engulfed in 1500 A.D. when it particularly struck in crowded population centers and among troops. Italy suffered an epidemic in 1505 A.D. and again from 1524 to 1530.

Labeled as gaol (jail) fever in England, it killed 510 people at Oxford, being transmitted from person to person among prisoners on trial. In early 1700 it was known as hospital fever in England because of outbreaks of the disease in that setting. In 1784 it was given still another title, factory fever because of the frequent outbreaks there. Finally after about 1800 it began to subside as a result of improvements in hygiene and sanitation.[53]

Epidemic typhus was common in wartime until World War II. After World War I large epidemics of typhus struck Poland, Russia and the Balkan states. During World War II the dusting of entire populations of some of the cities in Europe with DDT powder during invasions by the Allied forces prevented outbreaks of typhus among our troops. This was the first war in history when this scourge did not devastate the armies. Effective antibiotic treatment is now available, but the disease has been relegated to the back pages in most of the civilized world as a result of increased levels of personal hygiene. It cannot be transmitted without body lice.

SCRUB TYPHUS (Mite-Borne Typhus, Tsutsugamushi Disease)

Tropical Typhus is seen in the Asiatic-Pacific region encompassed by Japan, India, northern Australia and the New Hebrides. There are several islands in this region that are highly infested. Infection in humans is caused by *Rickettsia tsutsugamushi* and results from a chigger (mite larva) bite after the mites have fed on rural and forest rodents, including rats, voles and field mice. Symptoms begin in about 8 to 12 days and include a high fever (103° to 105° F), chills, severe headache and cough. Pneumonia may develop in the second week, as may inflammation of the heart muscle. The lymph nodes at all ports of the body are enlarged.

Some antibiotics are effective in treating scrub typhus, and as with Rocky Mountain spotted fever and other rickettsial diseases, it is important to get started early with these. Up to 60 percent of untreated cases may terminate in a fatality. It is far better to avoid the exposure, and insect repellents (DEET) applied to the clothing and exposed skin are effective. Protective clothing (see Chapter VIII) with permethrin sprayed on clothing and blankets will further diminish the risk. Visits to these regions should be planned carefully.

PLAGUE

The most dramatic and far-reaching epidemic ever to strike mankind was the **Black Death** or bubonic plague of the fourteenth century. This sweeping disease episode killed half of the population of England and at least one-fourth of the population of all of Europe. The pandemic ravaged the population of Asia and Africa, then spread to the Crimea. From Constantinople it spread to Turkey, Greece and Italy, them north and west until it had engulfed all of Europe and England by 1350 A.D. The death toll was over 60 million people. This great pandemic finally demonstrated the contagiousness of disease, and the biblical principles of isolation of the plague victim and everyone who came in contact with him were instituted. When a victim died his clothing and belongings were burned, and efforts to purify his house were taken.

The disease continued to strike at intervals until the end of the seventeenth century. The Great Plague of London in 1665 killed 69,000 of the population. In Vienna in 1679 it killed 70,000 people; in Prague in 1681, 83,000 died; in Italy in 1630, 500,000 people died as a result of that epidemic of plague. Russia was visited first in this pandemic, in 1601, and 127,000 people died in Moscow.[54]

The devastation of this catastrophic pandemic had profound social, political and religious consequences that changed the world forever. It resulted in diminished power of both the Church and civil authority. As one medical historian observed; *this terrible plague brought panic and confusion in its train and broke down all restrictions of morality, decency, and humanity. Parents, children and lifelong friends forsook one another, every one striving to save only himself and to come off with a whole skin.*[55] These observations may have implications for the epidemic that we currently face.

Bubonic plague continued to be spread from Hong Kong to the rest of the world from 1894 on. It was these epidemics of plague and cholera that forced public officials to assign attention to the development of public health agencies. Organizations were established in a few cities and locales throughout the world, mainly in port cities. The U.S. Congress established a National Board of Health in 1878 following a cholera and yellow fever epidemic. This agency expired due to a lack of funding, and its functions, which included quarantine responsibilities where no such local authority existed, were taken over by the U.S. Marine Hospital Service in 1883, the forerunner of the U.S. Public Health Service. When bubonic plague was introduced into San Francisco from Hong Kong in 1907-8 it was the experts of this Marine Hospital Service who diagnosed the disease, and brought the epidemic under control by destroying the rodents that carried the plague bacillus.[56] This action most likely averted a spread of the disease to other parts of the country. This was the first time that the entire rat population of a city was exterminated, a feat that we still do not fully appreciate to this day.

Untreated, the mortality of plague remains close to 100 percent, in spite of the fact that some antibiotics are effective. Streptomycin is the drug of choice, but it is no longer available in the United States, so other antibiotics must be substituted (see tuberculosis in Chapter XI). The most effective alternative drug is tetracycline, particularly doxycycline. These medications must be instituted early to reduce the mortality to about 10 percent. In plague pneumonia or septicemia effective antibiotic therapy must be started within 24 hours to avoid death. Unfortunately treatment is often delayed because the diagnosis is not considered. It is always much easier to arrive at a prompt diagnosis in the middle of an epidemic. In modern time, cases of plague arrive erratically and unexpectedly.

A vaccine for plague is available, and it was used in U.S. military personnel in Vietnam. The protection afforded by it is not absolute, however, as demonstrated in Vietnam between 1961-1971 when eight cases of plague were diagnosed among U.S. military personnel.[57] Serious reactions can occur following immunization. The vaccine is derived from a culture of the plague bacillus that has been inactivated by formalin. A series of three injections is required, the second injection 1 to 3 months after the first, and the third injection 5 to 6 months after the second. For travel to plague infested areas, therefore, immunization must be started at least 6 months in advance.

Plague is caused by a bacterium, *Yersinia pestis*, which is transmitted from wild rodents to humans by the bite of fleas. In the United States the wild rodents most frequently associated with transmission of the disease are rats, ground squirrels and rock squirrels (Colorado). However other squirrels, mice, chipmunks, prairie dogs and even rabbits can harbor the disease. Outbreaks of plague have increased in frequency over the past twenty-five years in the southwestern United States, due primarily to demographic trends. While cases of plague associated with rats in urban areas, the classic playground for the disease, have become rare, the threat is great in rural and suburban regions. This is especially the case in Los Angeles and Orange County, where the population has spread into the hills surrounding the city, where ground squirrels abound. The plague bacillus and the flea that transmits it are present among the squirrel population in that region.

As with typhus, one of the classic and very successful programs to control the disease has been to reduce the flea population by dusting the burrows of the rodent, rat or ground squirrel with DDT or other effective pesticide. In California an ingenious device that greatly increases the effectiveness of such control programs was developed. It consists of a length of tubing with a fabric at each end and an attractive bait in the center. The fabric is dusted with a pesticide. When the ground squirrels take their meal, they dust themselves at the same time, freeing themselves of their fleas. Their gratitude must be overwhelming, particularly considering that the alternative would be to eliminate the squirrel population. Poisoning of colonies of rodents such as prairie dogs, while effective and easily accomplished, is not routinely done because it releases the fleas into the environment to attack humans and domestic pets. Such "slaughter" would also be condemned by some irrational and confused souls.

While plague in the cities has been almost eliminated as a result of the control of the rat population, the number of cases acquired from rural and country rodents has been rising. These cases occur most frequently in the spring and summer, and very often among young people who spend more time venturing into the fields. The mortality among these cases is almost twice as high as normal because of the delay in diagnosis. Up to 20 percent of infected individuals develop plague pneumonia, which is almost always fatal unless treated vigorously. Plague pneumonia can readily be transmitted to other humans by droplet infection through a cough or sneeze. No such transmission has occurred in the United States since 1924. This in spite of the fact that plague pneumonia has occurred in 20 percent of the cases recorded. This is a testimonial to the proficiency of the medical treatment and management of cases.

Pet cats can catch and return plague-infested rodents to the home, or simply bring back the infected fleas. The fleas thus brought home can become established on mice or rats in the residential area. Cats can also transmit plague by a bite or scratch. Plague in cats is highly contagious and all of their secretions should be avoided. There have been cases of plague pneumonia in humans that were acquired by droplet infection (sneezing) from cats. The cat usually dies if it becomes infected. Dogs can similarly bring back the infected fleas, but they often recover if they become diseased.

In August 1992 a 31 year old man died in Tucson, Arizona as a result of pneumonic plague that he had contracted from a cat in Chaffee County, Colorado. He contracted the disease from a plague infected domestic cat that he had removed from a crawl space of a friend's home where he was visiting. This occurred on August 19. He became ill on August 22, was hospitalized on August 25 and died of plague pneumonia 24 hours after admission. The pneumonic form of plague can be rapidly fatal, as in this case, unless diagnosed early and treated aggressively. A dead chipmunk in the area where the cat lived was shown to be infected with plague. Other dead rodents were also found in the area.[58]

In 1996 five cases of plague in humans were reported in the U.S., two of which were fatal. One fatality was an 18 year old resident of Flagstaff, Arizona. He had become infected from fleabites while walking through a prairie dog colony. The other fatality was a 16-year-old resident of western Colorado who had acquired plague from a sick cat that she had cared for. The cat in turn had acquired plague from a prairie dog colony that was adjacent to the victim's property. Residents of areas where plague is known to be established in wild animals should avoid contact with any animal, wild or domestic, that appears to be ill. The areas of greatest risk have been New Mexico, Arizona, Colorado, Utah, western Nevada, California and Oregon. The disease can be expected to spread beyond these areas. Visitors to these regions should not take pet dogs or cats with them. Even with the greatest of precautions these pets face a serious risk of being exposed to fleas from wild rodents.

Plague seems destined to be with us forever. There is an abundant supply of wild rodents that harbor the bacterium. *Yersinia pestis* remains viable in the soil in the burrows of rats and ground squirrels for prolonged periods. Infected fleas also survive for long periods of time (months). The high point in the United States in recent times was in 1983 when 40 cases were reported. In 1984 there were 31 cases, in 1985 seventeen cases, in 1989 four cases, in 1990 two cases, and in 1991 eleven cases. This drop in spite of the greatly increased contact between ground squirrels and humans is a great testimonial to the control efforts of the public health officials.

Outside of the United States plague is well established in Russia, Indonesia, Burma, Vietnam, India and Africa where large populations of infected wild rodents abound. Large numbers of cases occur annually in Indonesia, Burma and Vietnam. Sporadic outbreaks occur in Peru, Bolivia and northeastern Brazil.

Education and modification of behavior of people will be necessary if this serious disease is to be kept under control in the areas where it is prevalent. Rodent populations must be kept under control by proper food storage and garbage/refuse disposal. Rodent fleas can be suppressed in relatively small areas of human use such as residential or recreational areas by insecticides, either by dusting the burrows or placing baited tubes near the burrows. It is essential to accomplish this before poisoning rodent populations. Otherwise orphaned fleas will come looking for humans as feeding stock.

Handling of dead rodents carries a high risk of contracting plague. Permitting pet dogs and cats to roam invites the infected fleas into the home and residential area. All dogs and cats that are in plague territory, either in residence or visiting, should be treated each week with an appropriate insecticide. The long acting polymer preparation should be effective for dogs, but it cannot be used on cats. (Review the precautions listed below under *Hantavirus*) Unfortunately the geographic range of plague has spread dramatically, and will spread even further.

HANTAVIRUS

During the Korean conflict in the 1950s thousands of United Nations military personnel, including U.S. troops, were infected with Korean hemorrhagic fever. This is a viral disease that is transmitted to humans from infected rodents, either by aerosol or direct contact with their excreta (urine and feces). The Korean virus was not identified until 1978 [59] and it has been assigned to the genus *Hantavirus* of the *Bunyaviridae* family. The *Bunyaviruses* are responsible for a variety of zoonoses, including California encephalitis. The *Hantavirus* group has been responsible for several epidemics and sporadic disease throughout Eurasia since the 1930s. Korean hemorrhagic fever continues to occur sporadically among United States military personnel training in Korea.

In the 1980s a *Hantavirus* was isolated from domestic rats in the inner cities of the United States and it was identified as the Seoul virus. This virus is associated with kidney damage and resultant hypertension. Less is known about the Prospect Hill virus, another *Hantavirus*, which is transmitted to humans from the meadow vole. These viruses had not been known to cause disease in the U.S. prior to this. In May 1993 cases of a serious acute illness began to be reported from the Four Corners region of the Southwestern United States (Arizona, New Mexico, Utah and Colorado). These cases began with flu-like symptoms, but rapidly involved the lungs and resulted in acute respiratory failure. Death occurred in fifty to seventy-five percent of the individuals afflicted with this *Hantavirus*. Investigation has revealed that these illnesses were caused by a newly recognized strain of *Hantavirus* that was transmitted from infected deer mice through aerosol from urine and droppings, or by direct contact with the excreta, perhaps through a scratch or other skin lesion.

Since the initial outbreak in the Four Corners region, additional cases have been identified in Texas, Louisiana, Nevada, California, Oregon, Idaho, Montana and North and South Dakota. As of May 28, 1999 there had been 217 confirmed cases of *Hantavirus* pulmonary syndrome in 30 states reported. Forty-three percent of these cases have died.[60,61,62] By 1995 *Hantavirus* infections had been reported in 23 states. There is no doubt that this illness will continue to spread to other regions of the United States, since the principal vector, the deer mouse, is present throughout the U.S. except for the Southeast.

The *Hantavirus* may well be transmitted to other rodent vectors also. It will be much more urgent in the future to prevent entry into homes of mice and other rodents. Where they are caught in traps, disposable gloves should be used in handling them, and the hands should be washed thoroughly afterwards. The droppings from these animals should be carefully vacuumed and disposed of, and the area should be disinfected with household bleach (chlorine). The nests and dead animals should be thoroughly soaked with a disinfectant prior to their removal to avoid aerosol transmission of the virus. *Hantaviruses* have lipid envelopes that render them susceptible to most disinfectants (see Chapter XV).[63] Placement of the dead animal in a sealed plastic bag helps to prevent subsequent exposure to the virus. This is a very serious illness with a high fatality rate.

In addition to exposure to rodents in the home and during camping and hiking, the disease has been contracted from planting and harvesting field crops, cleaning barns and other buildings and occupying previously vacant cabins. Children playing in areas infested with rats also have contracted the disease. The following precautions regarding rodents are important in guarding against *Hantavirus*, plague and other diseases where rodents serve as vectors.

• Keep all rodents (mice, rats, squirrels, chipmunks) out of the home and garage. Close all openings with concrete, mortar or steel wire. Trim tree branches away from buildings.

• Remove all trash or brush that may provide shelter or a nesting site for rodents.

• If traps are set, check them daily. If the trap contains a rodent, spray it and the surrounding area with a household pyrethroid spray to eliminate any fleas that might harbor the plague bacillus. Also spray nesting areas.

• Spray all dead animals until they are wet, the trap and the surrounding area with a 10 percent solution of fresh chlorine bleach before sweeping area or removing animal. Place the animal in a sealed plastic bag for disposal.

• Wear disposable gloves, disinfect them with bleach, and then wash hands carefully.

• Do not encourage any rodent species or rabbits to occupy your property by feeding them. Never entice them onto your porch or patio.

• When camping leave pets at home or in a kennel. If they deliver a disease to you or your family you will wish that you had. If they die from plague or other disease you will likewise regret having ignored this advice.

• When camping or hiking avoid areas that are inhabited by wild animals. Particularly avoid areas where rodent burrows are present. Sleep on a folding cot, never on the ground.

• Store all human and animal food, as well as garbage, in impervious, rodent proof containers.

• Avoid contact with sick or dead animals, especially rodents and rabbits. Give them a wide berth and report them to the proper officials.

• Wear appropriate clothing when hiking or camping; long sleeved shirts with pants tucked into socks or boots. Clothing should be treated with repellent (DEET) and permethrin (or other effective pyrethroid). Avoid skin contact. Reapply at appropriate intervals.

• If you live in an area where these diseases are endemic and you have pets, acceptable insecticide powders or shampoos should be applied to them at least once weekly. The long acting polymer is useful for dogs, but cannot be used on cats. Flea collars provide no protection from these diseases. The possession of pets in these areas presents some very serious problems, for which there is no entirely satisfactory solution.

• Seek professional veterinary care if a cat develops swelling and sores around the head, neck or mouth. Do not handle the animal without gloves and face protection.

• Skinning rabbits from these areas of endemnicity presents serious risks. In addition to the time-honored practice of wearing gloves as protection against tularemia, a face shield should also be worn as protection against splatter. It does not provide protection against aerosol transmission, however.

• Bites from any wild animal in any location should always receive the immediate attention of a competent physician. In addition to the many zoonoses discussed in this Chapter, tetanus is always a threat that needs assessment.

• Any onset of fever, chills, headache or general illness following any of the above exposures should prompt an immediate visit to the family physician. The incubation period of plague is short (2–6 days) and early treatment is essential (24 hours).

• Remember my cardinal golden rule of hand washing: It does no harm, is cheap, and may save you an unpleasant illness.

A recent report of the first Colorado resident to survive *Hantavirus* infection[64] suggests that early diagnosis and aggressive treatment may improve the chances of survival. This disease will require a high index of suspicion and prompt action on the part of both the victim and the physician.

CHAGAS' DISEASE (Carlos Chaga, Brazilian physician)

Chagas' disease is caused by *Trypanosoma cruzi*, another protozoan disease for which we have no effective treatment. The organism is transmitted to humans by the Triatomine bug, a member of the Reduviid family, and also called the "kissing," "cone-nose," and in error, the "assassin" bug. The true "assassin" bug is another member of the reduviid family. These insects feed on the blood of vertebrates, chiefly mammals and birds, mainly during the night. One of the most popular hosts is the opossum. They feed on humans wherever they can gain access to the home, and this occurs commonly in communities where housing is primitive. Spraying benzene hexachloride in these homes once or twice a year has been very effective in controlling the bugs. The bites occur around the mouth (thus the name "kissing" bug) and around the eyes.

The transmission of *T. cruzi* to humans is unique in that it is effected neither by the injection of infective saliva nor by contaminated mouthparts of the insect. The reduviid bug acquires the parasite in the process of blood-sucking an infected animal. The protozoan then passes through several stages in the intestinal canal of the bug, over a period of about 8 days. The infective forms are then passed in the feces of the bug, and deposited on the skin of humans when the bug feeds. Infection occurs only when these infective forms are rubbed into the bite wound. After the parasite enters the blood it is carried to other tissues, especially the muscle of the heart, esophagus and colon, where it causes permanent damage. Heart failure is a common sequela. The organism also can be transmitted by blood transfusions.

Chagas' disease, which is restricted to the Western Hemisphere, is prevalent in scattered areas of South and Central America and in some areas of Mexico. A few sporadic cases have been reported in Texas and California. The failure of this bug to transmit Chagas' disease as readily in the United States, even though it carries *T. Cruzi*, reportedly is due to the habit of the local species of bug of defecating after feeding, rather than during feeding as is the case in South and Central America.

Of greater concern than Chagas' disease in the southwestern United States where these bugs are established is the sensitivity that some people develop to the bite. This has resulted in severe anaphylactic reactions, and this trend is expected to expand. While the insect can gain access to any home, this is not common in modern construction, and the insect presents a greater threat when camping in the southwest than it does in the homes of the region.

MANGE (Demodex)

Human scabies (see Chapter XV) is not a zoonosis, but one form of mange in animals, sarcoptic mange, is the animal's version of scabies. The mites that cause this disease frequently inflict superficial bites in the skin of people when the animal is held. This particular mite does not burrow in human skin and thus does not cause disease, except for the bite. The same medication that has been given to dogs for heartworm since 1980, ivermectin, is also effective against this mite.

A less common type of mange in animals is caused by *Demodex folliculorum*, a larva shaped mite that is about 0.9 mm in length. These mites burrow into the sebaceous glands and hair follicles of humans, most commonly on the nose and to a lessor extent on the chin, forehead and scalp. Reproduction and egg laying take place in the pilosebaceous gland. Where few mites are present there may be no significant disease apparent. With many mites there may be a papular eruption and inflammation.

In some instances the infestation can produce a rosacea-like dermatitis. Although its role in the disease is controversial, the organism can frequently be found in patients with rosacea if it is looked for. This disease is usually seen only in people past 30 years of age, and rarely in children. It is an occupational hazard among veterinarians and pet groomers, only one among several.

The demodex mite can be expressed from the sebaceous glands by the same technique used on comedones, and then viewed under an ordinary light microscope. The classical treatment is the application of a 5 percent benzyl benzoate cream twice daily. (This is also the old classical treatment of scabies). Adding 5 percent sulfur increases the effectiveness of the treatment against Demodex. Kwell® (lindane) is a more potent agent but it is absorbed through the skin and is toxic to the nervous system. A five percent permethrin cream is the latest addition to our armamentarium. It is effective and safe, except for those people who develop sensitivity to it.

RAT BITE FEVER

This is an infection caused by a streptobacillus, the reservoir of which is the nose and mouth of rats. About one half of wild rats carry the bacterium, and laboratory animals may have a similar incidence; the disease has been contracted from bites in the laboratory. The infection may also be transmitted in contaminated food, and an outbreak in Massachusetts resulting from contamination of milk and ice cream was labeled Haverhill Fever, a dubious distinction for the town of this name. Fever and chills accompany this disease, and a rash is seen in most cases. It is readily treated with penicillin and other appropriate antibiotics.

Q FEVER

Query fever is a rickettsial (*Coxiella burnetii*) disease that is found in cattle, sheep and ticks. Most infections in humans result from inhalation of dust containing the organism; a single inhaled organism is adequate to initiate infection.[65] The organism is extremely resistant to inactivation in the environment, and can survive in dried dust for long periods. It is passed in the excreta of infected animals, and especially high concentrations occur in birthing areas. The organism is also more resistant to many disinfectants than most microorganisms. Chlorine (hypochlorite) solution in adequate concentration for a sufficient period of time is effective if blood or other organic material is not present.

There are several species of ticks in the United States that are naturally infected, including *Dermacentor andersoni*, which also causes tick fever. Tick feces, which contains large numbers of the organism, contaminates the hides of cattle and the wool of sheep. Workers who handle these are then infected when they inhale the infectious agent. Inhalation of dust from barns and pens of cows, sheep and goats is another source of infection. House cats may become infected and shed large numbers of the organism in their feces. Large numbers of the organisms are shed in the parturition products when any of these animals gives birth. Birthing for large herds of sheep should take place indoors in a special facility that can be disinfected afterwards with a phenolic compound (formerly Lysol before its change in formulation).

The organism is present in the milk of all of these animals when they are infected, and the disease may occasionally result from drinking unpasteurized milk, another affliction for those unwise enough to engage in this practice. As with virtually all of the pathogenic organisms found in milk, *Coxiella burnetii* is destroyed by both the flash and holding methods of pasteurization. It is not transmitted from one human to another, but the organism is present in the blood, presenting a hazard to health care personnel. An epidemic that persisted for six months occurred in a research laboratory in San Francisco in 1978 as a result of transporting sheep in an elevator in the building. Similarly, trucks transporting sheep have disseminated the disease to people on the street as they passed by.

In most instances Q Fever produces a pneumonitis, a mild flu-like illness, but it may produce a severe illness, with a temperature of 104° Fahrenheit. The illness is more serious in the elderly. It requires more intense and persistent treatment than most illnesses; doxycycline 100 mg twice daily for 15 to 21 days. Chronic infections require doxycycline combined with rifampin or trimethoprim-sulfamethoxazole for a minimum of 2 to 3 years.[66] Q fever also may affect the heart, and this sequela may occur many years after recovery. It is often fatal when the heart is involved, particularly in individuals who have valvular disease, as occurs as a result of rheumatic fever and congenital heart disease. Hepatitis is seen in about a third of the victims who have protracted disease.

Rickettsial diseases are transmitted to humans by mites, ticks, fleas and the body louse. Some of these diseases and their origins are listed below.

RICKETTSIAL DISEASES IN THE UNITED STATES

DISEASE	RESERVOIR	MODE TRANS-MISSION
Rocky Mountain spotted fever	Rodents, dogs	Tick bite
Rickettsial pox	Rodents, house mouse	Mite bite
Endemic typhus (murine)	Small rodents	Flea feces in broken skin
Epidemic typhus	Humans	Body lice feces into skin
Q (Query) fever	Sheep, goats, cattle	Inhalation of contaminated dust
Ehrlichiosis	Dogs	Tick bite

ECHINOCOCCUS

This parasite is uncommon in the United States, being seen mainly among sheep farmers who use dogs. The life cycle of the parasite requires both the dog and the sheep for maintenance. The eggs are deposited in the stool of the dog. When these ova are ingested by humans through contaminated food or hands, the embryo penetrates the intestinal wall and is carried by the circulation to the brain, liver, lung and kidney. In these anatomic locations, cysts are formed that slowly enlarge, producing pressure. The cysts are filled with infectious organisms. About 200 cases are reported in the United States each year, chiefly among Basque sheep farmers in California, the southwestern Indians, and sheep raisers in Utah.

GIARDIA

This protozoan disease causes intestinal infection in humans (diarrhea) and the organism is shed in the stool of infested humans and pets. It thus can be transmitted to humans by hands or by contaminated food. It is more commonly acquired by drinking contaminated water, either from wells in certain regions of the United States, or from natural bodies of water contaminated by animals, most notably beavers (see Giardia in Chapter V also). Outbreaks are common in mountain communities that derive their water supply from streams and rivers and fail to provide adequate filtration. The concentration of chlorine customarily used in municipal treatment plants does not kill the cysts of Giardia. Proper filtration is essential.

Giardia has become the most frequently recovered parasite in human stool specimens, occurring in over 7 percent of those examined in recent years. This incidence has almost doubled during the past decade, perhaps due to immigration from South America and Southeast Asia during that period.

CRYPTOSPORIDIOSIS

Cryptosporidium is a protozoan that can infect the intestinal tract of man and most other animals. Cattle, deer and sheep can carry both *E. Coli* O157:H7 and *Cryptosporidium* without any evidence of illness, and pass the organisms in their feces. The disease in humans, which was first observed in 1976, is usually acquired from water supplies that have been contaminated by human waste or that of animals. Cows are the animals that most frequently contaminate bodies of water. Calves with diarrheal disease are particularly hazardous. The *Cryptosporidium* spores are not inactivated by any of the conventional chemical means of treating water, and require more precise filtration than sand for control. *Cryptosporidium* is also discussed in Chapters V and XI.

CAMPYLOBACTER JEJUNI

Campylobacter has several features in common with *Giardia*. Many cases of diarrhea caused by this bacterium are acquired from drinking contaminated water from mountain streams or wells. *Campylobacter jejuni*, as well as other *Campylobacter* species, is present in the intestine of domestic and wild animals and poultry.

Excrement from these sources contaminates streams and water supplies. It is also found in contaminated milk or other dairy products, frequently from cattle that are carriers of the organism. Since 1983 several instances of *Campylobacter* illness have been reported among school children visiting dairies and consuming raw milk products in California, Michigan, Minnesota, Pennsylvania, Vermont, and British Columbia.

Prior to 1972 *Campylobacter* was not associated with intestinal infections, but by 1979 it had become second only to *Giardia* as a cause of water-borne diarrheal disease in the United States. Contamination of food by excrement from pets in the home is also a common source of *Campylobacter* infection. Puppies and kittens are a common source, particularly when they are sick. Infections have been seen frequently in slaughterhouse workers who are in contact with the intestines of animals. The diarrhea, which begins two to ten days after exposure, may be pronounced. It is accompanied by a fever, and bloody stools may be present, especially in children.

1. Bowie WR, King AS, Werker DH et.al. Outbreak of toxoplasmosis associated with municipal drinking water. *Lancet* 1997;**350**:173-177.

2. CDC. Encephalitis Associated with Cat Scratch Disease — Broward and Palm Beach Counties, Florida, 1994. *MMWR* 1994;**43**(49):909-916.

3. Drancourt M, Birtles R, Chaumentin G, et al. New Serotype of *Bartonella Henselae* in Endocarditis and Cat-scratch Disease. *Lancet* 1996;**347**:441-443.

4. Alkan S, Morgan M, Sandin R et al. Dual role for *Afipia felis* and *Rochalimaea henselae* in cat-scratch disease. Lancet 1995;**345:** 385.

5. Martinez S, Marr JJ. Allopurinol in the treatment of American cutaneous leishmaniasis. *N Engl J Med* 1992;**326**:741-4.

6. Dryden MS, Dalgliesh D. *Pasteurella multocida* from a dog causing Ludwig's angina. *Lancet* 1996;**347**:123.

7. CDC. Outbreaks of multidrug-resistant Salmonella typhimurium associated with veterinary facilities — Idaho, Minnesota and Washington, 1999. *MMWR* 2001;**50**:701-704.

8. Vinetz J. *Ann Intern Med* 1996; **125**:794-98.

9. CDC. Outbreak of Leptospirosis Among White-Water Rafters — Costa Rica, 1996. *MMWR* 1997;**46:**577-579.

310

10. CDC. Reptile-associated Salmonellosis — Selected States, 1996-1998. *MMWR* 1999;**48**:1009-1013.

11. CDC. Salmonella hadar associated with pet ducklings — Connecticut, Maryland and Pennsylvania, 1991. *MMWR* 1992;**41**(11):185-187.

12. Ohio Department of Health. Children, ducks and *Salmonella hadar*. *Preventative Medicine Monthly*, May, 1992.

13. Alavanja M, Brownson R, Berger E, Lubin J, Modigh C. Avian exposure and risk of lung cancer in women in Missouri: population based case control study. *BMJ* 1996;**313**:1233-1235.

14. Holst P, Kromhout D, Brand R. Pet birds as an independent risk factor for lung cancer. *BMJ* 1988;**297**:1319-1321.

15. Kohlmeier L, Arminger A, Bartolomeycik S, Bellach B, Rehm J, Thamm M. Pet birds as an independent risk factor for lung cancer: case-control study. *BMJ* 1992;**305**:986-989.

16. CDC. Human anthrax associated with an epizootic among livestock — North Dakota, 2001. *MMWR* 2000;**50**:677-680.

17. Rowe, PM. Anthrax continues to threaten human health. *Lancet* 1996;**348**:48.

18. Brachman PS. Inhalation anthrax. *Ann NY Acad Sci* 1980;**353**:83-93.

19. CDC. Update: Investigation of anthrax associated with intentional exposure and interim public health guidelines, October 2001. MMWR 2001;50:889-893.

20. Pini P. Anthrax continues to threaten human health. *Lancet* 1996;**348**:48.

21. Rowe, PM. Op. cit.

22. CDC. Update:Racoon Rabies Epizootic — United States, 1996. *MMWR* 1997;**45**:1117-1120.

23. CDC. Extension of raccoon rabies epizootic — United States, 1992. *MMWR* 1992;**41**(36):661–664.

24. CDC. Human Rabies — Texas and New Jersey, 1997. *MMWR*;**47**:1-5.

25. Petricciani JC. Ongoing tragedy of rabies. *Lancet* 1993;**342**:1067-1068.

26. CDC. Compendium on Animal Rabies Prevention and Control, 2001. *MMWR*;**50**:No. RR-8.

27. CDC. Human Rabies — Texas and New Jersey, 1997. *MMWR* 1997;**47**:1-5.

28. Feder HM, Nelson R, Reiher HW. Rat bite? *Lancet* 1997;**350**:1300.

29. CDC. Human rabies — Connecticut. *MMWR* 1996;**45**:207-209.

30. Wiktor TJ, Plotkin SA, Koprowski H. Development and clinical trials of the new human rabies vaccine of tissue culture (human diploid cell) origin. *Dev Biol Stand* 1978;**40**:3-9.

31. Burgoyne GH, Kajiya KD, Brown DW, Mitchell JR. Rhesus diploid rabies vaccine (adsorbed): a new rabies vaccine using FRhL-2 cells. *J Infect Dis* 1985;**152**:204-210.

32. CDC. Availability of New Rabies Vaccine for Human Use. *MMWR* 1998;**47**:12,19.

33. Talan DA, Citron DM, Abrahamian FM, et al. Bacteriologic analysis of infected dog and cat bites. *N Engl J Med* 1999;**340**:85-92.

34. CDC. Human Rabies — Washington, 1995. *MMWR* 1995;**44**:625-627.

35. CDC. Locally acquired neurocysticercosis — North Carolina, Massachusetts, and South Carolina, 1989–1991. *MMWR* 1992;**41**:1-4.

36. *The Australian*, April 12, 2001.

37. Brunetti R, Fritz RF, Hollister HC. An outbreak of malaria in California, 1952— 1953. *Am J Trop Med* 1953;**3**:779-88.

38. Maldonado YA. Nahlen BL, Roberto RR et al. Transmission of *Plasmodium vivax* malaria in San Diego County, California, 1986. *Am J Trop Med Hyg* 1990:**42**(1):3-9.

39. CDC. Mosquito-Transmitted Malaria — Michigan, 1995. *MMWR* 1996;**45**-(19):398-400.

40. Manson-Bahr PEC, Apted FIC; *Manson's tropical diseases*, ed 19. Bailliere Tindall, London, 1988.

41. CDC. Update: Aedes albopictus infestation — United States. *MMWR* 1986;**35**:649-651.

42. Francy DB et al. *Science*, Dec 21 1990, **250**(4988):1738-40.

43. CDC. Arboviral diseases — United States, 1991. *MMWR* 1992;**41**(30):545--548.

44. National Center for Infectious Diseases, CDC, Division of Vector-Borne Infectious Diseases, Ft. Collins, Colorado, 80522.

45. CDC. Outbreak of relapsing fever — Grand Canyon National Park, Arizona, 1990. *MMWR* 1991;**40**(18):296–303.

46. CDC. 1992. Personal communication.

47. CDC. Lyme Disease — United States, 1999. *MMWR* 2001;**50**:181-185.

48. Schaffner W, Standaert S. Ehrlichiosis — in pursuit of an emerging infection. *N Engl J Med* 1996;**334**:262-263.

49. CDC. Rocky Mountain spotted fever and human ehrlichiosis— United States, 1989. *MMWR* 1990;**39**:281-284.

50. Anderson BE, Dawson JE, Jones DC, and Wilson KH. 1991. Ehrlichia chafeensis, a new species associated with human ehrlichiosis. *J Clin Microbiol.* **29**:2838–2842.

51. Dawson JE, Anderson BE, Fishbein DB, Sanchez JL, Goldsmith CS, Wilson KH, and Duntley CW. 1991. Isolation and characterization of an Ehrlichia sp. from a patient with human ehrlichiosis. *J Clin Microbiol* **29**:2741– 2745.

52. Anderson BE, Sumner JW, Dawson JE, Tzianabos T, Greene CR, Olson JG, Fishbein DB, Rasmussen M, Holloway BP, George EH and Azad AF. Detection of the etiologic agent of human ehrlichiosis by polymerase chain reaction. *J Clin Microbiol* 1992;**29**:2741—2745.

53. Garrison, FH. *History of Medicine.* ed 4. Philadelphia: WB Saunders, 1929.

54. Garrison FH. op cit.

55. Garrison FH. op cit.

56. Garrison FH. op cit.

57. CDC. Prevention of Plague: recommendations of the Advisory Committee on Immunization Practices. *MMWR* 1996;**45**(No.RR-14):1-15.

58. CDC. Pneumonic plague — Arizona, 1992. *MMWR* 1992;**41**(40):737–739.

59. Lee HW, Lee PW, Johnson KM. Isolation of the etiologic agent of Korean hemorrhagic fever. *J Infect Dis* 1978;**137**:298–308.

60. CDC. Update: Hantavirus Pulmonary Syndrome — United States, 1999. *MMWR* 1999;**48**:521-525.

61. CDC. Update: Hantavirus-associated illness — North Dakota, 1993. *MMWR* 1993;**42**:707.

62. CDC. Update:hantavirus pulmonary syndrome — United States, 1993. *MMWR* 1993;**42**:816-820.

63. CDC. Hantavirus infection — Southwestern United States. Interim recommendations for risk reduction. *MMWR* 1993;**42**(No.RR-11):1-13.

64. Posson SC, Told TN, Hollar GF. Recognition of *Hantavirus* infection in the rural setting: Report of first Colorado resident to survive. *JAOA* **93**:1061–1064.

65. Raoult D, Marrie T. Q fever. *Clin Infect Dis* 1995;**20**:489-496.

66. CDC. Q Fever Outbreak — Germany, 1996. *MMWR* 1997;**46**:29-32.

VIII

HAZARDS OF RECREATION

Only a fool would be content to view the sunset through another's eyes.
— DEW

ACCIDENTS

By far the greatest hazard of recreational activities is accidents and personal injury. The leading causes of accidental death in the United States, in descending order, are motor vehicle accidents, falls, drownings, and fires and burns. About 43,000 people are killed each year in the United States in motor vehicle accidents. Falls account for about 14,000 deaths, half of which occur at home. About 4,000 people die by drowning, approximately 700 of these in the home. Fires and burns kill slightly under 4,000 people each year, the majority of which occur at home.[1] There were 77 deaths and an estimated 19,400 injuries among young people under 16 years of age from ATVs (all terrain vehicles) in 1990. These young people account for 40 percent of all such deaths and injuries. All terrain vehicles are dangerous even when driven by adults, and should not be turned over to young people as a toy. About 20 people are killed by avalanches each year in the United States and Canada and about 120 in the Alps. Of the 17 deaths while skiing in the United States during the 1996-97 season, 10 resulted from collisions with a tree.

These are the statistics. They tell nothing of the emotional trauma of those who are touched by these deaths. They also do not assay the financial hardship of those who are left behind. They tell nothing of the cost to society, financial or otherwise. Most of these deaths need never happen. While death is inevitable for everyone, untimely death invariably leaves a deep scar and levies a heavy burden on those left behind.

Many recreational activities naturally carry an element of risk. Skydiving, for instance, carries a risk of parachute failure, which is not preventable in many instances. Many drownings, on the other hand, could be prevented if proper floatation devices were used religiously, and if greater swimming proficiency were acquired. The two hundred or so people who are killed by lightning each year in the United States might not be victims if they avoided seeking refuge under trees during a thunderstorm. Smoking in bed probably cannot be classified as a recreational activity, but many people die in fires as a result of this foolishness each year.

HEARING

Damage to hearing is related to both the loudness of the sound and to the length of exposure. High-pitched sounds are much more damaging than low-pitched tones. Hearing loss, therefore, is most frequently seen in the frequencies of 2,000 hertz (cycles per second) and above. Exposure to jet engine noise and rock music has resulted in loss of hearing in the high frequency range in many individuals. A single exposure may result in fatigue of the inner ear and a loss that may be temporary. Hearing may recover after a period of freedom from exposure to that noise source. If that sound is repeated, and if it is frequent enough, the hearing loss may become permanent due to the destruction of the cells in the inner ear. These cells are never repaired or replaced. Such a hearing loss may result from repeated exposure over a long period of time, or it may result from a brief exposure to very loud noise.

Noise induced hearing loss normally begins at 4,000 hertz and spreads to the frequencies above and below this. Audiograms of workers exposed to noise typically demonstrate a significant hearing loss between the 3,000 and 6,000 Hertz range. The human ear is much less sensitive to low-pitched sounds than high frequency sounds. The loss is invariably insidious, with the individual unaware that any change has taken place. Frequently the first evidence of a hearing loss is the inability to understand what has been said, even though the statement had been heard. This deficit in "discrimination" occurs because the hearing loss at the higher frequencies results in parts of words, usually the consonant sounds, not being heard.

In a recent routine health screen of 123 employees of a small company, over 70 percent of the employees demonstrated a significant hearing loss, chiefly in the high frequency range. Most of these were individuals in their forties, and the majority were not job related. Virtually none of these employees was aware of any hearing loss. A sampling of dentists in the Seattle area in 1987 revealed that 77 percent in the 40-to-50 year age group had a moderate to severe hearing loss as a result of exposure to the high dental speed drill.

Exposure to noise on the job and the resultant hearing loss is the most common occupational risk in the United States today. About eighty million dollars is paid each year in workers compensation claims for loss of hearing. This is a greater sum than is paid for any other occupational disease. These facts introduce a compelling financial incentive to take measures to reduce this morbidity. Governmental agencies charged with this responsibility have been aware of the problem for many years. Technology sophisticated enough to measure noise levels and the related hearing loss was not available until well after World War II. Standards were set and more precise controls outlined with the passage of the Occupational Safety and Health Act in 1970. The history of these efforts and their current status are discussed in Chapter X.

Significantly, much of the hearing loss in our society today results not from the job. While we have made much progress toward protecting the hearing at work, the loss of hearing at play has increased. The level of noise that we are exposed to in our everyday lives away from the work place is not at all appreciated. Some of these noise levels, measured in decibels, are listed in the table below. (The decibel is a logarithmic expression of sound pressure levels. Each ten-decibel increase represents a doubling of the sound pressure level at the ear.) Any exposure at 100 decibels or above entails a high risk of a hearing loss.

NOISE LEVELS WITH SOME COMMON ACTIVITIES

Conversation	65
Lawn mower	93
Diesel garden tractor	83–95
Chain saw	105
Grinding	115
Rock and roll band	110–130
Shooting a .44 magnum	140
12 gauge shotgun	140
Jet plane taking off	145
at 50 feet	130
Thunderclap, overhead	120
Pain threshold	100

Headphones with portable music sources are particularly insidious, for they deliver loud music directly to the ear, at a very high level in some instances. The lack of any apparent immediate adverse effect prompts individuals to discount any hazard. As discussed above, hearing loss is insidious, is not readily apparent, and is progressive over time. Ringing in the ears after such a noise exposure is a warning sign of the danger.

Noise levels below 80 decibels do not induce a hearing loss, whereas sustained noise levels of 85 decibels present a definite risk of hearing loss. Hearing protection should always be worn during activities that expose individuals to a noise level over 85 decibels for any period of time. This covers all shooting activities, and should include many other activities, obvious from the table above, where protection is never utilized. The human ear should never be exposed to a level in excess of 140 decibels. Repeated or prolonged exposure to noise levels below 140 decibels can produce significant hearing loss through fatigue of the muscles that dampen the movement of the tiny bones that transmit the sound to the inner ear.

Hearing protection is available in the form of earplugs and earmuffs. There has been significant progress in the development of these aids recently, rendering them more effective. They are rated on the basis of a "Noise Reduction Rating" which, by law, must be printed on the outside of the package that they are sold in. Although these ratings are given for various frequencies, the most important from a hearing conservation standpoint is the rating at 500 and 1,000 Hz. Properly fitted earmuffs generally offer better protection than earplugs, but are more expensive and less comfortable.

The effectiveness of earplugs has been improved significantly, especially those that now are built with a valve incorporated. This design permits the passage of some normal sounds, but closes when struck by a loud impulse. A combination of earplugs and earmuffs provides the greatest hearing protection, and this combination should be considered when involved in prolonged noise exposure. All of these hearing protection devices are available at any gun dealer and at most sporting goods sections of department stores where guns and hunting supplies are sold.

Hunting and shooting are two of the most common causes of a hearing loss. This loss is easily prevented by wearing hearing protection. I have seen an eardrum ruptured and virtually destroyed as a result of permitting a shooting partner to rest a .357 magnum on the victim's shoulder and fire it. The damage required reconstructive surgery. Damage to the inner and middle ear from such abuse may not be reparable. The blast from a handgun or other short-barreled gun is closer to the ear than is the case with a rifle or shotgun, and thus is potentially more damaging.

The noise level from a 12 gauge shotgun is listed at 140 decibels, but more sensitive modern equipment measures peaks as high as 176. If this blast rebounds off of walls of a range or hill this renders it more damaging to the ear. The more prolonged the noise exposure, the greater is the risk of hearing loss. It is clear that even the high noise levels measured with the equipment of the past present a greater risk to hearing than previously thought. Hearing protection should always be worn when shooting.

Some hearing loss with age is inevitable. This involves the higher frequencies more than the lower ones, and results in difficulty understanding conversation in a noisy room, or with background noise such as a television set. There is no cure for any hearing loss, and no absolute prevention for the loss that occurs with age. The latter can be developed sooner and made more severe, however, by unnecessary noise exposure. Hearing loss that results from noise exposure outside of the work place has received very little attention, and the general public is not aware of the danger. Ringing in the ears after a noise exposure such as shooting is a warning that hearing protection should have been utilized. Continual ringing in the ears, while frequently caused by drugs such as aspirin and certain antibiotics, may also be evidence of a noise induced hearing loss. Assessment of noise exposure, both at work and at play, should be undertaken when this is noticed.

Noise has been defined as any undesirable sound. In this vein, beauty is in the eye of the beholder. What is music to one ear is noise to another. The damaging effect of noise depends upon both the frequency and intensity. As stated above, the human ear is more sensitive to high-pitched sounds. Aside from damage to the hearing apparatus, loud noise can produce physical and psychological stress. Some studies have indicated that noise increases the pulse rate, elevates the blood pressure, causes constriction of the arteries and tensing of the skeletal muscles. Individuals chronically exposed complain of nervousness, sleeplessness and fatigue. The adverse effects of excessive noise have been appreciated virtually from the beginning of civilization as evidenced by the many laws that have been passed over the decades in an effort to control it.

The symptoms that result from excessive noise exposure are most frequently produced in the home by music of one form or another. Barking dogs are also a frequent contributor, and this is particularly offensive during the night. Sounds produced in the course of normal activity and play by children and teenagers can at times contribute to stress. All of these sources of noise, while usually well tolerated by the young individual with normal hearing, are not always well tolerated by individuals with a hearing loss, especially age-induced hearing loss. This is not merely a reduction in the hearing level, but a distortion of hearing that makes comprehension of speech more difficult.

Age-induced hearing loss (presbycusis) makes it much more difficult to listen to two different conversations at the same time. With presbycusis, attempting to carry on a conversation with background music or with the television set on is difficult and frequently stressful. This is what frequently accounts for the demands of the middle-aged parent to turn down the television set or music box when the telephone rings.

In the home, it is not practical to walk around all day wearing hearing protection. Much can be done, however, to control the sound level. Sound absorbing materials such as draperies can be used throughout the house. In new construction, sealing of all cracks reduces noise from the outside. Dual pane windows not only conserve energy but also reduce the noise levels transmitted from the outside. Insulation that is installed for energy conservation provides similar benefits in noise reduction. In apartments or duplexes, many measures can be taken to prevent noise transmission between units, such as staggering the studding in the walls between units. This architectural design does much to dampen noise transmission and should be used universally.

Builders are familiar with other sound insulating techniques that should be utilized when planning new construction or remodeling. In existing homes, noise can be isolated to a single room, to a degree, by installing sound absorbing tile or other material in that room. Acoustic tile on the ceiling, for instance, reduces noise transmission from the room where it is applied. In the extreme, the walls can be lined with acoustic tile or cork. The efficiency of sound absorption of various materials can be obtained from building supply dealers. Typically, these materials absorb seventy percent or more of the sound that strikes them.

Most people appreciate the fact that placing distance between them and the source of noise renders it more tolerable. For each doubling of the distance, sound is decreased by six decibels. Most homes do not provide enough space to utilize this principal to render noise acceptable, however.

Hearing loss, like the loss of other faculties, is subtle. As stated earlier, most individuals with a loss are not aware of it. Anyone who has had significant noise exposure should have a hearing test performed by a competent, qualified professional with accurate equipment. Individuals who are continuously exposed to noise on the job or otherwise, such as shooters, should have this test performed at regular intervals to detect any loss early so that appropriate preventative measures can be taken.

ULTRAVIOLET RAYS—SUN

One of the most serious hazards of recreation is excessive exposure to the sun. The major complications of long term exposure to ultraviolet radiation are premature aging of the skin with irreversible loss of the normal elasticity, skin cancers, which include squamous cell carcinoma and its precursor, actinic keratosis and malignant melanoma which is the most lethal of all cancers. These lesions are seen more frequently in sportsmen, farmers, ranchers, sailors and sun worshippers. All of these pathologies occur more commonly in individuals who demonstrate poor tanning, that is, those who have a fair complexion, light hair and light colored eyes. People of Celtic heritage have an ethnic predisposition to skin cancer for unknown reasons. Their known inherited deficiency in the melanin producing system in the skin may be the culprit.

It is known that a single severe sunburn early in life, prior to age twenty years, predisposes to skin cancer later in life. Ultraviolet radiation from the sun produces cellular damage, with alteration in the DNA (desoxyribonucleic acid), proteins, lipids and other cellular components of the skin. It is theorized that this

damage is responsible for the development of skin cancer subse
quently.

For a child born in the United States in the 1930s, the risk
of developing one of the skin cancers during his lifetime was one in
1500. That risk has increased fifteen-fold for children born today.
The risk now is one in one hundred. Between 80,000 and 100,000
individuals develop squamous cell carcinoma of the skin each year,
with 1,900 deaths occurring in 1985. Malignant melanoma develops
in 23,000 Americans each year, with 5,600 deaths recorded in 1986.
Melanoma accounts for 74 percent of all of the deaths from skin
cancer. The risk of contracting this lethal disease has increased
1,000 percent in the past fifty years. The increase in the incidence
of these cancers is not related in any way to atmospheric carbon
dioxide levels or changes in the ozone layer. Rather it is related to
the increase in the amount of leisure time that individuals in the
United States have to bath in the sun.

One severe sunburn in the first ten to twenty years of life
triples the risk of developing malignant melanoma later in life. This
results from the damage to the DNA by the ultraviolet (sun)
exposure and the latency of that damage. See Chapter XIII for a
description of the mechanisms of carcinogenesis and the involvement
of DNA therein.

The dramatic increase in the standard of living in the United
States during the past fifty years has given us much more time for
recreation. It has also given us the discretionary income to utilize
that recreational time in ways that were not available to us in the
past. This has resulted in a vast expansion of recreational activities
such as golfing, boating, water skiing and visits to the beaches. It
has become a popular national pastime to jet off to the beaches of
southern climates where the sun is in abundance during the winter
season. All of these activities have greatly increased our sun
exposure. On those days when the sun does not cooperate in our
efforts to cultivate the tan that everyone worships, we can skip down
to the neighborhood tanning parlor.

This entire spectrum of increased exposure to ultraviolet rays
has produced an alarming increase in the incidence of not only skin
cancers but other skin diseases associated with ultraviolet exposure
as well. These include actinic keratosis, elastosis (loss of elasticity),
premature aging of the skin and of course the skin cancers. The

tanning parlor will assure you that their UV-A radiation does not burn and damage the skin. These UV-A rays do penetrate the skin deeply, however, where they damage the collagen and elastic tissues as well as the blood vessels. These changes account for the premature aging of the skin manifested by wrinkles, dilated blood vessels in the skin and permanent redness.

UV-A has also been found to increase damage done by UV-B, particularly the damage that leads to skin cancer. Most of the tanning devices that produce UV-A also produce some UV-B, although efforts are being made to develop units that deliver pure UV-A. Approximately 700 burn injuries occur in tanning parlors each year in the United States.

It is ironic that the incidence of skin cancer that results from excessive exposure to the sun has increased so dramatically during an era when very effective sunscreens have been available. Use of a sunscreen with a sun protective factor (SPF) of fifteen enables us to remain exposed to the sun all day with no apparent effect on the skin, so long as the sunscreen is renewed to compensate for loss by perspiration, swimming, and wiping with towels. The SPF (Sun Protection Factor) is defined as *the number of MEDs (Minimum Erythema Dose) of radiation required to induce a burn through a thin film of the sunscreen cream or lotion.* The MED is defined as *the smallest amount of sunlight exposure necessary to induce a barely perceptible redness of the skin 24 hours after exposure.*

The sunscreen preparations that contain para-aminobenzoic acid (PABA) and its esters provide protection against UV-B but not UV-A. These products permit some tanning since the UV-A that reaches the skin provokes some melanogenesis (formation of added melanin). This increased melanin production lasts for about 2 weeks and provides some protection from subsequent sun exposure. The down side is that the irradiation of the cells of the skin by the UV-A adds to the risk of skin damage and skin cancer.

The products that contain benzophenones provide efficient protection against UV-A but not UV-B. Products that contain opaque shields such as titanium oxide, zinc oxide, talc and iron oxide provide protection against both UV-A and UV-B. These products reflect and scatter ultraviolet rays and are thus more effective. They are cosmetically less desirable, however. One such product containing titanium dioxide (plus methyl anthranilate) is A-

Fil®. Zinc oxide ointment USP, which is white, is available at pharmacies. Some companies have added dyes to provide a chic red or green cosmetic affect. The opaque sunscreens are what skiers, mountain climbers, pilots and people who live at 10,000 feet should use. They are not as cosmetically appealing as the "invisible" screens, however.

It is also important to note that SPF ratings apply only to UV-B. No rating scheme has been devised for UV-A. A new class of UV-A blocking sunscreens based upon the dibenzoylmethanes has been introduced into the United States. These were designed not for recreational protection against sunburn, but for protection against the photoallergic UV-A mediated reactions experienced by people with disorders such as lupus erythematosus, and people on certain medications. Two such products are Photoplex® and Filteray®

Repeated applications of sunscreens do not extend the protection beyond the factor listed on the label. In other words three or four applications of a product labeled fifteen still protects only for a period fifteen times as long as would be the case with no protection. From a practical standpoint, nothing is gained from protection extending beyond a true fifteen since that would extend protection into the darkness. Even preparations that are promoted as waterproof need to be reapplied after swimming. Sunscreens should be applied about an hour prior to sun exposure in order to permit penetration into the skin for maximum effectiveness. They should not be applied so close to the eyes that they might be inadvertently carried into the eyes. This is especially important in children who are even more prone to rub their eyes than adults are.

Sunscreen preparations are one of the few items on the shelf in the drugstore that do not carry expiration labels. The agents used as UV blockers are for the most part stable compounds. Exposure to freezing may cause a breakdown in emulsification in those products so formulated. Sunscreens should not otherwise lose their effectiveness if retained for 2 or 3 seasons. These products are not cheap and most people will not want to discard them needlessly as is done with many products carrying an expiration label.

While most sunbathing is done at beaches that are close to sea level, skiers need to be reminded that the closer that one gets to the sun, the stronger its effects are. At 5,000 feet the intensity of the sun is 20 percent greater than it is at sea level. Much skiing takes place at altitudes of 8,000 to 11,000 feet. The time period that the skier can be exposed to the sun safely is thus shortened significantly. Attention to protection of exposed skin becomes much more urgent at these altitudes. The risk of ultraviolet burns of the surface of the eye, keratoconjunctivitis, is also greater at higher altitudes, especially when snow is reflecting the sun. Sunglasses help to protect against this risk. Ski goggles offer the added protection of blocking the UV rays that are reflected around and behind conventional glasses. Some goggles are advertised to provide 100% protection from UV radiation.

Evidence has evolved recently that ultraviolet radiation also plays a roll in the development of cataracts. Plastic (CR-39 and acrylic) and glass conventional lenses screen most ultraviolet radiation. Contact lenses may screen 30 to 80 percent, depending on the type. This has offered a market for the promotion of both conventional and contact lenses that protect from ultraviolet radiation. The consumer has no way to measure the effectiveness of any of these products. You must rely upon the professional advice of your optometrist or ophthalmologist.

It is also important to keep in mind that most of the commonly marketed sunscreens do not protect against photosensitivity reactions that are invoked by certain medications. These medications include certain antibiotics, tranquilizers, diuretics and oral diabetic medication. Not all medications in any of these groups cause this reaction. Phenothiazines can provoke such a reaction if accidentally applied to the skin, and this problem has been seen in nurses and pharmacists. A similar phototoxic reaction can occur after ingesting furocoumarins (psoralens) that are found in parsley, celery, and limes. This reaction can occur after simply rubbing these substances on the skin, for they readily penetrate the skin. This has been observed in individuals handling produce in grocery stores, and in workers harvesting celery with pink rot disease. Photosensitization can also occur after ingestion of a tea brewed from Saint-John's-wort due to the presence of the poison hypericin.

Photoallergic reactions also can be provoked by the antibacterial agents incorporated into common household hand soaps, one being tribromosalicylanilide (tribromsalan). Most companies have now substituted triclocarban for tribromsalan (Safeguard®, Dial®). Triclocarban is less likely to provoke a photoallergic reaction. Hexachlorophene also carries this risk. Sunscreens that contain 6-methylcoumarin can also cause a reaction. Coumarins (psoralens) as a group are notorious for causing photoallergic reactions. They are also of concern because they enhance the carcinogenic activity of ultraviolet radiation. Some individuals develop a sensitivity to some of the chemical constituents in the sunscreen products. This occurs on rare occasions with PABA. If this occurs, switching to a different preparation with different ingredients may resolve the problem.

Coumarin is one of a group of substances derived from essential oils, so named because they contain the essence, that is the odor or flavor, of the plant from which they are extracted. Some of the more common such oils are lemon, lime and orange, cedarwood, sandlewood, lavender and musk. All of these can produce photoallergic reactions. This becomes particularly important when they are used in perfumes.

Photosensitivity reactions are provoked by the UV-A fraction of the sun, against which the commonly used sunscreens do not protect, as mentioned above. As a result reactions can be provoked by sun irradiation through a window or an automobile glass. Although UV-B is blocked by glass, UV-A is not. UV-A, even though it is a less potent cause of sunburn, is no less potent in causing skin damage including aging and cancer. UV-A radiation reaches the earth's surface fairly constantly throughout the day, whereas very little UV-B does so before 10:00 A.M. and after 3:00 P.M. It is thus possible to experience exposure to UV-A for twice the period each day as for UV-B. This exposure is not noticed because less erythema is produced.

Snow and white sand reflect UV radiation very effectively, and a burn can result even in the protection of an umbrella or other source of shade. A thin cloud cover also permits 50 percent or more of the UV radiation to penetrate. The security felt under these circumstances is frequently unwarranted.

Total avoidance of the sun is mandatory with some acquired and familial diseases. Lupus erythematosus is perhaps the most common example of one such disorder that individuals are born with. Others include phenylketonuria (PKU), albinism and the porphyrias. Forms of the latter two can also be acquired later in life. Some red or sandy-haired individuals of Celtic ancestry have deficient melanin producing systems, and cannot achieve tanning without the risk of a severe sunburn. Efforts to achieve a tan should be avoided by these individuals because of the adverse long-term effects of ultraviolet radiation.

If a sunscreen is to be relied on by these people it should be one of the so-called broad- spectrum products that contain protection for both UV-A and UV-B. The opaque screens such as zinc oxide and titanium oxide offer better protection. The use of these products cannot offer total protection. Avoidance of sun exposure to the fullest extent possible is still the wisest course of action with these diseases. The herpes virus is also frequently activated by sun exposure due to the immunosuppressant action of UV-B. This is mediated through several mechanisms including suppression of lymphocytes.

PHOTOTOXIC OR PHOTOALLERGENIC AGENTS

Coal tar (anthracene, phenanthrene)	Para-aminobenzoic acid
Creosote	Chlorothiazide
Carrots	Phenothiazines
Celery	Griseofulvin
Dill	Benzophenones
Lemons, Lime	Quinine
Parsley	Nalidixic acid
Parsnip	Tetracyclines
Buttercup	Sulfonamides
Mustard	Tribromsalan
Cedarwood oil	Hexachlorophene
Sandlewood oil	Saccharin
Lavender oil	Optical whiteners
Musk	Epoxy resins
Coumarins (psoralens)	St. John's wort (hypericin)

TEMPERATURE DISORDERS

Many recreational activities expose the individual to excesses of heat or cold that threaten serious consequences. These disorders are covered in Chapter IX and that information should be reviewed before undertaking recreational activities in extremes of heat or cold. Familiarization with these disorders of heat and cold exposure will permit individuals to avoid some serious and painful consequences. This is particularly important for those individuals who are past their prime years of the thirties.

The adaptive mechanisms of the body for both heat and cold become less efficient after our youth, a process that progresses with age. Some activities, such as strenuous running, especially in hot weather, have resulted in publications of descriptions of special disorders that are merely variations of previously recognized heat stress diseases. Runners should become thoroughly familiar with the information on heat disorders before embarking on their adventures.

ALTITUDE (MOUNTAIN) SICKNESS (MONGE'S DISEASE)

José d'Acosta, a Jesuit missionary, first described mountain sickness in 1590. The illness results when people travel from sea level or the altitude of the cities of the Midwest (700 to 800 feet) to an altitude of over 8,000 feet in a short period of time. This classically happens when skiers travel by jet to one of the popular resorts in the Rocky Mountains. In the milder form the only symptoms are headache, nausea, loss of appetite, weakness, shortness of breath with exertion and a general feeling of malaise (sickness). The symptoms are provoked by a sudden drop in the amount of oxygen available to the blood. This stimulates deeper and more rapid breathing, which alters the acid-base balance and results in a respiratory alkalosis. Breathing is diminished during sleep, further aggravating the oxygen deprivation. At the cellular level throughout the body an imbalance between sodium and potassium ions occurs which disrupts the water balance and interferes with normal function.

In a sudden ascent to 12,000 feet 50 percent of the people will experience headache, about 10 percent will suffer severe headache and nausea and vomiting. At this elevation altitude sickness is usually mild and clears in a day or two. Activities should be restricted and moderate in nature for the first day or two. Salt should be restricted and a concerted effort to increase water intake should be made.

Individuals who have preexisting pulmonary or heart conditions who attempt any physical exertion such as skiing on the day of arrival may end up in the hospital. At 17,000 feet the air entering the lungs provides only half of the oxygen that it does at sea level. The reduced atmospheric pressure compounds this deficiency by decreasing the force that drives oxygen from the lungs into the bloodstream. Even in a rapid ascent to only 9,000 feet (Midwesterner flying into Denver, driving to Winter Park) at least 20 percent of individuals will experience evidence of mountain sickness with headache, nausea, fatigue, shortness of breath and some loss of appetite. These normally subside in one to two days.

Altitude sickness tends to be more common and more severe in women during menstruation. Women who have less than optimal hemoglobin levels (14.5 gm/Dl) as a result of excessive menstruation, will also suffer more pronounced symptoms. Efforts to correct this deficiency through iron replacement and adequate protein intake will prove to be beneficial. Frequently, one month of such therapy prior to ascent to altitude will prevent or at least minimize the symptoms of altitude sickness.

After arriving at altitude, activities should be restricted and moderate for the first 1 to 2 days. Drinking adequate quantities of water while avoiding alcohol and salt (sodium) is beneficial. Sedatives and sleep medication should also be avoided since they further impair lung function during sleep. Dramamine® (dimenhydrinate), meclizine or cyclizine (Marezine®) provides relief from the symptoms. Acetazolamide (Diamox®) has long been known to ameliorate the symptoms of mountain sickness, especially if taken prophylactically before ascent.[2] It acts in the kidney to correct the respiratory alkalosis that is associated with altitude sickness by increasing the excretion of bicarbonate. Acetazolamide is used in acute cases, sometimes along with dexamethasone, and some experts recommend that it be taken prophylactically the day before, the day of and the day after arrival at altitude. A small dose, 50 to 125 mg taken three times daily at 8-hour intervals for the three days described above will provide relief for most people. It effectively corrects periodic breathing or sleep apnea that is almost universal when sleeping at high altitudes.

Acetazolamide should not be taken when pregnant, or when pregnancy is a possibility. Caution is needed also in cases of liver or kidney dysfunction. It is a member of the sulfa family, so should not be taken by those who are sensitive to this class of drugs. Although side effects are uncommon, it should be taken only after approval by the family physician. This medication is available by prescription only, for good reason.

In the severe form of altitude sickness fluid accumulates in the lungs. Bleeding into the lungs also occurs in some instances. Accumulation of fluid in the brain sometimes accompanies the pulmonary edema. Even the administration of pure oxygen at high altitudes does not rectify the crisis. The reduced atmospheric pressure does not permit the adequate transport of oxygen from the lungs into the blood. Fatalities occur every year at resorts that are located at altitudes above 8,000 feet. Sleeping below 8,000 feet would avoid these deaths. Newborn infants should not be taken to these altitudes until they are at least two weeks old, since their lungs are not completely expanded.

The same precaution for newborn infants applies to air travel, since the immature lung may not be able to compensate for the reduced oxygen level in the cabin. Commercial airplanes are reputedly pressurized to 8,000 feet, but this can not be assured at all times. Even when it is this reduction in cabin pressure from most regions where people reside (700 feet) results in a 30 percent expansion of gas in the stomach and intestines.[3] Consumption of carbonated beverages increases this expansion even more. Under these circumstances it is surprising that there is not a greater incidence of perforation of ulcers and diverticula.

The only certain prevention for altitude sickness is to spend a minimum of two days at an altitude of about 7,000 feet before attempting skiing at 11,000 feet. If staying at an altitude of 11,000 feet it is better to drive in, where some acclimatization is made automatically by the trip, than to fly in where no adjustment period is provided. For those climbing to even higher altitudes, the experts recommend a gradual climb of 2,000 feet per day above 5,000. No amount of cardiovascular or muscular conditioning prior to the trip prevents this problem. Living and sleeping in an altitude chamber for three or four days prior to the trip would provide the necessary transition, if you have one accessible.

Chronic mountain sickness (Monge's disease) is common in regions such as the Andes, where it has been labeled soroche (antimony), through a mistaken belief that it was due to inhalation of that metal. The disease is caused by hypoventilation along with the decreased oxygen content of the air. The complexion takes on a distinctive reddish hue that turns to cyanosis with even minimal exertion. The condition occurs primarily in those past the age of 40, and returns to normal upon descent to sea level. Most of the residents of these high altitude civilizations develop compensatory mechanisms after a period, such as polycythemia (an increase in the number of red blood cells and a hemoglobin level above the normal), an increased volume of blood in the capillaries in the lungs, increased diffusion capacity in the lungs, and an increased heart output. These mechanisms take a long time to develop, and are not available to most skiers.

The issue of health risk during skiing is especially pertinent in older individuals (anything past 38 years can be "older"). About one-third of the skiers who invade the slopes in Colorado (9,000 to 11,000 foot altitude) who are over 45 years old have some level of coronary artery disease. In these individuals the decrease in oxygen available to the body is compounded by the exertion inherent in this activity. The reduced oxygen supply in itself increases the heart rate and causes the heart to work harder. At the same time the work capacity of the heart is reduced by about 30 percent at the altitude of the slopes. Some of this capacity is regained after a few days of adaptation by the body, so prudence would dictate no strenuous activity for at least 2 to 3 days at altitude. Approximately 500,000 people die of ischemic heart disease in the United States each year. It is the leading cause of death, and some of these will occur at ski resorts. Of course there is an increased risk in these people, but the level of risk varies. It is obviously significantly higher in those who are overweight, who smoke and who are "out of shape".

Even those in excellent health should "tone up" before a skiing trip. Brisk walking or an exercise unit can accomplish this. It is especially important to tone up the thigh muscles (quadriceps). For the individual who is overweight, in poor shape and past mid-life it will take more than a few weeks to prepare for a ski trip. It may take 6 months or more, depending upon the level of overweight and poor muscle tone.

About 400,000 people die unexpectedly in the United States each year. Most of these are cardiac deaths. Some of these are going to occur on the slopes, but that is not to say that the event would not have happened had the individual stayed at home. Many cardiac deaths occur each year while snow shoveling and hunting. Skiing is excellent exercise and is beneficial to the heart-lung machine. It should not be undertaken as the first step in a physical fitness program if you are past 50 and overweight, however.

Physicians can assess the status of the coronary arteries but the tests are not infallible. The issue of skiing and climbing is an especially difficult problem in those who have had a previous myocardial infarction or who have undergone a coronary bypass operation. The status of the lungs is just as important as the heart, especially in smokers. Anyone on medication should consult with the family physician regarding the wisdom of traveling to high altitude or skiing.

Hypertension per se is not a contraindication to skiing. The blood pressure is not adversely affected by altitude. If the hypertension has contributed to the development of coronary artery disease, the coronary disease is the problem to be considered. Statistically, in the studies that have been done, very few individuals who have climbed to higher altitudes have suffered cardiac problems. While it will be safe to continue most medications, some can pose a serious threat. An individual who is on anti-coagulants and who falls striking his head (not unheard of in skiing) is at risk of hemorrhage in the brain. Even aspirin consumption increases the risk of internal hemorrhage in the event of an injury, and thus should be avoided during skiing.

Aside from the problem of altitude sickness, visitations to high altitudes such as are encountered when skiing may also result in additional problems with contact lenses. The reduced oxygen content of the air results in even less oxygen being available to the cornea. In addition the increased loss of fluid by the body that results from the low humidity of the ambient air and the reduced atmospheric pressure also produces greater drying of the lens and the cornea. Periodic moistening of the contact lens and cornea with an acceptable wetting agent will minimize this problem.

BITES AND STINGS

INSECTS

For most people a sting by a bee, wasp or hornet is a painful experience. For the many people who have become hypersensitized it may be fatal as well. Three times as many people die each year as a result of bee stings as from snakebites. Death results from anaphylaxis (shock) due to an allergic reaction. Sensitive individuals should carry a kit that contains epinephrine that is marketed for this purpose. These individuals should consult with their family physician regarding the use of the kit, and other recommended procedures. The stinger should be gently teased out by scraping rather than by pulling, to avoid injecting additional venom into the skin. Perfumes and bright colors attract bees, and should be avoided when in bee territory. Desensitization for bee venom is available and is effective.

A new dimension has been added to the risk of bee stings with the invasion of the Africanized honeybee. A scientist in Brazil brought the African honeybees to his laboratory for study because of their reputation for greater honey production. Some of the bees escaped from his laboratory in 1956, and have since killed more than 2000 people. They traveled through Central America into Mexico, and were detected near Hidalgo, Texas in October 1993. The bees continued to advance 100 to 300 miles per year, colonizing the hives of domestic bees as well as forming new hives in the wild. They spread into New Mexico and Arizona, and in 1999 they were on the doorstep of Los Angeles and San Diego. Africanized honeybees are much more aggressive and are more likely to attack than domestic bees. They also attack in large numbers, resulting in massive envenomation. This causes rhabdomyolysis, hemolysis and acute kidney failure. Survival requires aggressive, sophisticated therapy (e.g. hemodialysis) and even then kidney function may not return to normal for months.

Both the red and black imported fire ant were brought into the United States from South America in cargo shipped through the port of Mobile, Alabama in the early 1900s. By the 1950s they had been distributed through nine southern states in nursery stock. By 1989 they had spread throughout Florida, South Carolina, Georgia, Alabama, Louisiana, Mississippi and eastern Texas. The fire ant has displaced all other ants in these regions for the most part.

Recent studies have revealed that a hybrid has evolved from the two species, and that it survives colder temperatures than the 10° F. that restricted the spread of the original imports. In view of the increased tolerance of colder weather it is projected that the hybrid fire ant will spread further to Arizona, California and coastal Washington and Oregon.

The fire ants have had no natural enemies in the United States, and are resistant to most pesticides. Heptachlor was used effectively as a control in the 1960s, but it is related to chlordane chemically and was removed from the market. Mirex was then used successfully, but the discovery that it degrades to chlordecone (Kepone), which is toxic to the liver and brain in man, led to a ban on it also. Treatment of the mound nests with diazinon or chlor-pyrifos (Dursban) clears the center of the nest temporarily, but survivors from the periphery soon repopulate it. There currently is no means of controlling this pest. In 1996 researchers began studying a South American fly, the Phorid fly, that may help to control fire ant populations. This fly attacks only South American red fire ants, injecting its eggs into the body of the ant. When the eggs hatch, the larva consumes the ant from the inside, destroying it. This control was planned for release in 1997.

Fire ants build large mounds that interfere with farming and damage machinery and equipment. More serious is the ferocity with which they attack humans. Although these ants do bite, the chief reaction is to the venom that is injected through a pod on the ant's abdomen. Each ant may sting 3 or 4 times in rapid succession. Large numbers of ants usually attack, and they move very swiftly. As many as 3,000 to 4,000 stings have been tabulated on a single person. In addition to the serious and unpleasant local reactions, severe allergic reactions are not uncommon, some resulting in death. The stings may result in a severe vesiculation (blistering) of the skin with necrosis (decay). Infection is common following these bites. The ants have invaded houses and attacked humans, especially during rains. During a flood the ants float on the water, and attack anyone they come in contact with.

Bites of ticks, chiggers, mosquitos and deerfly may result in disease in addition to the local discomfort. These diseases, including Lyme disease, are discussed in detail in Chapter VII. Wearing appropriate clothing and using insect repellents such as diethyl-meta-toluamide (DEET) when in the field or woods will minimize these risks. The combination of DEET and permethrin, applied to clothing only, offers even greater protection, since permethrin kills ticks on contact. The pants legs should be tucked into the tops of boots or socks. Hunting or boot socks serve this purpose well. If this does not fit your dress style, some alternate system to prevent ticks from crawling up your pants legs should be devised (perhaps leggings).

Whenever in any area where ticks might be encountered, the body should be inspected daily, more frequently with extended exposure, for their presence. This task has become much more urgent since the appearance of Lyme disease, and at the same time more difficult. The Lyme tick is very small, about the size of a pinhead, and it is difficult to spot (see Chapter VII). When ticks are found they should be removed by careful traction, taking care to not leave the head of the tick behind. If the head remains lodged in the skin, it should be surgically excised, for it can continue to migrate deeper into the tissues. Care should be taken to not compress the body of the tick to avoid injecting disease-producing organisms that may be harbored there. The hot cigarette technique for persuading the tick to dislodge has been abandoned, for it causes the tick to regurgitate, thus injecting more of its toxic and infectious materials.

A more recent technique for tick removal is the application of a cream or shampoo that contains permethrin or one of the other pyrethroids and piperonyl butoxide to the tick until it releases its grip. In the case of seed ticks they may be simply washed off after they become paralyzed. This preparation is sold without prescription for the treatment of head and body lice. A 5 percent permethrin cream (Elimite™) that is available only on prescription is equally effective.

INSECT REPELLENTS

Insect repellents are one of the most valuable discoveries of our era. During my younger years we applied citronella liberally, burned rubber tires or anything else that would produce smoke and noxious fumes, but still were eaten alive by mosquitos. Diethyl-meta-toluamide (DEET), which is the only truly effective repellent, is remarkable in its effectiveness. Products that contain 25 to 50 percent of DEET are more effective and last longer than the less concentrated preparations. Applying these preparations to the clothing rather than to the skin is always preferable. The stronger products are also more effective against the black fly, which is the ultimate challenge.

Products that contain 98 percent of DEET are now available, but are not normally needed. They also increase the risk of sensitivity and toxic reactions even more. Diethyl-meta-toluamide is absorbed through the skin, and has been reported to produce toxic reactions in the nervous system of children. Some children have died, usually after excessive use. Skin contact in children should be avoided, especially in the very young. It also has been reported to produce skin rashes in some individuals. This has usually occurred after heavy applications.

In using the more concentrated preparations these adverse reactions become more probable. A new long acting preparation that contains 35 percent DEET along with a polymer that inhibits both evaporation and skin absorption should be very useful. This promises to do much to reduce both the sensitivity problem and the nervous system reactions. Another new product designed to repel ticks has been marketed under the name of Permanone® Tick Repellent. This product contains the pesticide permethrin 0.5%, a synthetic pyrethroid (see Chapter XIV), and is for application to the clothing, not the skin. Field trials by the Air Force and others have demonstrated that when both DEET and permethrin were used on clothing, protection was virtually 100 percent. This dual application to the clothing will be very useful in the battle against Lyme disease, and indeed all of the tick-borne diseases.

In view of the prolific use and abuse of DEET over a period of many years, it is remarkable that so few problems have surfaced. We should, however, exercise much greater caution in applying this chemical to the skin. It is safer to apply it to clothing, where it also lasts much longer. Perspiration shortens the period of effectiveness. Wearing of long sleeved shirts and pants, and spraying the repellent on them, provides more safety and better protection. This procedure is mandatory for protection against ticks. The pump spray bottles are safer and more economical than the aerosol cans.

In using the aerosols keep in mind that they are flammable, and should not be used in the presence of a lighted cigarette or open flames. They should never be sprayed into the face; rather the repellent should be sprayed onto the hand, then applied to the face and ears, avoiding the eyes and mouth. A recent study has discovered that DEET works by interfering with the receptor cells in the mosquito that respond to the lactic acid that is excreted through our skin. This discovery opens the way for the development of additional substances to thwart this mechanism.

COLORADO TICK FEVER

This is a viral disease that replicates in ticks and is not transmitted from animals. It has been identified in Colorado, Idaho, Nevada, Wyoming, Montana, Utah, Oregon, Washington and California. It has been misdiagnosed as Rocky Mountain spotted fever, partially because it outnumbers that disease by twenty to one in Colorado. It occurs mainly in May and June (March through September for the full season). About one week after the bite of a tick the victim experiences fever of 102 to 104 degrees Fahrenheit, chills, severe aching and headache. There is rarely a rash. The symptoms last from one to three weeks, depending upon age. There is no effective treatment, and recovery is almost universal.

RELAPSING FEVER

Relapsing fever is an infectious disease caused by one of several species of spirochetes that are transmitted from ground squirrels or other small rodents to man through the bite of a soft-shelled tick. It is endemic in the western mountain states where individual infected ticks may live for decades. The ticks infest the nests of rodents that are built above the ceilings and below the floors in cabins in this region. In an outbreak of relapsing fever among visitors to the north rim of the Grand Canyon in 1973, 62 cases were identified.[4] This outbreak was associated with an epidemic of plague among the rodents of the region that decimated the population. This resulted in a much higher attack rate of humans by the ticks that were left with a shortage of rodents to feed on.

Another outbreak among visitors to the Grand Canyon North Rim occurred in 1990. During that summer 19 persons who had stayed in the cabins there were identified as victims of the ticks. Inspection of the cabins revealed rodent nests. Although officials at the park now take measures to control ticks, such as removing nests and spraying the cabins, visitors should be alert to this danger.

Insect repellent should be applied day and night when staying in that region, and cans of pyrethroid sprays should be part of camping gear and vacation equipment. This should not be applied to the skin of course, but to clothing and the cabin surfaces. Pets and children, as usual, will require careful and regular scrutiny.

The tick is a nocturnal biter, and feeds on inhabitants of mountain cabins while they sleep. Most victims are unaware that they have been the subjects of these nocturnal raids. The ticks are active in the spring and summer, with less of a risk during the skiing season. Untreated, the mortality rate ranges from 30 to 70 percent. With antibiotics the mortality rate is reduced to less than 1 percent. As always, prevention is far preferable to relying on a cure.

ROCKY MOUNTAIN SPOTTED FEVER (RMS)

Rocky Mountain Spotted fever is caused by a rickettsia that is transmitted to humans by the bite of a tick. It was so named because it was first detected in the Rocky Mountain states, but few cases are seen in that region today. It has been reported throughout the continental United States except for Maine and Vermont, with an average of 600 cases per year reported to the Centers for Disease Control. The largest number of cases has occurred in North Carolina. Ninety percent of reported cases occur between April and September.

In 1987 four cases occurred among residents of New York City, none of whom had been outside of the city for the previous three weeks. There appear to be ticks in residence in the parks of the city. This development, along with the discovery of ticks that cause Lyme disease on lawns of suburban homes, forces us to alter our previous concept of tick-borne disease as a risk only in the woods or fields.

Ticks are the natural reservoir for Rocky Mountain spotted fever. They live off of the blood of small animals such as ground squirrels and rodents. Adult ticks can survive for two years without feeding. The female tick transmits the rickettsia to subsequent generations of ticks through the eggs that it lays. Ninety-five percent of the cases each year are reported between April 1 and September 30, the period when ticks are active and when people are in tick country. The disease may be seen throughout the year in the south.

The onset of symptoms in Rocky Mountain spotted fever occurs about seven days after the tick bite. Typical onset is a fever of 103 to 104 degrees Fahrenheit, chills, muscular pain, and a pronounced headache. A rash appears on the fourth day of the illness in over 80 percent of the cases. It appears first on the wrists, ankles, palms, soles and forearms, then spreads to the rest of the body. Only about 65 percent of the victims can recall a tick bite. When a tick bite is recalled, typically it occurred within the preceding two weeks. Untreated cases may progress to pneumonia and circulatory failure with brain and heart damage. Encephalitis may develop. Early treatment with appropriate antibiotics has significantly reduced the mortality, which was formerly about 20 percent, much higher than that in patients past fifty. Mortality in children under 10 years of age is still 2 to 3 percent, usually because of delay in diagnosis and treatment.[5] There are no significant sequelae if early treatment is instituted. Doxycycline is the treatment of choice, and penicillin and most broad-spectrum antibiotics are not effective.

There is no vaccine for RMS; prevention is the best control. Prevention is accomplished by wearing proper clothing and by application of an effective insect repellent. The diagnosis is not considered in some cases, primarily due to the absence of a rash. A significant percentage of cases (about 20 percent) never develop the rash.

As with all tick-borne diseases, a careful search of the clothing and exposed portions of the body for ticks every two hours should be routine whenever in the woods or brush where ticks are present. Wearing light colored clothing greatly facilitates this task, especially when dealing with small ticks. Any ticks that are found on clothing should be disposed of before entering the home. Those found attached to the skin should be removed carefully by steady, gentle traction with tweezers. If the head is left behind, it must be removed surgically as mentioned above to prevent migration deeper in the skin. The bare fingers should not be used to remove ticks.

Protective clothing should be worn, with bands around the ankles, to protect against ticks. Insect repellent (DEET) is effective and should be used. The new permethrin clothing spray mentioned previously, Permanone Tick Repellent®, should also be used with DEET. This provides virtually 100 percent protection against ticks. These measures should bring about a reduction in the incidence of Rocky Mountain spotted fever as well as Lyme disease, and indeed all tick-borne illnesses.

DDT and dieldrin are effective in controlling tick populations in wooded and bushy areas around rural homes, but are no longer available. Diazinon is currently marketed for this use, and some of the other organophosphates should be effective. Chlorpyrifos (Dursban®) for instance is effective against ticks, and it can be applied as a spray in areas of known tick habitation. These are agents with a significant toxicity, however, and should not be applied where children will be exposed to them or where they might be tracked into the home. Controlling the tick population is particularly important for those homes that are in regions where Lyme disease, babesiosis, Rocky Mountain spotted fever and tick paralysis are reported (see Chapter VII).

With the widespread cultivation of litigation as an income producing industry, and with the current hysteria regarding pesticides, it becomes more and more difficult to obtain effective agents to control the disease vectors that cause disease and death in humans. It is even more difficult to get objective information on this subject. Environmental extremist organizations have become very wealthy by cultivating fear and hysteria in the public through lies and false propaganda. They have been able to extract immense sums of money from a gullible public who have been led that these people are their saviors. The organizations have been aided and abetted in this plunder by corrupt bureaucrats such as the EPA.

PLAGUE

The dread "Black Death" of the middle ages, which killed more than 60 million people, lives on in the United States today, albeit at a much lower incidence. The advent of effective antibiotics that control the disease in most cases lessens our risk. Antibiotics must be started early in the course of the disease, however, and frequently plague is not considered at first. The most important factor in the reduction of the incidence of this serious disease has been the control of rat and other rodent populations that have been the reservoir for the bacterium that causes it.

It is believed that plague arrived in the United States from Asia about 1900 during the last great pandemic. It became established in the ground squirrels in the San Francisco Bay area, and spread south and east from there. It is of particular concern in and around Los Angeles because of the great increase in the human population there, and the building of homes in the countryside among the ground squirrels.

Plague was first seen on the east slopes of the Colorado Rockies in the early 1940s. It is firmly established there now in various species of ground squirrels, including the rock squirrel, as well as in chipmunks, prairie dogs and wood rats. It also can be seen in the fox squirrels that have been imported into the city parks and residential areas of the Front Range. It even can be contracted from rabbits. Plague is transmitted from the rodents to humans by the bite of fleas, which transmit the bacterium. Even with prompt treatment the mortality rate is about 10 percent. This is a disease to avoid.

The areas of the United States where plague currently is a risk include New Mexico, Arizona, Colorado, Utah, Nevada, California and Oregon. Visitors to these regions should not take pet dogs or cats with them. Even if they are kept indoors, they face a serious risk of acquiring fleas from wild rodents. During recreational activities in these geographic regions the precautions against attacks by fleas that were described previously should be taken.

Pets such as dogs or cats should not be taken into the field or woods in regions where plague is endemic. Even if kept indoors they risk picking up fleas from wild rodents in the vicinity. Every precaution should be taken to assure that they do not bring these fleas or ticks back to the automobile or living quarters. This poses a serious problem, but you do not want plague, for you or your family. Although we tend to think of fleas as firmly attached to the dog or cat, it must be kept in mind that they live much of their life cycle off of the animal. This means that in order to eliminate fleas you have to treat not only the animal but also the yard where the animal strolls, the kennel, the carpet, the furniture, the crevices in the house, etc.

There are a number of products that are effective in killing fleas. The objective is to kill the fleas and not the dog or the kids.

Some agents that are acceptable for use on the lawn should never be used indoors, especially if you have a child crawling around on the carpet. There are new flea and tick preparations on the market that combine the active ingredient with a polymer. This combination is supposed to adhere to the hair of the dog, and remain active for 2 weeks against ticks, 60 days against fleas. These products CANNOT be used on cats because of their cleaning and grooming habits.

Pets, especially cats, can also contract plague and then transmit it to humans through scratching, biting or sneezing. If a cat appears ill during a visit to these areas, immediate medical attention for the family should be obtained. The incubation period for plague is usually 2-6 days, so illness is likely to begin during the vacation.

Observation of visitors to recreational areas such as Rocky Mountain National Park does not give encouragement to efforts to evoke responsible behavior from the tourists. All of the signs and bronze plaques warning of the dangers of feeding the native animals are universally ignored. Children are encouraged by their parents to feed the squirrels and chipmunks, even enticing them to accept hand held food. The residents of the U.S. have been so brain-washed by the humanization of animals on television and in movies that they are totally oblivious to the dangers of trying to feed and pet wild animals. They actually have been educated into ignorance by the entertainment industry and the mass media, and by the misplaced priorities of the education establishment. Skills such as condom application have taken precedence over more mundane studies like health.

For further information on plague see Chapter VII. The precautions listed there for plague and Hantavirus infection should be reviewed carefully before vacationing to the western one-third of the United States.

TYPHUS

Murine (endemic, flea-borne) typhus fever is another disease that is transmitted by way of fleas from rats and mice to humans, the same flea that transmits the plague bacillus. U.S. military personnel in Vietnam suffered many cases between 1961-1971. It has been reported in virtually every state of the United States, but it is more common in seaports and near food storage facilities. Murine typhus is prevalent in the southeastern states and along the Gulf Coast. The incidence in the United States has been greatly reduced by taking measures to deny access to grain and food stores by rodents. Although this form of typhus produces a pronounced illness, it is treatable with antibiotics and has a low mortality rate. Recreational trips to the regions of greatest incidence, or in areas where rats and mice are in evidence, should prompt the same preventative measures as describe above for plague. Pets will be a major factor in bringing this disease home.

Epidemic (louse-borne) typhus fever, on the other hand, is uncommon in the United States. It is transmitted from human to human by the body louse, and the causative organism, *Rickettsia Prowazekii*, dies out with the demise of the body louse. It has been transmitted from flying squirrels by their fleas, however, to at least 33 people in the U.S., mainly in Ohio, Indiana, Illinois and West Virginia. It is more prevalent in Mexico, and Central and South America. Scrub (mite-borne) typhus is found in countries of the Pacific Rim, and is very prevalent on some islands in the region of the New Hebrides. These diseases are discussed also in Chapter VII.

HANTAVIRUS

The most recently discovered disease that is transmitted from wild rodents to humans is a viral respiratory illness that results in death in approximately two-thirds of the cases. The first cases were reported in May 1993 in the Four Corners region of the United States (Arizona, New Mexico, Utah and Colorado). Other cases have been reported since in Texas, Louisiana, Nevada, California and North Dakota. The virus is spread from infected rodents (initially the deer mouse) both through aerosol and direct skin contact with the saliva and excreta (urine and feces).

The Hantavirus does not appear to cause illness in the rodent. Exposure to the virus may occur during recreational activities such as hiking and camping in regions inhabited by infected rodents, or by staying in a cabin or other quarters that have been invaded by rodents. Little is known about this new disease as yet, but it has been discovered that rodents other than the deer mouse can carry the virus.

In hiking and camping it would be prudent to avoid areas that are occupied by rodents. This would be obvious if burrows are present. All food should be stored in impervious containers to prevent contact with rodents or their excreta. Campers should also sleep on a cot, never on the ground. More detailed precautions for Hantavirus disease are listed in Chapter VII.

MOSQUITOS

There is nothing more consistently disruptive of the pleasures that we derive from recreational activities than mosquitos. From family picnics, to Boy Scout encampments, to a simple evening on the patio, they inevitably arrive to interrupt an otherwise memorable occasion. During most recreational activities we have to deal with the elements and, with the exception of skiing trips, mosquitos. There are very few geographic locations on earth that are not plagued by these pests. In many parts of the United States we have always considered them to be merely a nuisance, rarely carrying disease. Increasingly, however, they are expanding their disease-transmitting role in the United States.

Aside from the annoyance factor, mosquitos also introduce the specter of disease during recreational, a factor that seldom occupies our minds on these occasions. As stated in Chapter VII, diseases transmitted by mosquitos have killed more of the earth's human inhabitants than all of the wars in history combined have. The level of the risk of disease, and the seriousness of the disease, varies somewhat with the geographic location in the U.S. where the activity takes place. Both the geographic area of risk and the seriousness of the disease presented have been greatly enlarged since the introduction of *Aedes albopictus*, the Asian tiger mosquito, into Houston, Texas in 1985 (see Chapter VII). *A. albopictus* is much more aggressive than the native species that we have been accustomed to doing business with. The fact that it has become established in such a wide area, including Ohio, Indiana, Illinois, Kentucky, Tennessee, North Carolina, Maryland, Delaware and most of the southern states, has serious implications for recreational activities in these regions.

Since *Aedes albopictus* is capable of transmitting the encephalitis viruses, it will undoubtedly increase the incidence of these diseases. It is expected that it will transmit all four of the types of encephalitis seen in the United States, and will very likely increase the incidence of eastern equine encephalitis, which has a particularly high fatality rate. The discovery in 1990, in *Aedes albopictus*, of ten strains of a virus previously seen only in Africa make it clear that we will be faced with new and more serious diseases during recreational activities.

It has thus become more urgent than ever before to take every precaution to protect oneself from attacks by mosquitos when on recreational outings. It is essential to become thoroughly familiar with and faithfully use an effective insect repellent program. Please review the section on insect repellents above. For a more detailed discussion of diseases transmitted by mosquitos and ticks see Chapter VII.

In the United States mosquitos are also responsible for the transmission of malaria in Florida and in California. Several outbreaks of malaria that was transmitted from an individual carrying the parasite in his blood have occurred in Florida and California. These are reviewed in Chapter VII. To avoid the risk of malaria, as well as encephalitis, dengue fever and other as yet not identified diseases, protection against mosquitos for you and your family is urgent when undertaking recreational activities in these areas.

When camping, netting on tents is essential. Some mosquitos will gain entry as a result of repeated passage by children during the day. These can be eliminated before retiring for the night by spraying the tent with a household pyrethroid aerosol 30 minutes to one hour before bedtime. Exit the tent after spraying to avoid inhaling the aerosol.

EHRLICHIOSIS

Ehrlichiosis is a new and serious disease that is transmitted to humans by ticks. First reported in the United States in 1986, many of the early cases were misdiagnosed as Rocky Mountain spotted fever. Tests for *Ehrlichia canis*, an infection of dogs, proved to be positive in humans with this new disease. It was thus assumed that this was the same disease, transmitted from dogs to man by ticks. Further study isolated the causative organism as a new species of *Ehrlichia*, *Ehrlichia chaffeensis*, which is closely related to *E. canis*. Although it is known that the organism is transmitted to man by tick bites, the natural resevoir of this new disease is not known.

Ehrlichiosis ranges from mild to severe, even fatal and is characterized by fever, headache, nausea and confusion in the more severe cases. This newly discovered disease provides an added incentive for travelers to these regions to exercise precautions against ticks. It is essential to prevent tick acquisition by any member of the family. The children and pets will require particularly close scrutiny.

SANDFLIES

Also called biting midges, these are related to mosquitos and other blood-sucking flies. They are about one to four millimeters in length, about the same size as the dog flea. They can penetrate ordinary screening. Their attacks are rapid and aggressive. Severe itching may follow a bite, and the treatment is antihistamines by mouth and topical cortisone cream to the bites. DO NOT apply cortisone products to the face. Sandflies do not transmit disease to humans in most regions of the United States. They are common vectors of some significant parasitic infestations in Africa and the Mediterranean region. They inoculate the protozoan of leishmaniasis into the skin of humans in Central and South America, Mexico and south central Texas. This parasite is transmitted from dogs and rodents to humans by the fly. Sandflies also transmits sandfly fever, a viral disease, in Africa, the Mediterranean region and Panama.

Sandflies presented their very unpleasant and unwanted gifts to the United States armed forces personnel during their deployment to the Persian Gulf during the war in 1991. Please see the discussion of leishmaniasis and sandfly fever in Chapter VII.

BLACKFLIES

Blackflies are small (about five millimeters in length) highly aggressive biting flies that attack throughout the day and in the open. They are encountered in huge numbers during the late spring and early summer in northern climates, such as Canada, where they extract a heavy penalty for a day of fishing. They have invaded Michigan recently in lesser numbers. In Africa, South America, Guatemala and southern Mexico these flies transmit the parasitic worm *Onchocerca* to humans, causing "river blindness" and filariasis. Fortunately they do not transmit this disease in the United States. As with most parasitic diseases there has been no successful treatment.

In 1989 ivermectin was shown to be effective and safe in the treatment of a variety of roundworm and mite infestations in humans in Germany. It has been used in the United States to control heartworm and sarcoptic mange in dogs since 1980. It has become the treatment of choice to control *Onchocerca*. It does not kill the adult worm in the body, however, killing only the microfilaria that the worm releases. Treatment must be repeated once or twice yearly therefore to prevent these newly released microfilaria from lodging in the eye. Although the safety of this medication in humans has been well demonstrated since 1989, it still is not approved for general use in the United States.

CHIGGERS

Chiggers (trombicula mites) are the larval form of the harvest mite, which feeds on vegetation, not man. The mite lays its eggs in fields where the larva hatch, then climb vegetation to lay in wait for a victim. A change in the carbon dioxide level of the air signals them to drop onto passing animals including humans. The larva, which is 0.5 millimeters in length, then attaches to the skin, usually at the ankle or higher, and ascends until it encounters tight clothing such as socks or the belt. It then penetrates the skin and secretes a tissue digestant, which causes intense itching. The itching and inflammation, which begins within a few hours after the larva invades the skin, may persist for weeks.

The larva feeds for three or four days before dropping off. A physician can remove any organisms that are found still feeding. An old folk remedy was to apply kerosene to the area of penetration to eliminate the larva. A more recent recommendation has been the application of lindane (Kwell®), which should be effective in killing the larva. The toxicity of this agent must be kept in mind, however, as well as the prohibition against applying lindane to the skin of children. A more recent treatment and the preferred one is a five percent permethrin cream discussed above for tick removal. It is effective in killing the mite without the toxicity of lindane.

It should be remembered also that the intense itching is caused by the secretion of the tissue digestant that persists after the chigger has departed. This itching can be relieved by antihistamine tablets and by the application of a topical cortisone cream to the inflamed area. Secondary infection may result from scratching. Bites by chiggers can be prevented by taking the same precautions as for ticks, wearing pants legs tucked into boots or socks, tight clothing and application of an effective insect repellent, which means diethyl-meta-toluamide (DEET). Application to the clothing of the newer mixture of diethyl-meta-toluamide and permethrin should be even more effective.

SPIDER BITES

Black widow spiders, Latrodectus mactans, are found in virtually all areas of the United States. In the fifties and sixties bites on the scrotum were reported each year, acquired while visiting outside privies. Progress in the installation of indoor plumbing seems to have reduced this risk. Severe muscle cramping follows the bite, and abdominal cramping may mimic an acute abdomen such as appendicitis. These bites are more serious in children, where convulsions may be seen, and in people over sixty years of age.

The brown recluse or violin spider, *Loxosceles reclusa*, was identified only in 1940, and was introduced into the southern United States around 1960. It is a light brown color with a dark brown violin-shaped marking on the cephalothorax extending from the eyes toward the rear, as viewed from above. It had been seen chiefly in the central and midwestern states, particularly in Missouri, Arkansas and Oklahoma. More recently the spider has been found as far north as Minnesota and Maine, thus debunking the belief that they could not survive in colder climates. In 1990 physicians reported almost 500 bites in S. Carolina where they were thought to not exist. This spread will continue as the spiders are transported in moving vans as well as in other cargo.

A similar dissemination of other species of *Loxosceles* has been observed in Central and South America. At least one South American species has been imported into Central America as well as into Massachusetts and California. It now appears that at least three different species of *Loxosceles*, all of which share the violin marking, are responsible for bites in the United States. As with the importation of the *Aedes Albopictus* mosquito, the importation of these spiders demonstrates that increasingly we in the United States will be sharing in the some of the diseases and afflictions of the rest of the world that we have heretofore been spared.

The brown recluse is uniformly described as "shy" because of its proclivity to remain hidden from view. Many bites have occurred when inserting a hand into a glove where the spider was residing, especially gloves that are kept in garages or outdoor sheds. Similarly, donning a jacket or any item of clothing that has been hanging in the garage, or even basement, presents the risk of a bite. It would be prudent to store gloves and clothing in the house, rather than leaving them in the garage or outbuildings. Bites also occur when the spider's web in a garage or outdoor building is disturbed.

This spider produces a potent toxin that produces not only tissue necrosis, but hemolysis as well. The toxin also contains an effective spreading substance. The result is often extensive tissue destruction and sloughing. Excision of the bite early, if identified, has been advocated by some, but this practice has always been controversial. In 1983 dapsone, an antibacterial agent that has long been used in the treatment of leprosy, was used at Vanderbilt University Hospital to treat a victim of a brown recluse bite with excellent results. The use of dapsone in this application was considered on the basis of its pharmaco-physiologic actions. It was used in this patient only after studies had been conducted on laboratory animals.

Further studies have demonstrated that whereas victims treated surgically experienced delayed healing and extensive scarring, those treated with dapsone healed much more rapidly and with less tissue destruction and scarring. This is an impressive example of intelligent deductive logic leading to a significant advancement in medicine. If you suffer a bite from the brown recluse, don't expect or demand this treatment however. Not every victim requires such treatment, and the drug has some potentially serious side effects. The decision will require a careful analysis by a knowledgeable physician, on a case by case basis.

In the event of a bite, it is important to identify the spider, since bites by other, less toxic spiders may mimic the bite of the brown recluse. A mild stinging is experienced at the time of the bite. This is followed a few hours later by an extreme pain that may require medication to control. A reddened area surrounding a central bleb follows the bite. This reddened area may be irregular in some cases, or may give the appearance of a target in others. The center enlarges, fills with blood and eventually becomes ulcerated. It is important to not simply observe and delay treatment as these changes progress, especially when the other symptoms are also worsening. If a physician fails to recognize the urgency, seek another opinion, preferably from someone who has seen such a bite.

Some victims experience chills, nausea and vomiting. Fatalities are rare, even in children. The chief risk from these arachnids is the necrosis, loss of tissue, and prolonged healing with scarring. Hemolysis and kidney failure can occur also, however. Bites by a brown recluse have been dismissed as trivial, even by physicians, to the point that severe destruction of tissue resulted. The new protocol of dapsone and antibiotics appears to render this outcome less likely. It is important, however, to not delay treatment following a bite from a brown recluse.

As with all such serious events, prevention is far better than treatment. There are several other members of the Loxosceles genus of spiders that vary in size and shape. All have the characteristic violin marking, but this is not prominent on some. It is wise to assume that all spiders are harmful and to keep the home and garage free of them and their nests. This can be accomplished by spraying the insects and their nests with one of the pyrethroid house spray (containing either resmethrin, permethrin, or tetramethrin). The nests and eggs should then be vacuumed and removed from the house before they hatch in the vacuum cleaner. Never use more toxic pesticides such as chlorpyrifos in the house. They are not needed and simply introduce an additional risk. (See Chapter XIV)

When vacationing, eradicate spiders from the vacation premises by the above procedures. Shake out all clothing and shoes before donning, for this is a favorite habitat for these spiders. This precaution also applies to gloves and clothing stored in garages and outbuildings at home.

SCORPION BITES

The only species of scorpions in the United States that present a threat to humans are found in Texas, New Mexico, Arizona and southern California. Considerable pain and discomfort follow the sting. There is generally no threat to life, however, except in young children, the aged and the debilitated. The sting, which is inflicted by the tail, may be accompanied by a burning pain and swelling. In some species a numbness and tingling follow the burning sensation. The entire arm or leg may become numb, and nausea and vomiting may ensue. Coma, convulsions and death may follow the initial hyperactivity. The venom produced by scorpions is more toxic than that of snakes, but only a small amount is injected. No tissue destruction is seen. Antivenom is available and should be used if symptoms are pronounced.

Scorpions are nocturnal creatures and seek refuge in shoes, clothing and bedding. The sting results from an accidental encounter. Precautions should include shaking out shoes and clothing in the morning before donning them. The same precautions should be taken before using towels and washcloths.

RABIES

Rabies is a viral disease that is 100 percent fatal without treatment, and people continue to die from it in cases where there is no known exposure. A high level of awareness must be maintained during all recreational activities where exposure to wild animals, either by humans or by pets, is a possibility. Virtually all domestic dogs in the United States are immunized, and thus are unlikely to bring rabies home to you. This is not true of cats, however. Cats are by nature a hunter, an animal of prey, and as such they are much more likely than dogs to encounter wild animals with rabies. The number of cases of rabies in cats now outnumbers that in dogs. It does not take a lot of imagination to see the risk from this source even at home, much less on outings.

Rabies is commonly found in skunks, raccoon, bats and fox. It has been found in bats in every state except for Alaska and Hawaii. Bats have caused rabies in at least 24 humans in the United States.[6] If your recreational activities include cave exploration, a risk of rabies exposure definitely exists. Rabies is rampant in the skunks in central California where they roam in great numbers. Rabies was found in the skunks living underneath a school, and in proximity to where the children played, in the Bay area in 1978. Raccoons are common in many residential communities in the United States, living among the human residents.

The potential for contracting rabies lies not only in being bitten by a rabid animal, but by coming in contact with it otherwise, either alive or dead. Rabies can be contracted through a scratch or abrasion on the skin while handling an animal with the disease, or by inhaling the virus. Public awareness of these means of transmission should be expanded. A nationwide effort to vaccinate cats must be undertaken, and it must succeed. We have been very fortunate that our children have been spared exposure through this route thus far.

Rabies is widespread among the wild dogs of Africa, and is common in India, the Philippines and Southeast Asia. If you are planning a trip to these areas and plan to be in the field, out of contact with modern medical care, please review the section on rabies in Chapter VII and consult your physician about your needs.

AQUATIC

Jellyfish stings in the United States produce pain and burning, swelling and redness at the site of contact. The victim may experience muscle cramps, nausea, vomiting and pulmonary edema. Some victims have died within a few minutes, although most survive, fortunately. Drowning is a significant risk following these encounters. In those who survive, all of the symptoms except for the local pain, swelling and redness dissipate within several hours. Victims of the Pacific box jellyfish of Australia, considered the most dangerous marine creature in the world, have not been as fortunate. Sudden death following envenomation from these creatures is common.

The **Portuguese man-of-war**, which is found in the coastal waters of the Gulf of Mexico, is somewhat less toxic than the jellyfish. The treatment for stings of both is immediate washing in salt water to dilute and remove as much venom as possible. DO NOT RUB the sting area, as this will inject additional venom from the tentacles left behind. These tentacles with their venom should be inactivated by sprinkling baking soda over the area for jellyfish and vinegar or isopropyl alcohol for the Portuguese man-of-war. The remaining tentacles should then be gently scraped off, taking care to not force further venom into the skin. This task is best accomplished by a physician experienced in the procedure. Rinsing in freshwater, using ammonia and rubbing with sand all tend to result in the deposition of additional venom into the skin.

The **stingray** delivers the most common toxic fish sting in the United States. It lives mostly along the California Coast, where several hundred stings are reported each year. These encounters occur primarily in shallow water. The habit of the fish of remaining buried in the sand increases the possibility of an accidental encounter with humans. Many stings on the hands occur among fisherman during attempts to dislodge fishhooks from stingrays when they are caught accidentally.

The wound from a stingray is caused by the tail of the fish, which is composed of a bony spine with a skin-like covering. The tail is lashed into the victim, sometimes penetrating an inch or more. Venom is deposited into the wound, and portions of the bony spine may break off in the wound. The skin like sheath is usually deposited in the wound even when none of the bony spine is left behind. It is indeed ironic that these "friendly little animals" that are petted by many people in the tank at the Epcot Center so commonly inflict so severe an injury on humans.

Severe pain and whiteness are the immediate findings following a stingray attack. This is followed by redness and swelling of the area of the wound. Systemic symptoms of muscle cramps, weakness, excessive salivation, heart rhythm irregularities, seizures and death can occur but are uncommon. Treatment is to apply a constricting band, taking all of the precautions to avoid the damage of prolonged tourniquet applications, and irrigating with saltwater to remove as much of the sheath as is feasible. The wound should then be immersed in water as hot as can be tolerated without inflicting a burn, for up to one hour. The venom is readily inactivated by heat. The wound frequently requires surgical debridement and suturing.

Several fish contain venom that can be deposited in the skin of humans by a fin or spine. These include the catfish, dogfish, bullhead sharks and lionfish. The latter species contains the most venomous fish in the world, the stonefish. There is an immediate severe pain at the site of envenomation, followed by swelling. This is followed by necrosis and extensive tissue destruction, especially with the catfish and lionfish. Muscle weakness, heart irregularities, hypotension, seizures and paralysis may follow. Treatment again is to immerse in hot water for one hour until the symptoms subside, to inactivate the venom. Infection commonly follows with these stings, and appropriate treatment should be instituted if this occurs. The indicated tetanus prophylaxis should always be administered with these wounds. This requires an assessment and judgement by a knowledgeable physician.

SNAKEBITE

The majority of poisonous snakes in the United States are pit vipers, which includes copperheads, cottonmouths and various species of rattlesnakes. Coral snakes, the other group of poisonous snakes, are found in Arizona, New Mexico, Texas, Arkansas, Florida, Georgia, Alabama, Louisiana, Mississippi, and North and South Carolina. Approximately 7,000 people are bitten by snakes each year but only about a dozen fatalities are recorded, mostly in children.

The impact of an attack by a snake can be minimized by wearing long trousers and boots whenever afield in snake habitat. Avoiding such well-known risks as stepping over a log or sticking one's hand into likely snake retreats also lowers the odds. Children should not be allowed out in the woods in snake country barefoot and in shorts.

The amount of venom deposited in human tissues after a snake strike varies considerably. No poisoning occurs in about twenty to thirty percent of strikes by pit vipers. A physician experienced in treating such bites can anticipate the degree of envenomation by the appearance of and reaction at the wound. There is no universal agreement upon what constitutes the best treatment, and any consensus that does exist changes from time to time. There is agreement, however, that the victim should seek medical help as soon as possible after being bitten.

Appropriate specific antivenom is available through medical facilities, but must be administered within four to six hours. It is derived from horse serum, and its administration carries a significant risk of reaction, shock and death unless appropriate precautions are taken. There is no disagreement upon the need to keep the victim quiet, avoiding panic. The bitten extremity should be splinted and kept in the horizontal position. Activity speeds the spread of the venom through the general circulation.

Tourniquets are discouraged in snakebite because their effectiveness has been called into question, and because of their potential for causing gangrene. The effectiveness of incisions over the points of venom deposition is also currently questioned, partially because the venom is usually injected deeper than most people are willing to cut. Making such incisions also runs the risk of damage to underlying nerves and blood vessels. If done at all, it must be done immediately to be effective. This measure is of no value in coral snakebite. Application of cold increases the extent of tissue destruction in snakebites, and such destruction may be considerable anyway.

Identification of the snake is important to subsequent treatment. Saving the snake, preferably inactivated, is more reliable than one's memory under such circumstances. All snakebites must be treated as puncture wounds. Appropriate tetanus prophylaxis is imperative. Other bacterial infections are also common, and should be prevented or treated if they ensue.

POISON IVY

Exposure of the skin to an oily substance produced by certain varieties of ivy, oak and sumac produces a characteristic reaction in some people. It represents a sensitization to the chemical, and this sensitization may occur at any time in life. The absence of a reaction to contact with these plants is no assurance that sensitization will not develop at a later date. It is important to keep in mind also that these reactions may occur in the winter as a result of wearing a sweater that had previously come in contact with the plant. It similarly can be acquired from a dog's coat after it had been out frolicking in the woods and brought back the oil with it. Contact is also made not infrequently from firewood that has vines adhered to it.

The reaction is heralded by itching, redness and a typical fluid filled vesicle. One can frequently see the linear distribution where the vine made contact with the skin. Reactions on the face and eyes can be the result of direct contact, or can be the result of the substance being carried to that location by the hands after they have come in contact with the plant. The fluid from the vesicles cannot spread the involvement. Thorough washing of any contaminated portion of the body with an effective soap will remove the oil, and this should be done as soon as possible after exposure. This will not guarantee against an eruption but it does diminish the risk. All contaminated clothing should also be thoroughly laundered or dry-cleaned.

Small, localized areas of eruption may be treated successfully with cortisone creams. It will be necessary to apply these more frequently than the four times daily that is recommended, usually at least six to eight times daily. These applications must also be replenished any time that the area is washed, or after perspiration has washed the cream off. These preparations should NOT be used on the face, especially in children. Itching is relieved to some extent by antihistamines such as chlorpheniramine (CPM), if the drowsiness can be tolerated. Scratching must be resisted to avoid the possibility of a secondary skin infection. More extensive or stubborn reactions will require injections of cortisone preparations. For those individuals working in areas where these botanicals are found, desensitization injections are available. Hunters who spend much time afield sometimes elect this approach.

FUNGAL INFECTIONS

Fungal infections are seen much more frequently in the summer, and in warm climates, since the organisms grow much more readily in warm, moist conditions. For the same reason they occur more frequently in areas of the body where skin folds are found, such as the groin, between the toes, the anal folds and underneath the breasts. These organisms are frequently acquired at swimming pools and in public showers. Simple household bleach (sodium hypochlorite) is very effective in destroying the fungi in these locations.

Athlete's foot is caused by a variety of strains of fungi and is seen most frequently between the toes. A rash on top of the toes and feet in the absence of involvement between the toes is most likely a sensitization reaction to the dyes or tanning agents in shoes, and not a fungus. Athlete's foot can be avoided by wearing slippers in public bathing facilities and by drying the feet well. A hair dryer is useful for this purpose. Changing socks daily also helps. Shoes with the uppers made of leather or nylon mesh are generally favored by foot and sport specialists.

If a chronic or recurrent problem exists, one may have to wear cotton socks, avoiding all synthetics such as Orlon, Dacron and nylon. Cotton is not always easy to find. It seems to be in fashion at the whim of the designers. In addition to the measures to dry the feet mentioned above, it might be useful to powder the feet prior to putting the socks on. Corn starch may be used, but Tinactin® is more effective, since it destroys fungi. Micatin® (miconazole) is even more effective, but it is more expensive. It is also helpful to leave the feet bare at home whenever possible, wearing sandals, NOT walking barefoot through the house to share the infection. When a full-blown eruption develops, with inflammation and cracking between the toes, nothing is more effective than the above measures. The Micatin powder should be applied four times daily, rather than just twice daily.

Jock itch is a fungal infection in the folds of the groin, appearing as a reddened area that may become extensive. It also may be caused by a variety of fungal organisms. The treatment is the same as outlined above for athlete's foot.

Itching and inflammation of the vulva is more commonly due to monilia (yeast) but can be caused by a distressing multitude of microorganisms. These may occur singly, but more commonly they are found in combinations of two or more different varieties. Successful treatment requires identification of the organism(s), since the treatment varies with each different class. The marketing of agents such as miconazole that have a much broader spectrum have simplified the management of this problem.

In the event of repeated or stubborn fungal infections anywhere on the body, either the proclivity toward or overt diabetes should be considered. Overt disease can usually be discovered by a well-timed blood test. Incipient disease may require a more complex glucose tolerance test.

SWIMMING

Swimming is excellent exercise, beneficial for high blood pressure, as well as for the heart, lungs and general circulation. It carries virtually no risk, outside of drowning, but ear infections are a frequent problem. In public pools, the bacterial count is generally well controlled. An otitis media (middle ear infection) can occur in this setting, however, because it commonly is not an infection at the onset. Individuals prone to develop this problem can minimize it by the same precautions taken when flying. Taking a decongestant tablet such as phenylephrine and chlorpheniramine, and spraying the nose with one-quarter percent phenylephrine solution before swimming will lessen the risk.

Swimming in lakes and ponds results in actual bacterial infections of the ear canal, and these require aggressive treatment. This is a common problem, due to the universal contamination of the lakes commonly used for recreation, including water skiing. Infections of the skin due to a variety of organisms occur in addition to the ear infections. The most troublesome infections of the skin and ear are those due to *Pseudomonas* bacteria. These are resistant to virtually every antibiotic that has been developed. An increasing number of these recreational waters are being contaminated by Giardia so we are seeing cases of diarrhea as a result.

Infections of the eyes (conjunctivitis) occur in the same settings for the same reasons. The most recent eye infection to evolve is that caused by *Acanthamoeba*. This serious infection does not respond to any of the conventional treatments and may result in a corneal transplant or loss of an eye. It is a particular danger for contact lens wearers. Contact lenses should never be worn when swimming; this practice carries a risk of a serious eye infection. Farm ponds carry some additional risks, including leptospirosis (see Chapter VII). Recreation in any of these bodies of water carries significant health risks that should be avoided.

A more serious amoebic infection that results from swimming in bodies of fresh water is meningitis caused by *Naegleria fowleri*. When contaminated water enters the nasal passages the *Naegleria* migrate to the brain by way of the olfactory nerve. The resulting meningoencephalitis is virtually always fatal, usually within one week. Over 100 cases have been reported in the United States, many more throughout the rest of the world. This organism is found most commonly in warm bodies of fresh water in the southern states, as well as in water that has been warmed by the discharge from power plants. It is also resident in the hot sulfur springs in Yellowstone National Park.

As with *Acanthamoeba* it can be acquired from hot tubs and spas also if they are not properly maintained. It is the general consensus that *Naegleria* are not a threat if adequate chlorine concentrations of 2 ppm are maintained. Proper maintenance of the filter with periodic hyperchlorination will also help to protect, but is not sufficient by itself. The smallest form of the organism is between 6 and 9 microns, which places it in the same category as *cryptosporidium*. Sand filters cannot therefore be relied upon to remove either of these organisms. Diatomaceous earth filters, which are purported to remove particles as small as one micron, must be used. Even with these great care must be exercised in changing or flushing the filters. Contamination has occurred during this process. Great care must be taken also to avoid the fine powder of diatomaceous earth, since inhaling it presents a serious risk of silicosis. No case of naegleriasis is known to have been acquired from a properly maintained, chlorinated swimming pool in the United States.

The emergence of E. Coli 0157:H7 (see Chapter V) has presented an additional risk with swimming or other recreational activities in bodies of water. There have been outbreaks of infection with this organism, as well as with Shigella, from inadequately chlorinated swimming pools. Other risks include hepatitis A, gastroenteric viruses such as rotaviruses, and cryptosporidium. Proper filtration and chlorination are essential, not only in public pools, but in private and housing complex pools to prevent transmission of these infections. Children with diarrhea and in diapers should be kept out of these facilities.

Swimmers itch, cercaria dermatitis, is caused by the penetration of the skin by larval forms of blood flukes (Schistosomes) that infest various migratory birds. The disease is acquired by wading or swimming in bodies of water that are frequented by ducks, geese and some shore birds. In the United States man is an end host. These cercariae in the U.S. never invade other organs after penetration of the skin, and do not mature in humans. In the United States the Great Lakes and some of the coastal waters of California are the most common source of this affliction. In many other parts of the world the cercaria do migrate to the liver in man where they mature, then disseminate to the bladder or intestine. These organisms produce the serious parasitic disease, schistosomiasis.

METAL TOXICITY

The most common metal toxicity encountered in recreation is that of lead. Even at low levels in the body lead causes damage to the brain, the kidneys and to other organs of the body. Young children in the household are particularly susceptible (see Chapter III).

A common recreational source of lead exposure is associated with casting of bullets or toys. Whenever lead is melted, high concentrations of lead fume accumulate in the local atmosphere. In addition, the dross (lead oxide) that forms on the molten lead results in dust contaminating the floor and surroundings. The formation of this dross can be greatly reduced by adding about 200 grains of pure tin to every 10 pounds of lead. If pure tin is not available, twice that amount of a 50–50 tin-lead solder will accomplish the same goal. This does not affect the hardness of the bullet and it improves the flow of the lead in the mold.

Lead may enter the body either by inhalation, through the skin or by ingestion. These projects are frequently carried out in a basement or garage workshop, without any ventilation. Even with an efficient exhaust fan, with adequate ventilation flow, high levels of lead and lead oxide form over the work. The average dust mask does not protect against this exposure. The 3-M Company markets a "Sanding Respirator" that is a more sophisticated dust mask. It provides better protection than the common dust mask, but the weak point is still the seal around the edge. Any leakage here permits the entry of hazardous particles into the lungs. These operations, therefore, call for great caution and care. The dross should be disposed of carefully in a closed container such as a plastic trash bag, and the work area should be vacuumed carefully. A central vacuum system is preferable for this job.

Ordinary solder has contained 50–60 percent tin and 40–50 percent lead in the past. A eutectic mixture, that which melts at the lowest temperature, is 63 percent tin and 37 percent lead. The soldering that is normally done around the home should not present a significant lead exposure. If an individual has a large wiring project that requires use of a molten pot of solder, or a similarly large plumbing project requiring a molten pot, he should avoid inhaling the fumes, and provide adequate ventilation. For soldering residential plumbing, federal regulations, prompted by the concern for lead leaching into the water supply, now require the use of a non-lead solder (see Chapter II).

Even more hazardous than lead in bullet casting is cadmium. This metal is not customarily added to lead for such purpose, since antimony provides the desired hardness in bullets. Cadmium is a frequent component of wheel weights, however, and they are sometimes collected for use in casting bullets. They should not be. Inhalation of cadmium fumes can produce a severe emphysema as well as damage to the kidneys. These fumes are extremely toxic and should be avoided.

MERCURY

This liquid metal and its salts are not as commonly encountered in recreational activities as they are on the job. The compounds have been used as fungicides on seed grain, however, and in paints and stains to inhibit mildew formation. The liquid metal has a low vapor pressure and toxic levels accumulate in the atmosphere from an open container. It seeps into concrete floors when spilled, and many laboratories are contaminated through this means. It then vaporizes and produces a hazardous level in the room air where it is inhaled.

Mercury should not be found in the home, but it frequently is. When this is the case, great care should taken to avoid spilling this substance on concrete floors or into cracks and crevices where it cannot be cleaned up. If spillage does occur, the mercury should be cleaned up carefully. If a vacuum cleaner is used the bag should be disposed of carefully. If some residual mercury persists in an inaccessible spot it can be amalgamated with tin metal foil and then vacuumed. A similar product for this use is marketed. There is no practical means to remove metallic mercury from concrete floors after it has permeated them.

Mercury is also discussed in Chapters V, X and XIII.

HOT TUBS

These oversized bathtubs are a recent addition to the recreational field, and some serious skin infections have resulted from communal sharing of them. The most serious of these skin infections has been produced by *Pseudomonas* bacteria, which have become notorious for being resistant to virtually every antibiotic available. Another serious infection that is acquired in hot tubs is *Acanthamoeba* eye infections, and this subject is discussed in Chapter XV. Contact lenses should never be worn in hot tubs. The most recent health risk associated with hot tubs was an outbreak of *Legionella* pneumonia that was acquired from a hot tub on display in a store showroom.

These infections are a serious problem that mandates much greater care in maintaining hot tubs. Every person entering the hot tub should bathe carefully before and after the activities. Every human body is host to a multitude of organisms that can cause serious illness. The organisms that seem to cause no harm in one individual can readily cause death in another. Careful cleaning and use of effective chlorine products periodically can minimize this risk. Instructions for the proper care and maintenance of these appliances accompany the purchase, and they should be adhered to strictly.

Alcoholic beverages should not be consumed prior to entering a hot tub. This is particularly imperative if you are entering the tub alone and unsupervised. Aside from the effect that these substances have on the temperature sensitivities and the cardiovascular system, people have drowned as a result of mixing these two pleasures. Sensible temperatures should be adopted and adhered to. The typical temperature is in the range of 102° F. but this must be individualized. This information accompanies the purchase, as does that on maintenance. Many people have suffered serious burns from hot pads because the sensory perception of the skin was dulled after a period of time. Since it no longer felt warm, the tendency was to turn the dial higher. A similar phenomenon occurs in a hot tub. The goal should not be to see how much heat could be tolerated.

TETANUS

Tetanus is a risk with many recreational activities. Contrary to popular belief it does not require a rusty nail. Tetanus spores are present in the soil all around us, where they can survive for years, and on most of the objects that penetrate the skin during recreational activities. Tetanus infection is a risk whenever a thorn from a rose or barberry bush penetrates the skin. Prevention is by far the best approach to this potentially fatal disease. Immunization is readily accomplished by a series of injections. This immunity can then be maintained by a booster injection every ten years. In the event of an injury a booster may be indicated at that time, depending on the injury and the length of time since the last booster. These are judgments to be made by the family physician.

Tetanus can carry a mortality of fifty percent once contracted, even with the best of medical care. The majority of people who suffer invasion by thorns and splinters do not succumb to tetanus infection. This fact is a graphic demonstration of the effectiveness of the immune and protective systems of the body. With the high mortality rate, however, and with effective immunization readily available at a reasonable cost at any family physician's office, this is a foolish risk to take. Not a single member of the United States armed forces in World War II died from this disease, although it killed many in previous wars. This is a remarkable testimonial to the effectiveness of immunization and to the diligence of the armed forces of the United States in executing immunization programs.

1. National Safety Council. *Accident Facts*, 1997 edition.

2. Evans WO, Robinson SM, Horstman DH, et al. Amelioration of the Symptoms of Acute Mountain Sickness by Staging and Acetazolamide. *Aviat Space Environ Med* **47**(5):512-516, 1976.

3. Woodward GA, Vernon DD. Aviation physiology in pediatric transport. In: Jaimovich DG, Vidyasager D, ed. *Pediatric and Neonatal Transport Medicine*. Mosby, St. Louis, 1996.

4. CDC. Outbreak of relapsing fever — Grand Canyon National Park, Arizona, 1990. *MMWR* 1991;**40**(18):296–303.

5. CDC. Consequences of Delayed Diagnosis of Rocky Mountain Spotted Fever in Children. *MMWR* 2000;**49**:885-888.

6. CDC. Compendium of Animal Rabies Control 1997. *MMWR* 1997;**46**:No.RR-4.

IX

HAZARDS OF TEMPERATURE EXTREMES

Simplistic solutions evolve from simple minds.   — DEW

HEAT STRESS

Humans, as with other warm blooded animals, are able to maintain their body temperature within a very narrow range in spite of wide variations in the environment surrounding them. These adaptive mechanisms have limits, however, and failure to recognize this fact and to take appropriate precautions results in many heat-related illnesses and many deaths each year. Most of these cases could be prevented by an awareness of the environmental conditions that lead to heat disorders, and by recognition of the early warning signs of impending illness.

Factors which influence the development of heat related disorders include the temperature of the air, the humidity of the air, the amount of air movement, thermal radiation, the level of physical activity being expended at the time, the age and physical condition of the individual, drugs, type of clothing worn and body build. These disorders occur much more commonly during periods of prolonged heat, and particularly when the humidity is high.

The chief mechanism by which the body dissipates heat is through sweating and the evaporation thereof. This mechanism becomes less efficient during periods of high humidity, because the sweat evaporates from the skin more slowly. Conversely, sweat is evaporated more rapidly when there is an appreciable air movement across the body, than when no such movement is present. When sweat is evaporated rapidly excess body heat is eliminated more efficiently. Short, stocky and obese individuals dissipate heat much less efficiently, both because of the increased body mass and the decreased skin surface area. More heat is produced in the greater body mass, and at the same time relatively less skin surface area is available for sweating and heat dissipation.

Age plays a significant role in the amount of heat stress that an individual can tolerate. This decreased tolerance to heat stress begins as early as the age of thirty-five years. After that age the amount of oxygen that is made available to the body is reduced by 25 to 30 percent. This results partially from a decrease in the functional output of the heart and circulatory system and partially from the reduction in the efficiency of oxygen transport in the lungs. Obviously this deficit, in both of these components, is much more severe in smokers. The greater the age, the more pronounced these physiologic deficiencies become. With age the muscles of the heart weaken and become less efficient as do the muscles of the body in general. These changes and their resultant deficiencies are precisely the reason that professional athletes begin to lose the ability to compete in strenuous sports during their late thirties.

The blood circulation also becomes less efficient with age, partially as a result of the weakening of the heart and partially because of arteriosclerosis. The result is that the heat produced in the body as a result of metabolism and muscular activity is not as readily transported to the surface for dissipation. Another factor making older individuals more at risk for heat disorders is that there is a delay in the onset of sweating and a reduction in the amount of perspiration produced. Both of these changes are age related. This results in greater heat retention within the body, and earlier onset of all of the heat disorders. The reduction in the efficiencies of these mechanisms also prolongs the recovery time for heat related disorders.

During periods of increased heat stress, with the accompanying increased perspiration, there is a significant increase in the amount of salt lost from the body. The resultant dilution of the body fluids results in a false signal from the region of the brain that normally conserves salt. The consequence is that the kidneys excrete additional quantities of salt as well as water. In order to avoid the serious consequences of these heat induced imbalances, it is necessary to increase the salt intake prophylactically. This is best done with meals.

Electrolyte solutions can be used to good advantage during periods of heat exposure if indicated. Balanced solutions that are designed to replace all of the fluids and electrolytes that are lost during heat exposure are marketed. The most urgent need, however, for prophylaxis and treatment of heat exhaustion is increased intake of water. Salt tablets should be avoided always, since they irritate the stomach. A simple solution of 1 teaspoonful of table salt, 8 tablespoonsful of sugar and 2 to 4 ounces of lemon extract in one quart of water provides a mixture that may be more palatable, and can be used as a supplement to plain water.

The quantity of salt supplementation needed is directly related to the amount of loss and can be calculated by experts using complex formulae. For recreational activities and tasks around the home such calculations are not practical, and are usually not necessary. In the extreme, as much as ten to fifteen grams of supplemental salt may be required over an eight hour period. Caution must be exercised in consuming supplemental salt, however. It would be rare circumstances where this quantity would be needed at home.

Under normal conditions any excess of salt and water consumed is controlled and eliminated by the kidney. This requires normal conditions of kidney function and normal water intake. Kidney function is commonly reduced in diabetes, in high blood pressure and in older individuals. It may also be reduced as a result of other diseases and as a result of exposure to toxic drugs and chemicals. The widespread use of illicit drugs has greatly increased the number of people suffering from chronic kidney failure. Several medications can also cause scarring in the filtering portion of the kidneys when they are taken for long periods. Some antibiotics such as methicillin can produce this, but analgesics are perhaps the most insidious.

Phenacetin is particularly hazardous, especially when combined with aspirin. Kidney damage from this drug is common in Australia, Switzerland and Sweden. Its use has been discontinued in the U.S., but one of its metabolites, acetaminophen, is still widely used here and it too causes damage in the kidney. The NSAIDS, non-steroidal anti-inflammatory drugs, also cause scarring in the kidneys, and they are given for long periods of time to individuals who are likely to have diminished function already because of age.

Thiazide diuretics, which are commonly taken for high blood pressure, also will be taken over long periods of time. Their role in controlling blood pressure is to deplete the body of salt and fluid volume. As a consequence they render the individual more susceptible to heat disorders. Supplementation of salt requires adequate intake of water at the same time. Prophylactic salt supplementation carries a particular risk for those individuals who have high blood pressure, because salt has a very deleterious effect on blood pressure. In these instances the quantity of salt consumed should to be monitored and balanced very carefully.

Lithium, even in the therapeutic range, and gold for rheumatoid arthritis, both commonly cause scarring in the kidneys. Individuals with high blood pressure, diabetes or any chronic illness should have their blood chemistries monitored regularly. Patients on any of the aforementioned medications also should be so monitored. Even with monitoring, when the serum creatinine or BUN (blood urea nitrogen) is elevated, it is not an early indication of damage. We have no simple blood test to give us an early warning of kidney damage. People with any chronic health problem and those on any of the medications listed should simply anticipate a greater risk of heat disorders and plan accordingly.

Alcohol consumption greatly increases the susceptibility to all of the heat disorders. It suppresses the hormone in the body that regulates salt and water excretion through the kidneys, leading to excessive water loss and dehydration. Excessive alcohol consumption several days before exposure to heat may result in this deleterious effect. Alcohol should be avoided, therefore, whenever recreational activities or home projects are planned, especially during periods of prolonged hot weather.

Physical conditioning improves the efficiency of the circulation and of the function of the heart in general. It also improves lung capacity and the efficiency of lung function. This improves heat tolerance to a degree, but it does not eliminate the need for acclimatization. Exposure to heat should be undertaken in steps in order to permit time for the physiological adjustments that take place with prolonged exposure to heat. These include an increase in the capillaries and in circulation and an increase in oxygen transport in the lungs. This acclimatization generally takes about four to seven days. It is somewhat analogous to the acclimatization in oxygen transport through the lungs to the blood that is required for activities at altitudes above 10,000 feet. In anticipation of recreational activities that might involve heat stress, particularly strenuous activities such as running, these principles should be applied during preparation for the event.

HEAT EXHAUSTION

This disorder is also called heat prostration, heat collapse and heat fatigue. It is the mildest form of heat disorder and the most common. It results from an excessive loss of fluid from the body after a prolonged exposure to high temperatures. It can occur indoors or outside. Although it occurs most frequently in individuals who are not acclimatized to the heat and who are involved in strenuous activities, it can happen to sedentary people. It is a common occurrence each summer, particularly during periods of high relative humidity. Strenuous exertion, poor ventilation and heavy clothing contribute to the development of this disorder. It is more common in and poses a greater risk for older individuals, especially those taking diuretics for high blood pressure or heart failure.

There is usually adequate warning that heat exhaustion is eminent through the development of increasing fatigue, weakness, anxiety and drenching sweats, but the symptoms may not be dramatic, and are often overlooked. Faintness usually develops following the above symptoms. Disordered mentation such as confusion may be seen. The body temperature is below normal, the skin is pale and clammy, the pulse is weak and slow and the blood pressure is lowered.

It is essential to recognize these early warning signs of heat exhaustion at the earliest possible moment, and to take steps to prevent progression to a more serious stage. These early steps include removal from the hot environment to a cooler one, even if only in the shade, or removal from a hot attic or roof. Discontinuance of physical activity, removal of heavy clothing and drinking cool fluids will all help to reverse this potentially serious condition. Once the heat exhaustion victim has progressed to the point where assistance is needed, these measures become more urgent. In addition to removing from the hot environment, the person should be made to lie flat or with the head slightly low.

HEAT STROKE

Heat stroke is also called sunstroke, but it is not necessary to be exposed to the sun to fall victim to this disorder. It is a stage beyond heat exhaustion and is life threatening. Aggressive measures are urgent. In this disorder, the body's temperature regulating mechanism fails. In most cases there is little or no perspiration, the skin is dry, hot and red. Some victims with fully developed symptoms continue to perspire, however. The pulse is rapid (160 to 180) and firm. Respirations are rapid and shallow. The blood pressure is usually low.

Constriction of the blood vessels prevents the transfer of heat from the body core to the surface. As a consequence the body core temperature rises rapidly to a level of 105 to 106 degrees Fahrenheit. If aggressive measures to reduce this are not taken, the temperature rise progresses to convulsions and death. Permanent brain damage may occur if the individual survives. Headache, weakness and dizziness are followed by a sudden loss of consciousness. Disorientation may be present and may progress to delirium.

Efforts to control the body temperature should be initiated immediately by immersing the victim in cool water or by wrapping him in cool moist blankets or cloth. It is essential that the body temperature be lowered as rapidly as possible. The victim should be hospitalized immediately. The outlook is less favorable for the aged, debilitated and alcoholics than is the case for young individuals in good health. Most heat related deaths are due to heat stroke. Individuals who have survived a previous episode of heat stroke are particularly at risk and should exercise the utmost care in avoiding excessive heat exposure.

Heat exhaustion and heat stroke occur with increased frequency during heat waves. Daily deaths due to these disorders double or triple during prolonged periods of high temperature. It is essential to decrease physical activities, increase fluid intake, especially water, and to stay in a cool environment. Fans and light, minimal clothing may be adequate in some cases. At temperatures of 95 degrees Fahrenheit and above, fans lose their effectiveness, however.

Air conditioning can be life saving during very hot periods. If air conditioning is not available at home, spending a few hours at an air conditioned shopping mall during the middle of the day is helpful. Nursing home patients are a group of individuals who are particularly at risk during periods of prolonged heat. The majority of cases of heat stroke occur in elderly people who have preexisting diseases such as arteriosclerosis and heart disease, especially those taking diuretics.

PRICKLY HEAT

Also called miliaria, this condition occurs when the ducts of the sweat glands become plugged with keratin and dead cells on the skin. The sweat retained in the glands bursts through the wall of the duct into the surrounding tissue. Here it causes inflammation, and sometimes infection. Frequent bathing, skin hygiene and clean clothing are the measures to take to prevent this condition.

HYPOTHERMIA

Hypothermia is a disorder that can occur in anyone with prolonged exposure to the cold. It occurs in the elderly, however, in circumstances where it might not be expected. Many of the aged die in their homes each winter, even when the temperature is only mildly cold, in the range of sixty-five degrees Fahrenheit. Among the factors accounting for this are impaired circulation induced by age, decreased vasomotor ability to compensate for exposure to lower temperatures, and a decreased perception of cold.

Decreased heat production through metabolic channels and poor heat conservation of the body in this age group also contribute to the increased risk. The tendency for older people, especially those who live alone, to neglect regular and adequate nutrition also increases the risk in this age group. Both by the aged and their families need a greater awareness of these risk factors. It is urgent that this population and those who care for them fully understand the risks and how to avoid them.

Once the body core temperature falls below 95 degrees Fahrenheit, the definition point for hypothermia, it continues to fall insidiously until death results. (A rectal temperature reading normally gives an accurate assessment of the body core temperature.) This condition carries a mortality rate of approximately 50 percent. About 700 to 800 people die each year in the United States from hypothermia. The number has increased in recent years due to the increase in the aged population, and to the increase in the number of people living without shelter.

Evidence of impending hypothermia is fatigue, weakness, lack of coordination, apathy and drowsiness progressing to confusion. When the body core temperature falls below 90 degrees Fahrenheit, these symptoms progress to stupor and coma. Anyone who has been in a cold environment will have cold extremities, but older individuals who are at risk of hypothermia will present a cold abdomen that is not normally seen. The lack of shivering in this age group can be misleading.

Shivering increases heat production in the body and is a natural defense mechanism in hypothermia. Its absence in older people compounds the danger. The presence of hypothermia in these people may be overlooked since the standard thermometer measures only to 94 degrees, and it must be diligently shaken to get it to that level. Thermometers that measure lower are available, and should be used when checking for hypothermia. In rewarming older people suffering from hypothermia, it is important to not rewarm them too rapidly, since hypotension (low blood pressure) can result.

Alcohol increases the risk of hypothermia at any age. It interferes with the constriction of blood vessels that is the natural defense mechanism of the body in conserving heat. It also decreases the individual's perception of cold so that normal precautions are not taken. Alcohol should be avoided by everyone during activities that involve prolonged exposure to cold, such as skiing, camping, hunting and hiking. Drugs that depress the central nervous system such as tranquilizers, sleeping medications and so called "recreational drugs" may also increase the susceptibility to hypothermia. Hypothermia can occur under these altered circumstances when the outdoor temperature is only moderately cold.

Immersion in cold water brings about hypothermia much sooner due to the rapidity of heat loss from the body. A very lean person will suffer a life threatening lowering of the body core temperature sooner than will an obese individual. Heart irregularities are common with hypothermia and are a common cause of death. These are all the more serious by virtue of the fact that when the temperature of the heart muscle is lowered it responds much less readily to resuscitative measures.

FROSTBITE

This affliction also can affect any age, old or young. The risk is greater in the aged and in the very young, however. There also is an increased risk in those individuals who have impaired circulation, such as with diabetes, heart disease and arteriosclerosis. The decreased perception of cold and the diminished efficiency of vasomotor control, as described above, account for the increased problem in the aged. The risk is also increased with the use of alcohol, impairment of consciousness from any cause, exhaustion and hunger. The windchill factor also influences the risk, and thus it is greater with wet clothing. Contact with metal greatly increases the risk of frostbite. Many B-17 gunners during World War II suffered frostbite of the fingers and hands when they removed their gloves to work on jammed machine guns. Flying at 28,000 feet they were exposed to temperatures of minus 50°F.

With frostbite, ice crystals may form in the tissues, and the small blood vessels may thrombose (clot), leading to gangrene. Where the frost damage is superficial, the tissues will be firm, cold and white. The areas most commonly involved are the face, ears, fingers and toes. The skin may peel or blister one to two days after frostbite occurs. Pronounced permanent damage to the blood vessels may occur, with resultant hypersensitivity to cold.

Where the cold damage is deeper, a loss of feeling is noted in addition to the cold, hard, white tissues. These areas become red, blotchy, swollen and painful as they rewarm. If the damage is severe enough, gangrene results. The frozen tissues should be handled gently to avoid additional damage. The involved areas should be rewarmed as rapidly as practical, without further damaging the tissues by excess heat. Rewarming is best accomplished by immersion in warm water, starting at 60 to 70 degrees Fahrenheit. The temperature of the water can be gradually increased to 80 to 90 degrees Fahrenheit. It is important to keep in mind that these areas have no feeling, and the temperature of the water must be monitored for the victim.

Frostbite is frequently seen in hands and feet even though the body core temperature remains normal. If hypothermia is present also, the first priority should be to raise the core temperature. It accomplishes nothing to rewarm frozen feet and hands if the victim expires from hypothermia. Medical attention should be sought as soon as possible. Special techniques and equipment, such as peritoneal dialysis, intravenous solutions and monitoring of blood gasses, pH (acidity) and potassium all may greatly improve survival.

Cigarettes absolutely must be avoided during the recovery period. Infection and gangrene are common complications of this condition.

As mentioned previously, the elderly are at increased risk of all of the temperature disorders, both elevated and lowered temperatures. This fact is due to physiologic changes of aging that reduce the efficiency of the body in temperature regulation. The mechanisms that increase heat production during cold exposure, both shivering and other physiologic mechanisms, are reduced in the aged. There is also a decrease in the sensory perception so that these individuals don't feel the temperature changes as readily as younger people do. The age at which these changes occur is variable. Certainly they have taken place by the age of eighty, but they can occur in the fifties in some individuals. Illnesses such as diabetes invoke these changes at a younger age. These changes take place gradually over time, not overnight.

Another physiologic change that takes place in the aged that accounts for the impairment of adjustment to temperature extremes is a reduced ability of the autonomic nervous system to bring about constriction and dilation of the blood vessels. Sweating, which is the major mechanism whereby the body dissipates heat, is markedly impaired in the aged. Sweating does not commence in older people until a higher temperature is reached, and the amount of perspiration is greatly reduced.

Illness and disease also contribute to these impairments in adjustment to temperature extremes. Diabetes, arteriosclerosis, heart disease and any chronic illness that results in debilitation increase the risk. Malnutrition and poor hydration are common in this age group. Malnutrition in particular reduces the heat production in the body. This coupled with the reduction of circulation resulting from arteriosclerosis greatly increases the risk from cold exposure. Also adding to this risk is the reduced mobility brought about by arthritis, stroke, heart disease and degenerative joint disease, especially in the hip and knees.

Either heat or cold disorders frequently result in kidney failure which leads to death, even if the temperature disorder is successfully treated. Successful treatment of temperature disorders is much less likely in the elderly, however, than it is in younger, healthy victims. A high index of suspicion and observation during periods of temperature extremes is essential. The older age group should avoid going outdoors in periods of cold. Adequate clothing is essential, especially a hat, for 30 percent of the body heat is lost through the head. During extended periods of heat, older people should avoid being out in the sun, they should wear light clothing and develop a habit of drinking adequate fluids, chiefly water, on a regular basis, not responding merely to thirst. Fans and cool baths help avoid heat disorders.

MALIGNANT HYPERTHERMIA

This condition occurs in individuals who are unfortunate enough to inherit genetic disorders that render them susceptible to most of the common inhalation anesthetics. These include ether, halothane and cyclopropane. The condition is also precipitated by succinylcholine chloride, which is routinely used for muscle relaxation during surgery. The acute hyperthermia that is provoked by the administration of any of these medications invokes a serious medical emergency, and can result in death. Early recognition of the reaction and prompt, aggressive treatment is essential to survival. A family history of such a disorder provides forewarning. This history should be acquired before pregnancy and before any surgery is contemplated in anyone. Tests are available to identify the inherited trait.

X

HAZARDS OF THE WORKPLACE

No man is an island, entire of itself; every man is a piece of the continent, a part of the main.   — John Donne 1573-1631

HISTORY

The association between certain occupational exposures and the development of disease was documented as early as the fourth century B.C. when Hippocrates described the toxicity of lead to workers mining it. In the first century A.D., Pliny the Elder (23-79 A.D.) noted the sickness of the lungs that afflicted slaves who worked with asbestos. He also wrote about the health hazards that accompanied working with zinc. He described a protective mask made from the bladders of animals that he had observed workers who were mining and processing cinnabar (mercuric sulfide) wearing.

In the second century Galen, a Greek physician who practiced in Rome (he was physician to Marcus Aurelius), documented the adverse effects of acid mists in copper mines. Herodotus made similar observations regarding other exposures. None of these observations were accompanied by any advocacy of protection for the workers, who for the most part were slaves.

In the intervening period there is no documentation of any further interest in occupational hazards until the fifteenth century. In 1473 Ulrich Ellenbog published a pamphlet describing the adverse effects of lead and mercury fumes. He included recommendations for limiting the risks involved. The observations of Paracelsus and Agricola were published in the sixteenth century. Agricola's *De Re Metallica*, which is a scholarly work consisting of twelve books, was published in 1556, one year after his death. In it he not only described the hazards associated with mining, and with the associated smelting and refining of gold and silver, but also outlined preventative measures such as ventilation of the mines and masks for the workers.

Agricola also noted that "in the mines of the Carpathian Mountains women are found who have married seven husbands, all of whom this terrible consumption has carried off to a premature death." This "consumption" probably included silicosis, tuberculosis and/or carcinoma of the lung. Paracelsus also wrote about the health hazards associated with mining, and his work was published in 1567 after his death. It described the disease associated with the inhalation of mercury fumes. He was employed as a physician in a smelting plant in Tyrol, Austria and had traveled widely not only in Germany and Austria, but in Hungary, Denmark and Sweden as well. He was killed in a tavern brawl in Salzburg in 1541.

Born 100 years later, Bernardino Ramazzini, an Italian physician and the "Father of Occupational Medicine" published *De Morbis Artificum Diatriba* in 1700 at the age of 67. He was awarded a chair at the University of Padua during the same year. In the first chapter of this work he described the "pneumonokoniosis" of stone masons and miners, based upon findings at autopsy. He was the first to advocate documenting the occupation as a routine part of the patient's record, suggesting that this question be added to those recommended by Hippocrates. He outlined many precautions to reduce the risks that he observed in occupational exposures.

Sir Percivall Pott published the first documentation of an association between cancer and an occupational chemical exposure in 1775. He described in detail the cancer of the scrotum that afflicted young chimney sweeps and its spread to the testicle and abdomen. He accurately incriminated the soot that accumulated in their clothing as the cause. He also corrected the misconception of his colleagues that it was a venereal disease. Through his efforts the Chimney Sweepers Act of 1788 was enacted in England. Child labor laws were non existent at the time, and the abuse of children such as chimney sweeps was not only primitive but also barbaric. It was common practice for children aged 7 or 8 years, both male and female, to be indentured for twelve years in mines and in factories. They would arrive at work at 5:30 AM and labor until 7:00 in the evening.[1]

In 1820 John Ayrton Paris described skin cancers among workers in copper smelters in England, and correctly ascribed the disease to arsenic exposure. In 1894 Unna described actinic keratoses of sailors as being premalignant, and related them to occupational exposure to the sun. In 1895 Rehn made the association between cancers of the urinary bladder and occupational exposure to coal tar dyes. This association has been confirmed many times since. Cancer of the nose among workers exposed to chromate production was reported in 1890. Lung cancer from the same exposure was noted in 1912. Cancer of the lung and the nasal sinuses was related to occupational exposure to nickel in 1932.

Butlin, in 1892, demonstrated that pitch, tar and mineral oil that accumulated on clothing caused cancer of the scrotum. Several cases of other skin cancers resulting from occupational exposure to coal tars, paraffin, pitch and mineral oil were recorded subsequently. The synthesis in the laboratory of two of the carcinogenic components of these oils and tars in 1930 (dibenz[a,h]anthracene and benzo-a-pyrene)) made it possible to study this relationship in detail.

In 1942 Dr. Wilhelm C. Hueper published the first comprehensive text on occupational cancer. In *Occupational Tumors and Allied Diseases* he described the relationship between occupational exposure to certain chemicals, metals and minerals and the subsequent development of cancer. The National Cancer Institute's environmental research program was established in 1948 under his direction. He subsequently published a book on occupational and environmental cancers of the urinary system in 1969 and the carcinogenic properties of chromium, nickel and arsenic in 1962. He published an article on environmental cancer hazards in the Journal of Occupational Medicine in 1972.

INJURIES

The full extent of workplace injuries has not been known, primarily because many were not reported and thus not tabulated. Reporting requirements that have been put in place by OSHA and the accompanying forms have resulted in more complete data and thus more accurate statistics. This has resulted in greater efforts toward prevention. About ten million workers suffer traumatic injuries on the job each year. Approximately 30 percent of these are severe, with about 6,000 fatalities annually currently. These result from falls, blows, crushing injuries, fires, explosions and electrocution. Approximately eight percent of workers in the United States in a given year suffer injuries that require treatment. About three million workers each year suffer severe disabling injuries on the job, and about 70,000 of these disabilities are permanent. Over

20,000 amputations occur on the job each year, 93 percent being fingers, usually caught in machinery, belts, saws or other cutting devices.

Many of these events could be prevented, perhaps even the majority. Even when management installs protective devices, such as the harness to prevent finger damage from presses, the workers find these cumbersome, and take them off. Perhaps one of the most innovative safety device was a one legged stool provided to operators who controlled the apparatus for making nitroglycerin. If the operator got sleepy the loss of balance would awaken him.[2] These risks have been greatly reduced, both in magnitude and in number, since the passage of the Occupational Safety and Health Act by Congress in 1970. Some serious risks have been eliminated entirely, and progress continues year by year on the remainder.

CHEMICALS

While injuries and accidental death account for the majority of job related events, exposure on the job to agents that cause cancer is perhaps the most feared. Many substances, both naturally occurring and man made, are capable of causing cancer in man. Many, many more are capable of causing cancer in animals but apparently not in man, at least under normal circumstances. Some substances cause cancer only when they are bio-transformed in the body. Others cause cancer only in the presence of another chemical or physical agent. The mechanisms are complex, and seldom absolute with any given chemical (see Chapter XIII).

In 1970 the Occupational Safety and Health Administration was established, charged with establishing safety standards in industry. With respect to chemicals, this agency has established permissible exposure levels and handling techniques. It has published a list of substances that cause cancer in man, and a list of "suspected cancer agents". It must be kept in mind that inclusion on this list is influenced by court decisions. For instance MOCA, 4,4-methylene bis(2-chloroanaline), was removed from the list for such reason, even though it is clear that it causes tumors in the urinary bladder in humans.

Given these ground rules, there have been fourteen categories of substances that were listed by the Occupational Safety and Health Administration (OSHA) as CANCER SUSPECT AGENTS. All work areas where exposure to these substances is possible, and the entrance to these areas, must be identified by a sign reading **CANCER SUSPECT AGENT**. Mandatory guidelines for the handling of these substances, including eating and showering facilities, are published by OSHA. The substances identified by OSHA as cancer suspect agents are:[3,4]

4-Nitrobiphenyl	4-Aminodiphenyl
alpha-Naphthylamine	beta-Propiolactone
Methyl chloromethyl ether	Ethylenediamine
3,3-Dichlorobenzidine (and its salts)	2-Acetylaminofluorene
Bis-Chloromethyl ether (BCME)	4-Dimethylaminoazobenzene
beta-Naphthylamine	N-Nitrosodimethylamine
Benzidine	*Vinyl chloride

* Vinyl chloride currently (2001) has been removed from this list although it has a well established record of having caused angiosarcomas of the liver in humans.[5,6] (IARC S.7, 1987).

While these are labeled only as cancer suspect agents, any reasonable person would operate under the premise that exposure to them does pose a risk of cancer. The rules mandated by OSHA for handling and working with these agents reflect such consideration. Any biologic contact through inhalation, ingestion or through the skin should be avoided.

Listed clearly as cancer hazards are inorganic arsenic, benzene, coke oven emissions, acrylonitrile, ethylene oxide and 1,2-dibromo-3-chloropropane (DBCP). Listed as a potential cancer hazard is formaldehyde.

Even in circumstances where we might feel certain that a substance causes cancer in humans, as a result of observations of those exposed, it is difficult to make an absolute declaration. In the strictest scientific sense any such statement must be preceded by controlled studies that follow established protocols. Obviously we can't do such studies in humans where serious consequences, such as cancer, are involved. It is for this reason that we see such equivocation. A decision to label any substance as carcinogenic is necessarily based upon prospective, epidemiological evidence.

It is also important to keep a proper perspective regarding the incidence of occupational related cancers as compared to those not related to the job. Studies in 1981 demonstrated that only about 4 percent of all cancer deaths in the United States could be attrib-

380

uted to occupational exposures.[7] With the stringent controls that have been instituted, exposures have been markedly reduced, and that percentage is probably lower now. It is obvious that we should be directing attention to those factors that might be contributing to the other 96 percent, such as sun exposure and tobacco. Chemicals and viruses that are associated with cancer are discussed in Chapter XIII.

WORKPLACE CARCINOGENS

SUBSTANCE	APPLICATION	AFFECTED ORGAN
Arsenic	Wood preservative, Ag chems	Skin
Asbestos	Insulation, brake & friction	Lung, pleura, peritoneum
Benzene	Solvent, many other	Blood (leukemia)
Benzidine	Dyes	Urinary bladder
Bis(chloromethyl)ether	Ion exchange resins	Lung
Chromium	Smelting operations, other	Nose, sinus, lung
Coke oven emissions	Iron ore extraction	Lung, kidney
2-Naphthylamine	Dyes, rubber (discontinued)	Bladder
Thorium dioxide (radioactive)	Gas mantles, optical glass*	Liver cancers
Vinyl chloride	Plastics, building materials	Angiosarcoma of liver
Wood dust**	Furniture, home building	Nose & sinus

* Also tungsten filaments, welding electrodes, high temperature ceramics & crucibles and as catalyst. Has been discontinued as radiopaque x-ray medium. Thorium, as with uranium, is a naturally radioactive substance.
** Western red cedar, mahogany and oak

Aside from cancer, there are literally hundreds of chemicals that cause damage to the liver, kidneys or brain and nervous system. Virtually every job in industry exposes workers to some of these chemicals, or to the physical agents such as dusts, that may cause harm. Harmful effects most often result from breathing the vapors or fumes, or from skin contact with the substance. Most of the toxic chemicals are readily absorbed through the skin and thus are harmful to the internal organs through this route as well as when inhaled.

Some of the toxic chemical exposures on the job result from the manufacture of specific chemicals. Thus the vinyl chloride monomer gas used in the production of polyvinyl chloride induces a rare tumor in the liver (angiosarcoma) in workers exposed to it. This association was first made when a plant physician observed three workers with this affliction between 1967 and 1973, and noted that they all cleaned reactor vessels as part of their job in the plant.[8] Several subsequent studies have demonstrated the association of vinyl chloride with other cancers.[9,10]

One study evaluated the excess lung, brain and liver cancer, but was able to show a relationship only with angiosarcoma of the liver.[11] Other studies have demonstrated that even low levels of exposure to both vinyl chloride and to ethylene dichloride, which is extensively used worldwide to produce vinyl chloride, damages the liver.[12] It has also been identified as a causative agent in the development of scleroderma. Vinyl chloride is now used only in closed systems in order to eliminate exposure. BCME (bischloro-methyl ether), used in the manufacture of resins for water filters, carries a similar risk for lung cancer, even among nonsmokers. Inhalation of this substance and skin contact with it must be avoided.

Other chemical exposures in industry result from ancillary processes, and are thus seen outside of plants that manufacture chemicals. The use of chlorinated hydrocarbon solvents for degreasing is a common example, since this process is used in every plant where machining, stamping and shearing or shaping of metal takes place. Trichloroethane is the substance commonly used today, and it is well absorbed through the skin as well as the lungs. It is very difficult to avoid exposure, and it produces a significant toxicity in the liver as well as the nervous system. Both chlorine and ammonia gas may cause severe irritation of the lungs and bronchi. Exposure to either may be fatal, depending upon the concentration and the duration of exposure. Hydrogen sulfide gas has killed a number of workers in sewers and in sewage treatment facilities.

Many organic solvents such as acetone and ketone can produce muscle weakness, irritability, memory loss, changes in per-sonality, difficulty concentrating and other nervous system disor-ders. There have been several reports of connective tissue disorders such as scleroderma being produced by heavy exposure to halogenated solvents such as trichloroethylene. Such cases must be uncommon, if they do occur. No organized study of this association has been undertaken. A more common and insidious toxic effect of the inhalation and dermal absorption of the organic solvents is solvent myopathy. This is a weakness of the skeletal muscles that results from degenerative changes in the cellular components of the muscles.

Trichloroethylene and carbon tetrachloride have been replaced in the workplace because of their liver toxicity and other toxic effects. The substitutes continue to demonstrate their own toxicity, however. Dimethylformamide (DMF), a solvent that is widely used in the manufacture of polymerized films, fibers and coatings (acrylic fabrics), produces a chemical hepatitis when it is inhaled. Careful attention to adequate ventilation is essential where it is used.

Organic solvents are commonly encountered in glues and adhesives, paints and lacquer, dyes, plastics, printing inks and in degreasing and cleaning operations. Adequate ventilation is essential in minimizing the exposure to these chemical substances. This requires properly engineered booths and ventilation systems as mandated by the Occupational Safety and Health Administration. Ordinary respirators provide no protection against vapors. An appropriate charcoal canister filter does offer protection, if it is well fitted and properly maintained. Adequate design and engineering controls provide a safer approach in the workplace. If hand immersion is required, special solvent resistant gloves and aprons are necessary. These solvents penetrate most gloves, but materials such as Viton provide some protection. Manufacturing systems that avoid all contact are preferable.

Methylene chloride (dichloromethane) is an organic solvent that is widely used in industry in a variety of products. It is often included in products such as furniture strippers because it does not present a fire or explosive risk. It causes damage to the central nervous system, as do most of the organic solvents. It produces "fatty liver" changes but does not cause the death of liver cells that is seen in such solvents as carbon tetrachloride and chloroform. Inhalation of any of these solvents may cause problems in patients with heart conditions. The greater risk with methylene chloride may relate to the findings that it causes cancer in rats and mice. This concern prompted OSHA in early 1992 to propose a marked reduction in the allowable exposure level for workers involved with this chemical. The proposal would also require medical evaluation and monitoring of workers who are exposed to a given level. As of 2001, however, the ACGIH had not revised its TWA exposure limit of 50 ppm for methylene chloride.[13]

With every toxic substance exposure one must be mindful of the interaction with other agents. It takes much less alcohol to damage the liver, for example, after that organ has been exposed to trichloroethane and similar agents. Exposure to asbestos increases an individual's risk of developing lung cancer by a factor of 6 to 8, but if that person smokes cigarettes, the risk is increased to at least 80 times the normal. Similarly, a welder who smokes cigarettes carries a much greater risk of developing lung disease than does a welder who does not smoke.

CUTTING OILS

Insoluble cutting oils (neat oil), which are used in low speed cutting and grinding operations, have long been known to produce acne, inflammation of hair follicles and cancer of the scrotum. The exact mechanism or culprit is not known, but cancer of the scrotum in young chimney sweeps, resulting from the tars collected during their work, was reported by Sir Percivall Pott in 1775. Butlin reported similar cancers in England as a result of exposure to pitch, tar and mineral oil in 1892. Fifteen polycyclic aromatic hydrocarbons (PAH) that might be found in these substances are known to be carcinogenic.[14]

More recently it has been found that nitrosamines, among the most potent carcinogenic agents known, are formed in soluble cutting oils. This reaction between nitrites and amines may result from the bacteria that are known to reproduce in these oils. Soluble cutting oils are used in high speed cutting and grinding operations. They are oil and water emulsions, composed of chlorinated or sulfurated oils, which are more likely to provoke skin reactions. In addition they contain detergents and emulsifiers that are potentially irritating. Preservatives in these oils, such as ethylenediamine, cause eczematous skin reactions.

Where the oil is aerosolized, as it frequently is with machining operations, and more so when compressed air is used to remove the oil from the parts, pulmonary reactions are common. The normal pulmonary protective system, the mucociliary escalator, cannot remove aerosolized oil that is inhaled, and this can result in a lipoid pneumonia. The agent provoking asthma may be the ethylenediamine in one worker, and microorganisms growing in the oil in another worker. Workers exposed to these oils and their additives can lessen their risk by changing clothes daily, laundering these clothes well, and by showering thoroughly every day after work. Wearing of an impervious apron offers some additional protection.

HYDROQUINONE

Loss of the pigmentation of the skin can result from contact with hydroquinone and related compounds. This phenomenon was first reported forty-five years ago in workers wearing rubber gloves. It continues to be a risk in rubber workers today as well as in those who come in contact with printing inks, lubricating and cutting oils, germicides and photochemicals. The loss of pigmentation is permanent, and there is no cure for it. This presents a serious problem with sun exposure, both because of the risk of sunburn and of the development of skin cancers.

CHLORACNE

This is a very resistant form of acne. It results from exposure to chlorinated hydrocarbons such as PCB (polychlorinated biphenyls) and PBB (polybrominated biphenyls) that are used as a fire retardant in the manufacture of paper, plastics and electrical and electronic components. They also are present in biphenyls that are used in herbicides. Most of these substances are now processed in closed systems to avoid contact. Contact still occurs due to trace contaminants and in handling cables where lubricants contain chlornaphthalene and biphenyls. Chloracne associated with TCDD (dioxin) is described in Chapter XIV.

Under federal and state Right to Know Laws, workers must be apprised of potentially harmful chemical and physical agents to which they are exposed. Labels must be on the containers, and the hazards must be listed. It is very foolish for a worker to not acquaint himself with these substances and their risks. Some management individuals have little concern for the health of their workers. Some workers, on the other hand, insist upon exposing themselves in spite of the best efforts of management. Both positions are to be condemned. Gambling should be reserved for the casinos, and it should never involve health.

PESTICIDES AND HERBICIDES

The hazards related to exposures to pesticides, herbicides and fungicides are covered in detail in Chapter XIV and this should be reviewed for their occupational consequences. Occupational exposures to these agents occur in their manufacture, in farming, among grounds keepers, commercial growers and harvesters and during aerial application (including the pilots, mixers, loaders and flagmen).

A unique occupational exposure that is reflected by the affluence in our society is the serious toxic symptoms reported in pet groomers that resulted from skin contact with organophosphate flea dips. These were first reported in 1986, and included head-ache, nausea, dizziness, tiredness, blurred vision, sweating, confusion and a feeling of being "spaced out."[15,16] These symptoms are well recognized, for they have been common in aerial applica-tors of pesticides for many years. Both individuals who treated pets in the flea dips and pet groomers suffered poisoning from the pesticides. The two agents incriminated in the preceding reports were chlorpyrifos and phosmet, both organophosphates. This group of pesticides should not be permitted to come in contact with the skin, and should not be applied to pets, to be carried home to the children.

An example of an unanticipated occupational exposure is the cleanup of the spill of 19,000 gallons of a pesticide when a train tanker car derailed and overturned in northern California. The substance was metam, a soil fumigant used in commercial farming. The breakdown product of metam, methylisocyanate, is known to be a skin irritant. An outbreak of dermatitis occurred among 76 percent of the cleanup crew who had worked in the water removing dead fish.[17] It is imperative to avoid skin contact with all pesticides, as with chemicals and solvents in general. When contact does occur, the skin should be washed well as soon as possible and clean clothing should be donned

TOXIC METALS IN THE WORKPLACE

Aluminum	Gallium	Platinum
Antimony	Gold	Selenium
Arsenic	Indium	Silver
Barium	Lead	Tellurium
Beryllium	Lithium	Thallium
Bismuth	Magnesium	Tin
Cadmium	Manganese	Titanium
Cobalt	Mercury	Uranium
Copper	Molybdenum	Vanadium
Chromium	Nickel	Zinc

Not all are of equal toxicity. Some are toxic chiefly in the form of their compounds.

METALS

LEAD

Several metals produce significant toxic effects in the body, lead being perhaps the best known. Lead is commonly encountered in many jobs in industry. It carries a very high risk to the developing fetus, resulting in mental retardation among other effects. It is well absorbed from the stomach, so any dust that is inhaled and swallowed, or accidentally introduced into the mouth through smoking or eating, produces a risk. As a consequence, any woman who might become pregnant should have no exposure to lead. This often poses a dilemma for both management and the worker. It places an unfair burden on women, but perhaps the burden to the developing fetus is even greater.

Some areas of employment where lead exposure is encountered are:

Auto manufacture
Battery makers: lead-acid storage batteries
Battery reclamation
Brass and bronze foundries
Ceramic and pottery makers, dinnerware
Chemical manufacturer, various
Glass workers
Insecticide manufacture
Lead burners (soldering & welding with lead)
Lead shields for x-ray and other radiation devices
Lubricant manufacture
Match manufacturer

Paint and enamel manufacture
Petroleum refining
Painters
Plastic pigments (manufacture and use in formulating plastics)
Plumbers
Solderers

The exposures to lead on the job are many and varied. Some of the sources of lead poisoning are obvious as in the manufacture of lead acid batteries and in the processing and recycling of depleted batteries. In other jobs the exposure is not so obvious. As of May 1, 1992 laboratories in 18 states were required by law to report elevated blood levels in adults to the respective state health department.[18] OSHA has had standards limiting and controlling lead exposure in the workplace since 1978. Many cases of serious exposure to lead have occurred since that time, however.

In 1990 a laboratory in New Jersey reported elevated blood lead levels in 13 individuals to the state health department. All of the individuals worked in a small foundry that produced brass and bronze valves. The blood lead level was above 60 μg/dL in six of the workers, and was 277 μg/dL in one. The upper limit of normal has been set at 25 μg/dL, and levels above that should prompt removal from exposure. As is frequently found, these cases were associated with an accumulation of lead dust in the workplace.

Recycling of lead acid batteries generates considerable quantities of lead oxide and lead sulfate dust from the plates. Industrial batteries require torches to cut open the outer steel cases, which generates lead fumes. Workers in these operations are frequently found to have blood lead levels well above safe limits. Battery reclamation operations had been permitted more generous standards than other lead industries, but a court ruling effective in July 1993 eliminated this variance. Even so, the OSHA regulations still permitted blood lead levels that are harmful to health. Chronic exposure to the levels commonly seen in this industry can be expected to produce significant damage to the brain and kidney. It will not be easy to eliminate the lead dust hazard in these operations.

Another occupation with heavy lead exposure is lead burning. This occupation includes all those who solder or weld with lead. An example is a construction site where a crew of 17 lead burners was lining the interior of two large steel tanks with lead sheets. This operation required coating the interior of the tanks with solder first, then sealing lead sheets to the solder. The lead level in the air in the tanks during these operations was obviously high. Protection depended upon respirators, but for these to be effective they must be well fit and properly maintained. From the blood levels obtained it was obvious that the protection was less than adequate in some of the workers. In this industry, as with all occupations that involve heavy lead dust levels, stringent precautions must be taken to avoid carrying dust home on shoes and clothing, and thus exposing other members of the family.

A more obscure lead exposure occurs in the plastics industry. Lead chromate is widely used as a coloring pigment in plastic products. The pigments are mixed with plastic, then heated and formed into pellets. These pellets are then sold to manufacturers of plastic products to use in coloring the various products. Workers who are exposed include those who mix and formulate in both the pigment and plastic manufacturing operations, as well as workers who are involved in heating, molding and cutting of the plastic parts. These frequently are jobs where lead exposure would not be suspected.

CADMIUM

Another metal that matches lead in toxicity if not in diversity of exposure is cadmium. Cadmium is distinctive in that it has been used industrially only since about 1935. In that short period it has achieved very extensive use in diverse industries. Perhaps the most important use is in electroplating of metals and screws to protect against corrosion. It is also used in pigments for paints and the plastic industry. Cadmium sulfide provides yellow pigments while cadmium selenide yields red pigments. Cadmium red (cadmium sulfoselenide) caused many cases of sore throat when it was used in lipstick. Its use was banned in 1938. Cadmium is also used in the manufacture of nickel-cadmium batteries. Cadmium is obtained as a by-product of lead and zinc mining and smelting, and is thus encountered in these operations.

The serious toxic effects of cadmium became painfully obvious after the epidemic of "Itai-Itai-byo," ouch-ouch disease, in

Japan during and after World War II. With the increased industrial activity the smelting plants produced heavy pollution of copper, zinc and cadmium in the streams and rivers. This resulted in contamination of the rice crops, which take up cadmium more readily than lead and the other metals. Shellfish such as mussels, scallops and oysters also accumulate cadmium in significant concentrations from the water. Large numbers of postmenopausal women emerged with excruciating back pain. The cause was unknown for a long time, until autopsies demonstrated high concentrations of lead, copper and cadmium in all of the internal organs. The cadmium produced a pronounced decline in the internal architecture and integrity of the bones, accounting for the pain in the vertebra (spine).

Cadmium is extremely toxic when inhaled or ingested. Working in an atmosphere where dust containing any of the compounds such as pigments is present, or where fume from welding or silver soldering is present, is particularly hazardous. When inhaled cadmium causes a bronchitis that progresses to fibrosis resulting in profound emphysema. In workers who smoke cigarettes the courts will very likely blame the cigarettes and not the occupational exposure for the disabling emphysema.

When cadmium is ingested it is deposited in all of the internal organs, but serious damage results in the kidneys. The renal tubules are severely damaged with many profound metabolic consequences in the body, one of which is the osteoporosis and osteomalacia demonstrated in Itai-Itai. This damage to the kidneys is reflected by the presence in the urine of a protein that is not normally found there, beta–2–microglobulin. This provides a diagnostic test for exposure to cadmium. There is also evidence that cadmium contributes to the development of prostate cancer.

Some of the occupational exposures to cadmium are listed in the table that follows. A serious risk would be encountered in welding, soldering, blending, grinding, smelting, recycling or many other manufacturing operation in these areas.

OCCUPATIONAL CADMIUM EXPOSURES

Alloys	Electroplating and galvanizing (dipping)
Aluminum solder	Jewelry
Batteries (lead-acid & nickel-cadmium)	Lithographers
Bearings (ball and roller)	Paints; manufacture and spraying
Brazing and silver soldering	Pesticides
Cables	Plastics; pigments, manufacture & blending
Ceramics	Printers; inks, pigments
Copper alloys	Torch cutting cadmium plated and galvanized metals
Dental amalgams	Welding cadmium plated and galvanized metals
Electric wires and cables	Zinc and lead; mining, smelting and refining

BERYLLIUM

Beryllium also produces some very dramatic and profound toxic abnormalities in the body. It also is an invaluable and irreplaceable industrial metal, but extensive controls and precautions have sharply reduced the incidence of deaths and disease it causes.

Poisoning from exposure to beryllium dust was noted and reported in Europe in 1936, but it attracted little attention. A great increase in the number of workers exposed, and the number of reactions to the metal occurred during World War II. In 1946 a diffuse fibrosis in the lungs of workers in the fluorescent light bulb industry was reported. Sometime after this the public was advised to break these bulbs only under water, and to avoid inhaling the dust from inside the tubes.

In 1949 the industry agreed to discontinue the use of beryllium phosphors in fluorescent tubes. Strict engineering controls and personal hygiene procedures were instituted to eliminate exposure on the job, and to avoid carrying the dust home on clothing. These measures, adopted in all industries where beryllium is involved, have virtually eliminated occupational berylliosis. Only sporadic cases have been seen since.

In 1952 the Beryllium Case Registry was established at the Massachusetts Institute of Technology for the purpose of registering cases, collecting data on and study the course of the disease. A total of 887 cases were listed in the registry between 1952 and 1977. The registry was moved to the National Institute for Occupational Safety and Health in Cincinnati in 1978, where it remains today. From 1978 to 1983 only 10 additional cases were registered. No cases resulting from air pollution or from dust on clothing taken home have been reported since 1949. No acute case has been reported in the United States since 1968.[19,20]

Air pollution from a plant in Lorain, Ohio that produced beryllium resulted in beryllium lung disease in 13 residents who lived within three-quarters of mile of the plant. Sixteen cases similarly occurred in people who lived in the vicinity of a plant in Reading, Pennsylvania, but some of these had exposure to clothing from workers in the plant. One case occurred in a woman who lived across the street from a fluorescent lamp plant.

Inhaled into the lungs, beryllium produces an acute inflammation followed by a pronounced fibrosis. Little is understood about the reaction, and it is felt to be a sensitization, immune reaction. Death is common in the acute cases. There is a latent period of 10 to 15 years before the development of the disease in chronic cases. When beryllium is deposited in a cut in the skin a similar granulomatous lesion or an ulcer appears. The wound may not heal. About 60 percent of the reported cases resulted from exposure to the phosphors. Some feel that the chief risk is exposure to beryllium oxide, and that cold working alloys that contain less than 2.5 % beryllium involve little risk. This issue remains unresolved.

Beryllium has been used extensively in industry and that use has expanded greatly during the past fifty years. The success in virtually eliminating additional cases is all the more remarkable in view of the increase in potential exposure. Beryllium is irreplaceable in producing copper and brass alloys with elastic properties for switches and contact points. Beryllium-copper alloys are the standard materials used in dies and molds for the multitude of plastic parts and ornaments in the automobile industry. It is widely used in the spacecraft industry, and is used in windows on X-ray units. Its use in foundries has resulted in some of the acute cases of poisoning seen in the past. Four cases of berylliosis were seen in 1983 in a plant in Connecticut where copper-beryllium scraps were being smelted for recycling.

MERCURY

Individuals who are working in any setting where any form of mercury is present face a significant health risk unless appropriate precautions are taken. This has been dramatically and tragically demonstrated on many occasions, some of which are described in Chapters V, VIII, and XIII. In any facility where mercury or any of its salts are manufactured, stored or applied to seed grain, everyone is at serious risk. Inhalation of dust in such facilities has resulted in death, including two female stenographers who worked in a warehouse where diethylmercury was stored. They had no suspicion of any danger.

Even in settings where liquid metallic mercury is present, a serious threat exists. Mercury has a low vapor pressure and toxic levels in the room atmosphere accumulate from an open container. These fumes are not visible, but when illuminated by an ultraviolet lamp they can be seen, giving the appearance of steam arising from a boiling pot. Even more insidious is when mercury is spilled, particularly onto a concrete floor or into cracks and crevices where it cannot be cleaned up. It seeps into concrete floors from which it then escapes into the ambient air. These floors should be covered by tile or sealed by an impervious material to prevent seepage of mercury into the concrete. When mercury is spilled, it should be cleaned up carefully and disposed of in a safe manner.

Lewis Carroll characterized the serious consequences of exposure to mercury compounds in 1865 in *Alice's Adventures in Wonderland*. The Mad Hatter portrayed the behavioral changes and the tremors that reflect the damage to the nervous system that was characteristic of workers in the felt hat industry of the day. The tremors were assigned the name the "Danbury Shakes," in honor of Danbury, Connecticut. Mercuric nitrate is still used in the felt hat industry today for the same purpose, but with some improvement in controls.

These toxic effects of mercury have been recognized since medieval times. Ellenbog described the effects of lead and mercury fumes in a pamphlet in 1473. Paracelsus and Agricola followed with the publication of their observations in the sixteenth century. Ramazzini published his comprehensive work, *De Morbis Artificum Diatriba,* in 1700 A.D. The observation of the dire consequences of this occupation lead to the practice of assigning only slaves and convicts to such labor.

Although much of the mercury used industrially in the United States today is imported, it is still mined in Alaska, California, Idaho and Nevada. The red colored ore is cinnabar, mercuric sulfide, which has been used throughout history as a pigment. It has been found in the ruins of a number of ancient civilizations, including those of Egypt and Babylon. It was widely used by the Romans for writing books and for decorating statues, tombs and walls. It was also used to coat copper objects with gold.

When the expanded Roman Empire encompassed Spain the Romans acquired the mercury mines at Almadén, which remains the largest single producer of mercury today. Pliny the Elder wrote about this mine and the various uses of mercury during that period. He also described some of the adverse effect the miners suffered from that exposure. Ramazzini (see above) described the disability and suffering that afflicted those who worked in the mines and those who worked with the metal.

Mercury in cinnabar is refined by distillation, heating the crushed ore to a temperature in excess of 1,000° F. The boiling point of mercury is 675° F. and it remains liquid to about minus 102° F. The distillation process vaporizes the mercury, which is then collected and cooled to the liquid state. The concentration of mercury vapors in the work environment during this process is much higher than would be seen with the mercury at room temperature, which is risk enough in itself. The only safe process for distillation of mercury ore is a closed system that permits no mercury vapors to escape to the room air. Even the cooled mercury in open vats presents a significant exposure.

Mercury compounds have long enjoyed wide use in medicine in spite of the serious neurological disorders that were described by Lewis Carroll in 1865. Their use for skin disorders was recorded as far back as the twelfth century, and their popularity continued to modern times. Mercury is one of the chief ingredients in dental amalgam, and many dentists suffered mercury poisoning during the long era when the amalgam was mixed in the palm of the hand. Mixing machines with capsules to hold the mixture have eliminated this risk, and dispensers for the mercury lessened the risk of spills onto the floor.

In spite of the fact that the dire consequences of exposure to mercury were well known in the 40s, it continued to be used as a medicine. Calomel, mercurous chloride (not to be confused with mercuric chloride), was a favorite diuretic and cathartic until about 1940. Its use in medicine is recorded as long ago as 1595. Calomel was readily available and was used by many parents as a general remedy for many mild illnesses, including intestinal worms. It is still used in some skin creams for some mysterious reason. Mercurochrome® (merbromin) was introduced as a skin disinfectant in 1919. Merthiolate® (thimerosal) was introduced later for the same application. Neither has any application as an antiseptic today. Mercuhydrin®, a bivalent organic mercury compound, was the only potent diuretic available for some forty years, but safer and more effective agents have supplanted it now.

In the past mercury compounds were commonly used in teething lotions for infants. This application resulted in a condition known as acrodynia or pink disease. This is characterized by irritability, a rash and swelling with a pink discoloration of the fingers and toes. These symptoms can be mistakenly diagnosed as Kawasaki's disease, a much more common affliction. As with other cases of mercury poisoning, loss of teeth may also occur in older children. Some individuals will promote and sell anything to the unsuspecting public, regardless of the disastrous toxic effects that it may produce, until prevented by law. Then we trade one master for another, for the resultant bureaucracy is no less of a tyrant, and produces at least as many problems as it was charged to solve.

Mercuric chloride (bichloride of mercury, corrosive sublimate) was used extensively to sterilize instruments and it was very effective, and very deadly. Accidental ingestion of this substance results in severe abdominal cramps and bloody diarrhea, the result of corrosive ulceration or the gastrointestinal tract. This usually results in shock and death. If the victim survives for 24 hours kidney failure results from severe damage to the filtering tubules.

Phenylmercuric salts were used formally as a rinse in laundries and especially for diapers, where they were very effective bactericides. They also produced acrodynia as described for teething lotions above. Thimerosal, also a mercurial, is still used as a preservative in some medicines and cosmetics, although it is a common cause of sensitization and reaction (see Contact Lenses in Chapter XV). Ammoniated mercury ointment is still available and it is used by some for acne and other skin problems. It also causes sensitivity reactions and more serious toxicity when it is absorbed through skin lesions. Better medication is available.

Mercury and its compounds are very widely used in industry. Some examples of applications where it is encountered follow:

Aluminum alloys, some
Barometers
Batteries, dry cells
Catalysts in some chemical processes
Dentistry
Dyes
Electronics
Fireworks, pyrotechnics
Fluorescent lamps (activated by mercury vapor)
Fungicides for seed grains
Gold mining
Herbicides
Mercury vapor lamps
Paints and pigments
Percussion caps for explosives
Plastics manufacture
Silent light switches
Tattooing
Thermometers
Thermostats
Ultraviolet lamps
Wood preservatives

The toxic consequences of exposure to mercury in settings other than the workplace are discussed in Chapters V, VIII and XIII.

ARSENIC

Arsenic occurs abundantly in the earth's surface, ranking twentieth in frequency among the elements. It is therefore found in most of our water supplies in small quantities. Environmental contamination comes from industrial emissions from smelters, fossil-fuel-burning power plants (from coal) and from geothermal power plants. Serious contamination of the soil in the communities surrounding Anaconda, Montana resulted from fallout from the copper smelting plant there (see Chapter XIII). All of these sources contribute to air, soil and water levels.

Pesticides contribute significantly to the level in the soil, and result in a reduction in plant growth of as much as 50 percent when a certain level is reached. Tobacco contains significant quantities of arsenic as it does cadmium, both taken up from fertilizer. Waste disposal sites contribute further to contamination that can reach the underground aquifers where conditions permit.

Occupational exposures occur mainly in smelting, refining and production activities involving both copper and lead, orchard spraying and sheep dipping. The route of exposure in occupations is most frequently the respiratory system. This results in a higher incidence of lung cancer in those exposed. The increased incidence of deaths from lung cancer has been tabulated in workers in pesticide manufacture as well as those exposed to copper smelting, where arsenic is present. Exposed workers who smoke cigarettes experience lung cancer at a rate five times that of cohort workers who do not smoke.

The production of skin cancer by arsenic exposure has been well documented over the past 20 years. Arsenic has a predilection for skin, hair and nails, and can be identified in these tissues after exposure. Thickening of the skin of the palms of the hands and the soles of the feet is common as is darkening of the skin from hyperpigmentation.

The near universal replacement of redwood and wood preservatives with treated lumber, most frequently chromated copper arsenate (CCA), has added a widespread occupational exposure to arsenic. Workers in the treatment plants, in the lumberyards and carpenters building the decks, porches and stairs that are universally made from this material all have significant occupational skin exposure. Sawing presents an added risk from inhalation and ingestion of arsenic in sawdust. Lumber treated with CCA remains quite wet for some time, certainly during the period that it is in the lumberyard and during construction.

The trivalent forms of arsenic represent the toxic compounds, with little toxicity noted with the pentavalent substances. Arsenicals were popular as a medicinal in the 1800s, and some writers suggest that Napoleon was being treated with them at the time of his death.

Fowler's solution, potassium arsenite, was one such commonly used remedy. Sir Jonathan Hutchinson, in 1913, reported skin cancer resulting from long term use of this substance in England. Agricola reported the toxic effects suffered by miners and smelters of an arsenic ore in *De Re Metallica*, published in 1556.

CHROMIUM

Chromium is an essential industrial metal with very diverse applications. The metal itself is important for its role in stainless steel and in plating for its ornamental benefits and corrosion protection. Sodium dichromate is used in the production of pigments for paints and plastics, in the production of chromium salts that are used for tanning leather, and in wood preservatives. It is also used as an anticorrosive in boilers and in oil drilling mud.

Cancer of the nasal passages and sinuses and the lungs in workers in smelting and refining operations, as well as in chrome pigment production has been reported for a long period. Cancer of the lung was reported in Germany in 1936, resulting from exposure to chromium dust. The major toxic effect aside from cancer is to the kidney, where it produces acute tubular necrosis. Ulceration of the nasal septum is also seen in these workers. Allergic skin reactions are common in occupational exposures to chromium. The hexavalent compounds produce the toxicity, rather than the trivalent forms found in natural deposits.

NICKEL

Nickel is the other essential metal in stainless steel, and it is also used to plate other metals for corrosion protection. It is, of course, a component in nickel-cadmium batteries. Nickel also produces cancers of the respiratory tract (the nasal passages and the lungs). Richard Doll reported on these cancers among workers in nickel refining in 1977. Several subsequent studies have confirmed these findings.

The most common method of refining nickel produces nickel carbonyl, the substance that was suspected to be responsible for the epidemic of Legionnaires disease in Philadelphia. This compound is extremely toxic; exposure results in severe, acute symptoms, with death not infrequently. Headache, nausea, vomiting, cough, fever, and cyanosis follow exposure. The more severe cases progress to pneumonia, respiratory failure and death. Autopsy reveals the greatest concentration of nickel carbonyl to be in the lungs, with smaller quantities in the kidney, liver and brain.

Nickel dermatitis is one of the most common forms of allergic contact dermatitis, seen frequently from contact with jewelry. Nickel is used not only in stainless steel (watch backs) but also in white gold and other jewelry alloys. White brass contains 25 percent nickel. It has been suggested that the ingestion of foods that contain quantities of nickel increase the risk of developing skin sensitivity to it.

THALLIUM

Thallium and its compounds are commonly encountered in industry. It is produced as a by-product in the refining of lead, iron, zinc and cadmium. It is used as a catalyst in many organic chemical reactions, including the production of certain dyes and pigments. It is used in bromoiodide crystals in the manufacture of lenses, plates and prisms in infrared optical instruments, in photo-electric cells, alloyed with mercury in low temperature thermometers, in switches, optical lenses, semiconductors and fireworks. It is also used in making artificial diamonds. Alloyed with silver it makes a stainless alloy. Alloyed with arsenic and sulfur it produces a low melting point glass.

Thallium was formerly used in the manufacture of rodenticides but this use was banned in the United States in 1955 (see Chapter XIV). This metallic element is extremely toxic and is absorbed through the intact skin. The powder is toxic when it is inhaled. Eating, smoking and chewing gum must be prohibited in any occupational setting where thallium is found.

Thallium poisoning presents a diagnostic challenge because the symptoms resemble those seen in advanced diabetes or chronic alcohol abuse. It is cumulative in the body, making chronic exposure hazardous. Serious damage to the peripheral nerves produces a burning pain in the extremities. A prominent loss of hair is a clear clue to the diagnosis. The mental confusion that is commonly associated with the nerve damage may result in a failure to obtain a history of hair loss. The confusion may also be misdiagnosed as a mental disorder. The damage to the nervous system can be permanent and irreversible. Thallium also causes damage to the liver and kidney. Inflammation of the optic nerve has led to blindness. Thallium is not included in the customary screening tests for poisoning and must be specifically requested. First it must be considered.

No successful treatment has been approved for thallium poisoning, although Prussian blue is effective.

ALUMINUM

Aluminum has not been associated with toxicity in the workplace, and most occupational health authorities have assigned little risk to workers in this field. During World War II, however, German workers exposed to aluminum powder in the manufacture of explosives, incendiary powder and paints did develop pneumoconiosis. Workers in England and the other countries participating in the war, involved in the identical occupations, did not suffer this disability. It has been suggested that the heavy dust exposures in Germany, with inadequate ventilation, accounted for the difference. It is also possible that the dust contained other fibrotic material, such as silica.

In Canada in 1947 workers exposed to bauxite fumes (Al_2O_3 – $3H_2O$) in the process of making corundum, an artificial abrasive, developed a pneumoconiosis. This condition was labeled Shaver's disease after one of the two men who first made the observation. However, the material that the men were exposed to contained up to 7 percent of silica, and some have suggested that this element was responsible for the pulmonary fibrosis. There is precedent for this hypothesis, for a similar situation existed among carbon workers who similarly developed pneumoconiosis. This has occurred in other industries as well. At any rate the issue is still contested.

In studies in other operations where exposure to aluminum dust exist, such as grinding aircraft propellers, no lung pathology has been found. Some authorities suggest that the risk depends upon the type of flake produced. In producing pyro powder for fireworks the flakes are of a different and characteristic shape. Workers in this industry have developed pulmonary fibrosis. The moral of the saga is that the lungs should be protected from any form of dust, to the greatest degree possible.

TIN

Inorganic tin (metallic tin, some tin salts) is relatively non-toxic, partially because of very limited absorption, even after ingestion. It has long been used to plate food cans and containers where the lack of toxicity has been apparent. Elemental tin is also used as a component in solders, bronze and brass. Long term inhalation of tin dust causes a benign pneumoconiosis that presents a characteristic appearance on x-ray.

Organic tin compounds, on the other hand, are more readily absorbed and distributed within the body. Their toxicity has been well demonstrated, particularly that of triethyltin and tributyltin. Bis{tributyltin} oxide is an organic tin compound sold in a 25 percent solution to be added to paint as a mildewcide. It was previously incorporated into marine paints to inhibit the growth of marine life on boats. This use has been discontinued due to its potent toxic effects and the dispersion of the compound into the marine environment. Poisoning resulted not only from the manufacture of the paint but during its application.

Bis{tributyltin} oxide and some other organic tin preparations, notable triethyltin, are very toxic when ingested, producing serious central nervous system (brain) symptoms. They are also readily absorbed through the intact skin with the same risk of brain damage. Skin contact should always be avoided. Pronounced irritation can occur, even if washed immediately. Industrial exposure has produced visual disturbances and headaches. Abnormal electroencephalograms have demonstrated the toxicity to the central nervous system.

SELENIUM

Selenium is encountered in the workplace less frequently than the metals discussed above, but presents no less of a toxic hazard. It is used in some metallurgical applications, in the glass and ceramic industries, and in the cosmetic industry in anti-dandruff shampoos. It is used in a specialty pesticide to control aphids in growing carnations. Its most common use is in electronics where its photovoltaic properties make it valuable for use in photoelectric cells and in rectifiers.

The body permits only a very narrow range of selenium before toxicity develops. Serious toxicity has occurred in individuals who took dietary supplements of selenium (see Chapter XV). Many of its preparations are well absorbed through the skin, and some, such as selenium oxychloride, cause severe blistering as well. Chronic exposure to selenium and its compounds results in damage to the liver, the spleen, and the nervous system. Loss of hair and nails and an anemia also are part of the picture. Irritation of the nasal membranes and the lids of the eyes, manifested by redness of the lids, results when absorption causes general toxicity. The toxicity of selenium is also discussed in Chapter XIII.

METAL FUME FEVER

Exposure to metal welding fumes can result in "metal fume fever." This is an influenza-like illness with chills, fever, rapid pulse (100-120), nausea, muscle aches, dry throat, cough, weakness and lassitude. Fine crepitant rales can be heard in the lower lung fields. Some have suggested that it is an immunologic disorder, but this has not been proven. Welding of galvanized steel with the production of zinc oxide fume has been the most common cause, but exposure to welding fume from copper and other metals can also initiate the process. Welding of stainless steel has been demonstrated to produce both acute and chronic lung damage because of the nickel and chromium content.[21] Inhalation of zinc chloride fume is uncommon in industry except during accidents, but it leads to death as a result of pulmonary edema and respiratory collapse.

PHOTOCOPIERS

The contribution of photocopiers to contaminants in the air in the workplace has come under scrutiny in recent years because of respiratory complaints from workers in proximity to them. The ozone produced by these machines has been shown to be responsible for some of these symptoms. The toners used in copy machines have been of greater concern because some of the components used were shown to be mutagenic. Safer non-mutagenic substitutes are now in place, and this is reflected in current (1999) Material Safety Data Sheets. Several cases of serious lung fibrosis have been reported, however, as a result of inhalation of silicon and copper in the toner dust.[22] Siderosilicosis from inhalation of silicon and iron in the toner dust has also been reported.[23] This serious disease has been seen chiefly in miners, welders and foundry workers in the past. Clearly people who operate photocopiers, and those who work in proximity, are at risk of pulmonary fibrosis. This risk can be reduced, but not eliminated completely, by adequate venting of the machine. Redesign of photocopiers to accomplish this is urgently needed.

OCCUPATIONAL ALLERGIES

Allergies are a very common and disabling problem in the workplace. They involve chiefly the skin and the lungs. Individuals who have a past history of allergies are more predictable victims, but the majority of reactions occur in people with no past problem with the offending agent. Once sensitization has developed it is unlikely that the individual will be able to continue in that job unless successful desensitization can be accomplished. Some of the allergies commonly encountered in the workplace are listed below.

OCCUPATIONAL ALLERGIES

CLASS OF AGENTS	INDIVIDUAL AGENTS, ACTION
Industrial Chemicals	Isocyanates (TDI, HDI, MDI), phthalic anhydride and trimellitic anhydride sensitize in plastics, paint & varnish and electronics.
Vegetable Gums	Acacia, tragacanth, guar and karaya are used in printing, pharmaceuticals, carpet mfg and adhesives industry.
Latex	Health care workers become sensitized to latex proteins.
Hospital and Lab Antigens	Ethylene oxide, formaldehyde, ispaghula, drugs, & animal proteins.
Molds and Thermoactino-mycetes	Farmer's lung and ventilation pneumonitis.
Antigens in Food Industry	Papain & other enzymes, egg proteins, soybean flour, coffee bean dust, mold proteins.

Occupational asthma is a term applied to a common reaction to a class of chemicals that are widely used in paints, varnishes and the plastics industry. The classic culprit is toluene diisocyanate, TDI. It has been replaced by MDI, diphenylmethane diisocyanate, which itself causes asthmatic reactions, but at a lesser incidence.

Several other isocyanates are in common use in industry and they share the toxicity of MDI for the most part.

Asthmatics who react to pollens, molds, dust and animal dander will of course be troubled by these agents whether on the job or at home. More troublesome is the multitude of previously healthy individuals who develop a hypersensitivity pneumonitis. This is an allergic reaction in the tissues of the lung to inhaled organic dust from a variety of sources. The first recorded cases were due to grain dusts, described by Ramazzini in 1713, and they remain a common offending agent today.

Perhaps the best known example of hypersensitivity pneumonitis is farmer's lung, caused by inhaling dust from hay that contains spores of actinomycetes mold. Continued exposure with chronic hypersensitivity pneumonitis over a long period of time can result in scarring and reduced pulmonary function. A large number of agents that are responsible for this reaction are encountered in a wide diversity of occupations. Some that have been tabulated are listed at the end of this chapter.

Occupational skin reactions are even more numerous than the lung disorders, and are caused by just as wide a diversity of substances. Aside from accidents and injuries, skin problems account for about one-half of all occupational illness. These are by no means all allergic in nature. Solvents such as acetone, toluene, trichloroethane and alcohol serve to degrease the skin as well as the products that they are used on for this purpose. This will result in irritation and cracking. Soaps and detergents also serve to remove the protective lipids of the skin and additionally may cause irritation from chemical components. In general alkaline substances such as ammonium hydroxide and Portland cement are more irritating to the skin than are acidic compounds.

The most troublesome skin reactions result from sensitization, which results in an inflammatory response whenever the skin comes in contact with that substance. With some substances such as poison ivy or oak a chemical bond with the skin proteins accompanies the reaction. With other substances such as nickel, cobalt and chromium salts the reason for the sensitivity is unknown. Gold does not cause a skin reaction, but its salts used in arthritis medication frequently do.

Regardless of the type of skin reaction or the cause for it, prevention requires protection of the skin from contact with the offending agent. In some operations this may be accomplished by designing systems that do not require that the hands be immersed in the work. Where this is not possible, protective gloves may be necessary. Virtually no glove provides absolute protection, however, as permeability tests have shown. The common materials of vinyl and latex provide very limited protection. In addition, many people develop an immunologic response to the protein in latex that is very serious in some.

The degree of protection provided by any glove material is influenced by both the thickness of the material and the length of time in contact with the chemical.

Virtually any chemical or solvent can serve as an irritant and produce redness, cracking or other reaction of the skin. Some of the common sensitizers encountered are listed below.

Rubber accelerators, antioxidants	Thimerosal
Epoxy resins, hardeners	Benzocaine
Phenolic resins	Neomycin
Formaldehyde resins	Parabens
Acrylic resins	Ethylenediamine
Dyes	Hydroquinone
Nickel	Fragrances (numerous)
Chromates	Cashew oil
Mercury salts	Poison ivy, oak, sumac
Beryllium salts	Citrus oil

AIR QUALITY

Since about 1979 there have been an increasing number of incidents of complaints of respiratory symptoms such as burning throat, cough, nasal congestion, and burning of the eyes in the workplace. These incidents have invariably occurred in offices, where such complaints have not been common in the past. Numerous investigations have been undertaken to identify the culprit in these mini-epidemics. In most cases, the usual and expected agents have been measured, frequently without success. Particulates (dust), carbon monoxide and formaldehyde have been implicated in some cases. Formaldehyde finds its way into the home and office through insulation, urea foam padding in furniture and in adhesives in plywood and particleboard. It is an irritant to the eyes and respiratory system and is suspected of causing cancer.

Some of the highest levels of formaldehyde have been found in mobile homes. The levels in these units have exceeded by many fold the level recommended by the American Conference of Governmental Hygienist of one part per million. In new buildings the elution of various gases from the building materials and furnishings has been identified as the source of many complaints.

Some of the gases that have been identified in new buildings are 1,1,1-trichloroethane, toluene, styrene, xylene and benzene. Benzene has been associated with the development of leukemia, and styrene causes concern because of its structural relationship to vinyl chloride, a known carcinogen. These substances are less readily identified and measured than particulates and carbon monoxide. Some of the complaints seem to abate after about six weeks, with virtual disappearance of problems after four to six months. Delay of occupancy in new buildings, with adequate ventilation to air the building out, would appear to be a prudent measure to take to avoid these problems.

In many outbreaks, absence of the usual culprits prompted a search for other irritants. In cases where the complaints included fever, chills, fatigue, chest tightness, cough and wheezing, hypersensitivity pneumonitis was suspected. Many of these outbreaks were traced to the presence of actinomycete or other fungi in the circulated air. It was discovered that these organisms were growing in the moisture or water pools in the air conditioning units or in humidifiers. It was thus that the term "humidifier fever" was coined. Other organisms such as amoeba and bacteria have also been isolated as causes of this syndrome. Persistence of these symptoms over a period of time can produce pulmonary fibrosis with permanent lung disability.

The presence of the *Legionella* bacteria in air conditioners and humidifiers was first identified after the death of American Legion members attending a convention at a hotel in Philadelphia. Several outbreaks of *Legionella* pneumonia have occurred subsequently, including one in a hotel at the Detroit airport in June 1985 that resulted in three deaths.

In sixteen large studies, 281 cases of humidifier fever were traced to *Actinomycetes*, *Bacillus subtilis*, *Flavobacterium* or

Cephalosporium. These were found in the humidifier systems, in the ventilation ducts and in air filters. In these cases anywhere from a few to seventy percent of the occupants of a given facility were affected. Through investigation of such outbreaks, it has been established that whenever thirty percent or more of the workers in a facility complain of symptoms that clear up within eight hours after leaving the job (particularly noticeable on weekends), the problem lies with the work environment.

The marked increase in the frequency of complaints of the "sick office syndrome" has been traced to energy saving measure of the past decade. These have resulted in much tighter buildings and in a marked reduction in the circulation of outside air. It has become customary for ninety percent of the indoor air to be recirculated, with only ten percent of fresh air being introduced from outdoors. The result has been the recirculation of the air and all of its accumulated contaminants.

These recirculated contaminants include carbon monoxide, carbon dioxide, dust, bacteria, ozone and other vapors from the resin in the toner in photocopiers, formaldehyde and other gases from building materials, furniture and carpeting, cigarette smoke and detergent residues (sodium lauryl sulfate) from improper carpet cleaning techniques. In submarines such unhealthy accumulations are taken care of by sophisticated filters and air scrubbers. No such precautions are taken in office buildings.

A source of irritant totally overlooked until recently is cigarette smoking. In the past it has not been the practice to measure hydrocarbon levels that result from smoking. When this finally was done, some surprises were in store. In one study the hydrocarbon level of the outside air was measured at 210 micrograms per cubic meter, while the level indoors in the work area, where only 15 percent of outside air was being introduced, was measured at 1627 micrograms. When the system was reset to circulate 100 percent outside air through the work area, the hydrocarbon level fell to 364 micrograms.

This one case graphically demonstrates the logical solution to most cases of "sick office syndrome," simply providing adequate ventilation. It has been determined that four times as much outside air must be introduced into ventilation systems in offices where smoking takes place as has been the custom. It is recommended that at least twenty cubic feet of outside air per occupant be introduced to accommodate for smoking, rather than the customary five cubic feet that is required by most building codes. In 1991 ANSI (American National Standards Institute) recommended that the five cubic feet requirement be tripled to fifteen cubic feet. This solution has been resisted because of the increased cost of heating and cooling such outside air brought in. The savings in wages and salaries due to lost work time would go far toward compensating for such increased costs.

In addition to increasing the quantity of outside air introduced to ventilation and heating systems, proper air balance is also essential to bring this benefit to all areas in the work place. This requires a professional assessment and adjustment of heating and cooling ducts and distribution systems. The current trend toward eliminating smoking in the workplace altogether will do much to mitigate the problem of contamination of the air. The compromise solution of merely designating certain areas as smoking areas does nothing to solve the problem unless a sufficient exhaust is provided to remove the hydrocarbons and other noxious and toxic contaminants from the smoking area to the outside.

Complaints of skin rashes and itching in the workplace have been traced to fiberglass or mineral wool fibers from faulty ventilation systems. The simple solution is to install efficient filters in the ventilation system or outlet ducts, and to keep them maintained properly. Fibers imbedded in contact lenses are a tip off to this problem. Fibers are readily detected in particulate sampling, a simple procedure for any competent industrial hygienist. A further clue to the cause of this problem is the clearing of symptoms after showering, and relief from the complaints after a period away from work, as over a weekend or during a vacation.

ASBESTOS

One of the most serious and most frequently encountered risks in the workplace is that of the mineral fiber, asbestos. Asbestos is the term applied to a group of minerals composed of silicates of iron and magnesium. They are one of the most versatile and useful elements in the industrialized world because of their virtual indestructibility. The fibers possess excellent insulating properties and are impervious to both heat and acid. They are superb products for brakes, clutches and other friction devices. The other, man made, mineral fibers provide poor substitutes in the manufacture of these latter products.

The seriousness of exposure to asbestos lies in the propensity that it has to bring about a severe and disabling fibrosis of the lung. In this characteristic it is similar to silica sand. The inhalation of asbestos fibers also carries a significant risk for the development of cancer. One of the cancers that develop as a result of inhaling asbestos fibers is mesothelioma, a cancer of the lining of the lungs (the pleura). This has been a rare cancer in the past, but it has been increasing in frequency in recent years, reflecting not only the great expansion in the use of asbestos, but the latency period as well.

Mesothelioma does not develop until thirty to thirty-five years after the exposure to asbestos. It does not require prolonged exposure for this cancer to develop; a single exposure may result in cancer thirty years later. This is one of the very few cancers where cigarette smoking plays no role. The incidence is the same regardless of the smoking history. This is a very insidious cancer and there is no cure or treatment. Very few people survive for two years after it is diagnosed and one-half of them are dead in six months. Crocidolite, which is the type of asbestos mined in South Africa (Cape Blue), carries the greatest risk for mesothelioma. Amosite, also from South Africa, which has been used in insulation in the United States, also carries a significant risk, however. Both are members of the amphibole family of asbestosis, which is the most resistant to heat and acid.[24,25]

Many of the studies and much of our knowledge of these risks has come from surveys of insulation workers by Selikoff and his coworkers.[26,27] Chrysotile (white asbestos, member of the serpentine family), which has coiled fibers rather than straight, needlelike fibers, is felt to carry a much lesser risk for the development of mesothelioma. It is the type most widely used, and it is the type of asbestos fibers that was discovered in the public water supply of San Francisco and the Bay area in 1978. It has been mined predominantly in Quebec, Canada.

The water supply for the San Francisco Bay area comes from reservoirs in the nearby hills where the rocks contain deposits of chrysotile asbestos. This discovery caused great concern and consternation, but it is generally felt that this presents no significant risk to the residents of the area. This discovery was made at a time when it was discovered that public water supplies throughout the United States contained asbestos fibers that were being leached out of the concrete pipes that carried the water. Asbestos has long been used in concrete to strengthen it, and it has been assumed that the fibers were firmly imbedded in the concrete. The leaching of fibers out of the concrete occurs more readily in areas where the water is acidic.

The risk from asbestos fibers in drinking water lies in the ability of these fibers to migrate to virtually every organ in the body. They have been found often in the ovary in association with cancer there. Mesothelioma occurs in the lining of the abdomen (the peritoneum) as well as the pleura. It is not known what if any other adverse reactions may be seen. It is not known why or how the asbestos fiber causes cancer. It is not through chemical reaction, as is the case with chemicals that cause cancer. Asbestos in an inert mineral that is virtually indestructible, at any temperature. That property has made it very valuable in a multitude of applications.

Some of the areas where workers have been exposed to asbestos fibers are:

Mining, manufacturing, bagging, handling and processing of asbestos
Plumbers, pipe fitters and insulation workers
Vinyl asbestos floor tiles, manufacturing and sanding
Asbestos papers and felt
Friction materials, brake pads and clutches
Asbestos-cement building materials, water pipes
Lining of furnaces and kilns and insulation of boilers
Spray on materials for sound, fireproofing and insulation
Reinforced plastics
Dry wall construction and spackling (done prior to 1975)
Shipyard workers, maritime crews, U. S. Navy personnel
Stationary power plants
Schools, public buildings

The use of asbestos in dry wall and spackling compounds was banned in 1975. It was routinely incorporated prior to that, so that any remodeling or repair in those homes puts the worker at risk. Workers using these materials prior to 1975 must worry about the long latency period (30 years or more). Many of these workers were young people, many in their first jobs in their late teens or early twenties.   Most of them smoked cigarettes.   All of these individuals should have regular, careful physical examinations, especially beginning twenty years after their exposure.

The combination of asbestos and cigarettes is about the most potent risk for lung cancers (excluding mesothelioma) that has ever been observed.   Workers who are exposed to asbestos get lung cancer (other than mesothelioma) seven to eight times as frequently as those not exposed.   For those workers who are exposed to asbestos and who smoke cigarettes, the risk is seventy to eighty times as high as individuals who are not exposed.   These cancers are either of the squamous cell or adenocarcinoma variety.   There is a latency period of at least twenty years before these tumors show up.   In many cases it is longer.   The lung cancers that resulted from asbestos exposure among shipyard workers in World War II (mostly smokers) began showing up in 1978, some thirty years later.

The other serious consequence of inhaling asbestos fibers is asbestosis, a severe and disabling fibrosis of the lungs.   It was first reported in 1907.   In 1930 Merewether and Price reported that 80 percent of the workers who had spent 30 years or more in a British plant with exposure to asbestos had x-ray evidence of asbestosis.[28] In 1955 Richard Doll reported that the lung cancer risk in asbestos workers with 20 years or more exposure was 10 times as high as the population in general.[29]   It is quite apparent that we were aware of the problem and of the risks long before we became concerned enough to take action.

Doll also will be remembered as the researcher who in 1955 reported the high lung cancer risk among smokers.   Many, many subsequent studies since have confirmed and reinforced these findings.   While we may have taken some action, we certainly have not taken the cure.

Asbestosis, unlike mesothelioma, is related to the length and intensity of exposure.   The longer and the heavier the exposure, the greater is the chance of developing the disease.   All types of asbestos will produce this disease, although not equally so.   The disease has developed in wives and children of workers who carried the fibers home on their clothing.   It has also been seen in clusters in neighborhoods surrounding a factory where asbestos was discharged into the surrounding air.   Anyone who has a history of asbestos exposure, especially if it was twenty years ago or longer, should have an examination for this disease at least once yearly. A skilled physician with a stethoscope will detect the disease before it shows up on x-ray.

While asbestos has been removed from dry wall materials, and efforts have been made to substitute fibers such as fiberglass in some materials, it has not been substituted in many applications. The reason for this, very simply, is that there does not exist a satisfactory substitute in most cases. Asbestos is a remarkable substance of great and diverse use. Fiberglass does have the advantage of not provoking the serious lung diseases associated with asbestos. Recent studies have confirmed this.[30,31,32]

OTHER SILICATES

Talc, also called soapstone, is a hydrated magnesium silicate, and thus similar to asbestos. Natural deposits in mines contain between 1 and 17 percent free silica, and thus present the risk of silicosis to miners.[33] It is frequently found in association with dolomite, another reason to avoid that source of calcium for dietary supplementation. Talc has been used in the manufacture of paints, tires and other rubber products, ceramics, paper, asphalt products, insecticides, dusting powders and cosmetics. Inhalation of talc during the manufacture and handling of any of these products can result in a serious fibrosis in the lungs. This has been most clearly demonstrated in the rubber tire industry. Disabling pneumoconiosis (including silicosis and asbestosis) has also been demonstrated widely in the mining and processing of talc.

Micas are complex aluminum silicates combined with either potassium, magnesium, iron or calcium. Natural deposits contain 0 to 10 percent free silica. In some studies pneumoconiosis developed in 10 to 20 percent of workers who were exposed to dust generated by grinding mica, even in the absence of any free silica.[34] Its unique characteristic of translucency and its resistance to high temperatures makes it useful in constructing windows for furnaces and similar devices. It is a poor conductor of electricity, which makes it useful in making the windows of fuses and in other electrical applications.

Vermiculite is the name applied to a group of hydrous silicate minerals, usually resulting from alterations of mica, which greatly expands when it is heated. It has had wide application in insulation and as a soil conditioner in gardening. In natural deposits it is accompanied by tremolite asbestos, and workers in these mines have developed the usual asbestos related illnesses, asbestosis, lung cancer and mesothelioma. Care should be taken to avoid inhalation of any airborne particles when this is used as a soil conditioner.

SILICOSIS

The severe fibrosis in the lung that results from inhaling particles of silica sand (silicon dioxide) has some similarities to asbestosis. Both cause disruption of the cell wall of the macrophages that engulf the foreign particles. This releases enzymes into the lung tissue that results in damage and fibrosis. This process has been demonstrated in silicosis long ago, and only recently in asbestosis. Individuals with silicosis commonly succumb to tuberculosis, and these people should be skin tested for this disease. Those who present with a positive test should be placed on prophylactic medication.

Silicosis is the oldest, commonest and the most studied of all occupational diseases. The problem was covered in 1546 by Georg Agricola in his *De Re Metallica,* in which he discussed the need for ventilation in the mines, and the value of human health over financial gain. Bernardino Ramazzini, the Father of Occupational Medicine, published his first edition of *De Morbis Artificum Diatriba* at the age of 67 in 1700, the same year that he was awarded a chair at the University at Padua. In the first chapter of this work he described the "pneumonokoniosis" of stone masons and miners.

Ramazzini was the first to advocate the inclusion in the patient history of the simple question, "what is your occupation." By the 1830s early death from silicosis was recognized to be associated with the grinding of knives and needles, work in foundries, makers of pottery, mining of virtually all minerals and in stone cutters working on sandstone, but not on limestone (calcium carbonate).

During the depression in the United States, in the 1930s, the Hawk's Nest tunnel was cut through a sandstone mountain at Gauley Bridge, West Virginia, for a hydroelectric power plant. Workers, who came from many different states, worked with no protection and no efforts to control the dust. An appalling 476 of these workers died of acute silicosis, and an additional 1500 contracted the disease by the time the tunnel was completed. Many of the workers were buried in cornfields nearby with no ceremony.

Strenuous efforts were made to cover up this tragedy, but a congressional inquiry brought the facts to light and prompted the initiation of measures to control such exposure. If you visit this area for the white water rafting, or skiing, or merely to stop at the turnout to enjoy the view, you may see the plaque commemorating the great engineering feat that was accomplished. There is no memorial to those who gave their lives, however.

The use of silica sand in sandblasting was banned by law in Great Britain in 1949 and in Europe in 1955, but continues to be used in the United States today. Substitutes such as shot or carborundum are available but are more costly, in monetary terms. The incidence of silicosis as a result of sandblasting has actually been increasing in the United States. Sandstone grinding wheels were gradually replaced by carborundum (silicon carbide), alumina or emery starting in 1923. Natural emery may contain small amounts of silica, and the pure aluminum oxide, alumina, is safer. This transformation not only markedly reduced the incidence of silicosis, but also the incidence of crushed chests and skulls from broken wheels.

Sandstone wheels are still used in some areas in Nigeria because they are cheap and locally available, and cases of silicosis still occur in that country as a result. Silica is also present in talc (magnesium silicate) in an amount up to 5 percent. Talc is commonly used in the rubber industry, and an increased incidence of chronic obstructive lung disease is associated with it. Fortunately talc is being removed from baby powders and being replaced by cornstarch, the substance that was commonly used on infants fifty years ago (see Chapter XV).

An unusual source of silica is diatomaceous earth, which is mined and processed for use in filters, abrasives, some soaps and to control some insects such as cockroaches. It is also used as a desiccant to protect against moisture in some pharmaceutical products, and in the storage of various items. A diatom is a microscopic form of algae that has a wall of silica, unusual in that the structure of most such marine forms incorporates calcium rather than silica. The accumulation of deposits of the shells of the many species of diatoms is what forms diatomaceous earth. Mining and processing of these deposits in Santa Barbara County, California produced silicosis in 68 percent of the workers.[35] Silica, being the most abundant and widely dispersed mineral on earth, is so widely encountered in occupational, recreational and even household activities, that it is impossible to assemble a complete list of exposures without omissions. Some of the more common exposures are listed below:

Mining of coal, gold, silver, tin, lead, copper, nickel, uranium
Quarrying, except in pure limestone or marble
Tunneling
Sandblasting
Foundries, making and cleaning molds, grinding castings
Glass manufacture
Pottery, ceramics and china
Kilns, furnaces, boilers (lining and scaling)
Stone masons, monument grinders
Scouring powders, soaps, abrasives
Diatomaceous earth, processing of for filters, soaps, abrasives
Slate, processing for furniture, billiard tables and ornaments
Shipbuilding
Construction
Optical lens grinding
Tire makers, commercial talc lubricant in tire molds
Commercial mica and talc contain both silica and asbestos.

ACUTE SILICOSIS

The acute form of silicosis results from a brief, very heavy exposure, as may occur in sandblasting. The first cases described occurred in workers mixing silica for abrasive soaps in 1929. The exposure that precipitates acute silicosis may vary from a few weeks to a few years. A cough develops, accompanied by fever, shortness of breath and weight loss, all of which are progressive. Death from respiratory failure may occur within two years. There is no treatment and no cure.

CHRONIC SILICOSIS

The symptoms of chronic silicosis are again cough and shortness of breath, but evidence of the disease usually becomes evident only after fifteen years or more of low dose exposure. With heavier exposure, the disease may become manifest sooner. It is normally progressive, even if exposure is discontinued, due to the continued presence of silica particles in the lungs and its continued destructive process there. Sandblasting, grinding and packaging of silica and the blending of this product in abrasive soaps carry the highest risks.

There is no cure for the chronic form of silicosis either, and little remedy for the symptoms. The disease slowly progresses to death. If a positive tuberculin test evolves, prophylactic medication should be instituted and continued for life, due to the continued risk of active tuberculosis. Some treatment is available to mitigate the bronchitis and heart complications that accompany the disease. Continuous medical monitoring and care will be required.

Modern technology makes it possible to eliminate most exposures to silica. Substitute materials are available in many cases. Engineering controls could prevent virtually all exposures that result in silicosis. It is very difficult to justify the continued existence of this disease as an occupational hazard today.

CONTACT LENSES

This innovation in corrective lenses merits special consideration. Individuals who wear soft lenses are aware of the necessity to keep these lenses scrupulously clean, clear of protein and other deposits. Not everyone appreciates the fact that soft lenses, which are thirty-five percent water at a minimum, and up to seventy percent in some, absorb and concentrate many chemicals. This precludes wearing these lenses in any atmosphere where these chemicals, such as ammonia and organic solvents for example, are present.

Silicone spray will coat contact lenses and interfere with the normal uptake of water. Hair spray will similarly leave a residue on the lens. Optometrist frequently find handcreams on contact lenses. Hands should always be washed well with a soap that is free of oils and greases, and rinsed before handling lenses. The problem of fiberglass particles imbedded in lenses was discussed previously. (See Chapter XV for a complete discussion of contact lenses.)

HEARING

Virtually all factory work settings have a high noise level and thus present the threat of a hearing loss. Studies have shown that exposure to noise levels below eighty decibels do not present a risk of a hearing loss (see Hearing in Chapter VIII for a further discussion of noise and hearing). Studies by the National Institute for Occupational Safety and Health (NIOSH) have indicated that twenty-five percent of individuals age fifty-five years and over who have been exposed to an average of ninety decibels in their employment have developed a significant hearing loss due to occupational noise exposure. Approximately eighty million dollars per year is paid in workers compensation for hearing loss. This is a greater amount than that paid for any other occupational disease.

Everyone working in a noisy environment should have a baseline audiometric test, preferably before starting work. In the event that no pre-employment test has been done, it should be done as soon as possible. A periodic test should then be done to monitor any change. Follow-up tests should be done every one to two years, at least until stability has been established. Hearing loss that results from repeated noise exposure invariably is not recognized until it becomes profound. When a hearing loss is detected, an assessment of noise exposure should be made not only on the job, but at home and at play as well. It does little good to expend great effort to reduce the threat of hearing loss at work if the individual spends all of his time away from the job listening to rock music through headphones at 100 decibels.

The risk of hearing loss on the job has long been appreciated by people concerned with worker protection. The Walsh-Healy Public Contracts Act, passed in 1936, mandated that companies working under contract to the federal government must provide safe and healthful working conditions for employees. The onset of World War II greatly increased the number of such contracts, and thus the scope of the act. The stipulation of precise standards for noise was hindered by the limited availability of technology to measure and assess this risk on the job.

Standards to regulate noise exposure on the job were finally adopted in 1969 when the Walsh-Healy Act was revised. The American Conference of Governmental Industrial Hygienists (ACGIH), which was established in 1938, published recommended limits for noise exposure on the job in 1969. These formed the basis for the standards adopted in the Walsh-Healy Act.

The Occupational Safety and Health Act (Public Law 91-596) was signed into law in December 1970. The provisions of the Walsh-Healy Act were incorporated into this new law, and the published recommendations of the ACGIH were added. The initial limit for noise exposure on the job was set at 90 decibels for an eight-hour day. The Occupational Safety and Health Administration lowered the action level for permissible noise level on the job from 90 decibels to 85 decibels in 1985. All workers who are exposed to noise levels in excess of 85 decibels must have their hearing assessed and monitored in accordance with specified standards.

Since its inception the National Institute for Occupational Safety and Health worked to reduce this occupational noise induced hearing loss. These efforts led to the regulations that were issued by OSHA as outlined above. The noise level permitted, averaged over an eight-hour day, remains at 90 decibels. Workers who are exposed to levels above 85 decibels must be identified, however, and their hearing must be monitored in accordance with OSHA rules. Wearing hearing protection in noisy operations will substantially reduce hearing loss on the job. Wearing efficient, well-fit earplugs designed for this purpose will reduce effective noise levels by 10 to 15 decibels.

Absolute noise levels can often be reduced by engineering controls, and this is the preferred approach where it is feasible. Machinery can be installed on mounts that absorb and prevent transmission of sound to the foundation and building, much the same way that motor mounts are used in automobiles. Enclosures constructed of sound absorbing materials can isolate noisy operations from the remainder of the workplace. Machinery itself can be redesigned so that it produces less noise as a by-product of manufacturing.

All of these measures are costly and are frequently deferred for this reason, especially in the current era of cost consciousness. The adversarial tug of war between labor and management over who is responsible for hearing protection may provide entertainment, but it is small comfort to the worker who has suffered a profound hearing loss. Prudence dictates that the individual accept the responsibility for protecting his hearing. This can be accomplished by wearing personal protective devices in any work environment where the noise level exceeds eighty decibels.

Management and labor have the responsibility to work together to reduce the level of noise whenever feasible. Both parties gain by working in cooperation. Both parties lose when an adversarial relationship exists. Having someone else to blame seems little comfort for the loss of a possession as valuable as hearing.

The hazards of noise in recreational activities are discussed in Chapter VIII. A table listing the noise level in decibels of some commonly encountered sources can be found there.

DIESEL EXHAUST

In August 1988 the National Institute for Occupational Safety and Health (NIOSH) released a Current Intelligence Bulletin in which they recommended that diesel exhaust be classified as a potential occupational carcinogen. This release contained summaries of recent studies regarding the carcinogenic effect of diesel emissions.

Studies of the content of diesel exhaust were conducted as long ago as the 1950s and 1960s, in both the United States and Great Britain. In November 1977 the Environmental Protection Agency (EPA) announced that it was initiating a study of the potential health hazards of diesel exhaust emissions. The explanation for this action was that several of the seven fractions that had been identified in these emissions had been found to be positive in the Ames test, an indirect test for mutagenicity.

PEDCO Environmental, Inc. conducted a study for the EPA and it was reported to that agency in March 1978. The findings were in agreement with studies carried out by Daimler-Benz and others, namely that diesel exhaust does contain small amounts of polynuclear aromatic hydrocarbons that are known to cause cancer. This is also true of gasoline fueled engines.

The other substances in diesel exhaust that are of concern are sulfates, nitrogen oxides and ozone. The sulfate emissions are directly related to the quality of the engineering design of the engine and the quality of the fuel. This is also true of the level of emissions of nitrous oxides. Mercedes Benz recommends fuel with a sulfur content no higher than 0.5 percent. Number 2 diesel fuel marketed in Michigan by both Union Oil and Amoco claim a sulfur content below 0.1 percent. Studies have verified that levels above 0.3 percent are unusual in most areas of the United States. With low-grade fuel, sulfate emissions and the quantity of particulate "soot" are greatly increased. With poor maintenance both these and nitrous oxides are increased. This is very evident when following some of the municipal buses and poorly maintained tractor-trailer rigs.

Occupational exposure to diesel exhausts occurs among those who work in maintenance garages for autos, trucks and buses, in mines, in tunnels, on railroads, on loading docks and on farms. The risk that is outlined by NIOSH is that of lung cancer, which it concludes is associated with inhalation of diesel exhaust on the job. One of the major problems with making such an assessment is the frequency of cigarette smoking, which is the most common cause of lung cancer. It has also been well established that cigarette smoking potentiates the carcinogenic risk of many other substances.

In addition to the cancer risk, chronic exposure to diesel exhaust, and indeed the exhaust of gasoline engines, carries a risk of the development of pulmonary fibrosis and emphysema. Nitrogen oxides, ozone and many particulates are irritating to the lung, and over a period of time can produce pathologic changes in the lungs. These changes occur more frequently and more rapidly in those who smoke cigarettes. It is imperative that exhaust emissions from any engines be kept to a minimum by proper ventilation and by ducting exhausts directly to the outside whenever possible.

HEAT DISORDERS

Exposure to elevated temperatures that present a threat to health are encountered in a wide array of occupational settings, and involve a large number of people. Human beings possess a remarkable degree of adaptability to temperature extremes. This ability has its limits, however, and exposure to heat on the job causes much illness and many deaths each year. Most of the fatalities and many of the cases of heat-related illness could be prevented by monitoring the worker and the environmental conditions surrounding him. The application of some well-known principles and procedures would augment any prophylactic program.

Disorders caused by heat are related to the temperature of the air, the humidity of the air, the amount of air movement at the job site, thermal radiation, the level of physical activity required by the job, age and physical condition of the worker, drugs, type of clothing worn and body build. Short, stocky and obese individuals dissipate heat much less efficiently, both because of the increased body mass and the decrease in skin surface area. More heat is produced in the greater body mass, and at the same time relatively less skin surface is available for sweating and heat dissipation. Heat disorders occur more frequently in non-acclimatized workers. They also occur more often in individuals who are past forty and in those who are taking diuretics for high blood pressure or heart failure. Alcohol consumption renders workers much more susceptible to all of the heat disorders. These disorders occur much more commonly during periods of prolonged heat, and particularly when the humidity is high.

The early symptoms produced by heat disorders are not always dramatic and are often overlooked. The chemical and physiological imbalances that accompany the condition (see Chapter IX) result in a clouding of the mental faculties resulting in less vigilance and in increased risk of injury. Impaired performance results from decreased function of both the nervous system and muscles. Poor job performance and decreased productivity become apparent. As the condition progresses, weakness, dizziness, headache, nausea, vomiting, loss of appetite and faintness appear. These proceed to collapse if the appropriate remedial steps are not taken.

It is important to recognize the threat of this disorder at the earliest possible signs, and to take measures to prevent progression to a more serious stage. These early steps include removal from the hot environment to a cooler one. In the factory the worker should be moved to an air-conditioned location. This would usually be the plant medical facility. Discontinuance of physical activity, removal of heavy clothing and drinking cool fluids will all help to reverse this potentially serious condition. Once the heat exhaustion victim has progressed to the point where assistance is needed, these measures become much more urgent. In addition to removing from the hot environment, the person should be made to lie flat or with the head slightly low.

The most urgent need for the prevention of heat disorders is an increased intake of water. Electrolyte solutions as described in chapter IX can be used as a supplement to water to replace lost fluid and salt. Salt tablets should be avoided, however, since they are irritating to the stomach. The quantity of salt supplementation needed is directly related to the amount of loss and can be calculated. In rare circumstances where a significant loss occurs over an eight-hour day ten to fifteen grams per day of additional salt are required. In most occupational circumstances much less is adequate. A greater quantity is required during periods of acclimatization than during maintenance.

Any supplementation of salt requires adequate intake of water at the same time. Prophylactic salt supplementation carries a particular risk for those individuals who have high blood pressure, because salt has a very deleterious effect on blood pressure. In these instances the quantity of salt consumed should be monitored and balanced carefully.

Several formulae and criteria have evolved in an effort to predict the levels at which heat stress occurs. These are complex and require trained personnel as well as specialized apparatus. They attempt to factor in the various environmental conditions such as absolute temperature, air movement, wet bulb reading and humidity, as well as physiologic factors. For the individual, the best indication of impending heat stress is the body core temperature (rectal temperature) and the heart rate. The latter varies with age, and a higher rate is acceptable in younger workers than in those who are past forty years of age. These two measurements give a clear indication when it is time to remove the worker from the hot environment, and to initiate remedial action. They are less helpful in predicting the length of time that a given worker will be able to work in a hot environment.

HEAT CRAMPS

Heat cramps are characterized by spasms and pain in the muscles of the arms, legs and sometimes of the abdomen after prolonged exposure to heat. The muscles that are in use on the job are particularly affected. These symptoms are caused by an excessive loss of salt, with the resultant flow of water into the cells of the muscles. In some cases albumen may show up in the urine. These symptoms may not develop until after the worker is away from the job. The body temperature is usually normal. This condition frequently results from drinking water in response to thirst and fluid loss on the job, without accompanying salt. The water dilutes the fluids in the body, sending a false signal from the pituitary which reduces the hormone that would normally reduce water and salt loss.

Heat cramps can occur very unexpectedly in hot dry climates, since the profuse sweating evaporates so rapidly that it is not noticed. It can also occur in people at work or at play in cold climates if they are over dressed. Heat related disorders are seldom considered in these settings. Prevention of this painful condition requires supplementation of the appropriate quantities of salt and water when the loss of these substances is excessive.

HEAT RASH

Heat rash is manifested by small raised red blisters accompanied by a prickly sensation during exposure to heat. It is caused by a retention of sweat in the sweat glands when plugs of keratin and cells obstruct the ducts. The retained sweat bursts through the wall of the sweat glands into the surrounding tissue and this results in inflammation, and sometimes infection. It occurs primarily after prolonged exposure to heat when the humidity is high. The evaporation of sweat is thus impaired, leaving the skin constantly wet. The inactivation of the sweat glands produces a pronounced reduction in heat tolerance due to the loss of this valuable mechanism for the dissipation of heat. Bathing, skin hygiene and clean clothing are important in preventing skin infections when this condition occurs. Prevention of heat rash is accomplished by limiting exposure under hot, humid conditions, and allowing the skin to dry periodically.

HEAT SYNCOPE

Fainting with exposure to heat occurs when the worker stands in one place for protracted periods with minimal or no movement. It results from the pooling of blood in the skin and legs due to dilation of blood vessels. It occurs more readily in the non-acclimatized worker. Treatment is accomplished by removal to a cooler location and having the worker lie down with the head slightly lower than the legs. It can be prevented by acclimatization and by taking brief steps periodically and regularly in order to stimulate the venous return from the legs to the heart.

OCCUPATIONS WHERE HEAT DISORDERS ARE ENCOUNTERED

Bakeries
Boiler operators
Cannery workers
Chemical plants
Coke ovens
Construction workers
Cooks
Dry cleaners and press operators
Factories, especially in hot weather
Farmers
Forge hammer operators
Foundries
Furnace operators
Glass manufacture and blowing
Iron and steel mills, rolling
Kilns
Metal casting
Mining, deep mines
Outdoor jobs, summer
Roofers
Ships and shipyard workers
Smelters
Textile industry
Tire and rubber manufacture

HYPERSENSITIVITY PNEUMONITIS

DISEASE	SOURCE	ANTIGEN
Bagassosis	Moldy sugar cane	Thermoactino-mycetes
Bird fancier's lung; chicken, turkey raisers disease	Pigeons, parrots, other birds; chickens, turkeys	Serum, feathers, droppings
Byssinosis	Cotton bract	Undetermined material
Cheese washer's lung	Moldy cheese	Penicillium casei
Coffee worker's lung	Coffee bean	Thermoactino-mycetes
Detergent worker's lung	Detergents containing enzymes	Bacillus subtilis (alcalase)
Dog house disease	Moldy straw	Aspergillus versicolor
Farmer's lung	Moldy hay	Thermoactino-mycetes, Micropolyspora
Furrier's lung	Animal hairs	Proteins

Hard metal lung disease	Tungsten carbide	Cobalt
Humidifier fever	Water reservoirs	Various bacteria and fungi
Malt worker's lung	Moldy malt and barley	Aspergillus clavatus, fumigatus
Mushroom worker's lung	Compost (manure and straw)	Micropolyspora faeni, Thermoactinomyces vulgaris
Paprika splitter's disease	Moldy paprika pods	Mucor stolonifer
Papuan lung	Moldy thatch dust of huts	Various fungi
Pituitary snuff taker's disease	Bovine and porcine pituitary snuff	Pituitary antigens
Red cedar lung	Red cedar wood	Plicatic acid
Rodent handler's disease	Rats and gerbils	Urine proteins
Sequoisis	Redwood sawdust	Graphium pullaria
Sisal worker's disease	Bag and rope dust	Thermoactinomyces
Suberosis	Moldy cork dust	Penicillium frequentus
Wheat weevil's disease	Wheat flour	Sitophilus granularius
Wood pulp worker's disease	Moldy wood pulp	Alternaria, Aspergillus

1. Hunter D. *The Diseases of Occupations*. 6th ed. London: Hodder and Stoughton, 1978.

2. Ibid, p. 562.

3. 29 CFR 1910, Code of Federal Regulations, Occupational Safety amd Health Standards, Title 29, §1910, Washington, DC. Rev. July, 1991.

4. 29 CFR 1910.1003 as posted on OSHA website May, 2001.

5. National Toxicology Program. Ninth Report on Carcinogens, 2000.

6. International Agency for Research on Cancer (IARC), S.7, 1987.

7. Doll R, Peto R. *The Causes of Cancer*. Oxford University Press, Oxford, 1981.

8. Creech JL Jr, Johnson MN. Angiosarcoma of the liver in the manufacture of polyvinyl chloride. *J Occup Med* 1974;**16**:150-151.

9. Selikoff IJ, Hammond EC, eds. Toxicity of vinyl chloride-polyvinyl chloride. *Ann NY Acad Sci* 1975;**246**:1-137.

10. Hiatt HH, Watson JD, Winsten JA, eds. *Origins of human cancer*. New York: Cold Spring Harbor Laboratory, 1977.

11. Wu W, Steenland K, Brown S, et al. Cohort and case-control analysis of workers exposed to vinyl chloride: an update. *J Occ Med* 1989;**31**(6):518-523.

12. Cheng TJ, Huang ML, You NC, et al. Abnormal liver function in workers exposed to low levels of ethylene dichloride and vinyl chloride. *J Occ Med* 1999;**41**(12):1128-1133.

13. ACGIH, *Threshold Limit Values for Chemical Substances and Physical Agents and Biological Exposures*, American Conference of Governmental Industrial Hygienists, Cincinnati, OH, 2001.

14. U.S. Department of Health and Human Services, Public Health Service, National Toxicology Program. *Report on Carcinogens*, Ninth Edition, 2000.

15. CDC. Organophosphate toxicity associated with flea-dip products — California. *MMWR* 1988;**37**(21):329-335.

16. Ames RG, Brown SK, Rosenberg J, Jackson RJ, Stratton JW, Quenon SG. Health symptoms and occupational exposure to flea control products among California pet handlers. *Am Ind Hyg Assoc J* 1989;**50**(9):466-472.

17. CDC. Dermatitis among workers cleaning the Sacramento River after a chemical spill — California, 1991. *MMWR* 1991;**40**(48):825-827.

18. CDC. Surveillance of elevated blood lead levels among adults — United States, 1992. *MMWR* 1992;**41**(no.17):285-290.

19. Eisenbud M, Lisson J. Epidemiological aspects of beryllium-induced nonmalignant lung disease:a 30-year update. *J Occ Med* 1983;**25**(3):196-202.

20. CDC. Beryllium disease among workers in a spacecraft-manufacturing plant — California. *MMWR* 1983;**32**:419-425.

21. Sobaszek A, Boulenguez C, Frimat P et. al. Acute respiratory effects of exposure to stainless steel and mild steel welding fumes. *J Occup Environ Med*. 2000;**42**:923-931.

22. Armbruster C, Dekan G, Hovorka A. Granulomatous pneumonitis and mediastinal lymphadenopathy due to photocopier toner dust. *Lancet* 1996;**348**:- 690.

23. Gallardo M, Romero P, Sanchez-Quevedo M, Lopez-Caballero J. Siderosilicosis due to photocopier dust. *Lancet* 1994;**344**:412-13.

24. Zenz C, ed. *Occupational Medicine*, ed 3. St. Louis, Mosby 1994.

25. Morgan WK, Seaton A. *Occupational Lung Diseases*. Ed 2. Philadelphia: WB Saunders, 1984.

26. Selikoff IJ. The occurrence of pleural calcification among asbestos insulation workers. *Ann NY Acad Sci* 1965;**132**:351.

27. Selikoff IJ. Cancer risk of asbestos exposure, in Hiatt HH, Watson JD, Winsten JA eds: *Origins of Human Cancer*. Cold Spring Harbor Laboratory, 1977.

28. Merewether ERA, Price CV. Report on effects of asbestos dust suppression in the asbestos industry. Part I. Her Majesty's Stationaery Office, London, 1930.

29. Doll R. Mortality from lung cancer in asbestos workers. *Br J Ind Med* 1955;**12**:81

30. Marsh GM, Youk AO, Stone RA et al. Historical cohort study of US manmade vitreous fiber production workers: I. 1992 Fiberglass cohort follow-up: Initial findings. *J Occup Environ Med*. 2001;**43**:741-756.

31. Marsh GM, Gula MJ, Youk AO et al. Historical cohort study of US man-made vitreous fiber production workers: II. Mortality from mesothelioma. *J Occup Environ Med*. 2001;**43**:757-766.

32. Youk AO, Marsh GM, Stone RA et al. Historical cohort study of US man-made vitreous fiber production workers: III. Analysis of exposure-weighted measures of respirable fibers and formaldehyde in the nested case-control study of respiratory system cancer. *J Occ Environ Med*. 2001;**43**:767-778.

33. Zenz C. Ed. *Occupational Medicine*, ed 3. St. Louis: Mosby, 1994.

34. Raffle P ed. *Hunter's Diseases of Occupations*, ed 8. London; Boston: Arnold, 1994.

35. Ibid.

XI

HAZARDS OF SEX

Generosity should never exceed ability
                    — Marcus Tullius Cicero (106–43 B.C.)

SEXUALLY TRANSMITTED DISEASES

Perhaps it would have been more appropriate to include this material in the chapter on recreation. Sex seems to have joined football and baseball as great American recreational activities. It was not left for our society to discover it, however, and perhaps it only seems that we have carried the sport to a new high. After all the Romans had their day.

Prior to 1960 the only two sexually transmitted diseases (STD) that promiscuous individuals risked were syphilis and gonorrhea. Currently there are more than twenty, many with serious consequences. This is the result of the sexual revolution and the liberation of individuals from all responsibility and self-restraint. In our modern enlightened society sex is as easy to obtain as milk in the super market; it just isn't pasteurized. The ready availability and widespread use of abortion as a means of terminating unwanted pregnancies has freed women of that complication of promiscuity, but at the same time it has increased the spread of sexually transmitted diseases. As a result about 20 percent of the U.S. population is infected with at least one of the sexually transmitted diseases. The percentage is even higher in the population under 25 years of age. Currently (2001) about 8,000 teenagers in the U.S. acquire an STD every day. One of the great tragedies of the sexual revolution has been the introduction of sexual activity on a wide scale among not only adolescents, but also children even younger. The United States has the highest adolescent pregnancy rate among the developed countries of the world, with over 800,000 teenagers becoming pregnant each year (Centers for Disease Control, September 2000).

Many of those individuals who are infected with STDs harbor more than one disease, some have several. During 1995 among the 55 infectious diseases that were required to be reported to health departments, sexually transmitted diseases predominated[1] and they were reported among all age groups. The three most frequently reported infectious diseases were chlamydia, gonorrhea and AIDS in that order. Even salmonella food infections were surpassed by these sexually transmitted infections. This is less a testimonial to our success in decreasing the transmission of infectious diseases than it is to the disgraceful deterioration in the morals and ethical standards in our society. The misinformation presented in the multi-billion dollar campaign by the United States government and the public schools bears much of the blame for this national catastrophe. No amount of money can undo the tragedy that has ensued.

The true incidence of sexually transmitted diseases in the United States is not known because many cases, perhaps even the majority, are not reported. Indeed many cases of chlamydia and the various vaginal infections are not diagnosed. Many of these resolve into a chronic infection that is shared with subsequent sexual partners. Many sexually active males harbor pathogenic organisms in their urethra that may be transmitted to sexual partners even though they themselves experience no symptoms.

Since the 1940s every state health department has had organizational procedures and trained personnel to investigate cases of sexually transmitted diseases, which, as stated previously, were primarily syphilis and gonorrhea until the 1970s. These activities were executed under the legal authority of statutes enacted by the various legislatures. The procedures, which were both routine and effective, involved interviewing individuals who had been diagnosed with syphilis or gonorrhea as a means of identifying contacts, and thus other individuals who might be at risk of also contracting these diseases. These sexual contacts were then interviewed and referred for treatment where needed.

The rationale, of course, involved humanitarian as well as public health considerations in that both diseases have serious consequences if not diagnosed and treated early. Gonorrhea can progress to severe pelvic infections with attendant scarring in both sexes, and sterility in the female. It can further be disseminated to the remainder of the body, particularly the joints where it will produce a septic (infectious) arthritis.

The sequelae of syphilis infection are even more devastating and grave. It can progress to involve the heart and aorta where serious damage leads to an untimely death. Left inadequately treated syphilis invades and destroys the brain and other portions of the central nervous system. This results in impairment of motor functions (walking, talking, any use of hands, arms and legs) and mental illness. The more serious of these complications do not become evident until twenty to thirty years after the acquisition of the disease. The ultimate disease of the nervous system is dramatic in appearance and certain in development. No amount of treatment can reverse these consequences once they occur.

SEXUALLY TRANSMITTED DISEASES AND PATHOGENS

DISEASE	AGENT
§Syphilis	Treponema Pallidum (bacterium)
§Gonorrhea	Neisseria gonorrhea (bacterium)
AIDS	HIV (virus)
Herpes	HSV-1, HSV-2 (virus)
Hepatitis B	Hepatitis B virus
Condyloma (warts)	Human papilloma virus (HPV)
Molluscum contagiosum	Molluscum contagiosum virus
§Chancroid	Haemophilus ducrei (bacterium)*
§Lymphogranuloma verereum	Chlamydia (bacterium)*
§Granuloma inguinale	Calymmatobacterium granulomatis*
Vaginitis, balanitis	Bacteria, protoaoa, fungus**
Pelvic inflammatory disease	N. gonorrhea, Chlamydia, Myco-plasma
Urethritis	N. gonorrhea, Chlamydia, Myco-plasma
Epieieymitis	Neisseria gonorrhea & Chlamydia
Cancer (cervix)	Human papilloma virus

Enteritis	Shigella, Salmonella, Campylobacter, Giardia, Amoeba ***
Pediculosis	Crab louse
Scabies	Sarcoptes Scabei (mite)

§   The five historically defined as Sexually Transmitted Diseases
*   Uncommon in the United States
** Bacteria include Gardnerella and other species, protozoan is Trichomonas, and fungus is Candida.
*** Primarily in male homosexuals

Even more tragic are the children born to mothers who have these diseases. Congenital syphilis produces numerous malformations and mental retardation. The progression of the disease may be arrested with adequate treatment, but the developmental abnormalities that have occurred in the children cannot be reversed. Gonorrhea can produce an infection in the eyes of the newborn, which can lead to blindness if not treated. It was to prevent this tragedy that the states passed laws mandating routine treatment with silver nitrate drops to the eyes of every newborn infant. (These laws were amended in the 1980s to permit treatment with other substances such as penicillin).

Preventing all of these tragedies is reason enough to justify intervention by public health authorities and the medical profession in general. The far greater imperative in terms of magnitude behind the public health laws and attendant intervention and control measures, however, was the enormous consequences of taking no such action. It was recognized in the earliest days of medicine that one individual with a communicable disease could transmit that disease to many others. These individuals thus infected could in turn transmit the disease to a much larger population. It is thus that epidemics are born.

With every case of a sexually transmitted disease that emerges, there is at least one other individual with that disease. These infections are not acquired from door handles or from plumbing faucets as may occur with other communicable diseases. They similarly are not transmitted by food or water. Even with all of our control efforts and the development of effective antibiotics the sexually transmitted diseases continue to be the most common communicable diseases in the world.

In the case of smallpox, measles, scarlet fever and other serious communicable diseases, quarantine was an effective measure to prevent dissemination and the resultant epidemics. Public health officials had the authority under state statutes to impose and enforce these quarantines. With the advent of antibiotics and widespread routine immunization of the population, quarantine for many of these diseases is no longer needed. A modified form of quarantine is still routinely used when large outbreaks of influenza strike a community; the schools are closed until those infected are no longer communicable.

In the case of sexually transmitted diseases such as syphilis and gonorrhea quarantine certainly would have been effective, but enforcement would have required a jail cell. The system of interview and case investigation and follow up is more practical and has proven to be effective. If we had not had public health departments, if we had had no statutes authorizing and mandating these measures, we would have had many widespread epidemics. We would have institutions full of syphilitic mental patients, many of them children. We would have even larger numbers of disabled individuals requiring public assistance than is currently the case. Such a situation would be a great tragedy and a national disgrace. It would also be an enormous financial burden on the taxpayers.

Strangely enough, when the AIDS (acquired immunodeficiency syndrome) problem surfaced, these public health measures which had been well established and proven over the previous eighty years were not applied to this new sexually transmitted disease. The social stigma of the disease has often been cited as an excuse for treating HIV (human immunodeficiency virus) infected individuals differently than those with syphilis or the other sexually transmitted diseases. However, no disease ever presented more of a social stigma than did syphilis. From the very onset of the AIDS epidemic strong political pressure was exerted to tie the hands of public health officials and the medical profession. This action was even supported by some local and state health departments and by the Centers for Disease Control. What makes this malfeasance even more repugnant is the fact that this new disease initially involved only a very select and easily identified group of people that represents less than three percent of the general population.

First, laws were passed which prohibited physicians from obtaining routine tests, as had been done with all other sexually transmitted diseases in the past, and prohibiting public health officials from identifying contacts who would be at risk of contracting the disease. Because of the combined forces of state legislatures, ineffective and irresponsible members of Congress, lawyers and self serving individuals in Congress and other seats of power, the established, effective, common sense measures that should have been applied to help control this horrendous and fatal disease were totally prohibited. Now that the disease epidemic is totally out of control these pressure groups and their allies in Congress are screaming for more money to solve the problem. Even at this late date, the measures that could have held the epidemic in check are still forbidden.

The consequences of this neglect and political manipulation of the medical community are very obvious. Thousands of people have become infected needlessly and we have an epidemic of a disease that is 100% fatal, that runs a very protracted course and that produces many ancillary infections along the way. Many of these infections, which are communicable, have been very uncommon or even rare prior to the advent of this new disease. The result for the infected individual is many years of anguish, suffering and depression. The result for the society as a whole is the exposure to and threat of not only AIDS, but also a long list of infectious diseases that have not previously been a threat. Most of these are diseases for which we have no control.

An additional problem for society is an enormous financial burden through taxation that could reach unsustainable levels. The financial burden imposed through taxation to support current welfare and social programs is already onerous. These added financial demands were unloaded upon the population at a time when the magnitude of the costs of bailing out the savings and loans and banks raised serious questions about the financial survivability of our society. Irresponsible expansion of government programs with extravagant expenditures and waste continues unabated into the new millennium, with no promise of restraint.

No one can foresee the ultimate outcome of this epidemic. Initially it seemed that it would inevitably become a pandemic that would rival the "Black Death" bubonic plague pandemic of the fourteenth century. That episode killed half of the population of England and at least one-fourth of the population of all of Europe (see plague in Chapter VII). The forces that came into play to ultimately control the plague pandemic will not come to our rescue in the case of the AIDS epidemic. With the plague, as the rats died off, the major reservoir of the infection disappeared with them.

We are led to believe by our politicians and the elite news media (both of which are rarely accurate or objective about anything) that a cure is only a short distance down the road. We are told that at the very least we can expect a vaccine that will prevent the spread of AIDS. The very powerful AIDS lobby is constantly screaming for more money from the public coffers to speed that day of deliverance. Enormous sums of such public funds (tax dollars) have already been diverted from other health endeavors by these vocal and powerful political forces and vested interest groups. Funding for HIV vaccine research by the National Institutes of Health increased from 100 million in 1995 to 194 million in 1999.

The overwhelming majority of these funds, disbursed in order to assuage a vocal minority, disappear down the proverbial black hole. In spite of our voluminous experiences during the years of the Great Society, during which time billions of dollars have been poured down such black holes, there has been no change in the practice of throwing money at social or medical problems to attempt to solve them. No amount of federal expenditures will solve this serious problem, however.

The sober reality is that a review of all that we have learned about the human immunodeficiency virus indicates that we will not develop a cure for AIDS, or any vaccine to prevent it in the foreseeable future. The AIDS virus mutates readily, and because of its genetic structure there are thousands of possible variants. We have developed two different classes of drugs that interfere with the metabolism of the virus at different sites, but again the virus adjusts to this challenge and becomes resistant to these weapons. There is virtually no possibility of developing a vaccine for this virus.

This reality has started to dawn upon some of the most enthusiastic researchers in this endeavor. Results of tests in monkeys of a weakened version of HIV-1 over a six year period reported in February 1999 that a large proportion of the animals were either sick or dead. Other trials have yielded similar findings. Plans for trials in humans have been put on hold. Public remarks by these researchers have been muted out of a fear of losing grant funding. On March 17, 1999, however, the executive director of UNAIDS publicly stated that a vaccine for HIV is still 10 years away, and that "prevention remains the only option."

In November 1999 the United Nations and the World Health Organization reported that during the previous year an additional 5.6 million people worldwide had been infected with HIV. They reported that 2.6 million people had died during that year, the highest total for any year since the onset of the epidemic.[2] At the time of that report there were 32.4 million adults and 1.2 million children living with HIV/AIDS. A total of 16.9 million people had died of the disease since the beginning of the epidemic. The previous year (1998) had seen 5.8 million new infections, with half of these in people 15-24 years of age.[3] HIV is still infecting 16,000 new people each day worldwide. Ten percent of the adult population in South Africa is infected with HIV. In some African countries 20 percent of the adults are infected. The disease has reached alarming epidemic proportions in Russia, where the health care system has been under a severe strain. Even though deaths from AIDS have dropped in the United States as a result of effective drugs that prolong life, the rate of new infections has not declined.

The litany of diseases that the medical experts of the world have failed to find a cure or prevention for would fill volumes. Multiple sclerosis, amyotrophic lateral sclerosis (Lou Gehrig's disease), lung cancer, breast cancer, cervical cancer, uterine cancer, ovarian cancer, and indeed most cancers, are but a few examples. We know that some of these cancers are associated with viruses (cervical cancer for example), but we have no means of preventing these viruses from invading the body (other than avoidance). We further have no means of eradicating them once they gain entrance and little or no means of controlling their activities once they are established therein.

The only hope of a cure for the cancers produced by these viruses, or even any significant control, is early detection and total surgical excision. These grim facts are not surprising when one understands the nature and properties of viruses, their modes of operation and their ability to readily mutate. (See viruses in Chapters V and XIII). It should be clearly understood that once an individual is infected with one of the viral sexually transmitted diseases such as herpes or one of the several papilloma viruses, it is a permanent infection. We have never developed an antibiotic or chemotherapeutic agent that will kill these viruses within the body. This is a significant factor in the association of these infections with the development of cancers.

In only a very few instances have we developed a vaccine that is effective in preventing viral infections. Smallpox is one of the rare exceptions, and one of the great successes in medicine. The polio vaccines are another great achievement, although they were not without their dark side. They have certainly markedly reduced the incidence of polio, but they also transmitted a simian virus (SV-40) to millions of people who received them through contamination from the monkey cell cultures. SV-40 has been found recently to be associated with the development of brain cancer, and perhaps multiple sclerosis. The full ramification of this is not yet known.

The time and effort invested in the development of the Salk and Sabin vaccines vividly demonstrates the formidable task medicine faces in attempting to control viral diseases. Success required the development of a vaccine against three different strains of poliovirus. This success in developing the vaccines for poliomyelitis was achieved by diligence and perseverance by physicians in research laboratories. It was not accomplished merely by Congress shelling out huge sums of money to solve the problem. There remain many other similar enteroviruses for which no control exists. Almost seventy different types have been identified thus far, with more yet to come. Some of these are listed in the table below.

DISEASES OF MAN CAUSED BY ENTEROVIRUSES

DISEASE	NUMBER OF VIRUS STRAINS CAUSING
Meningitis, encephalitis	18
Pericarditis, myocarditis	11
Rash	20
Herpangina	6
Epidemic myalgia	9
Conjunctivitis	5
Respiratory	13
Hand, Foot and Mouth	2
Gastroenteritis	3
Paralysis other than polio	13

SYPHILIS

Syphilis is a disease that has enjoyed a prominence in much of recorded history. It left its mark in many societies among both the lower classes and the aristocracy. Several writings of the sixteenth century described syphilis as an entirely new disease, brought by Columbus's sailors to Barcelona, Spain from the West Indies, specifically from Haiti. Peter Lowe published an essay on the "Spanish Sickness" (syphilis) in 1596. That story provides an interesting parallel to the current epidemic of AIDS in our society. In 1999 scientists established a diagnosis of syphilis in a 200-year-old skeleton from Easter Island, Chile by PCR (polymerase chain reaction) amplification of DNA.[4] The skeleton had deformities of the tibia that are typical of syphilis.

Syphilis remains a very serious disease today both because of its incidence and its serious impact on virtually the entire body. It's ravages of the heart and the brain are perhaps the most devastating legacies of the disease. The actual number of cases may well be four to five times the reported figures since many cases are not reported. Many are not seen by a physician, and are thus not diagnosed. In 1943 over 575,000 cases of syphilis were reported in the United States. This incidence fell to about 65,000 by 1977, due mainly to intense public health measures and the development of penicillin. Following this there was significantly less organized control measures and a corresponding increase in the disease resulted. Over 50,000 cases of primary and secondary syphilis were reported in 1990, and in excess of 3,000 new cases of congenital syphilis were reported each year from 1990 through 1993. More than one-half of the cases of syphilis reported occurred in homosexual men. Happily there has been a steady decline in the number of cases reported each year since then, so that 6,657 new cases of syphilis were reported in 1999, and 556 cases of congenital syphilis.

The radical change in the mores and social education of our population was largely responsible for the great increase in not only syphilis, but also all of the sexually transmitted diseases. This is particularly evident in the increase in these diseases among the teenage population. A major factor in the explosive increase of syphilis, as well as other sexually transmitted diseases, has been the widespread use of illicit drugs, especially crack cocaine. Individuals are far more willing to undertake any type of sexual activity while detached from reality by cocaine or other drugs. Additionally they frequently trade their bodies for access to the drug.

The corresponding increase in syphilis among the newborn has been particularly distressing. About 800 new cases were reported to the CDC each year through 1998. Even those numbers are misleading, however, for many cases are not reported. New York City alone reported an estimated 900 to 1,000 cases of congenital syphilis for 1989. This represented an increase from 57 cases in 1986 and 357 cases in 1988.[5] Many pregnant women with syphilis have stillborn infants. The true number is not known because syphilis as a cause of stillbirths has not been recognized, and thus not reported. It has been estimated that in pregnant women with untreated syphilis, 40 percent of infants will die before or shortly after birth.

All of the tragic cases of congenital syphilis could have been prevented simply by treatment of the mother with penicillin. A blood test for syphilis is required during pregnancy in all 50 of the states, but many women do not seek prenatal care and thus are not tested early in pregnancy. Considering that the causative organism can live outside the body for only a few seconds, that the only natural reservoir is man, and that the disease is one hundred percent cured with penicillin, one would think that eradication of this plague from the face of the earth could be achieved. Such an achievement would require additionally a serious modification of the sexual habits and mores of people, however. A tall order indeed.

Syphilis is caused by a bacterium, a spirochete, *Treponema pallidum*, which is fragile and cannot live outside the human body for more than a very brief time as mentioned previously. It cannot be contracted from door handles, dinnerware, drinking cups, towels or bathtubs. As we were taught in the military during World War II the disease cannot be caught from a toilet seat. The Treponema organism cannot be viewed through the light microscope using ordinary staining techniques as can be done in the case of gonorrhea and most other bacterial infections. It can be seen with the light microscope using a special technique called darkfield microscopy. This requires a special light attachment that is mounted underneath the stage of the microscope. The light is then directed obliquely through the specimen, which renders the corkscrew shaped bacterium visible.

A specimen from an active lesion is required for such visualization, however. Correct identification of *T. pallidum* by this technique requires both skill and experience. The organism cannot be grown on any artificial culture media as can be done with most other bacteria. This makes the diagnosis much more difficult. Unless the organism can be demonstrated by darkfield microscopy of specimens from active lesions we must rely upon indirect blood tests. These tests may not become positive until three to six weeks after the initial infection, so they must be repeated at that interval. Additionally the usual screening test does present the possibility of a false positive, requiring a confirmatory test when that occurs.

Most disease-causing organisms require a break in the protective skin barrier in order to gain access to the body. The *Treponema pallidum* spirochete, however, is able to penetrate the mucus membrane lining of the urethra, genitalia and mouth, the lining of the rectum and even the intact skin. Once through these barriers it spreads rapidly throughout the body, within hours. Syphilis is truly a systemic disease, infecting every organ and tissue in the body. It invades the brain and all of the central nervous system very early even though the evidence of the damage there does not appear for 5 to 10 years.

Syphilis is transmitted primarily through sexual contact, whether it is vaginal, oral or anal or through the penis. A reddened papule usually appears at the site of inoculation within about four weeks. This progresses to an ulcer, which is painless and has a firm base. This lesion is known as the chancre. In untreated individuals this chancre will heal in about an additional four to six weeks. The chancre classically appears on the penis, the vulva or the cervix, but may also be seen on the tongue, lips, inside the mouth, the rectum and even the fingers. It is not unusual for the lesion to be ignored while it heals spontaneously without treatment. This describes the primary stage of syphilis.

If a diagnosis is not made and proper treatment instituted, the disease progresses to the secondary stage, with the bacterium multiplying and producing destruction in virtually every tissue in the body. This destruction takes place in the heart and blood vessels, the brain, spinal cord, eye, kidney, liver, spleen, bones, joints and other tissues. A skin rash usually appears about six to ten weeks after infection. This is accompanied by fever, headache, nausea, loss of appetite, swollen glands, and sore throat. Syphilis has long been labeled the great imitator, and for this reason its diagnosis is frequently delayed. The patient presenting to the physician's office may appear to have any one of a long list of diseases, and treatment may be instituted for the apparent disease. In spite of the multiplicity of symptoms and the extensive nature of the disease at this point, it can still be cured with appropriate antibiotic therapy.

In the absence of treatment of secondary syphilis the symptoms gradually subside and the individual feels and appears reasonably normal, particularly after the second year. The disease may still be transmitted to others through sexual contact, and through pregnancy to the newborn. During this latent period syphilis continues to damage the many organs of the body. About one-half of the victims suffer damage to the aortic heart valve, the coronary arteries or the aorta, with aneurysm (ballooning) of the latter. These changes become apparent ten to thirty years after the initial infection.

Symptoms of syphilitic infection in the brain, such as headache, dizziness, poor concentration, mental confusion, insomnia, difficulty in speech, seizures, and blurred vision may become apparent in anywhere from a few months to ten years. Weakness in the muscles of the arms and legs may also appear during this period, but the more serious weakness and paralysis of these areas may not appear for twenty years. Destruction of the nerve tracts in the spinal cord results in serious impairment of coordination of walking and periodic attacks of severe pain in the legs. This characteristically occurs about 25 to 30 years into the disease.

Many of the symptoms of syphilis at this stage do not evoke consideration of this disease in the diagnosis. Many of the later manifestations, however, are strongly suggestive, and some are very characteristic. Treatment at this late stage of the disease must be much more intense than that which is applied in the earlier stages, but no amount of therapy will reverse the damage already done. Treatment does afford some relief for some of the more troublesome symptoms. Individuals being treated at this stage of the disease require regular and periodic assessment for a prolonged period to assure that the disease has been arrested.

Remarkably the *Treponema pallidum* organism of syphilis remains fully susceptible to penicillin. In the early stage of the disease a single injection of long acting penicillin cures about 95 percent of the cases. Later stages of the disease require increased doses over more prolonged periods. In every instance it is essential to recheck blood tests over an adequate period of time to be assured that a cure has been achieved. Failure to persevere in this follow-up may result in progression to advanced stages of the disease. Individuals with HIV infection who contract syphilis are more difficult to cure, and require more intensive investigation and treatment.

It is essential that all sexual contacts of individuals who have been diagnosed with syphilis be identified, tested and treated adequately. This is a very sensitive and difficult undertaking. It is not always accomplished and the consequences are tragic. It is very sad to discover a positive test for syphilis as part of routine pre-surgical evaluation in a woman whose husband has passed on. A great laxity in pursuing the long established and proven control measures has developed in recent years.

In 1988 the Centers for Disease Control, concerned about the increase in the incidence of syphilis and congenital syphilis, urged a return to the traditional practice of interviews and sex partner notification. Screening for sexually transmitted diseases in high-risk populations was also recommended. These should be standard procedure for all sexually transmitted diseases. To exempt any STD from these measures is foolhardy and irresponsible. In 1866 the British Parliament passed the Contagious Diseases Act which mandated that prostitutes who worked near military or naval facilities must receive periodic medical examinations, and further mandated treatment for venereal infections when found. Perhaps we could take a lesson from history.

GONORRHEA

Gonorrhea is caused by a bacterium, *Neisseria gonorrhea,* which is easily identified under the light microscope after proper staining. The organism is present in discharges from infected areas (the urethra, cervix and rectum). The discharge may be absent in chronic infections of the cervix, pharynx and larynx. Gonococcal infection in the rectum and pharynx is common in male homosexuals, and may be asymptomatic. About one-half of women infected with gonorrhea have no symptoms, or at least not pronounced enough to prompt them to seek treatment. Culture is required to identify these chronically infected individuals. Culture is simple and easily accomplished, but requires specific techniques that frequently are not adhered to strictly. Because of this many cultures are falsely reported as negative. In about 20 percent of women with gonorrhea the infection ascends to the fallopian tubes to produce salpingitis that results in sterility.

The acquisition of any of the sexually transmitted diseases is frequently associated with a concomitant infection with another STD. For this reason the other diseases should be screened for. The test for syphilis should always be performed when any sexually transmitted disease is diagnosed. It should be repeated two to three months later, since it may take that long for the test to become positive.

Symptoms of gonorrhea in men characteristically begin on the third to fourteenth day after sexual contact with an infected individual. Burning with urination is followed by a yellowish discharge, which is a reliable indication of the infection. The infection in the urethra may be followed by epididymitis, with pain, swelling and inflammation in the scrotum. In women the symptoms are generally about one week later in presenting and they may be less pronounced. The infection involves the cervix and associated glands as well as the urethra. Salpingitis, infection in the fallopian tubes, is a common complication. Gonorrhea is responsible for about one-half of such infections, which frequently result in sterility.

Sadly gonorrhea must be looked for in young girls who present with a vaginal discharge. The incidence of this infection in young girls has increased with the increase in the incidence of crime and sexual abuse of children in our society.

Gonococcal infections in the pharynx and rectum have become common in recent years. In either of these infections symptoms may or may not be present. It has become common practice to routinely obtain a culture from the rectum when obtaining cervical cultures. A rectal culture for gonorrhea should also be obtained from men with a rectal discharge or suspicious symptoms.

As is the case with all sexually transmitted diseases, all sexual partners should be examined and treated. Failure to do so not only guarantees a recurrent infection that may not be as readily treated, but also assures further transmission of the disease to other noninfected individuals. In the 1950s all cases of gonorrhea could be readily cured by penicillin. Since that time strains of the organism that are resistant to not only penicillin but to alternate antibiotics as well have evolved, presenting a serious challenge. By 1999 strains of *Neisseria gonorrhea* that were resistant to not only penicillin, but also to the newer fluoroquinolone antibiotics were being increasingly reported.[6] The continued transmission of gonorrhea at a high rate greatly increases the risk of further development of resistant strains. Gonorrhea is the most common reportable infectious disease in the United States, with 690,000 cases reported in 1990, and 620,478 in 1991. Estimates at that time placed the actual number of people infected at 3 million. The number of cases reported has since declined steadily, but about 340,000 cases were still reported in 1999. As has been the case with other STDs many cases are not reported.

GENITAL HERPES

Genital herpes is a viral infection that can occur anywhere on the genitalia or around the rectum in either sex. The most common site in women is the cervix and vagina; in men the glans penis. The responsible virus is herpes simplex virus, type 1 (HSV-1) and type 2 (HSV-2), which can be distinguished by their DNA and antigenic differences. Type 1 is seen principally in or around the mouth, but about 5% of genital infections are caused by HSV-1. HSV-2 produces the predominance of genital cases. The disease is contracted through sexual contact, producing itching and redness of the skin or mucosa about 4 to 7 days after exposure. A cluster of small painful blisters then appears which progress to small ulcers. These are particularly painful when they are located in or around the urethra. Healing is usually complete in two weeks or less. At that time the virus has established itself in the nerve cells (ganglia) where it resides for the lifetime of the individual. It remains latent for variable periods, descending periodically to cause recurrent lesions. The frequency of these recurrences varies from rare to three or more a year in different individuals. Reactivation is initiated by stress, menstruation and exposure to ultraviolet light (sun). Recent studies have revealed that viral shedding continues even in the absence of an overt recurrence of lesions.

Cervical infection with herpes has been associated with the subsequent development of cervical cancer. The more immediate threat is to the fetus during a vaginal delivery. If the infection is active during delivery there is a high incidence of infection in the newborn. With untreated encephalitis and local involvement such as the eyes and mouth the mortality rate in the infant is 60 percent. In untreated disseminated infection in the newborn there is a mortality rate of 85 percent. At least 95 percent of those who do survive demonstrate severe neurological damage, which may not become apparent until 2 to 3 years of age. Appropriate antiviral (acyclovir) treatment may improve survival rates but does not eliminate the neurological consequences. In those treated infants who do survive only 40 percent develop normally. The virus may spread to many other organs and tissues of the infant with a 60 percent mortality rate when that occurs, even with antiviral treatment. Ninety percent of those infants who have involvement of the internal organs suffer subsequent complications.

In adults the virus can be spread from the genital lesions to the finger. It may also be spread to the eye and may invade the brain and cause encephalitis. The virus can be identified by taking a specimen from an active lesion, using appropriate care and techniques. It can be transmitted to others even in the absence of any evidence of infection. The clear message is that the current epidemic of genital herpes presents grave consequences for our society and future generations.

GENITAL WARTS (Condyloma Acuminata)

All warts in humans are caused by one of the more than 63 strains of human papillomavirus (HPV) that have been identified.[7] The source for all of these DNA viruses is another human; there is no other natural reservoir. On the skin they gain entrance through an abrasion or other break in the epithelium. The virus invades and dominates the metabolic processes of the cell nucleus, where it replicates. This presents the potential for abnormal cell growth, and indeed squamous cell carcinoma of the finger and around the nail has been found to be associated with chronic common warts.[8,9] This finding would seem to indicate that all warts should be treated, replacing the laissez faire attitude of the past. It is also of note that warts respond to treatment more readily early than they do when they have been established for a long period of time.

Genital warts are caused by six or more different strains of HPV. They have been associated with the development of cervical cancer, even when they occur on the external genitalia. HPV types 6 and 11 are the types that most frequently cause genital infections, and they are almost always associated with benign external warts. Types 16 and 18 on the other hand, which generally do not cause external genital warts, have been shown to cause anal and genital cancers. Carcinogens that are present in cigarette smoke have been found in the mucus on the cervix and smoking increases the risk of the development of cervical cancer in the presence of HPV.[10,11] Several studies have demonstrated that HPV is the primary cause for virtually all cases of cervical cancer.[12] HPV has also been implicated in the development of cancers of the tonsils and oropharynx.[13]

It is now known that cervical cancer is a sexually transmitted disease, caused by infection with the human papilloma virus.[14] The risk is directly related to the number of sexual partners that one has during her lifetime. The risk also is higher in women who first have intercourse at a young age. As a result of the sexual revolution in the 1960s the risk of cervical cancer is fourteen times greater in women born in the early 1960s than in similar women who were born before 1935.[15] In the 1930s cervical cancer was the most common cause of cancer deaths among women in the United States. Both the incidence of and the mortality rates from cervical cancer declined dramatically following the institution of routine screening utilizing the Papanicolaou preparation.[16] Human papillomaviruses are transmitted by sexual activities and can be found anywhere on moist genital surfaces such as the cervix, vagina, the penis and foreskin, in the urethra and in and around the rectum. HPV infection in male homosexuals who have HIV has been associated with a high incidence of anal carcinoma. As in the cervix, the area affected is the squamo-columnar juncture, the transition zone. The warts appear at about 2 to 3 months after inoculation, but this period varies.

The incidence of genital warts has increased greatly since the mid 1970s, another reflection of the so called "sexual revolution." The CDC estimates that about 24 million people in the U.S. are infected with genital HPV. The warts present a challenge in treatment because of the multiplicity of the lesions and because many infected areas are not visible to the eye. The infection may be extensive throughout the vagina and/or rectum. There is no systemic medication that can be taken to eradicate the virus. As with the herpes viruses, once the papillomaviruses become established in the body there is no way to eliminate them. The fact that the virus integrates with the DNA in the cells within the body has serious implications. Treatment of genital warts entails repeated visits to the office, usually on a weekly basis.

Multiple genital warts, especially within the vagina or rectum, will require more extended periods of treatment. This may be done with podophyllin, laser, cryosurgery, or bichloracetic acid. There is no way to ascertain whether or not the virus in the wart has been completely eliminated, and recurrence of genital warts is common with all treatments. Given the alarming increase in the incidence of both genital herpes and condyloma, it seems certain that the incidence of cervical cancer will increase in the future. The need for periodic and regular Papanicolaou smears is even more urgent now than ever before. It also is very urgent that these specimens be collected carefully and properly, which they frequently are not. Any specimen that does not collect endocervical cells, as verified on the report from the pathologist, risks missing an existing cancer.

MOLLUSCUM CONTAGIOSUM

This poxvirus infection is characterized by small, pink tumors that have an appearance similar to warts. These may occur on the face, arms or buttocks, on any area of direct contact. The lesions also may be spread from inanimate objects such as towels and barber's capes and instruments. It has been less common than the other sexually transmitted diseases, but with the increase in sex as a recreational activity it has been on the increase, especially among the young. The virus is much more difficult to identify than the herpes virus, and much less is known about its long-term implications. Although you may avoid the risk of sexual transmission, it is important that you assure yourself that your barber understands and meets the minimal hygienic precautions. Not all of them do, and this has been a route of transmission of the virus.

CHANCROID

Chancroid is a sexually transmitted bacterial infection caused by *Hemophilus ducreyi*. In 1947, 9,515 cases were reported to the Centers for Disease Control. This number declined as a result of antibiotics and public health efforts so that an annual mean of 878 cases was reported between 1971–1980. An epidemic among foreign workers in Orange County, California in 1981 initiated an upward trend in the disease, peaking in 1987 at 5,035 cases for that year. Cases during the epidemic were spread primarily through prostitution, and this remains a principle source of the disease in the general population. Exchange of sex for drugs is another major source of spread of the disease. Over 4,000 cases are reported to the Centers for Disease Control each year currently.

A study conducted by the Centers for Disease Control in 1990 suggested that many cases of chancroid are not diagnosed, and thus not reported.[17] A definitive diagnosis requires the culture of *H. ducreyi* from lesions on suspected patients, but culture media for this purpose is not commercially available. Even more disconcerting was the finding that of the 115 sexually transmitted disease clinics surveyed (operated by city or county health departments), less than half had laboratory facilities adequate to differentiate between chancroid, syphilis and herpes, the three diseases most likely to cause genital ulcers. The study revealed some serious deficiencies in diagnostic capabilities of many STD clinics.

Chancroid is ushered in by the appearance of small, painful papules on the genitalia at the site of contact about 3 to 5 days after inoculation. These then ulcerate, increasing the risk of contracting

HIV infection, as is the case with all venereal sores. Infection spreads to the inguinal lymph nodes causing tender enlargement followed by abscess formation. Antibiotic therapy has been effective in the past, but the organism has developed an increasing level of resistance. It is common for such antibiotic resistance to develop in bacterial infections that are inadequately diagnosed and treated repeatedly.

LYMPHOGRANULOMA VENEREUM

This STD, caused by another strain of *Chlamydia trachomatis*, is one of the less frequently seen in the United States; about 300 cases are reported annually. It is more common in homosexual males in the U.S., in whom rectal infections, accompanied by considerable pain, are common. The disease is endemic in Asia, Africa and Latin America. It is likely that we will see an increase in the incidence of lymphogranuloma venereum in the U.S. in the future. In addition to fever, chills, headache and joint pains, the inguinal lymph nodes become swollen. It can be treated successfully with doxycycline, but treatment must be continued for a long time.

VAGINITIS

Vaginitis is an extremely common infection, caused by a variety of organisms. During the past generation it seems to have become an almost universal disease. The majority of cases are sexually acquired, as any physician who has struggled to cure these cases can attest to. Even under the best of circumstances it is not possible to cure a case unless the sexual partner(s) also receive(s) treatment. It is very difficult to convince a man who has no symptoms that he should be treated, however. It is also very difficult to bring treatment to all of the sexual partners in many cases.

Trichomonas vaginalis, a protozoan, accounts for between one-third and one-half of all cases of vaginitis. It is harbored in the prostate of an unknown percentage of men, only rarely producing any noticeable symptoms. This undoubtedly accounts for the high re-infection rate among women. The organism has a distinctive appearance and is readily recognized in specimens collected from infected women. Collection and transport to the laboratory require some attention to detail, however, as with gonorrhea, herpes and chlamydia. A culture technique is now available that relieves the medical personnel of some of this burden, and improves the chances for an accurate diagnosis.

Protozoan infections are difficult to treat; no antibiotic is effective. Prior to 1960 no effective treatment was available for trichomoniasis. We are currently fortunate to have metronidazole (Flagyl®), which is very effective in both males and females. Unfortunately some resistance to the drug has developed recently, and this can be expected to become a major problem. Both (all) sexual partners must be treated to cure this disease. Obviously this would be a challenge in a harem or a brothel.

Chlamydia trachomatis, anothe cause of vulvovaginitis, is a bacterium that behaves more like a virus in that it is an obligate intra-cellular parasite. This means that the organism can exist and reproduce only inside cells of the host. It cannot be grown on the usual culture media but can be cultivated on appropriate tissue cultures. Collection techniques must be very specific. For these reasons *Chlamydia* was not recognized as the culprit in urethritis and some other diseases until recently. It is now recognized to be the most common of the sexually transmitted diseases in the United States, with about four million cases annually. Ascending infections with *Chlamydia* result in as many as 500,000 cases of pelvic inflammatory disease each year and account for much of the increase in the incidence of infertility in women in recent years.

Chlamydia produces urethritis in males and cervicitis in females. The symptoms in both resemble gonorrhea, but the characteristic discharge of gonorrhea is absent. The disease produces no symptoms in some individuals even though they are capable of transmitting it to others. This disease in men was classified as non-gonococcal urethritis (NGU) for many years because no organism could be demonstrated. Advances in culture techniques finally revealed the culprit. The infection may spread to the contents of the scrotum in the form of an epididymitis. In the female it may spread to the fallopian tubes, causing infertility.

Newborn infants may acquire chlamydia eye and lung infections in their passage through the maternal birth canal. The routine treatment instilled in the eyes of all newborns does not assure resolution of these eye infections. The tetracyclines are effective in treating most of the infections caused by *Chlamydia*, another characteristic separating them from viruses. The newer fluoroquinolones and azithromycin also are effective. With the frequency of *Chlamydia* infections, and the large number of people being treated, it is very likely that resistant strains will emerge.

Bacterial vaginitis is common, but the cause is frequently obscure. *Gardnerella vaginalis (Hemophilus vaginalis)* is the most frequently found bacterial organism, but often others are present. Very often a "cocktail" of microorganisms is found. Infections due to *E. coli* from the intestinal tract occur in young girls and in women who are careless in cleansing techniques after a bowel movement. Young girls can also acquire vaginal infections from sitting on the ground. Factors that alter the normal protective environment of the vagina appear to play a part in infection. Diagnosis of bacterial infections can usually be made by examination of stained specimens under the light microscope. Characteristic "clue cells" identify *Gardnerella* infections. *E. coli* can be identified with a Gram stain. Treatment is directed at the specific organisms involved and includes efforts to lower the pH (increase the acidity) of the vagina to encourage growth of the normal bacterial flora. Bacterial vaginitis during pregnancy is associated with an increased incidence of miscarriages and infections after childbirth.

Candida albicans (yeast) infections occur more frequently in diabetics, post-menopausal women and in cases where the normal vaginal milieu has been altered. Tight, nonabsorbent underclothing contributes to this as well as bacterial infections of the vagina, especially in the presence of poor hygiene. *Candida* can be readily diagnosed under the light microscope, but several simple and convenient culture systems are available to any physician. One of the antifungal suppositories or creams e.g. miconazole is effective, but the underlying contributing factors must be corrected in order to avoid recurrence.

PELVIC INFLAMMATORY DISEASE (PID)

PID is a bacterial infection of the fallopian tubes and surrounding structures. It virtually always spreads from the uterus to the tubes, usually from a cervicitis that is sexual in origin. Introduction of infection into the uterus is always a risk during surgical procedures, including insertion of an intra-uterine device

(IUD). Scrupulous surgical aseptic techniques are mandatory for these procedures, and carelessness can readily yield infection. The most common organism causing PID in the past was *Neisseria gonorrhea*, but currently it shares the spotlight about evenly with *Chlamydia trachomatis*. In view of the significant increase in the incidence of tuberculosis in our society, infection in the tubes from that organism, more common in the past, may enjoy a resurgence. Teenagers and promiscuous women are at greater risk of tubal infections as a complication of STDs than are older women. The major sequelae of PID are infertility and ectopic pregnancy, both of which result from scarring in the fallopian tubes. The incidence of ectopic pregnancy, a serious and life threatening condition, increased six-fold between 1970 and 1997 as a result of the increase in sexually transmitted diseases

Treatment of PID is best approached as a hospital procedure, and must be directed toward the offending organism(s). Follow-up cultures should be done to confirm successful eradication of all organisms involved. Treatment of PID has notoriously presented a high rate of failure. This may be due in part to failure to correctly identify all organisms properly, or to reinfection. As with all sexually transmitted diseases, all sexual partners must be treated, and treated adequately. Barrier contraceptive devices provide some protection against the infections that result in PID, but the protection is far from absolute. Great care must also be exercised whenever douching to avoid forcing infection into the uterus and tubes. Obstructing the outflow in order to distend the vagina is a risky technique that should never be practiced.

URETHRITIS

Females are particularly prone to develop infections in the urethra, partially because of the anatomy of the structure, and partly due to the anatomic proximity of the urethral opening to the anus. Poor hygiene further enhances this risk. Sexual intercourse also facilitates the introduction of organisms into the urethra by the mechanical massaging inherent therein. *E. coli* from the intestinal tract is the most common causative organism. Pain and burning with urination accompany the infection. If the infection spreads to the bladder, pain above the pubic region is added along with urgency and frequency of urination. Antibacterial treatment should be directed at the offending organism after it has been identified.

EPIDIDYMITIS

Infection in the epididymis in the scrotum results from the spread of infection from the urethra or the prostate. The infecting organisms in men 35 years of age and under are *Neisseria gonorrhea* and *Chlamydia trachomatis*. Significant pain and swelling in the scrotum usually prompts the individual to seek medical attention and helps to make the diagnosis apparent. Appropriate antibiotic therapy along with scrotal support results in a resolution of the infection. In the case of a recalcitrant prostatic infection recurrence can be expected.

CERVICAL CANCER

As discussed previously, the revelation by recent studies that cancer of the cervix is almost invariably the sequelae of infection with the human papilloma virus, it must be considered a sexually transmitted disease. Six of the strains of human papilloma viruses have been incriminated in the development of cervical cancer. The herpes simplex virus, even when the initial infection is on the vulva rather than the cervix, also has been incriminated in the subsequent development of cervical cancer. Even though the infection clears, these viruses remain in the nerve ganglia, latent, indefinitely. The integration of these viruses into the DNA in the cells not only explains the mechanism of the malignant transformation, but also would seem to guarantee against any system to eradicate the organisms from the body.

SCABIES and PEDICULOSIS

Pediculosis (head and body lice) and scabies, parasitic afflictions that have increased greatly in incidence in the past 25 years, can also be shared during sexual encounters. Pediculosis can be acquired by simply crawling into a bed where the louse has been left behind. Scabies requires bodily contact. Both of these problems are discussed in Chapter XV.

HEPATITIS

Viral hepatitis is another relatively new addition to the listing of sexually transmitted diseases. This is not because the disease is new but simply because the incidence of the disease has increased so dramatically. The hepatitis A and hepatitis E viruses are shed in the stool and are transmitted by the fecal-oral route. They can also be transmitted by needles, as is the case with hepatitis B and C. Aside from drug users, however, hepatitis A and E are transmitted by getting fecal contaminated food, water, ice, hands or other objects to the mouth.

Hepatitis A is not transmitted by conventional sexual intercourse. During 1991, however, there was a significant increase in the number of cases of hepatitis A reported among homosexual males in New York City, San Francisco, Denver, Toronto and Montreal. No such trend was observed among the heterosexual population. This increase is interpreted as a reflection of sexual practices that favor fecal-oral transmission, rather than any change in the virus or the means that the disease is transmitted.

Hepatitis B **IS** transmitted by conventional sexual practices. Both the semen and saliva are infectious, and sexual contact with people who either have active disease or who are carriers presents a very real, almost certain, risk of contracting the disease. Transmission of hepatitis C by sexual contact appears to occur, but studies done thus far indicate that this is infrequent, and that it is transmitted primarily by needle stick, blood products and by IV drug use.[18,19] Unlike hepatitis A, hepatitis B and C are not commonly spread through the feces because of their lipid capsule.

Hepatitis B is also spread through the placenta from the mother to the infant. Ninety percent of these newborns that acquire hepatitis B from the mother are infected during the birth process rather than through the placenta, however. The risk of this means of transmission of hepatitis C appears to be much less. Most infants born to mothers who have active hepatitis B, or who are chronic carriers, will acquire the disease. Ninety percent of these infants will become carriers of the hepatitis B virus and about 25 percent of these will die in adulthood of cirrhosis or cancer of the liver. All infants who are born to mothers who test positive for the hepatitis B virus should receive both immune globulin and hepatitis B vaccine immediately after birth to prevent these tragic sequelae. No vaccine is yet available for hepatitis C.

Individuals who have active hepatitis B or who are carriers can and do transmit the disease to sexual partners. The only adequate protection against the acquisition of hepatitis B from sexual activity is immunization. The only vaccine for hepatitis B that is currently marketed in the U.S. is a recombinant bioengineered product. It is not derived from blood and is both safe and effective. Sexual partners of people who have active hepatitis B, or who are carriers of the disease, should receive the vaccine. As mentioned previously, no such vaccine for hepatitis C has been developed as yet and there is no simple effective treatment for it (see chapter XV). It carries a much higher incidence of chronic hepatitis and cirrhosis than does hepatitis B. The success in developing a vaccine for hepatitis B has spurred the search for a similar vaccine for hepatitis C. The fact that there are a number of different strains of the hepatitis C virus has hindered those efforts, however. See Chapter XV for a more detailed discussion of hepatitis.

AIDS

Acquired immunodeficiency syndrome (AIDS) is the term applied to the symptom complex of opportunistic infections that develop as a result of infection with the human immunodeficiency virus (HIV). The criteria for the definition is set forth by the Centers for Disease Control in Atlanta, and has been subject to modifications as time progresses and our knowledge of the disease expands. Unfortunately political pressure from special interest groups has also influenced the selection of criteria more recently. Classification as an AIDS patient can result in generous financial support. Various government programs, including Medicaid, Social Security, and those of the National Institutes of Health, the CDC, HUD, the Veterans Administration and the Agency for International Development spend in excess of $7 billion each year in welfare payments to HIV infected individuals and other support programs.

The opportunistic infections (e.g. pneumonia from *Pneumocystis carinii*, and infections from cytomegalovirus, cryptococcus, candida, cryptosporidium and others) are caused by microorganisms that are present in our everyday environment but which do not ordinarily gain a foothold in our bodies because of our natural defense mechanisms (the immune system). When this defense system is compromised and rendered less effective these organisms are able to set up shop and to reproduce. The microorganisms that are able to invade the body when the immune defenses are lowered include bacteria, fungi, viruses and protozoa. One unfortunate consequence of this new chapter in infectious diseases is that the thousands of immunodeficient individuals with these unusual diseases are cultivating strains that are more virulent and resistant to the agents that we have used to control them. They have already begun to share these new strains with the general population.

Most homosexual men exhibit a mild suppression of the immune system even in the absence of HIV infection, but the CD4 lymphocyte counts and ratios remain within the normal range. On the other hand, certain drugs such as those used to prevent the body from rejecting organ transplants, and to treat malignant neoplasms (cancers), significantly suppress the body's immune system. Other conditions that also result in a compromised immune system in the body are leukemia, Hodgkin's disease, multiple myeloma, and aplastic anemia. Cortisone medications suppress the immune system, and this often prevents their use in conditions where they would be useful. All of these conditions that depress the body's immune system increase the risk of opportunistic infections becoming established. These cases, as well as congenitally acquired immunodeficiency states, are excluded from the definition of AIDS.

The epidemic of immunodeficiency among AIDS patients began about 1980. The causative agent of AIDS is the human immunodeficiency virus (HIV). When it was initially isolated in 1983 it was referred to as the human T-lymphotrophic virus Type III (HTLV-III), but once characteristic differences between it and HTLV were recognized in the latter half of 1986, the terminology was changed. Both are retroviruses in which the genetic code is incorporated in RNA within the virus, rather than in DNA, as is the case in other viruses. In order for replication to take place it is necessary for the virus to make a DNA copy of this code. Retroviruses contain an enzyme, reverse transcriptase, which accomplishes this after the virus invades the cells of the victim. The discoverers of this enzyme and this unusual process were rewarded with the Nobel Prize for Medicine in 1975.[20] Each time the host cells divide, new copies of the virus are produced.

Four human retroviruses have been identified at present, and these are divided into two separate groups, HIV-1 and HIV-2 in one group, and HTLV-I and HTLV-II in the other group. The human T lymphotrophic virus, HTLV-I, is responsible for adult T-cell leukemia/lymphoma. HTLV-II is closely related to HTLV-I, and is probably associated with a myelopathy and possibly some forms of leukemia. The extent of diseases associated with HTLV-II has not been fully established as yet. These two viruses have been identified only recently (HTLV-I in 1979), and relatively little is known about them.

The paucity of investigative studies is surprising, particularly in view of the fact that we know that these viruses are transmitted in blood. This factor alone should assign a high priority to research into their properties and control of their transmission. We also know that they are sexually transmitted, at least in some societies. We have known since 1988 that approximately 1,000 units of donated blood each year are infected with HTLV-II. A number of cases of cutaneous T-cell lymphoma mycosis fungoides that resulted from blood transfusions have been reported since 1991. This has been a rare disease, but the number of cases following transfusion is growing. Increasingly, certain religious prohibitions against blood transfusions appear to have been prudent after all.

The highest prevalence of HTLV-I infection in the world is in the southwestern district of Japan, primarily in Kyushu. There is also a high prevalence in the Caribbean Islands and the surrounding countries. The Japanese have studied the infection and its sequelae in some depth. They have concluded that HTLV-I is the direct causative agent of adult T-cell leukemia, a disease entity that was first identified in 1977. The virus was then identified in 1979,[21] and it was the first known human retrovirus. HTLV-I is also associated with other diseases such as uveitis, chronic lung disease, chronic renal failure, opportunistic lung infections, cancer of other organs, spastic paresis and others.[22]

These studies have suggested that there are three modes of transmission of HTLV-I, all requiring contact of infected lymphocytes with lymphocytes of the victim. Sexual transmission from husband to wife occured frequently, but rarely from wife to husband. Transmission also occured by transfusion of infected blood, but the Japanese have eliminated this route since 1986 by

456

testing all transfusion blood for the presence of the virus. We could learn from this example. The third mode of transmission was through breast-feeding. HTLV-I positive mothers are discouraged from breast-feeding. All of these findings may bear significantly on HIV infections and transmission.

Prior to 1996 commercial blood tests to detect and differentiate HTLV-I and HTLV-II were not available. The newer test kits now available provide enhanced detection of HTLV-II in blood supplies. PCR techniques also are now available to differentiate the two. Availability of these tests is important because of the linkage of HTLV-I with leukemia/lymphoma, and because intravenous drug users have been shown to test positive for it. A reliable test would provide an additional surrogate test for a group of donors known to also have a high incidence of hepatitis B and HIV infection.

These facts, taken in conjunction with the cavalier attitude demonstrated by some blood collection centers in collecting from donor groups known to be infected with the AIDS virus, lead us to the inevitable conclusion that large numbers of people have been infected with viruses through blood transfusions. This was graphically demonstrated in 1987 with the discovery of the hepatitis C virus, and the realization that it has been transmitted to millions of people through blood products. The true extent of this hazard from blood products is not known because all of the appropriate studies have not been undertaken. Intimidation by the militant organized homosexual lobby has discouraged serious interest in such studies.

The second group of human retroviruses, the human immunodeficiency viruses HIV-1 and HIV-2, are responsible for AIDS. They are members of the lentivirus subfamily of retroviruses, and like all retroviruses they are RNA viruses. Virtually all of the cases of AIDS in the western world are caused by HIV-1. HIV-2 is much less common and has been identified as a cause of AIDS primarily in Africa. It is considered to be a less potent cause of disease than HIV-1. The two can be readily distinguished and categorized by virologists on the basis of certain characteristics. These processes are far more complex than the methods that are used to classify bacteria, however (staining characteristics, reaction to and utilization of certain culture media in the case of bacteria). To complicate matters further, mutations in HIV-1 can produce thousands of different variations, thus thwarting efforts to develop a vaccine. Many different variants of the virus can be found even in a single infected individual. This feature also permits it to become resistant to the few drugs that have been developed to control it.

Simian immunodeficiency viruses (SIV) are closely related genetically and antigenically to HIV-2. They produce an AIDS-like illness in some primates, including some that are commonly used for research. This infection has been transmitted to laboratory workers, both from contact with the animals and from blood and serum of the animals. In one case the infection was transferred not by a needle stick or bite, but merely through a skin rash. The positive blood test in these individuals could not be differentiated from HIV-2. The long-term significance of these events is unknown. A similar transmission of the human immunodeficiency virus (HIV-1) to a laboratory worker through a skin rash has been documented.[23]

It has been proposed that HIV-1 in humans evolved from a simian virus in Africa, supposedly the green monkey, or from a subspecies of chimpanzee. One scientist who has presented this implausible thesis to the public is fully aware of the impossibility of any such evolution. This is the virologist at the National Cancer Institute who claimed credit for the discovery of the virus and for the development of the HIV blood test, for which he has been receiving royalties of $100,000 annually. After the Pasteur Institute challenged his patent, lengthy investigations by several bodies, both government and private, disclosed that he had indeed used cultures of the virus from the Pasteur Institute for his alleged discoveries. In spite of the facts that were uncovered the United States Government expended every effort to cover-up and suppress the evidence. Reports from outside experts in the scientific community were ignored.

A deluge of articles were then published in the scientific journals in the early 1990s denouncing this case and other cases of scientific fraud. Some of these cases involved major academic institutions, and resulted in a re-evaluation of the rules governing ethical conduct in science. The results did not reflect favorably upon some academic institutions. The documentation of lies and deceit at the National Institutes of Health are a testimonial to the dishonest, immoral and devious character of some of the corrupt individuals who have infested the government health agencies, and

458

the U.S. government in general, for a long period of time. The disinformation campaign to deceive the American people about the origin of AIDS follows the pattern of previous unethical and criminal experimentation on U.S. civilian and military personnel. The pattern has been repeated most recently in the lies and deception regarding the Gulf War Illness mentioned previously. Experts are certain that the AIDS virus, HIV-1, did not evolve from any animal; it still cannot be found naturally in any animal species.

Although a suitable candidate for the evolution of HIV-2 has been found in a simian immunovirus in sooty mangabeys (monkeys) in West Africa, none has been found for HIV-1. Moreover while HIV-1 will replicate in chimpanzees when they are experimentally inoculated, it will not do so in any species of monkey. These factors are presented as evidence by some scientists that HIV-1 was in fact cultivated by the National Cancer Institute and the World Health Organization (WHO) in their laboratory at Fort Detrick in Frederick, Maryland. Research done by Dr. Theodore A. Strecker, one of the world's leading scientists in AIDS research until his assassination on August 11, 1988, suggests that the virus resulted from combining the bovine leukemia virus and the sheep visna virus, both retroviruses, and growing them in human tissue cultures. The result was the human retrovirus, HIV-1.[24]

Such efforts were known to be taking place in 1974 when the National Academy of Sciences urged scientists throughout the world to discontinue experiments attempting to link animal viruses. During the same year the World Health Organization suggested that a virus thus developed could be included in a vaccine for a mass immunization program as an experiment to study patterns of subsequent transmission. It is common knowledge that the vaccinia virus used in smallpox vaccination is still being considered as a vehicle for introducing foreign genes into selected populations. This appears to have been the mechanism for the introduction of HIV-1 during the WHO's smallpox immunization program in Africa, Haiti and Brazil.

The connection between the smallpox immunization program and the onset of AIDS was reported on the front page of the *London Times* in its May 11, 1987 issue. Scientists have pointed out that if HIV-1 had evolved from a single source in Africa, and spread in the manner that outbreaks are known to multiply, we would have at most several thousand cases today. In order to have instead the millions of cases that we know exist, many people had to be inoculated at the same time. This would have occurred in the early 1970s, during the period of the WHO smallpox vaccination program. The geographic pattern of the HIV-1 epidemic in those countries also coincides with that program.

The World Health Organization has been caught in several unsavory and unethical activities. In 1996 the Philippine Medical Association discovered that the tetanus toxoid vaccine that the WHO was administering in that nation included an abortifacient agent that had been added covertly. The program, designed and administered by WHO, was offered only to women aged 15 to 45, the group most likely to be pregnant, and was denied to men and to children. The goal was to precipitate an abortion in those women who were pregnant. The WHO carried out the same program in Mexico and Nicaragua. There is an obsession that borders on paranoia among these New World Order elite regarding over-population of the earth. Introduction of AIDS into Africa through the smallpox vaccination program could wipe out 75 million of what these people term "useless eaters."

Some scientists dispute the "conspiracy theory" that HIV-1 was cultivated in the laboratory, pointing to recent findings of foreign retroviral DNA hidden in the DNA of normal cells in humans. They theorize that this material is a residual from generations ago, but nobody knows the facts behind the origin of this material, or its significance. It is possible that the virus existed in a less virulent form before the development of the newer detection tool of PCR, discussed later. The expansion of rampant, wholesale anal sexual promiscuity, with many different partners each night, in homosexual communities such as San Francisco certainly would have been conducive to the cultivation of a more virulent strain of a virus. This is especially true of a virus that mutates as frequently as HIV-I. The sudden eruption of AIDS in thousands of persons over wide and divergent geographic areas could not have occurred under any such evolutionary scheme, however. Some people continue to insist that HIV-1 was transmitted to man from a monkey, but this contradicts present scientific knowledge and facts.

Although the Human Immune Virus, HIV-1, was not isolated until the end of 1983, two years after the first case of AIDS was recognized, retrospective studies of stored blood samples suggest that it appeared in the blood supply of the United States in 1978. It is not present in any of the stored blood samples that were collected before that year. The subsequent spread of the disease in the U.S. was again explosive, incompatible with the transmission from Haiti explanation offered by some authorities. According to Dr. William Campbell Douglass the onset and spread of the disease in the United States mirrored the hepatitis B immunization program among the homosexual population.[25] He reported in 1991 that 100 percent of the population that received hepatitis B vaccine in that program were infected with the AIDS virus. He also reported the strange administration of that program by a recent Polish-Russian immigrant who somehow became head of the New York City blood bank, who then set up the rules for the immunization program.

Those rules stipulated that the hepatitis B vaccine would be administered only to homosexuals who were promiscuous, thus guaranteeing the efficient spread of any virus that might have been surreptitiously incorporated into the vaccine. This is the same technique that was used by the World Health Organization in the tetanus toxoid program described previously, and in countless other unknown programs.

In 1984 the CDC published a report which was a smoke screen, attempting to deny the connection between the hepatitis B immunization program in New York City and the subsequent AIDS epidemic.[26] In the cover-up in the report they cited data from Denver rather than from New York City, where the transmission of AIDS actually occurred. All of the records of the New York City program, rather than being stored by the FDA or CDC as is customary, are being hidden by the U.S. Department of Justice. This is very curious and raises some serious and disturbing questions. The long history of lying, deceit and cover-up by our government and bureaucrats, especially those engaged in evil, nefarious activities, should make us all very skeptical of all of their tailor made excuses.

In the 1980s Kary Mullis, a scientist at Cetus Corporation in Emeryville, California, developed the PCR (polymerase chain reaction) technique for identifying a specific DNA or RNA structure. With this technique it is possible to look for evidence of HIV-1 and other viruses in stored blood and autopsy specimens from years past. Mullis won a Nobel Prize in 1993 for this discovery. Applying this tool, some claim that the earliest case of AIDS documented thus far was a British sailor who died in 1959 with a severe immune deficiency that was not understood at the time. Preserved tissue samples from a 17-year-old male homosexual who died in 1968 of strange opportunistic infections revealed "HIV genetic material." He had never been outside of the U.S. Preserved serum samples of IV drug abusers from the 1971 to 1972 period reveal that four percent were HIV-1 positive. These findings suggest that the virus has been around longer than we had believed previously, but whether or not it was the same varmint, with the same genetic structure and virulence is not known. The absence of evidence of transmission and spread suggests that it was not. The possibility of cultivation, modification and distribution of that virus remains.

In the 1980s HIV-1 spread rapidly, infecting one half of the high-risk populations of male homosexuals and IV drug abusers. This spread was facilitated by the promiscuity that resulted from the sexual-social revolution of the time, and the riots and demands from the radical homosexual groups that they be permitted complete and unfettered freedom to engage in any behavior that pleased them. The homosexual bathhouses flourished during this time. Dugas, the French-Canadian airline steward who has been labeled patient zero, is known to have had sex with at least 40 of the first 248 Americans to be diagnosed with AIDS by April 1982.[27] Of the first 19 cases of AIDS reported in Los Angeles, nine had had sexual contact with Dugas.

Two other viruses, unrelated to either HIV or SIV, can be acquired either directly from primates or from infected blood and serum. These are the Marburg virus and the Ebola virus. Both cause African hemorrhagic fever, a serious illness with a high fatality rate. It is readily spread to others and to hospital personnel from infected patients. The Marburg virus was first seen in Marburg and Frankfort, Germany and in Belgrade in 1967 among laboratory workers who had been exposed to African green monkeys. This may be where the advocates of the green monkey theory for the origin of AIDS got the idea, although as virologists they know that it is an implausible explanation. The Marburg virus may have been spread through respiratory droplet infection. One victim transmitted the virus to his wife through his semen in which the virus was detected for at least 61 days. Stringent quarantine measures for imported monkeys were instituted after this outbreak in 1967.

Ebola virus hemorrhagic fever was first seen in July 1976 simultaneously in epidemics in southern Sudan and Zaire. Spread of the infection among family members and hospital personnel was common, probably through contact with blood or secretions from seriously ill patients. Recent studies have recovered the virus not only from the cells in the lungs, but free in the alveoli.[28] It would be prudent to conclude from this that the virus can be spread by aerosol (coughing, sneezing), and precautions taken accordingly.

In the Sudan over 300 cases were reported, with 151 deaths. In Zaire 237 cases with 211 deaths were reported. In outbreaks it is assumed that 80 percent of the victims will die. No monkey had ever been found to be naturally infected with the Ebola virus prior to this epidemic. Where these two viruses came from in nature is still a mystery, in spite of extensive investigation. We know that the natural reservoir is not monkeys. Although researchers have spent much time in the jungles of Africa searching for these viruses they have not thought to look in the research laboratories such as at Fort Detrick. As with HIV some scientists believe that the Ebola virus was genetically engineered from the Marburg virus in laboratories.

In 1989 an outbreak of Ebola virus occurred in a government laboratory in Reston, Virginia among primates that had been imported from the Philippines.[29,30] The infection was transmitted to at least four humans, but the expected serious illness did not develop.[31] The virus was identified as the fourth subtype of the Ebola viruses, and it was concluded that it was less virulent to humans than the three African species had proven to be. Four additional episodes of Ebola virus infection among monkeys imported from the Philippines have occurred in the U.S. The latest episode was in a private quarantine facility in Texas in April 1996, and required the euthanizing of the remainder of the shipment of fifty animals.[32] The most recent outbreak in Africa occurred in Zaire in May 1995 with 296 human cases identified, 79 percent of which were fatal.[33]

In humans infected with the immunodeficiency virus, HIV-1, it is present in all of the body fluids that contain infected white blood cells. These fluids include not only blood but also semen, tears, vaginal secretions and saliva. The tragic case of transmission of HIV infection through artificial insemination is clear proof of the risk from semen.[34] Sweat and urine are suspected but not proven, for no serious studies have been undertaken to make this determination. Certainly in cases of urinary tract infections where white blood cells are present in the urine the virus would be present. It is also important to recognize that anyone who has been infected with HIV-1 can transmit the virus to others, regardless of the stage of his infection, even though he has not developed any symptoms of AIDS.

It is known that white blood cells are shed in feces, and it would seem logical that contact with excrement from infected individuals would present the opportunity for transmission of AIDS. This contact would occur frequently in changing diapers of infected infants, and in caring for adults in the terminal phase of AIDS. Anyone who has a proclivity toward dry, chapped or cracked hands will be at a much greater risk. This will especially apply to health care professionals, who wash their hands frequently, and usually with very efficient and very denuding agents.

HIV infected cells can produce infection in a noninfected individual by direct injection into the blood, or by aggressive contact with mucous membranes or the vaginal or rectal lining. Trauma or abrasion of these membranes facilitates transmission. The rectal lining is much more readily traumatized than is the vaginal lining by virtue of the nature of the cells of the respective tissues. The cells lining the rectum also are a much less effective barrier to the passage of microorganisms than are the cells lining the vagina. Erosion of the cervix, which is very common, as well as the inflammation and lesions associated with herpes greatly increase the risk of acquiring the virus from an infected individual.

There is a great reluctance on the part of the "authorities" to accept the fact that AIDS can be transmitted by saliva. The same people who would have us believe that HIV was initially transmitted to man by the bite of a green monkey insist that it cannot be transmitted through saliva. The incongruity of such a claim is obvious. The most tenuous sales pitch in the world is one that is based upon a lie. Even if saliva proves to be an inefficient transmission agent for the virus, aggressive kissing has already resulted in transmission of the disease. It has been clearly established that HIV-1 can be transmitted by a human bite.[35] This occurred during a seizure, and reinforces the mandate to keep the hands out of the mouth of any patient having a seizure.

It is not uncommon for the gums to bleed with brushing of the teeth, and the risk of HIV transmission under those circumstances is obvious. This phenomenon would also present the opportunity for transmission of the disease during oral sexual activity. It is not known how often this has occurred because no one has made an effort to find out. It is data that will be very difficult to acquire, and will not be even estimated until the event has occurred many times. Even then the data most likely will not be widely publicized.

It is thus obvious that transmission of the disease from male to female is more likely than the reverse, as has been the case in studies of HTLV-I in Japan. Since there is no procedure that can eliminate the virus from semen, transmission of AIDS during artificial insemination presents another risk for females.[36] Transmission from female to male is being reported with increasing frequency, however. A lesion on the penis, such as herpes, greatly increases the possibility of such a transmission. Similarly any inflammation of the glans of the penis such as frequently occurs, especially in uncircumcised men, facilitates the transmission of the AIDS virus from an infected woman. The presence of sexually transmitted diseases increases the risk of transmission of HIV by as much as a hundred times.

Since the first case of AIDS was reported in 1981 it has been the conviction of some authorities that transmission of the virus requires intimate contact of some form. This conviction has been based upon the assumption that the virus is not capable of actively penetrating the skin and other membranes, as is *Treponema pallidum* of syphilis fame. If we could be confident that this is correct we would indeed be fortunate, for this characteristic would greatly reduce the risk of casual transmission. If, on the other hand, it turns out as many physicians and scientists suspect, that the virus is far more resilient in the environment than has been reported, and is capable of significantly more modes of transmission than has been admitted to, then the projections of the number of new cases will have to be revised upwards drastically. It will also mean that the time to the apocalypse will be much shorter than anyone might have imagined.

Studies done by Dr. Braathen in Switzerland and reported in the November 7, 1987 issue of *The Lancet* have thrown a serious chill on the previous optimistic and complacent assumptions. He placed semen infected with the AIDS virus on intact skin. By using fluorescent tagging techniques he was able to demonstrate that the Langerhans cells in the skin quickly and efficiently attached to the virus and transported it through the skin. These findings, which have been confirmed by others, present us with obvious and ominous conclusions; there is a serious possibility that HIV infected blood on intact skin might transmit the virus. Additionally, Langerhans cells also are present in the nose, mouth and esophagus.

We know that health care personnel who have had AIDS contaminated blood splattered in their eyes and mouths have contracted the virus. This was graphically demonstrated in the case of Nashville surgeon Dr. Harold Dennison who contracted AIDS from blood that was splattered in his eyes. He became ill and developed an infection in the cornea that never healed. Even after a corneal transplant they never healed. He subsequently died in January, 1989.[37] Dr. Lorraine Day, who has been a leader in the fight to establish sound precautions against the transmission of AIDS during surgery, personally knows of 18 additional cases.

The risk of contracting AIDS after being stuck with a needle that has been used on an HIV positive patient has been listed as 1 in 300.[38] The risk is greatly increased if the puncture is deep or into a vein, if the needle has contaminated blood on it, or if the AIDS patient is in an advanced state. The concentration of the HIV virus in blood and tissues is much higher in patients who are in the more advanced stages of the disease. In reality the risk from a contaminated needle stick is much greater than that generally ascribed to it. We have known that a nurse or a physician who is stuck by a needle that is contaminated with blood from an AIDS patient will almost certainly test positive for the virus within six months to three years. It is not safe to conclude that no transmission has occurred when the health care worker tests negative after only six months or even one year.

The dramatic increase in the incidence of other sexually transmitted diseases which compromise the natural skin or other membrane barrier is bound to deliver a concomitant increase in the transmission of AIDS. This will increase the efficiency of disease transmission in both directions. It will be most notable in the number of cases transmitted from female to male. All of the STDs will play a role in this, but herpes will be in the forefront.

We have been told that the major modes of transmission of the HIV infections that have been reported have been sexual activities and sharing of needles by IV drug abusers. In fact the official position has been that these are the only means by which the disease can be "caught." It is now known, however, that the virus is transmitted to the fetus through the placenta by pregnant women and can be transmitted to infants in breast milk. Between 6,000 and 7,000 women with HIV infection give birth each year in the United States.

As is the case with hepatitis B, sharing a razor or toothbrush with HIV infected individuals presents a serious risk of transmission of the disease. Ear piercing, as well as tattoo and acupuncture needles present additional risks of not only HIV but also hepatitis B and C transmission. These carry the same risk as would be present with an accidental needle stick from a contaminated needle. Many practitioners now use sterile disposable acupuncture needles, as everyone should, but about half of them are reusing the needles. Such practice is gross misconduct and they should be prosecuted for criminal behavior if AIDS is transmitted thereby.

The sharing of needles by anabolic steroid abusers has recently come to light as a new risk for HIV spread. About one-half of individuals using these steroids do so by injection and they commonly share needles, as is the practice with other types of drug abuse. By sharing needles they are at risk of acquiring not only AIDS but hepatitis B and C as well. The first case of AIDS in a bodybuilder who had abused anabolic steroids was reported in 1984. In view of the long incubation period, and the fact that this population has not been screened for HIV, the true magnitude of this risk is not yet known.

One of the most certain means of contracting the AIDS virus in the past, and one of the most tragic, was through blood transfusions and administration of blood products that were contaminated with the HIV. Between 1978 and 1986 virtually all hemophiliacs were infected with HIV-1 through blood derived clotting factors. Even now at least half of the hemophiliacs in the United States are known to have been infected through the clotting factors derived from blood that have been vital to their survival. All of these people face an untimely and unpleasant demise. Factor VIII, for those suffering from hemophilia A, the most common type, became commercially available in 1965. It has been prepared from blood pooled from large numbers of donors by a process of lyophilization, that is by freeze-drying. The availability of this product increased the life expectancy among hemophiliacs to the point where it was almost normal by 1980.[39] It was soon discovered, however, that this product also delivered hepatitis B and C to virtually all of those who received it.

Heat-treated factor VIII products were developed in 1979 to eliminate this serious threat. In order to inactivate HIV the lyophilized blood products need to be treated at 154.5°F (68°C) for 72 hours. Unfortunately the cost of doing this is high, and the clinical trials that are required by the FDA delayed the availability until 1983. The routine use of blood products that were not heat-treated continued until 1985, at which time the FDA mandated that all blood products be heat-treated. In December 1992 the FDA approved a recombinant factor VIII that is not derived from blood, and thus is free of the risk of AIDS and hepatitis transmission. This factor VIII is arrived at by modifying hamster cells through biotechnology so that they produce it.

In spite of the availability of this safe product, blood derived factor VIII that was not heat-treated continued to be marketed in the U.S. as late as 1997. In late 1995 four cases of hepatitis A were reported among hemophiliacs who had been treated with blood derived products.[40] Similar outbreaks of hepatitis A had been reported previously in Europe (52 cases in Italy in 1994). Hemophiliacs who receive inadequately treated factor VIII almost universally exhibit chronic infection with hepatitis C (see Chapter XV for the complications of hepatitis C). Several manufacturers in Europe belatedly added the heat-sterilization method, but those in the United States continued to resist this added cost. As of March, 1996 only one manufacturer in the U.S. was using this method, and in that case only for factor IX, the remedy for hemophilia B.[41] There are about 4,000 individuals in the U.S. with hemophilia B. The continued use of these inadequately treated blood products is unfortunate and represents a continuation of the follies of the past.

The need for greater precautions in the collection and treatment of blood and blood products should have been obvious after the virus of AIDS was identified in 1984. In 1989, after the new higher purity factor VIII preparation had become available, the government's Health Care Financing Administration refused to pay for it on the basis that there was no proof that it was more effective. The risk of hepatitis and AIDS transmission from products produced with the existing system was not considered in the decision. In 1997 private insurance reimbursement was still set at the cost of plasma derived products. The balance of the cost for recombinant factors had to be born by the patient. A strong case could have been made at that time for the withdrawal of licensure by the FDA of all unsafe plasma derived products where more refined and safer products had been developed.

Retrospective studies of stored blood samples have revealed that some hemophiliacs had developed antibodies to the AIDS virus as far back as 1978. Similarly, recent studies of stored blood and plasma products, using new PCR testing, have revealed that they became contaminated with HIV in 1978. Because of the increasing mortality caused by AIDS, life expectancy among hemophiliacs began a sharp decline after 1984, and by the early 1990s it was at the lowest level than at any time since before World War II.[42]

The Centers for Disease Control reported that by 1990 new cases of AIDS among the hemophiliac population had risen to 1,316, with 837 having died. There are currently about 20,000 hemophiliacs in the United States, a figure that has remained stable during the past two decades. By 1994 one half of these were known to have contracted the human immunodeficiency virus through blood products. Deaths of those so infected numbered 2,799 as of December 31, 1996.[43] Attrition and improved safety of the blood products had reduced the total number of hemophiliacs with AIDS to about 4,000 to 5,000 in 1997. This tragedy could have been averted if responsible measures had been taken by the blood banks.

In the case of the AIDS virus, HIV, it is now known that it takes anywhere from 6 months to 3½ years after infection for an infected individual to develop antibodies. The only screening test that has been available to blood centers for the AIDS virus is an antibody test, which became available in 1985. It does not detect the virus in the blood. This means that every donor who was infected with AIDS but who had not yet developed antibodies would test negative, and their blood would be placed in the general blood pool. That blood would transmit the AIDS virus to those individuals who received it, either by way of transfusion or as one of the blood derivatives such as factor VIII (unless heat-treated adequately). Tests unilizing the polymerase chain reaction (PCR) technique detect both DNA and RNA from the virus. This test is more complicated and expensive and has not been used for routine screening. In 2001 some blood collection centers began using tests based upon PCR technology.

In addressing this serious threat to the blood supply, the blood collection agencies have developed questionnaires to guide donors in a "voluntary self-exclusion" program. They have also established prescreening interviews in some centers in order to attempt to identify high-risk individuals. Unfortunately studies have revealed that these efforts have been virtually useless in preventing HIV infected blood from being collected into the general pool. No one is going to admit to some of the confidential, sensitive activities sought in these interviews, or in the questionnaires for that matter. It is difficult enough for a physician with some established rapport with the patient to acquire some of this information. Other findings from these confidential studies include:

• Many donors who have heterosexual relations with IV drug users believe that they are not at risk of getting AIDS, and that their blood is safe.
• Studies have shown that donors who test positive for HIV, even after having read the literature on voluntary self-exclusion, do not believe that their activities have placed them at risk.
• IV drug users, a common source of donor blood, rely upon blood banks as a source of income, and disregard the guidelines.

• Even though a confidential ballot system has been used by blood centers since 1987, 95 percent of donors who test positive for HIV designate their blood for transfusion, rather than for restricted use.
• Some AIDS victims are driven by a desire to infect others. The classical example is the French Canadian male airline flight attendant, Gaetan Dugas, who purposely infected countless numbers of victims. This attitude is surprisingly common. It is reflected in the statement of the man arrested for raping a 12-year-old girl. He told police that it didn't matter what they did to him because he already had AIDS.

A number of AIDS victims have proclaimed that they plan to take as many people with them as they can. This vendetta is being demonstrated in an increasing number of HIV infected individuals. One of the most recent examples is a woman in Dallas, Texas who claimed that she contracted AIDS from a so-called male bisexual. She wrote to *Ebony* magazine expressing her anger and her determination for vengeance by taking as many others with her as she could before she dies. Most AIDS patients develop dementia at some point in their illness, and this is used to excuse the quest for vengeance. It is clear from the statements of many of these people, usually early after they are diagnosed, that their actions are deliberate and calculated, and not the result of dementia. An urge for vengeance in such circumstances is not uncommon in humans. There is reason to believe that Dr. David Acer, the Florida dentist who infected Kimberly Bergalis and at least four more of his patients with the AIDS virus, did so deliberately.

Certain blood collection agencies continue to this day to conduct blood drives in communities where it is known that 75-80% of the population is infected with the AIDS virus. The officials of these units insist that the voluntary self-exclusion program is protecting the blood supply. The facts demonstrate that this is not so. The issue is so politically explosive, with blood bank officials being threatened with "blood terrorism" (infected individuals will deliberately donate infected blood), that blood collection agencies are intimidated into taking no action. This policy is not only irresponsible, it is criminal.

In 1982 the Centers for Disease Control advised blood collection agencies to test all donors for hepatitis B antibodies as a means of identifying blood from HIV infected donors. It is known that the majority of HIV infected donors test positive for hepatitis B. This simple measure would have identified much of the AIDS infected blood and blood products that were subsequently administered to hemophiliacs and other patients. Failure to take this simple precaution, whether for economic reasons or for fear of offending a powerful political group, condemned most of the hemophiliac population to a prolonged and agonizing death. For a thorough review of the sordid history of the callous and needless infliction of HIV on countless individuals through contaminated blood, and the collusion of U.S. governmant agencies in covering up these crimes, read Judith Reitman's *Bad Blood; Crisis in the American Red Cross.* Kensington, 1996, New York.

The leader of one blood center related the fear of inciting hysteria as the reason for not revealing the newly discovered risk of HIV. Calculations placed this risk at 1 in 100 rather than the 1 in 100,000 that had been announced previously. Some blood bank officials currently assign the risk of contracting HIV infection from a transfusion at 1 in 45,000. It is obvious that we do not have an accurate estimate, and that many spokesmen are exercising nothing better than a guess, perhaps coupled with a prayer. During the period when hemophiliacs in the United States were infected with HIV through blood products, hemophiliacs in Germany were not so infected, even though much of their blood was acquired from the United States.[44] The difference was in the way that the blood was processed (heat-treated).

In addition to the hemophiliac population, tens of thousands of other individuals who received blood transfusions since about 1980 have been infected with the AIDS virus. The Centers for Disease Control estimates that 29,000 people might have been infected through blood transfusions between 1978 and 1985. Since 10 years is the general period that it takes for symptoms to develop, some of these victims have now started to appear. One well-known sports figure, Arthur Ashe, appeared on national television to explain how he had acquired AIDS from a blood transfusion nine years previously. He subsequently died in 1993. Thousands more are now due. Most will not want to appear on television.

We have known since long before the discovery of the hepatitis B virus in 1966 that other infectious agents were lurking in blood. Some of these such as the hepatitis C, E and G viruses have been revealed in the interim, but others have not been identified yet. One of these, a newly discovered DNA virus was reported in 1998 to be a cause of post-transfusion hepatitis.[45] Investigation revealed that the virus is common in the blood-donor population, and that transmission through blood products such as factors VIII and IX may have been extensive. Some blood collection centers now routinely test for abnormal liver function in an effort to detect active infection with viral agents.

The use of human blood is essential in serious trauma cases and certain surgeries. New technology that permits the salvage of blood during surgery has diminished the need for replacement by about one-half, but has not eliminated the need altogether. This presents us with a painful dilemma. Although great effort has been expended by the American Red Cross to screen donors more effectively, those individuals who are intent upon deception are difficult to unmask. We also know that there are infectious agents in blood that we have not identified yet. This was dramatically demonstrated once more in 1997 when the human herpesvirus 8 (HHV-8) that is associated with Kaposi's sarcoma was found in blood in the Irwin Memorial Blood Center.[46] It was traced to a donor who was healthy and had no evidence of either Kaposi's or HIV. This revelation was made possible by the new PCR techniques that have proven so valuable. There is no simple, reliable test to detect all of the possible pathogens that blood carries. Each one must be tested for individually, and each time a new one emerges or is discovered, the new test that is required adds to the cost of each unit of blood and its derivatives.

Adequate heat-treatment of blood products inactivates some viruses, and renders the product free of that particular risk. Other viruses are resistant to heat treatment and are best inactivated by the detergent/solvent process. This not only complicates processing but also makes it more costly. In the case of factor VIII the recombinant product is the obvious choice, but it is very expensive. The prions that cause Creutzfeldt-Jacob disease and the other spongiform encephalopathies such as the "mad cow disease" require autoclaving at 270° F. for at least one hour to inactivate the agent. They are not inactivated by heat, irradiation, chemicals (formalin) and all of the usual disinfecting techniques. We know that there are other viruses and agents in blood that we have not identified yet.

A new law in California forces the blood banks to permit individuals to avoid this risk by pre-donating their own blood or specifying donors among family or friends. The blood banks refused to permit this option prior to the passage of the new law. The law was enacted only after a ten-year battle with the legislature by Howard Jarvis who acquired AIDS from a blood transfusion. He has since died.

The PCR test that is capable of detecting the AIDS virus in blood became available in 1990. It does not rely upon the presence of antibodies to the virus. This test can detect the DNA and the RNA (genetic material) of viruses, then multiply it millions of times so that the laboratory can detect the presence of the virus itself. It makes it possible to detect the virus in the blood of an infected person very early. This test is new, is more complex and is expensive. It has not been used as a screening test until recently. In time it should become a routine procedure in all blood collection.

The issue of whether or not AIDS can be transmitted by insects is a matter of great concern to a growing number of people, and one that is very difficult to investigate. Certainly no controlled studies can be conducted. The very long latency period between infection and the appearance of the disease makes it very difficult to make the association with an insect bite. The association between the bite of a tick and the subsequent development of Lyme disease cannot be made in a substantial number of cases even though the incubation period is only 3 to 30 days before the appearance of the characteristic rash.

It has been known for decades that in addition to the very efficient transmission of encephalitis, dengue fever, yellow fever and the other diseases where replication takes place within the mosquito, the mouthparts of mosquitos that are contaminated by viruses as the result of feeding on infected hosts may serve to mechanically transmit those viruses to a noninfected human. It has been demonstrated that the *Aedes aegyptii* mosquito is able to transmit the chikungunya virus in Africa in such a fashion for up to 8 hours after feeding. This fact has a significant implication for the current AIDS epidemic, although this means of transmission is difficult to document even when it occurs.

It is currently the contention of the CDC that the AIDS virus cannot be transmitted to man by the bite of a mosquito. This issue was examined by the CDC in western Palm Beach County, Florida when 79 cases of AIDS were reported between July 1982 through September 15 1986. The possibility of mosquito transmission in this group of patients had been raised because of such a high concentration of cases in an area with a large mosquito population. The Florida Department of Health and the CDC conducted detailed studies of these cases.[47]

Some of the victims were IV drug abusers, and this was assumed to be the source of infection. Some were sexual contacts of patients with AIDS or with risk factors for AIDS. At least 13 persons had no risk factors for AIDS, and 10 of these died before the investigations were completed. The assumption was made that AIDS was acquired through IV drug use where this was identified, or through sexual contact with those at risk. A significant percentage of this group of infected patients had no demonstrable source for infection. This fact was more of less glossed over, and the possibility of mosquito transmission of AIDS in this group was dismissed as just unlikely. On the contrary it is very likely.

The investigators addressed the issue of mosquito transmission by testing the AIDS victims and other residents of the area for antibodies to five other viruses that might be transmitted by mosquitos. No association was found, so the mosquitos were ruled out as a possible vector. One weakness in this hypothesis is the assumption of an association between the transmission of the five other viral diseases. This is analogous to saying that any patient who develops an encephalitis that we know came from a mosquito, must also show evidence of dengue fever or one of the other viruses in the region.

This is not the case, however. A mosquito may feed on an AIDS patient who does not carry any of the other viral diseases, then transmit the AIDS virus to a noninfected victim by mechanical means through contamination of its mouthparts. The victims will not demonstrate any antibodies to any of the other viral diseases, and there will be no way to tell where the AIDS virus came from. When a patient in Florida or California acquires malaria we know that it came from a mosquito, transfusions being ruled out. Unfortunately, no such assumption can be made with AIDS. There is no way to rule out the possibility that a significant percentage of the

AIDS cases in western Palm Beach County resulted from mechanical transmission of the virus by mosquitos.

This is the most prominent episode in the United States where arthropods were suspected of playing a role in the transmission of AIDS. The answer is not at hand, of course, for it would be necessary to catch the culprit in the act. It would be necessary to trap a large number of mosquitos during the epidemic and test them for contaminated mouthparts. The epidemic in West Palm Beach County presented an ideal opportunity for such a study. In the absence of such a high concentration of cases, it would be like looking for a needle in a haystack. There is far more circumstantial evidence for mosquito transmission of AIDS in Africa. I believe that it would be possible to demonstrate the possible association, and Africa would be an ideal laboratory.

The other means by which AIDS can be spread have not been studied in any detail. It has been shown that the virus is present in aerosols such as those produced by instruments in surgery and in the dentist's office. It has also been demonstrated that the virus suspended in these aerosols can cause infection. The human papilloma virus is aerosolized when the lesions are treated with a laser, and the virus remains suspended in the smoke indefinitely. Surgical masks do not protect against inhaling these viral particles.[48] A number of viral diseases that are transmitted to humans principally by mosquitos, are also transmitted to humans by aerosols. Rift Valley Fever is commonly transmitted to humans in Africa by aerosols during the butchering of animals. The virus is also transmitted to veterinarian surgeons who are involved with dead animals. Blood-sucking flies transmit the Rift Valley Fever virus to humans by purely mechanical means through the mouth parts of the fly.

Butchering of infected animals also has resulted in the aerosol transmission of the virus of Crimean–Congo hemorrhagic fever on numerous occasions. European tick-borne encephalitis can be acquired by drinking the milk from an infected goat. The Junin virus of Argentine hemorrhage fever, first seen in that country in the 1950s, can be contracted by contact with excreta from infected rodents. Its sudden appearance was linked to an explosion in the population of field mice after widespread corn production was instituted there.

The virus of Venezuelan equine encephalitis can be acquired by humans by breathing suspended viral particles from the urine or feces of infected animals, and laboratory infections by aerosols are common. There has been no evidence of direct aerosol transmission of this virus from horses to man, but then man does not ordinarily butcher horses. Korean hemorrhagic fever is another viral disease that is transmitted by aerosols, directly from infected rodents through their urine.[49] In the 1950s thousands of United Nations military personnel were infected with this virus during the Korean conflict. A recently discovered related virus, labeled the Seoul-like virus, infects rats in the inner cities of the United States, and is suspected of causing kidney damage and resultant hypertension.

Both the Korean hemorrhagic fever virus and the Seoul-like virus belong to a family called Hantaviruses. In May 1993 an outbreak of a disease in the southwestern United States revealed the emergence of a new strain of Hantavirus in the Four Corners region (Colorado, Utah, Arizona, New Mexico). This outbreak has subsequently spread to other regions of the United States. By the middle of September 1993 thirty-six cases of acute illness had been confirmed, with at least twenty-one deaths.[50,51,52] The transmission of the virus to humans has been traced to excreta from deer mice, and possibly other rodents. The virus can be acquired either by direct contact with the excreta, or by aerosol from the droppings (see Chapter VII). This new strain, though very serious, lethal to many, appeared to lack the damage to the kidneys characteristic of the previous two strains. This event again reminds us of the dangers that we may face at any time from the emergence of new deadly viruses.

The first case of AIDS in the United States was reported to the Centers for Disease Control from Los Angeles in June 1981. The studies mentioned previously show that some hemophiliacs tested positive for the virus in 1978, and may have acquired the virus as far back as 1975. By the end of 1981 a total of 189 cases of AIDS had been reported from 15 states and the District of Columbia; 76 percent of the cases were reported from New York and California. Ninety-seven percent of the cases reported were in men, and 79 percent of these occurred in homosexuals. Since that initial report, the number of cases of AIDS reported has increased each year. From 1981 through 1987, 50,000 AIDS cases had been reported. By August 1989, 100,000 cases had been reported.

It had taken 8 years for the first 100,000 cases to be reported. It took only an additional 2 years for the second 100,000. Such logarithmic increase in the number of cases is characteristic of epidemics of communicable diseases. In 1990, AIDS cases were reported in every state in the U.S., with a total of more than 43,000 new cases, an increase of 8,000 cases over the previous year. By the middle of 1991 a total of about 180,000 cases had been reported in the U.S. About 63 percent of these (113,000) had died. By the end of 1991, 132, 071 new cases of AIDS had been reported for the year, bringing the total number of reported cases to 206,392. The total number of reported deaths at this point was 133,232.[53] By January 2001 the total cumulative reported cases in the United States numbered over 770,000, and again, 448,000 of these had died.[54] Hundreds of thousands of cases have not been reported. Homosexual men and intravenous drug abusers have accounted for about three fourths of the cases. Heterosexual transmission and transmission from mother to child have steadily risen in numbers however.[55]

As impressive as these statistics are, it must be kept in mind that they represent only the reported cases, the proverbial tip of the iceberg. With every infectious, communicable disease the number of reported cases does not reflect a true count of the number of people who are infected. With AIDS and its associated social stigma, many known cases will not be reported. The reported cases also reflect only the infected individuals who meet the criteria outlined by the CDC. Those who are ill with AIDS but who do not yet meet these criteria are not counted.

In 1992 the CDC broadened the criteria for the definition of AIDS. This added many additional people to the count. In the areas of high concentration of the disease it about doubled the numbers. As discussed previously, significant financial benefits accrue to those who are classified as having AIDS. In addition, many people, numbering in the tens of thousands, have not yet become aware that they have been infected. The long period between infection and the appearance of symptoms makes this feature of the disease inevitable. The screening test for AIDS does not become positive for six months to three years after infection.

By mid 1993 the World Health Organization estimated that at least 13 million adults and over 1 million children worldwide were infected with the human immunodeficiency virus. By 1994 over 4 million HIV infected adults had developed full blow AIDS, and most of these had died. AIDS has now (2001) become the leading cause of death among men 25 to 44 years of age in the United States. The vast majority of HIV infected individuals develop fatal opportunistic infections within ten years of their infection as a result of deficiencies in their immune systems induced by the virus. Prior to the availability of reverse transcriptase and protease inhibitors death occurred in most of these people about two years after the development of these opportunistic infections. These drugs have added 2 to 3 years of life to AIDS patients.

By the year 2000 the FDA had licensed sixteen drugs to fight HIV infections. These are all expensive and difficult to tolerate for prolonged periods. Many AIDS patients discontinue the drugs for one or both of these reasons. Even in those patients whose viral load had been successfully suppressed by these medications, the levels returned within 3 weeks after cessation of therapy.[56] In addition the emergence of strains of HIV that are resistant to these drugs is a serious and growing problem.[57]

The World Health Organization reported that at the end of 1998 there were 33 million people worldwide with HIV infection.[58] Estimates by others place the number at 110 to 120 million. It was estimated that by the year 2000, ten million children would have lost their mother or both parents to the disease. Over 90 percent of these estimated cases of AIDS will be in Africa, Asia, Latin America and the Caribbean. In view of the several features of the disease that have been reviewed previously, it seems inevitable that these estimates will be on the low side and the actual numbers will be much higher. Some experts believe that for every reported case of full-blown AIDS another 10 to 15 cases of asymptomatic HIV infected individuals exist.

There is no way to accurately assess the true numbers of AIDS cases worldwide. Many governments, if not most, have refused to address the issue. India had reported only 100 cases to the World Health Organization, but it was estimated that 1 million people in that country were HIV positive. In Bombay alone there are at least 100,000 prostitutes who service an average of 5 customers each night. At least 30 percent of the prostitutes are HIV positive, with the percentage rapidly increasing. This translates into 150,000 individuals each night being exposed to the AIDS virus in Bombay alone. Governments in Africa, Asia and elsewhere have similarly ignored the problem or deliberately underreported the number of cases. A former Surgeon General of the United States estimated that 100 million people would die as a result of AIDS in the decade from 1992-2002.

AIDS is a very ugly, unpleasant and prolonged disease. It is 100 percent fatal, a fact with devastating emotional impact upon its victims. Fifty to seventy percent of those who acquire an HIV infection experience an acute flu-like illness 3 to 6 weeks after the initial infection. They may recover from this and appear healthy for a variable period of time. The long tortuous battle that they ultimately fight, and the agony of their last days, particularly the last year, have not been made known to the public. AIDS dementia develops in two-thirds of patients with HIV infection, usually later in the disease. Initially the changes are subtle; inability to concentrate, forgetfulness, slowness in performing complex mental tasks and impaired attention. Decline in cognitive function is progressive. Difficulty in walking, unsteadiness and impairment of hand function follow. Personality changes are manifested by apathy, lack of interest, and at times agitation and hyperactivity.

Hollywood style presentations dramatize and glamorize the victim, grossly distorting the facts and hiding the true suffering. The physicians, nurses, medical technicians, as well as the remainder of the health care team, see the horror and suffering in its fullest. As the reality of the risks from this disease becomes more and more apparent, it seems inevitable that many of these people, so vital in this epidemic, will elect to not continue to expose themselves and their families to this grave risk. Their absence will be felt especially in the emergency rooms, the critical care units and in surgery, the areas where the risk is so great. This exodus will only be hastened by the deterioration that has already begun in our health care system, initiated and promulgated by a socialist government and its legions of Marxists cohorts in the media, large foundations and academia.

AIDS is the most profound event to occur in the field of medicine since the Black Death epidemic of the fourteenth century.

That epidemic resulted in the death of one-fourth of the population on earth (over 60 million people died). In Europe alone there were 20 million deaths (one-third of the total population). As the magnitude of the current epidemic approaches that of the Great Plague we may see some repetition of the behavior of that era. Parents abandoned children, children parents and friend abandoned friend. Panic, despair, depression and a sense of hopelessness drove people to abandon all standards of behavior and civilization, to abandon all of life's goals, work and other pursuits. Those who died were flung into huge pits without any rudiments of a service or memorial. Many fled to avoid the inevitable, terrible plague. But then we are a much more civilized society today.

The full-blown AIDS-related complex characteristically presents with Kaposi's sarcoma or a non-Hodgkin's lymphoma and an opportunistic infection. The most frequently seen opportunistic infection is *Pneumocystis carinii* pneumonia. Also common are cryptosporidiosis, toxoplasmosis, candidiasis (mouth, esophagus, bronchi, lung), histoplasmosis, cryptococcoses, *Mycobacterium avium* complex, cytomegalovirus (CMV) and recalcitrant herpes simplex that may involve many areas other than just the mouth (including the brain). All of these are infections that have not been seen in individuals with intact, functional immune systems in the past. By the mid 1990s they had begun to spill over into the general population, and this trend will accelerate. Prior to the current AIDS epidemic these were very uncommon diseases. Although some of these infections may be controlled initially, ultimately they expand out of control as the immune system continues to deteriorate. Such a scenario is invariably the cause of death in AIDS.

Tuberculosis: The most recent opportunistic disease to show up in HIV infected individuals is tuberculosis. During the resurgence of tuberculosis since 1985 (see Chapter III) new cases of active disease have been seen increasingly among immunosuppressed individuals with HIV infection. In the past, active tuberculosis in the U.S. has resulted primarily from reactivation of a latent infection. Healthy individuals who are exposed to active tuberculosis, and thus to the organism, normally contain this infection by surrounding the bacterium and walling it off. This is accomplished by the body's immune system, particularly the cellular immunity in the lungs. This process is imperfect in the case of TB, however, for the bacillus has the unique capacity to inhibit the mechanisms by which macrophages engulf and destroy bacteria. This feature of *Mycobacterium tuberculosis* is only now being clarified by research in cell biology.

Reactivation of tuberculosis customarily has resulted only during periods when the immune system was compromised, such as during pregnancy, alcohol abuse, administration of cortisone preparations and advanced years. Exposure to the disease is much more serious among infants, adolescents and immunosuppressed individuals. These patients must be treated very aggressively to prevent progression to active disease.

A primary exposure to the tubercle bacillus in individuals with HIV infection is much more likely to progress to active disease, and the progression is much more rapid than has been seen in patients in the past. This progression results from the failure of the cell mediated immunity in the lung, and from the severely impaired immune system of the body in general. The incidence of disseminated tuberculosis and tuberculous meningitis, both of which can be expected to be fatal, is thus much higher in AIDS patients following their exposure.

In residence facilities for HIV patients it has been observed that the HIV positive individuals contracted tuberculosis at a much higher rate than the HIV negative staff. The previously described accelerated progression to active disease was also observed. Similar observations have been made in substance abuse clinics. Intravenous drug users are another group of individuals who exhibit an increased susceptibility to and development of active TB. One man undergoing treatment at a residential substance abuse clinic in Michigan in late 1989 transmitted the disease to at least 15 other persons. The true number was felt to be at least 30, probably higher, but could not be documented.[59] This population is migratory and is very difficult to track

Early tuberculosis is also difficult to diagnose in HIV positive individuals because skin tests are ineffective. The erythema and induration of the skin that is characteristic of a positive skin test in individuals with early tuberculosis does not occur in the majority of HIV infected patients because of the diminished function of the immune system at the cellular level.

The increased transmission rate of tuberculosis in HIV infected persons results in a greater total number of patients with tuberculosis. The period during which HIV infected patients have an increased susceptibility to the disease is measured in years. This feature of HIV, coupled with the very rapid growth of the HIV positive population, will serve to significantly increase the numbers who develop active tuberculosis. These factors, coupled with the accelerated progression of the disease in this group, results in an increased yield of strains of the tubercle bacillus that are resistant to the anti-tuberculosis drugs. Drugs that are effective in controlling tuberculosis are few in number and have been very difficult to develop over the past sixty years.

There is also a tendency among AIDS patients to discontinue anti-tuberculosis drugs, to not complete the course of drug therapy because of their toxicity to the liver, a problem compounded by the other drugs that AIDS patients take. Three of the drugs available for the treatment of tuberculosis, isoniazid, rifampin and pyrazinamide, are all toxic to the liver. Periodic monitoring of liver function through blood tests is essential with all patients placed on these medications. The liver toxicity occasionally requires that these medications be discontinued even in patients who are not HIV positive. Their discontinuance is required even more frequently in HIV positive patients who are on zidovudine or other drugs for AIDS. The fourth drug for tuberculosis, ethambutol, can cause optic neuritis, which is inflammation of the primary nerve for vision, with resultant blindness.

Streptomycin, which was discovered in 1943, was the first drug that was effective in treating tuberculosis. It caused a high incidence of hearing loss and inner ear damage, however, and ultimately was discontinued after other drugs became available. Isoniazid was discovered to be effective in treating tuberculosis in 1945, and it is still the cornerstone of treatment and prophylaxis. Streptomycin has not been available in the U.S. during recent years, but in 1992 the CDC started acquiring it from overseas, and U.S. manufacturers made plans to resume production of the drug in the United States. It is currently available from one U.S. pharmaceutical company. We will desperately need new drugs before this new epidemic of tuberculosis can be brought under control.

Prior to the discovery of anti-tuberculosis drugs, isolation of patients with active disease was the primary means of preventing its spread. Before World War II sanitariums for this purpose were commonplace, but they have been closed. With the availability of effective drugs the period of isolation necessary to prevent spread has been shortened to a few weeks. This can be accomplished at home with many patients. Other members of the household are customarily placed on prophylactic isoniazid therapy, as are all other contacts. Isoniazid is the only drug that is effective in the prophylaxis of tuberculosis. This medication must be taken faithfully for six months for most, for 12 months for HIV positive individuals. Daily dosage is ideal, but twice weekly is an acceptable compromise for prophylaxis. Supervised administration (DOT, Directly Observed Therapy) for those with active disease is frequently necessary because failure to comply with the schedule risks not only the spread of the disease to others, but the development of resistant strains.

A persistent cough is the hallmark of active tuberculosis. It is spread by droplet infection, coughing, sneezing, talking and singing. Infection in the larynx is highly communicable. The tubercle bacillus remains suspended in the air for protracted periods, and it is dispersed widely. These features of the disease increase the spread to others, and greatly increase the risk of transmission. Those with active disease must be indoctrinated to cover their mouths when they cough, a practice that has been abandoned by many in our society in recent years.

Concern at the Centers for Disease Control over the recent trends in tuberculosis is already evident. We will see much higher numbers of people with the disease, primarily among those who are HIV positive and among intravenous drug users. It is inevitable that it will also spread to some other individuals, however, chiefly those who are at increased risk, e.g. the young, the elderly, abusers of alcohol and other drugs, and the malnourished. This spread will increasingly involve TB organisms that are resistant to our medications. Ultimately some Draconian measures may be called for. This epidemic, however, will not be neglected to the same extent that the AIDS epidemic has been. Health officials will be more diligent in their efforts to control this old scourge of mankind.

Interestingly, most of the laws needed to authorize the institution of control measures in the current epidemic are already on the books. Laws empowering public health officials to forcibly detain and treat uncooperative tuberculosis patients were adopted beginning in the early 1900s and continuing into the 1950s. The constitutionality of these laws was upheld in challenges all the way through the Supreme Court. Court challenges are again being threatened by civil libertarians who have a confused and narrowly focused mentality. It is difficult to imagine even the liberal courts of today reversing the previous rulings and turning these people loose to fan the flames of an epidemic that could easily spread out of control, however.

In major cities where the TB epidemic is spreading, with cases of resistant strains evolving rapidly, these laws are again being enforced. One hospital near Boston has established an 18-bed unit with locked doors to detain and treat TB patients who refuse to take their medication. In other areas these people are being treated in the hospital unit of the county jail. In 1991 the New York City Commissioner of Health ordered 44 tuberculosis patients who refused to comply with the treatment regime detained in hospitals until they were no longer contagious. Similar measures were taken in most of the cities where TB was becoming epidemic. We may even see the laws against spitting on the sidewalk enforced once again.

Tuberculosis has spread rapidly among AIDS patients and among the homeless, which includes many alcoholics and IV drug abusers. The disease could infect the majority of these populations in the not too distant future. As the resistance to drugs continues to emerge, the disease will spread even faster and to more distant populations. With no medications to control it, the disease will kill an even greater percentage of those infected. This will be especially true of those with malfunctioning immune systems.

Tuberculosis may become the primary cause of death in many AIDS patients, and it will shorten the life expectancy significantly. Some radical modification of the crowded homeless shelters will be required. It may be necessary to once again isolate TB patients to prevent further spread of the disease. Ironically, the population of mental patients that was freed to live in parks and subways by civil libertarians and misguided public officials may again be institutionalized, this time for a different and more ominous reason. Tuberculosis in children and adolescents is discussed in Chapter III.

OTHER OPPORTUNISTIC INFECTIONS

Involvement of the eye produces some of the most dramatic pathology in AIDS. The most common infection in the eye resulting from immunodeficiency is caused by the cytomegalovirus (CMV). The human CMV is the largest and most complex of the herpes viruses, all of which remain latent in man after invading the body. As many as 90 percent of adults demonstrate that they have acquired this virus at some time in their life. While the virus may cause abortion, stillbirth or death after birth, in adults it often produces no apparent symptoms. When the immune system is compromised in AIDS, the virus, which has been dormant in the cells within the body, is able to replicate (multiply). Unchecked it can produce serious infections in virtually any organ in the body. These infections began appearing among homosexual males in Los Angeles in 1981.

In the eye CMV produces an infection of the retina which leads to a reduction of vision, and may result in a complete loss of vision in those areas of the retina affected. This infection may spread rapidly over the retina in a few weeks, and early treatment is important. Treatment can arrest the infection, but it cannot reverse the damage that has already been done. There is a strong tendency for the infection to recur and it is necessary to remain on maintenance prophylactic medication. Serious toxic side effects of the medications (liver and kidney) frequently limit their usefulness. Retinal detachment occurs in about one-half of the individuals who have CMV retinitis.

Toxoplasmosis is another disease that may remain dormant in the body until the immune system becomes depressed. It may also be acquired after the depression of the immune system, however. *Toxoplasma gondii* is a parasitic protozoan that is commonly discharged in the feces of domestic cats (see Chapter VII). Exposure to the parasite among humans is widespread. The infection affects not only the eye but also the brain, heart, liver, lung, spleen, lymphatics and other tissues of the body. Neurological disorders ensue and encephalitis frequently leads to death. In the eye it produces a serious infection that results in loss of vision if it invades the optic nerve or central vision portion of the eye. As with cytomegalovirus, cortisone, which would normally be used to allay the inflammation in the eye, cannot be used in an immunocompromised individual.

Pneumocystis carinii, another protozoan which lies dormant in the normal lung and which causes pneumonia in immuno-compromised individuals, also infects the eye. It is a frequent cause of death in AIDS patients. Once a rare disease in our society, it is now seen as frequently as pneumococcal pneumonia. By 1981 pneumocystis pneumonia was being seen in large enough numbers among the male homosexual population in Los Angeles that physician reports caught the attention of the CDC. Treatment of the lung infection with aerosol pentamidine frequently controls the lung infection until the further deterioration of the immune system ensues. The eye may become infected in spite of such prophylactic therapy, however.

Kaposi's sarcoma is a vascular tumor that is now known (since 1994) to be caused by the human herpes virus 8 (HHV-8). It also has been demonstrated that it can be transmitted through blood transfusions as well as organ transplants. The lesions may appear anywhere on the skin, mucous membranes or internal organs. It may be seen in the lids and conjunctiva of the eyes. Involvement of the cranial nerves may cause crossed eyes and double vision. Once rare in the United States, Kaposi's sarcoma has reached epidemic proportions since the onset of the epidemic of AIDS.

One half of all patients with AIDS suffer from infections in the gastrointestinal tract that are frequently misdiagnosed as Crohn's disease or irritable colon. Most often the true cause is an opportunistic infection, frequently due to **giardia** or **cryptosporidium** (see Chapters V and VII). Cryptosporidium is a protozoan that can infect the intestinal tract in man and most other animals. It sheds small cysts in the stool, which are highly infectious and may remain active for up to six months after being passed. It can be transmitted to others through the fecal-oral route by contamination of food or water supplies. Cryptosporidiosis in humans was first recognized in 1976. Since then it has been seen with increasing frequency as a cause of severe, resistant diarrhea in AIDS patients. More recently it has spread to the general population, where thousands have been infected through public water supplies or swimming pools. The organism is not removed or inactivated by the conventional water treatment protocols. Diagnosis is difficult and no effective treatment is available.

Microsporidia, an intracellular protozoan, causes an infection in the conjunctiva and surface of the eye, in addition to infections in the liver and intestines. *Herpes simplex* causes similar infections of the conjunctiva and may be recurrent and recalcitrant. Herpes zoster, although seen less frequently, produces a similar picture.

No cure and no effective long-term control for HIV infection exists and none is on the horizon. There is virtually no possibility of developing a vaccine because of the unlimited mutations that take place in the virus. The many different isolates of HIV appear to be a broad range of related viruses rather than a single family. Even within each individual infected with HIV different genomes are found. There are 9,000 base pairs on the HIV genome, and the possible number of different viruses is this number carried to the fourth power. It has been observed for many years that the sheep visna virus continuously changes its antigenic presentation in response to the efforts of the host to develop antibodies against it.

Currently the only practical approach to attempt to control HIV infection in individuals is through agents that interfere with the viral cellular mechanisms. There are four drugs, including AZT and ddI (didanosine), which interfere with the reverse transcription that is necessary for viral replication. These drugs produce serious toxic reactions in the patients, however, as is usually the case with drugs used to control unwanted microbial growth in the body. In addition the virus develops the ability to overcome the roadblocks set up by these agents, through the mechanisms described previously. Drug resistant strains of the virus develop in most patients. In 1996 a new drug that works through a different mechanism, protease inhibition, was approved and marketed in the United States. These two types of agents are now used in combination. The World AIDS Conference in Geneva announced on July 1, 1998 that a new strain of the AIDS virus that is resistant to the protease inhibitors has been spreading among homosexual males. The game thus goes on.

Public health efforts to control the epidemic are centered on education, on modification of sexual behavior and so called "safe sex." The long history of sexually transmitted diseases clearly demonstrates the futility of efforts at sexual behavior modification. Control of syphilis and gonorrhea was not achieved until effective antibiotics were developed. Even with these tools the United States experienced an epidemic of syphilis in the latter half of the 1980s. "Safe sex" is a fantasy; it simply does not exist. Those of us who are old enough to recall the pregnancy rates prior to the discovery of oral contraceptives are well aware of how safe sex can be made. Pregnancy was possible only during about one half of the month. AIDS can be acquired during every day of the month.

Virtually all of the restraints of previous eras that limited sexual activity have vanished. Fear of pregnancy was eliminated with the arrival of the pill. The introduction of the intrauterine device, which was introduced in the United States in 1961, provided not only an alternative system, but a system that did not introduce hormones into the body. It's true that the trial lawyers eliminated the IUD from the American market in 1986, but one courageous company reintroduced a new model in 1989 (see Chapter IV). Parental wrath, which used to cause some hesitancy, has also vanished. This is partly the result of the general abdication of parental responsibilities, and partly the separation of parents from their authority by the courts and radical organizations working to destroy our constitution and our society. Added to these facts is the revolutionary change in the mores and attitudes of our society.

What those engaging in casual sex do not understand at all is that one's exposure is not measured by the number of direct sex partners. The additional sex partners of one's own sex contacts, the so-called "phantom sex partners," must be factored into the equation. Thus if an individual has sexual intercourse with 3 individuals, he has actually had contact with 7 partners. With 5 actual partners, the number reaches 31, and for 6 direct partners the number of actual contacts is 63 individuals. The actual risk of casual sex becomes more obvious when consideration is given to this facet of the sport. This risk applies not only to AIDS, but also to syphilis, gonorrhea, herpes, the human papilloma virus, hepatitis and indeed all of the sexually transmitted diseases. Very few people are able to comprehend this compounding of the risk, even when efforts are made to explain it.[60] Surveys have revealed that sexual relations with local residents or other casual contacts is common among travelers, both from the United States and Europe.

As for the application of the devices of safe sex, while they may reduce the risk during an individual encounter, if one plays Russian roulette often enough, the bullet will strike. One should also keep in mind that the acceptable failure rate for surgical gloves is 7 percent. That is the figure that the FDA sets for the number of gloves that may have pinhole defects during manufacture. Imperfections in the glove material (latex) that do not show up as pinholes, and that permit passage of chemical substances and viruses are even more numerous. These imperfections require more sophisticated equipment to measure than is required for pinholes. Surgical gloves do not provide absolute protection against disease. General latex gloves that are marketed without being labeled as "exam" gloves are not controlled at all by the FDA, and provide even less protection. Does your condom manufacturer do better? Condoms manufactured outside of the United States may be even less reliable, a reminder for those who travel and play.

In a study published by the FDA in 1992 in which condoms were tested on an artificial penis to simulate sex, the AIDS virus, HIV, penetrated the condom over 30 percent of the time. Latex condoms contain microscopic holes that are many times larger than the size of the AIDS virus. Condoms are not manufactured to the same standards as surgical gloves. The latex also deteriorates rapidly in storage, more rapidly at warmer temperatures. Any petroleum based lubricant or barrier cream causes a very rapid deterioration of the latex. Condoms provide a limited protection against syphilis and gonorrhea. They provide little protection against the AIDS virus. They are the only protection that the officials can attempt to sell to the public, however. Abstinence and responsible behavior do not sell well. Unfortunately condoms instill a false sense of security, and encourage people to engage in sexual activity that they believe to be risk free. The resultant increase in sexual activity, and especially risky behavior, coupled with the fact that condoms provide far from absolute protection, results in an increase in the incidence of sexually transmitted diseases. The results are just the opposite of what has been promised.

In our society, as has been the case in every society in the history of mankind, the penalty paid for sexual promiscuity is an epidemic of a destructive disease that takes a great toll on the members of the society. Many such episodes are recorded in the annals of mankind dating back to biblical times. Unlike previous societies, however, we have been visited by the greatest plague of all time. Any objective assessment of AIDS and attempts to project the future course produces no cause for optimism. The AIDS virus is a far more sophisticated organism than any of the bacterial pathogens that we have struggled to control.

AIDS is the first serious communicable disease where public health officials abandoned all of the effective control measures that have been routine for every other sexually transmitted disease. The result is the most massive epidemic of this century. It is not far fetched to suggest that this epidemic might exceed the great plagues of the middle ages in the numbers of people afflicted, and in the total number of fatalities. AIDS remains a 100 percent fatal illness. Every indication is that this will continue to be the case. The rapid replication of the virus and its ability to mutate, to select out strains that are resistant to the few medications that we have been able to develop to slow down the progress of the disease, present a discouraging picture for any efforts to bring the disease under control. It is very improbable that a vaccine to prevent the spread of the disease will ever be developed.

To argue about whether or not our religious faith dictates chastity is to beg the question. The fact is that the survival of a healthy society mandates monogamous relationships. This seems very obvious at this point. The great problem now is finding a healthy, uncontaminated mate with whom to establish such a relationship. Currently (2001) the average number of sex partners for individuals under 30 years of age in America is seventeen. Without a significant and radical modification of attitudes, ultimately everyone will become "unclean." Everyone who participates in sexual activities with multiple partners will ultimately acquire one or more of the sexually transmitted diseases. Those who acquire HIV will have a shortened lifespan, and an unpleasant end. Those women who acquire HPV will have to deal with the prospect of cervical cancer. So long as we encourage our children to partake of sex as long as it's "safe sex" we have not yet begun to address the problem.

1. CDC. Ten leading nationally notifiable infectious diseases — United States, 1995. *MMWR* 1996;**45**(41):883-884.

2. Ashraf, H. HIV/AIDS cases in 1999 set to keep increasing into the next century. *Lancet* 1999;**354**:1886.

3. Bradbury, J. Bad news for the young in AIDS epidemic update. *Lancet*, 1998;**352**:1760.

4. *J Infect Dis* 1999;**180**:2060-63.

5. CDC. Congenital syphilis — New York City, 1986–1988. *MMWR* 1989;**38**-(48):825-829.

6. CDC. *MMWR* 2000;**49**:833-837.

7. De Villiers EM. Heterogeneity of the human papillomavirus group. *J Virol* 1989;**63**:4898-4903.

8. Ashinoff R, Li JJ, Jacobson M, Friedman-Kien AE, Geronemus RG. Detection of human papilloma virus DNA in squamous cell carcinoma of the nail bed and finger determined by polymerase chain reaction. *Arch Dermatol* 1991;**127**:1813-1818.

9. Moy RL, Eliezri YD, Nuovo GJ, Zitelli JA, Bennett RG, Silverstein S. Human papillomavirus type 16 DNA in periungual squamous cell carcinomas. *JAMA* 1989;**261**:2269-73.

10. Burger MM, Hollema H, Gouw AH, et al. Cigarette smoking and human papillomavirus in patients with reported cervical cytological abnormality. *Br Med J* 1993;**306**:749.

11. Prokopczyk B, Cox JE, Hoffman D, et al. Identification of tobacco-specific carcinogens in the cervical mucus of smokers and nonsmokers. *J Natl Cancer Inst* 1997;**89**:868-873.

12. Walboomers JMM, Jacobs MV, Manos MM, et al. Human papillomavirus is a necessary cause of invasive cervical cancer worldwide. *J Pathol.* 1999;**189**:12-19.

13. Gillison ML, Koch WM, Capone RB, et al. Evidence for a causal association between human papillomavirus and a subset of head and neck cancers. *J Natl Cancer Inst* 2000;**92**:709-720.

14. Janicek MF and Averette HE. Cervical Cancer: Prevention, Diagnosis, and Therapeutics. *CA Cancer J Clin* 2001;**51**:92-114.2

15. Sasieni P, Adams J. Changing rates of adenocarcinoma and adenosquamous carcinoma of the cervix in England. *Lancet* 2001;**357**:1490-93.

16. Janicek MF and Averette HE. op cit.

17. CDC. Chancroid — United States, 1981— 1990: Evidence for underreporting of cases. In CDC Surveillance Summaries, May 29, 1992. *MMWR* 1992;**41**(No. SS-3):57–60.

18. Osmond DH, Padian NS, Sheppard HW et al. Risk factors for hepatitis C virus seropositivity in heterosexual couples. *JAMA* 1993; **269**:361–365.

19. Weinstock HS, Bolan G, Reingold AL, Polish LB. Hepatitis C virus infection among patients attending a clinic for sexually transmitted diseases. JAMA 1993;**269**:392–394.

20. Awarded to David Baltimore, Renato Dulbecco and Howard M. Temin.

21. Blattner WA. In Bennett JC, Plum F.; *Cecil Textbook of Medicine*, ed 20. Philadelphia: W.B. Saunders, 1996.

22. Yamaguchi, K. Human T-lymphotrophic virus type I in Japan. *Lancet* 1994; **342**:213-216.

23. CDC. Seroconversion to simian immunodeficiency virus in two laboratory workers. *MMWR* 1992;**41**(36):678–681.

24. Horowitz LG. *Emerging viruses:AIDS and Ebola; Nature, Accident or Intentional?* Rockport, MA: Tetrahedron, 1998.

25. Douglass WC. AIDS: Why its much worse than they're telling us. *Second Opinion Publishing*, Dunwoody, GA, 1993.

26. CDC. Hepatitis B vaccine: Evidence confirming lack of AIDS transmission. *MMWR* 1984;**33**:685-687.

27. Shilts R. *And the Band Played On: Politics, People and the AIDS Epidemic.* New York: Penguin Books, 1987.

28. Jahrling PB, Geisbert TW, Jaax NK et al. Experimental infection of cynomolgus macaques with Ebola-Reston filoviruses from the 1989-1990 U.S. epizootic. *Arch Virol Suppl* 1996;**11**:115-34.

29. CDC. Update: Ebola-related filovirus infection in nonhuman primates and interim guidelines for handling nonhuman primates during transit and quarantine. *MMWR* 1990;**39**:22-24, 29-30.

30. Jahrling PB, Geisbert TW, Dalgard DW, et al. Preliminary report:isolation of Ebola virus from monkeys imported to USA. *Lancet* 1990;**335**:502-505.

31. CDC. Update: filovirus infection in animal handlers. *MMWR* 1990;**39**:221.

32. CDC. Ebola-Reston virus infection among quarantined nonhuman primates — Texas, 1996. *MMWR* 1996;**45**:314-316.

33. CDC. Update: Outbreak of Ebola viral hemorrhagic fever — Zaire, 1995. *MMWR* 1995;**44**:468-475.

34. Matz B, Kupfer B, Ko Y, et al. HIV-1 infection by artificial insemination. *Lancet* 1998;**351**:728.

35. Vidmar L, Poljak M, Tomvažič J, et al. Transmission of HIV-1 by human bite. *Lancet* 1996;**347**:1762-63.

36. CDC. HIV-1 infection and artificial insemination with processed semen. *MMWR* 1990;**39**(15):249-256.

37. Day, Lorraine, MD. *AIDS:What the Government isn't Telling You.* Palm Desert, CA: Rockford Press:1991, 198.

38. CDC. Case-Control Study of HIV Seroconversion in Health-Care Workers after Percutaneous Exposure to HIV-Infected Blood — France, United Kingdom, and United States, January 1988–August 1944. *MMWR* 1995;**44**:929.

39. *Am J Hemat* 1988;**27**:7-12.

40. CDC. Hepatitis A among persons with hemophilia who received clotting factor concentration — United States, September–December 1995. *MMWR* 1996;**45**:29-32.

41. Haller, JD. Blood sterilization with high temperature terminal dry heat. *Lancet* 1996;**347**:827-828.

42. *Ann Intern Med* 1991;**114**:641-648.

43. National Hemophilia Foundation. Personal communication, November 20, 1997.

44. Schimpf K, Brackmann HH, Kreuz W, et al. Absence of anti–human immunodeficiency virus types 1 and 2 seroconversion after the treatment of hemophilia A or Von Willebrand's disease with pasteurized factor VIII concentrate. *N Engl J Med* 1989;**321**:1148-52.

45. Simmonds P, Davidson F, Lycett C, et al. Detection of a novel DNA virus (TTV) in blood donors and blood products. *Lancet* 1998 Jul 18;**352**(9123):191-195.

46. Blackbourn DJ, Ambroziak J, Lennette E et al. Infectious human herpesvirus 8 in a healthy North American blood donor. *Lancet* 1997;**349**:609-11.

47. CDC. Acquired Immunodeficiency Syndrome (AIDS) in Western Palm Beach County, Florida. *MMWR* 1986;**35**:609-612.

48. Garden JM et al. *JAMA* 1988;**259**(8):1199-1202.

49. Manson-Bahr PEC, Apted FIC. *Manson's Tropical Diseases*, ed 19. London: Bailliere Tindall, 1988.

50. CDC. Outbreak of acute illness—southwestern United States, 1993. *MMWR* 1993;**42**:421-4.

51. CDC. Update: outbreak of hantavirus infection—southwestern United States, 1993. *MMWR* 1993;**42**:441—3.

52. CDC. Update: Hantavirus-associated illness — North Dakota, 1993. *MMWR* 1993;**42**:707.

53. CDC. The second 100,000 cases of acquired immunodeficiency syndrome — United States, June 1981 — December 1991. *MMWR* 1992;**41**(2):28-29.

54. CDC. HIV and AIDS — United States, 1981-2000. *MMWR* 2001;**50**:430-434.

55. CDC. The HIV/AIDS epidemic: the first 10 years. *MMWR* 1991;**40**(22):3-57-369.

56. Harrigan PR, Whaley M, Montaner JS. Rate of HIV-1 RNA rebound upon stopping antiretroviral therapy. *AIDS* 1999;**13**:F59-F62.

57. Durant J, Clevenbergh P, Halfon P, et al. Drug-resistance genotyping in HIV-1 therapy: the VIRADAPT randomized controlled trial. *Lancet* 1999;**353**:2195-99.

58. World Health Organization, 1998. Geneva:Joint United Nations Programme on HIV/AIDS (UNAIDS): AIDS epidemic update: December, 1998.

59. CDC. Transmission of multidrug–resistant tuberculosis from an HIV–positive client in a residential substance–abuse treatment facility — Michigan. *MMWR* 1991;**40**(8):129–131.

60. Brannon LA, Brock TC. Letters to editor. *N Engl J Med* 1993;**328**:1352.

XII

HAZARDS OF DRUGS

All substances are poisons; there is none which is not a poison. The right dose differentiates a poison from a remedy.[1]

— PARACELSUS (1493-1541)

No more accurate or more astute an observation has ever been recorded. Even water, taken in excess, can cause death in humans. The human organism is a complex organization of a multitude of parts and systems, all carefully organized and integrated, working in close harmony. Disruption of the harmony in any one of these elements has an adverse impact on the others and upon the whole. The observation of this immutable natural biologic law provided the foundation for the philosophy outlined by Andrew Taylor Still, M.D. when he founded the American School of Osteopathy in Kirksville, Missouri in 1892.

The significance of the above statement by Paracelsus is well demonstrated by the many botanical poisons. Herbs and various plants were the only source of man's medicines until the twentieth century. The dose was determined by trial and error; it never occurred to early man to experiment with guinea pigs first. At some point some individual was astute enough to deduct that if one of the primates could consume a given plant, it would probably be safe for humans. This reduced the risk considerably.

In medical school, physicians are given comprehensive courses in pharmacology and pharmacotherapeutics. The former teaches the basic chemical systems of the body and the reactions of these systems to various classes of drugs. The latter teaches the appropriate doses and application of the many drugs, their interactions and the undesirable side effects. These courses instill a healthy respect for the undesirable and even hazardous actions of drugs as well as their beneficial effects.

We frequently hear talk of a "magic bullet" that will proceed from the mouth directly to the cancer cell and destroy it and it alone. There have been remarkable advances in approaching such specificity in genetic disorders through the use of recombinant DNA techniques. There has also been some success in designing some chemotherapeutic agents so that they concentrate in tumor cells. It seems unlikely, however, that we will ever be able to introduce a drug into the body without it being distributed to every organ and every tissue. Some drugs are not well distributed to the central nervous system, usually because their solubility characteristics inhibit their crossing the blood-brain barrier. Aside from this, drugs that are taken into the body are distributed throughout the body for the most part.

The serious side effects of cocaine so impressed me in my courses in pharmacology and pharmacotherapeutics that I never used it in over 40 years of treating patients. I have employed safer substitutes. These serious side effects resulted from merely applying cocaine to the mucous membranes of the nose. Medical use did not include injecting cocaine into veins or snorting a pile of the powder. I was particularly concerned when the widespread, indiscriminate use of cocaine by people who had never had any medical training became popular. I was amused by the disbelief expressed by these same people when somebody died unexpectedly while abusing cocaine. No one could believe that convulsions occurred during these recreational activities. There was universal shock to discover that young people could die of a heart attack or respiratory failure. These reactions and these deaths came as no surprise to the physicians who were familiar with the actions and hazardous side effects of cocaine.

There exists a very real risk of serious side effects with a single reasonable dose of many of the drugs discussed in this chapter. Where some supernatural sensation or emotional high is sought, a single dose is never enough. More is wanted, or there is a desire for the sensation of pleasure to go on forever. This cannot be, of course, and the repeated dose will of a certainty produce undesirable side effects, perhaps death. Some of these drugs, particularly cocaine, are taken to prolong the pleasant sensations associated with sex. Sex has always been a potent driving force in man, burying all reason and judgement. Under the influence of drugs this loss of judgement occurs sooner and more readily.

Aside from the serious risk of adverse reactions and death, the most serious consequence of drug abuse is dependence. Psychological dependence evolves from a desire to prolong the sensation of pleasure experienced during the visitation of the drug in the body. It produces an irresistible craving for the drug that results in compulsive use. Virtually all of the drugs commonly abused demonstrate this dependence. Physical dependence is more sinister in that withdrawal symptoms occur when the drug is withheld. These symptoms vary some in nature and in degree with the various drugs. They can be life threatening with some drugs. With cocaine and amphetamines withdrawal symptoms consist of depression, anxiety and a craving for the drug. With the opium derivatives the symptoms are much more intense and death can result in the absence of skilled management.

HISTORY OF SUBSTANCE ABUSE IN THE UNITED STATES

1800s	Opiates (opium, heroin and morphine) were legal and widely available through physicians, druggists and patent medicine peddlers.
Mid-1800s	Concept of "habitual inebriates" who were unable to control their drinking was advanced.
1885	Robert Louis Stevenson was treated for tuberculosis with cocaine, and wrote Dr. Jekyll and Mr. Hyde, reflecting his personal experiences from the drug, in three days.
1886	John Smyth Pemberton marketed an elixir of cocaine in combination with caffeine. Thus was Coca-Cola born.
1906	The Pure Food and Drug Act ordered the Coca-Cola Company to remove cocaine from coca leaves before using them in Coca-Cola.
1914	The Harrison Act prohibited physicians and druggists from dispensing opiates and cocaine to addicts. Opium use driven into black market.
1920-1933	Prohibition. Alcohol viewed as evil. Morality move was a failure.
1932	Federal Bureau of Narcotics established as part of Treasury Department.
1935	Alcoholics Anonymous established.

1937	Marijuana Tax Act required physicians, druggists and growers to pay a tax for prescribing, dispensing or cultivating marijuana. Prior to this marijuana was fully legal in the United States. Increasingly severe and restrictive legislation since. Currently possession is a felony in most of the states.
1943	Du Pont and Eastman-Kodak established first occupational alcoholism program.
1944	National Council on Alcoholism established.
1946	First scientific study of alcoholism. Dr. E. M. Jellinek conducted a survey of 1600 A.A. members.
1951	World Health Organization recognized alcoholism as a disease.
1956	American Medical Association recognized alcoholism as a disease. Al-Anon, support group for families of alcoholics founded.
1960	*Disease Concept of Alcoholism* published by Dr. Jellinek.
1960	Narcotics Anonymous founded, patterned after A.A.
1960s	Abuse of marijuana, LSD, cocaine became widespread nationally.
1964	Kemper and Wassau Insurance Companies provided coverage for alcoholism treatment.
Mid-1960s	Possession, manufacture or sale of psychedelic compounds (LSD) prohibited by federal law.
1971	Comprehensive Drug Abuse Prevention and Control Act of 1970 (PL 91-513) in effect on May 1. Established the BNDD, (later changed to DEA). Classified drugs according to potential for abuse. Began the "War on Drugs" (and on physicians).

Schedule I. High potential for abuse and no accepted medical use. Includes heroin, marijuana, peyote, mescaline and LSD. |

Schedule II. High potential for abuse, with psychic or physical dependence. Includes opium, morphine, codeine, methadone, meperidine, cocaine, amphetamines, amobarbital, pentobarbital and secobarbital.

Schedule III. A potential for abuse that is less than schedules I and II.

Schedule IV. A low potential for abuse, with limited physical or psychological dependence. Includes phenobarbital, benzodiazepines and propoxyphene.

Schedule V. A potential for abuse that is less than for those in schedule IV.

1986   Executive order by President Reagan initiated drug testing of federal employees. Many private companies subsequently established drug-testing programs for employees and applicants.

1988   Drug Free Workplace Act

1989   December 1, Department of Transportation issued rules for drug testing program in 49 CFR 40.

1991   October 28, Omnibus Transportation Employee Testing Act of 1991 (P.L. 102-143). Mandated drug testing, including alcohol, for workers who operate aircraft, trains, and commercial motor vehicles.

As can be seen from the above outline, drug abuse has had a long history in the United States as well as abroad. It experienced a great increase in the 1960s, however. This increase has been attributed to many factors; the arrival at adolescence of the large baby boom generation that followed World War II, the wide availability of drugs, etc. The latter was most likely the result of demand rather than the cause for it. Many social ills descended upon our society at about the same time.

It was more than coincidence that we had the government of the United States preaching to its citizens during this same period about all of the things in life that they had coming to them, all that they had been deprived of. The more that people came to expect of government, the more secure were the politicians and bureaucrats. It made empire building a cinch, and we witnessed an enormous expansion of government and its payroll. Individual responsibilities as an essential cornerstone of our society were abandoned. An era of widespread rebellion against society and all of its rules was ushered in. We are fortunate that we had a generation with enough sense of responsibility to rescue us from the tyrants of the world, such as Hitler and Stalin, before this new order became firmly entrenched.

As serious as the current drug abuse problem is in the United States, it is not unique to our culture and is not a new phenomenon. The history of the opium trade and of the opium dens of the orient has been the subject of numerous historical treatises. One example:

So great was the opium traffic that by 1836 it was causing a serious drain on the country's silver reserves. The balance of trade, once so favorable to China, had been dramatically reversed: in the eight years preceding, $38 million had flowed out of the imperial coffers. Alarmed at the harm being done to the nation's health and economy, Emperor Dauguang, a vigorous reformer who had come to the throne in 1821 (his name meant "Glorious Rectitude") ordered that all those convicted of opium smoking should be given 100 strokes with a bamboo rod and forced to wear the cangue— a heavy wooden collar through which the hands were fastened— for two months. Raids were also carried out on some opium dens and a number of dealers executed. One such execution in Canton provoked a near-riot among foreign merchants.

Such measures, however, proved totally ineffective, and in 1836, some of the emperor's advisers argued that the best course would be to legalize the importation of opium, tax it, and stop the outflow of silver bullion by making the drug salable only by barter.[2]

La plus ca change, la plus c'est la même chose (The more things change, the more they remain the same). I am in sympathy with the search for "mind altering" drugs. I have seen many minds that needed altering. Unfortunately no drug exists that will accomplish the task.

DEPENDENCE AMONG DRUGS COMMONLY ABUSED

DRUG	PHYSICAL	PSYCHO-LOGICAL	COMMENTS
Alcohol	yes	yes	Legal, socially accepted.
Marijuana (cannabinoids, THC)	no	some	Widely available, inexpensive.
Cocaine, crack cocaine	no	yes	Serious side effects.
PCP (phencyclidine, *Angel Dust*)	some	some	Unpleasant, undesirable effects.
Opiates (Heroin)	yes	yes	Develops rapidly.
Amphetamines	?	yes	Develops slowly.
Benzodiazepines	little	yes	Develops after about 40 days.
Propoxyphene (Darvon®)	little	yes	Related to methadone.
Methadone	yes	yes	Same as opiates.
Methaqualone	yes	yes	Develops after about 30 days.
Barbiturates	yes	yes	Develops after about 30 days.

ALCOHOL

Alcohol is a widely used substance and is the one that is most frequently abused. This is partially due to its widespread availability and social acceptability. It is universally believed to be a safe and innocuous material, and is not considered to be a drug by the general public. It is indeed a drug, however, and as with any drug it delivers deleterious side effects to various organs of the body.

The best known adverse effects of chronic alcohol use are those produced in the liver. The earliest changes noted are an abnormal deposition of fat in the cells in the liver, a condition known as "fatty liver." This progresses to the deposition of fibrous, scar tissue, replacing many of the normal cells in the liver. These changes diminish the ability of the liver to perform its normal functions, which are many, varied and vital. This advanced stage is known as cirrhosis and can be produced by drugs such as alcohol and methotrexate, by carbon tetrachloride and other chemicals and by Hepatitis B and C. It takes much less alcohol to damage the liver after that organ has been exposed to trichloroethane and halogenated solvents. Serious liver necrosis and death can result from the concomitant consumption of acetaminophen and even moderate amounts of alcohol. These two drugs should never be mixed. Taking acetaminophen in the fasting state can have similar deleterious effects. By far the majority of cases of cirrhosis are caused by chronic alcohol abuse. Cirrhosis of the liver is the third leading cause of death in the 45 to 65 age group, behind heart disease and cancer.

As with virtually all drugs taken into the body, alcohol produces affects on many different organs and tissues. Chronic abuse produces permanent and serious damage to the brain, manifested by memory loss, sleep disorders, psychosis and seizures. Atrophy in the cerebellum of the brain, as can be demonstrated by a CT scan, results in loss of coordination in walking. Neuropathies in the extremities reflect the nerve damage there.

Chronic abuse of alcohol also results in serious damage to both the skeletal muscle and to the heart muscle due to a direct toxic effect. A pronounced enlargement of the heart with diminished function develops in as short a period as 10 years. Irregularity of the heartbeat may accompany the cardiomyopathy. Heart failure ultimately develops and progresses to death. Chronic gastritis is common also in those who abuse alcohol. Both acute and chronic pancreatitis are produced by alcohol abuse, with pancreatic cancer developing in some victims.

The reason why some people become dependent on alcohol while others do not is not known. People who abuse alcohol also tend to be heavy smokers and tend to abuse sedatives and tranquilizers also. As with drug dependence in general there have been hypotheses advanced that alludes to the "addictive personality." Various personality traits have been identified as associated with alcoholism. These same characteristics are identified in individuals who become dependent on the other drugs of abuse. Many more people with these characteristic traits do not become dependent upon alcohol than do, however. Individual personalities certainly play a role. Genetic and biologic factors have been sought without success.

A history of alcohol dependence in a family is predictive of an increased risk for subsequent generations.

One of the most firmly established dictums of human behavior is that we learn by painful stimuli. At the age of 18 months my eldest son crawled to where I was using a soldering iron, reached out and placed his hand on it before I could react. He developed a large blister in the palm of his hand. He has known since that time that an object with that appearance is likely to inflict pain if approached too closely. Experience and intelligence, of course, allow us to modify or overrule these learned experiences. We are able to become thoroughly intoxicated at night even though we are well aware of the misery that we will suffer in the morning. This is called suppression and it is a device widely applied by humans.

Very often damage to various organs and tissues in the body results from substances other than the alcohol in beverages. Wormwood, *Artemisia absinthium*, a flowering plant, has been used in the preparation of a liqueur, absinthe. Extraction of the dried leaves and flowers produces a bitter oil, absinthe, thus the biblical significance of wormwood. The essential oil of *Artemisia absinthium* contains thujone, as does many other essential oils. Thujone is an aromatic terpene ketone, which is toxic, producing central nervous system damage with convulsions and death, as well as optic neuritis and heart failure. Consumption of less than one ounce of the essential oil can be fatal. The drink was very popular in Europe in the 19th century, especially in France. So many cases of poisoning occurred that it was banned in the United States in the early 1900's. Oil of wormwood is readily available currently, however, and is advertised on the Internet. A 31-year-old man was seriously poisoned in 1997 after consuming this substance, having purchased it on the Internet. Absinthe is currently a popular drink in the bars of Prague. Although wormwood was native to Europe, it was brought to North America and grows wild as far south as Pennsylvania.

MARIJUANA

Behind alcohol, marijuana is the second most commonly abused drug in the United States, being first among the illicit drugs. Cannabis is the active drug from the plant and the greatest concentration of this is found in the flowers. The dried resin from the flowers is called hashish. The remainder of the plant contains a number of cannabinoid substances, the most active of which is delta 9 THC. In the United States the leaves, flowers and stem are chopped up and smoked as a cigarette or in a pipe. Serious ill effects and even death have occurred when marijuana has been contaminated with herbicides (paraquat), *Salmonella* and fungus (*Aspergillus*).

Although the use of marijuana is popularly thought of as a discovery of the current generation the practice in reality is very old. It has been used for a long time even in the United States. The Marijuana Tax Act passed by Congress in 1937 required physicians, druggists and growers to pay a tax for prescribing, dispensing or cultivating marijuana. Marijuana produces a pleasant euphoria, or "high". Drowsiness follows, with impairment of concentration, learning and motor skills. This decrement in skills is very apparent in driving a motor vehicle and in flying an airplane.

The impairment in skills mediated by marijuana persists for at least 4-6 hours after a single dose. Experienced pilots in a flight simulator demonstrate impaired skills for at least 24 hours after smoking a single cigarette. Perhaps most alarming is the fact that these pilots were unaware of any of these effects. The impairments in skills are similar to those that occur with alcohol. When alcohol and marijuana are used together the effects are additive.

Larger doses of marijuana produce hallucinations, delusions, paranoia, confusion, disorganized thinking, restlessness and an anxiety that approaches panic. Long term use of marijuana produces changes in hippocampal neurons in the brain in test animals that persist for a long time. The relevance for humans of these findings is not yet known. Used during pregnancy, marijuana produces infants of lower birth weight, as does alcohol, and infants with malformations. It is known to be teratogenic. In men it lowers the testosterone levels in the body and inhibits the formation of sperm. The effect that it has on the quality of the sperm is not yet known. The quality of the sperm, of course, may well reflect the quality of the fetus.

Marijuana produces profound effects not only on the brain but also on the cardiovascular, hormonal and respiratory systems, particularly the lungs. It delivers many different compounds into the lungs and hundreds more are produced when it is burned. Several of these are the same cancer-causing compounds that are found in cigarette smoke. Smoking marijuana also produces the same deleterious effects on the clearance mechanisms in the lungs as does smoking cigarettes. Marijuana depresses the human immune system both at the cellular level and throughout the body. It also impairs the function of the T–lymphocytes. It is not an innocuous drug. Chronic use, as with chronic use of alcohol, leads to more frequent and more severe infections. Pneumonia is frequently the cause of death in young people in these circumstances.

With higher doses of marijuana, anxiety, mental confusion, delusions and hallucinations replace the euphoria. Chronic use can lead to impairment of memory, neglect of personal appearance, loss of interest in any achievement in life, mental dullness and apathy. Depression of ovarian and testicular function may diminish fertility. A decrease in the production of sperm has been measured. Withdrawal from marijuana produces irritability, sleep disturbances, decreased appetite, stomach complaints, salivation, sweating and tremors.

COCAINE

Cocaine is the second most commonly abused illegal drug and it has been responsible for many serious toxic reactions and deaths. It produces a euphoria ("high") identical to that produced by the amphetamines. It relieves fatigue and improves the performance decrement caused by sleep deprivation. The natives in the Andes chew the coca leaf while working to achieve these benefits, which are particularly appreciated at the high altitude at which they live and work. When these natives descend to the lower altitudes of the cities they have no problem abstaining from the drug. However the same people who live in the city and smoke a paste made from the leaves experience the typical toxic effects and a severe dependence on cocaine.

Individuals with an intrinsic anti-social personality are much more likely to develop a dependence on cocaine. It may be that these individuals are simply more intense in their abuse of the drug. Cocaine does amplify anti-societal behavior, however, which helps to explain the increased incidence of crime that has paralleled the increased use of cocaine. The cultivation of an increased number of anti-social personalities in our society during the past thirty years has accentuated the problem.

Among cocaine abusers, the practice of chewing the coca leaves, as do the people of the Andes, was replaced by a technique of snuffing cocaine powder into the nose, where it is absorbed from the mucosa. This cocaine hydrochloride powder can be converted to the "free base" by removing the hydrochloride radical. The resulting "crack" can be smoked and it is readily absorbed from the lungs. This produces a "high" much more rapidly, but it is shorter lived. This leads to repetitive dosing which not only leads to addiction sooner, but the higher levels in the blood and various body organs produce a higher incidence of lethal consequences.

Larger or repetitive doses cause mental confusion and paranoid delusions. These may progress to hallucinations and a fully developed psychosis. Repetitive dosing has become the rule with crack cocaine because the effects are short lived, lasting for only one-tenth the time seen with amphetamine. With the repeated dosing the serious side effects become more certain. Increasingly higher doses are required to achieve the same level of feeling. This is especially true when the drug is used to prolong sexual pleasure. This is somewhat analogous to racing an auto engine at top speed (high RPM, in the redline), in order to achieve more speed and performance. This works only until the engine self-destructs

A common effect of cocaine is a pronounced spasm in the smooth muscle lining the arteries. This results in coronary artery spasm and myocardial infarction. The same action in the arteries in and to the brain produces stroke and subarachnoid hemorrhage. In some cases dissection of the aorta occurs. Widespread clotting of the blood in the vessels throughout the body (disseminated intravascular coagulation) occurs. These diseases of old age are seen in young, healthy people. The occurrence of these events in young people is always a shock and surprise. These dramatic events are ordinarily seen only in older people. In pregnant women this arterial spasm results in spontaneous abortions in the first three months, and separation or infarction of the placenta later in pregnancy, with death of the fetus. In those infants who do survive, sudden death after birth is common. Birth defects as a result of arterial spasm and compromised blood flow to the fetus are also common.

Cocaine produces irregularities of heartbeat and an acute disease of the heart muscle similar to that seen with alcohol, resulting in dilation of the heart and heart failure. Inflammation of the arteries in the brain, seizures, and sudden death are common. Liver necrosis and massive disintegration in the skeletal muscles (rhabdomyolysis) are also common. This latter complication often leads to kidney failure and death. Rhabdomyolysis has also been seen frequently in abuse of alcohol, heroin, PCP and amphetamines. This is a very serious medical crisis that requires an astute physician to recognize and treat successfully. Many of these dramatic effects of cocaine were not taught in my pharmacology course in 1952. The findings have been derived from the volunteer research done since that time by thousands of individuals who have abused the drug.

AMPHETAMINES

Amphetamines are a class of medication that was widely used by the medical profession until some became popular street drugs. They had some very legitimate uses and were as safe as any other drug in our armamentarium. They had to be prescribed with the same wisdom and care as any of the other drugs that we used. There are still other drugs in use by physicians that carry every bit as great a risk if wisdom, knowledge and judgement are not employed. The amphetamines had the potential for abuse, as was the case with some other drugs that were used legitimately. This was not a widespread problem until the 1960s.

As a result of the street abuse, severe restrictions regarding the use of amphetamines and other "dangerous drugs" were placed on physicians in 1970. Public Law 91-513, The Comprehensive Drug Act, passed in 1970, imposing severe restrictions and onerous record keeping on physicians, was supposed to control the abuse of these drugs. The results are history. Patients are, in many cases, denied access to legitimate medications while amphetamines have been manufactured in garages and basements. The subsequent explosion in litigation served to further restrict the use of not only amphetamines, but also many other medications by physicians.

Some amphetamines are capable of producing euphoria, a "high" very similar to cocaine, but greater than customary doses must be taken. Serious risks are involved when amphetamines are

508

taken in these doses. Many of these adverse reactions are similar to those seen with cocaine. As with cocaine repeated dosing increases the risk, as the user attempts to maintain the "high." All good things must come to an end, however, and when the dosing is discontinued the user "crashes" into a deep sleep that lasts for 12 hours or longer. It is much easier to discontinue both cocaine and amphetamine than is the case with the opioids, however.

There is a subtle difference in the pharmacologic effects on the cells in the brain between cocaine and the amphetamines. There is a greater tendency to repetitive dosing with cocaine. As with cocaine, the higher doses of amphetamines commonly employed produce a psychosis that is quite similar to acute schizophrenia. Acute amphetamine intoxication is more common among neophyte users than among "experienced" users. This is characterized by dizziness, confusion, hallucinations, sweating, convulsions, a life threatening elevation of body temperature and shock. This package is quite different from the pleasant euphoria sought by the user. Chronic amphetamine use can cause permanent damage at the receptor sites in the brain (see excitotoxins below).

Methamphetamine or Methedrine®, called speed, has been the most popular member of the amphetamine class of drugs for abuse. Dextroamphetamine (Dexadrine™) was the form most widely used by physicians. This is another class of medications that the underground laboratories have had no problem providing, just as was the case with alcohol during prohibition.

Khat (*Catha edulis)* is a shrub cultivated in the Middle East and Africa for its leaves and buds that are a source of cathinone, a stimulant that is similar to amphetamine and is habituating. It is chewed or brewed as a tea, and has become a major social and economic problem in Yemen and other countries. Planes bringing in the daily supply from neighboring regions were widely viewed on television during the involvement of U.S. troops in Somalia. Since that time a derivative product, methcathinone, has been produced in clandestine laboratories in the United States for illicit use.[3]

Methylphenidate (Ritalin™) is a stimulant drug that is structurally related to amphetamine, and demonstrates similar properties and potential for abuse. It has been a very valuable replacement for dextroamphetamine in the treatment of attention deficit hyperactivity disorder (ADHD), which reflects an imbalance of neurotransmitters in the basal ganglia of the brain. It also has been very useful in treating narcolepsy. It is especially useful since its actions are primarily on the central nervous system, with fewer cardiovascular effects than dextroamphetamine. There has been criticism from elitist government bureaucrats recently regarding the use of methylphenidate. This medication provides invaluable relief to those afflicted with ADHD, and to their parents. It makes it possible for the victims to mature normally in their educational, emotional and social lives.

OPIOIDS

The term opioid includes all of the drugs derived naturally from opium, and the similar synthetic compounds that are manufactured in the laboratory. Opium is derived from the seeds of the poppy plant, and yields morphine, the most potent and most useful substance from a therapeutic standpoint. Heroin is diacetylmorphine and is not legally available for use in the United States. Codeine is methylmorphine, derived by a simple chemical modification of morphine. Other similar modifications produce hydromorphone (Dilaudid®), oxymorphone, hydrocodone and oxycodone, all licensed for therapeutic use in the United States. Fentanyl (Sublimaze) is a synthetic opioid that is primarily used for anesthesia, but has also gained popularity as a street drug, both in its licensed form and in the form of 3-methyl fentanyl, "China White." Fentanyl has been estimated to be 80 times as potent as morphine as an analgesic. Many fatalities have resulted from street use and abuse of both of these substances.[4] Meperidine (Demerol®) is a synthetic opioid with a long history of use in medicine. It and morphine have been the most valuable and most widely used medications for severe pain as seen with heart attacks, kidney stones and serious injuries. In relieving the pain and treating the accompanying shock in these conditions they have been life saving for many patients.

The opioids that are commonly used by physicians such as morphine, meperidine and codeine are entirely safe when used in the recommended dose, for a limited period. For most cases these medications are needed only for 3 to 4 days after surgery, perhaps 5 to 7 days for a heart attack. In the case of injuries, of course, the duration of the need depends upon the severity of the injuries, but in most cases 7 to 10 days is sufficient. Drug dependence or addiction does not develop during these short periods of use. For those individuals with the "addictive personality" the risk is greater of course, and this risk must be factored into the treatment regimen.

If someone decides that they like the way that they feel after a dose of one of these medications, they can elect to continue to take it, if they can obtain a supply of it. Most of us would not consider this because we have other things to do in life, like getting back to work to earn a living, family activities, golf, skiing, painting the house or a host of more pressing ways to invest our time. For the overwhelming majority of patients to whom opioids are administered for a medical need, reason and common sense prevail. A very small percentage of these patients fall into abuse of the drug. Those who do, frequently blame the physician for getting them "hooked." Americans have been indoctrinated to always look for a scapegoat, thus escaping personal responsibility. There are legitimate cases where the severity of injuries requires long term treatment, and dependency has developed in some of these cases. The responsibility for the cure falls upon those who have administered the treatment. As with any treatment, however, this requires the cooperation of the patient.

Methadone is a synthetic opioid compound that has been widely used as a substitute for heroin in drug treatment programs. Physical dependence is so great in heroin addiction that withdrawal is very difficult and can be life threatening. Methadone is useful because it substitutes for heroin in preventing these severe withdrawal symptoms. It also can be taken orally, simplifying administration, and it has a long duration of action. It can be given as infrequently as a single dose every 72 hours. It must be viewed as a temporary measure, however, as a step in the cure of heroin addiction.

Unfortunately most addicts do not want to be cured, and do not progress beyond the methadone step. The overall abuse potential for methadone is about the same as for morphine and other opioids. Physical dependence develops as it does for all of the opioids. It is available only through treatment centers. Strict controls have been formulated to prevent routine dispensing and unregulated widespread use. It is meant to be used only as a tool in curing addiction. For these and other reasons, the use of methadone in long term treatment programs as a substitute for the opioids has been controversial.

Most physicians learn early in the game that it is impossible to cure a patient who does not want to be cured. This certainly applies to those who abuse drugs or any substance. Anyone who has spent any significant length of time in practice has tasted the frustration of attempting to modify behavior relative to alcohol, food and tobacco.

Propoxyphene (Darvon®) is chemically related to methadone and has similar analgesic properties. It is about one-half as potent as codeine for pain relief and delivers more side effects. It gained popularity largely because of the stigma of prescribing codeine, further propagated by government bureaucrats and police bodies who are not knowledgeable about medicine and drugs in general. This new force of the seventies was layered on top of an already unhealthy and unjustified paranoia in the medical profession about creating drug addicts. It has been historical practice in the United States for the past fifty years to routinely deny pain relief beyond 2 to 3 days for post-operative patients because of this paranoia.

In spite of the limited value of propoxyphene, and the disproportionate unpleasant side effects, it has been abused by many. This abuse has never made much sense and it is a clear demonstration that some individuals will abuse anything. Propoxyphene requires 5 to 10 times the normal dose to achieve any semblance of pleasurable effects. These must be balanced against the risk of delusions, hallucinations and confusion, all of those great benefits of drug abuse. Respiratory depression is a serious side effect and this is made worse by alcohol or any other sedating drug. This has accounted for the many fatalities that have occurred with propoxyphene.

Tolerance does develop with propoxyphene, which explains the patients that I have seen who had been taking 6 to 8 times the customary daily dose for months. The potential for addiction with propoxyphene is not as strong as with some of the other opioids discussed above, however. The symptoms of overdose in general are the same as for the other opioids. These include drowsiness, mental cloudiness, mood changes, including euphoria, and respiratory depression that can be life threatening. Larger doses produce coma with a drop in blood pressure and shock. All of the opioids have been widely abused.

SEDATIVES-TRANQUILIZERS

PHENCYCLIDINE (PCP): Phencyclidine is a drug that was widely used in veterinarian medicine, but is no longer available legally. It is easily synthesized in illicit laboratories and that is the source for those who still abuse it. It is used much less today than in the past because of the wide diversity of severe and undesirable mental symptoms produced. It was tested for use in humans in the 1950s but was abandoned because of the severe anxiety, delusional and frank psychotic reactions that followed its use.

PCP is a white powder ("angel dust") and is most frequently smoked but may be injected or taken by mouth. At lower doses waves of anxiety, feelings of detachment, disjointed thinking and visual distortions follow the initial euphoria. Symptoms may mimic acute schizophrenia. Vomiting, convulsions, stupor, coma and death follow higher doses. A prolonged psychosis that threatens suicide or violence to others may follow use of PCP. Chronic use has led to severe mental and behavioral changes and to chronic schizophrenia similar to that produced by LSD.

BARBITURATES: This group of medications is used far less in medicine today than it was thirty years ago. The introduction of the benzodiazepine tranquilizers provided safer and more effective agents with fewer side effects. The routine use of a barbiturate in hypertension that was the practice in the fifties was rendered unnecessary with the advent of very effective anti-hypertension medications. Similarly the barbiturates have fallen out of popularity as drugs of abuse in favor of the agents that evoke more dramatic responses.

For most people dependence with the barbiturates developed only after they had been taken for a while and only after they had increased the dosage beyond what had been prescribed. Dependence was not a risk when they were taken at customary, prescribed doses. Problems ensued when the dose was increased significantly above that prescribed, usually 2 to 3 times the prescribed dose. Tolerance, which permits this increased dosage, can be developed. It develops more readily in some people than in others.

Some people seem to be more susceptible to abuse and dependence (the abusive personality). These same people often abuse alcohol and/or other drugs. Barbiturates, like all sedatives, depress the respiratory and other vital centers in the brain and ultimately result in death. Concomitant consumption of alcohol or other depressant drugs is particularly hazardous with barbiturates and can easily result in death. Many people have moved on to the great beyond through this mechanism.

BENZODIAZEPINES

This class of tranquilizers includes Valium®, Ativan®, Serax®, and Xanax®. They are widely used for anxiety and other less severe emotional states. They are very safe and effective when properly used. They do not activate liver enzymes that affect other drugs, as did the barbiturates. They can be and have been abused, however. They produce a mild sense of well being, and people who experience emotional distress frequently want to maintain and prolong this relief. This leads to repeat dosing and increases in the dose with subsequent tolerance and habituation. Some of these agents are transformed in the body to metabolites that persist for long periods, and this prolongs their effects. This is most pronounced after 1 to 2 weeks of continuous use.

Once tolerance and habituation have developed, withdrawal symptoms can occur. The severity of these symptoms is proportional to the extent and duration of the abuse. These usually include muscle aches, restlessness, irritability, insomnia and anxiety that may be pronounced. In more serious cases delirium and seizures may occur.

METHAQUALONE (Quaalude®):

This drug, which was popularly abused in the recent past, is particularly dangerous because of its narrow safety range. It has been removed from the market and is no longer available legally.

HALLUCINOGENS

There are three different chemical classes of hallucinogens. Mescaline, obtained from the peyote cactus, psilocybin from mushrooms and lysergic acid which is derived from a fungus that grows on wheat and rye as well as on morning glory seeds. The peyote cactus, psilocybin from mushrooms and morning glory seeds were all used by the Aztecs as a means of gaining entrance to what they believed to be another existence. Various other cultures in the past have valued hallucinogens for similar experiences, some believing that they were communicating with "the gods." LSD, lysergic acid diethylamide, is the hallucinogenic drug currently used on the street in the United States, and it is synthesized. Its property of producing a schizophrenic state was discovered in 1947 and this prompted some research in the hope of learning more about this psychosis, and finding a cure for it. An epidemic of abuse of LSD in the 1960s caused an abandonment of all such research, and legitimate manufacture was halted. Stocks of LSD for abuse were readily supplied from the same basements and garages that manufactured the amphetamines.

LSD produces the most dramatic and profound mental alteration of any of the drugs abused, sharing the spotlight only with PCP. It produces a mental state that mimics schizophrenia and does so with a very small dose. The profound mental changes include euphoria with gross distortion of reality, delusions and hallucinations as to who the person is and where he is. Distortions of judgement have led individuals to make decisions that resulted in serious accidents or death. Acute anxiety often develops into a panic state that may last for 24 hours after a single dose. In some individuals use of LSD resulted in a permanent psychotic state resembling schizophrenia, with impaired memory, learning and judgement. Flashbacks are a troubling characteristic of LSD, sometimes being precipitated by alcohol, marijuana or barbiturates. Stress and fatigue are other precipitating events, but sometimes the flashbacks occur spontaneously. LSD, like PCP and mescaline, causes a vasospasm of the arteries in the brain. This is a prominent pharmacological property of ergotamine, which is also produced by mold growth on rye. Gangrene of the fingers and toes results from the vasospasm that is precipitated by ergotamine poisoning.

These troubling and severe side effects were largely responsible for the dissipation of enthusiasm for LSD abuse as a form of recreation. Its use currently is limited to a small number of young people.

DESIGNER DRUGS

After the Comprehensive Drug Abuse Prevention and Control Act of 1970 was passed, clever people began to develop modifications of the controlled drugs in illicit laboratories. It has always been standard practice to study modifications in the basic molecular structure of a drug to find a form that produced better results with fewer side effects. In this instance the goal was merely to find suitable substitutes that would still produce cloud nine, and yet would not be described in the law. The efforts were successful at first, until the law was extended to cover the newcomers. This was yet another demonstration of the resourcefulness of people and the limitation of laws.

One unanticipated result of the back alley chemistry was unwanted side effects and deaths. It has been the rule that modifications in the molecular structure, perhaps the addition of a chloride radical, may increase the potency significantly. This generally reduces the range of safety, and when you're getting bombed with a drug, losing much of your judgement, you may need a very wide range of safety. Predictably the derivative of fentanyl (3-methylfentanyl, China White), presented great potency and several deaths, as discussed previously. Another such "designer drug" with serious consequences, including toxic hepatitis, is "ecstasy" (3,4-methylenedioxymethamphetamine, MDMA), which became popular in the mid-1980s. As with other designer drugs it was not listed in the Controlled Substances Act for a period of time. It was thus sold legally, and manufactured in private facilities. It is metabolized to methylenedioxyamphetamine (MDA) in the body, and has both psychedelic properties and those of amphetamines. More recently it has been discovered that MDMA destroys certain serotoninergic nerve endings in the brain. This results in a deficit of serotonin in the brain, that may cause mood disorders and memory loss.[5] This damage may result after a single dose and is increased by the use of alcohol and/or other drugs. These findings explain some of the disorders of mood and memory observed in drug users.

One congener of meperidine turned out to contain a contaminant that was a neurotoxin, producing permanent brain damage and Parkinsonism. In their search for everlasting euphoria and pleasure, many people have been condemned to a living hell instead. Since the state and county governments have closed down their mental

516

institutions at the insistence of the ACLU, many of these brain-damaged individuals become street people. Many of these are incarcerated in local jails, many times repeatedly. The closing of institutions that formerly provided care has not served these people well. Their disability qualifies them for public support, which is a greater financial burden to the taxpayer than the mental institutions would be.

EXCITOTOXINS

Every action of the body, from picking up a spoon to purely mental activities such as reading a book, involves chemical reactions in the nervous system. An imbalance in any of these chemical reactions causes disorders of varying degrees. War nerve gases for instance interfere with the chemicals that are essential to muscle activity, including breathing. Chemicals that produce similar imbalances in the nerve cells in the brain may cause headache, seizures, memory loss or impaired learning. Glutamic acid and aspartic acid are amino acids, neurotransmitters that transfer messages across the neurons in the brain and spinal cord. They are essential to the normal functioning of the nervous system, and subsequently the body as a whole. Research has demonstrated, however, that an excessive level of these substances and their analogues can produce undesirable reactions, up to and including death of the nerve cell. Substances that are capable of inducing excessive stimulation of neuronal transmitters have been labeled "excitotoxins."

Studies have shown that a number of excitotoxins, including both aspartic acid (from the sweetener aspartame) and glutamic acid (from MSG or monosodium glutamate) induce an influx of an excess of calcium into the cells of neurons in the brain. This influx results in an excess of free radicals in the cells, which kills them.[6] The extent of cell death is related to the quantity of any of these agents that is consumed, and to the length of time exposed to them. The effect is increased when multiple agents are consumed at the same time, as would be the case with drugs, alcohol and certain dietary substances. Damage from these excitotoxins has been associated with the development later in life of Parkinson's disease, Alzheimer's dementia, Huntington's disease and Amyotrophic Lateral Sclerosis. (See also Chapters IV and XV)

Several naturally occurring and man made substances produce a reaction in these nerve cells in the brain that is similar to glutamic acid and aspartic acid. The best known such reaction is the "Chinese restaurant syndrome," produced by consumption of large quantities of monosodium glutamate, MSG. Glutamate is the main chemical for the transmission of nerve impulses in the brain. MSG continues to be widely used in food even though research has clearly shown that it can destroy nerve cells in the brain.

Among the naturally occurring substances that have been recognized to be excitoxins is domoic acid, which is found in green algae and in some marine protozoa. Certain shellfish ingest these algae and thus accumulate domoic acid in concentrated amounts. Ingestion of these shellfish by humans then results in poisoning that has produced brain damage, including permanent memory loss, due to the destruction of neurons, and death in some instances.

Amanita muscaria mushrooms also contain an excitatory amino acid, ibotenic acid, which is 3 to 10 times as potent as glutamic acid. It is used in research to study the excitatory mechanisms of glutamate transmitters. Some species of peas contain an excitotoxin, an analogue of glutamate, which has caused permanent brain damage in both cattle and humans. When peas of the genus *Lathyrus* are consumed in significant quantities over a long period of time they produce lathyrism. This disorder is characterized by sudden onset of weakness or paralysis in the legs as a result of the destruction of (upper motor) neurons in the spinal cord. The severe spastic muscle weakness is followed by atrophy of the muscle. The chickling pea (*Lathrus sativus*), which is widely used as food in Africa, produces this disorder in the indigenous population. The disorder is also common in other tropical countries, in India, and in southern Europe, where this genus of pea is common.

The cycad nut, which is discussed in Chapter XIII for its content of a carcinogen, cycasin, also contains an excitotoxin, L-BMAA, that has been demonstrated to be the cause of the amyotrophic lateral sclerosis-dementia outbreak that occurred on Guam in the 1940s and 1950s. It was found that immigrants from Guam in the United States who had been away from the cycad diet for thirty years demonstrated a delayed onset of amyotrophic lateral sclerosis at a high incidence (ten to fifteen times the rate seen in U.S.

residents). Follow-up studies of the residents on Guam discovered that many also developed neurological disorders that are characteristic of Parkinson's disease and Alzheimer's dementia. Degenerative changes in the neurons throughout the brain and spinal cord were seen in these individuals.

Monkeys that were fed a diet high in cycad for several weeks developed the same disease that was seen in the natives of Guam. They were found to have the same degeneration of the anterior motor cells in the spinal cord that was seen in the humans. Additionally it was found that if these animals were fed the diet for a longer period, past thirteen weeks, they developed the shuffling gait and mask-like expression on their face that is seen in Parkinson's disease.

A species of seaweed in Japan contains an excitotoxin, kainate, which is a hundred times more toxic than glutamate. Although scientists such as Dr. Olney have been studying this area of brain chemistry for more than twenty years, the toxicity of many of these excitotoxins has evolved only in recent times.

INHALANTS

In an effort to experience euphoria and an intensified feeling of pleasure people have inhaled just about any substance that would pass from the container to the nose. The classical trick that all parents are familiar with is the brown paper bag and glue. Inhaling any of the organic solvents in this fashion will result in permanent damage to the nervous system, especially the brain, permanent damage to the skeletal muscles and damage to the liver and kidney. In the case of gasoline, the benzene also causes leukemia. In addition to gasoline and glue, paint thinner and aerosols from cans have been popular.

Nitrous oxide, an old and much used anesthetic, was also discovered by the enterprising and adventurous souls. It was safe in the hands of trained and experienced physicians and dentists, but they recognized its narrow range of safety and always had equipment and medication for resuscitation at hand. One of the most basic principles of anesthesia is to always stay within a range that permits the patient to wake up. The skill, training and experience that enable the anesthesiologist to be able to do this require many years of formal education.

Amyl nitrite was used in medicine in years past to dilate the arteries to the heart. Since newer and longer lasting medications became available this volatile liquid has been passed on to the amateurs. They have found pleasures in it that physicians overlooked during all of the years of use. Aside from a headache and rapid heartbeat the one significant side effect is that the user may "mess his pants."

TOBACCO

Columbus and his men were the first people to learn of tobacco and the pleasure of smoking it in a pipe. It is interesting to note that when Columbus introduced this commodity to his world there was intense opposition to its use, and severe penalties were invoked for doing so.

Until recent times nicotine was considered to be non-addicting. More recent laboratory studies have demonstrated that test animals do self administer nicotine as they do other addicting substances. This stimulus is less powerful than it is with amphetamines and cocaine, however. The withdrawal syndrome seen with cessation of smoking varies with the individual. There is a craving for tobacco for weeks, longer in some than in others. Common symptoms are irritability, anxiety, restlessness and difficulty in concentrating. Some people experience an increase in appetite, headache, insomnia and loss of memory. These symptoms are accompanied by demonstrable changes in the electroencephalogram. A decrease in both the heart rate and blood pressure accompany the elimination of nicotine from the body and there is an increase in skin temperature as the peripheral blood flow improves.

The nicotine chewing gums provide only partial relief from the above symptoms with smoking cessation, but they do eliminate the risks associated with the chronic carbon monoxide exposure of smoking. Since they rely upon absorption in the mouth they should be chewed slowly, and swallowing should be avoided as long as possible. Switching to a low nicotine cigarette invariably results in an increase in the number of cigarettes smoked. Switching to high nicotine cigarette results in a reduction in the number smoked. Interestingly, the smoker adjusts in order to maintain the same level of nicotine in the body.

There are definite and specific receptors in the brain that are responsible for the stimulant effects and an increase in some mental functions. Nicotine suppresses the appetite for certain foods, affecting weight. The weight of smokers is about 5 percent below that of comparable nonsmokers. Nicotine evokes nausea and vomiting by stimulating the vagal nerve reflexes. Cigarette smoking diminishes fertility in women, increases the incidence of spontaneous abortion, premature placental separation and premature rupture of the membranes. It also produces infants of low birth weight, a higher incidence of death at or shortly after birth and sudden death in infants later.

In excess of 4,000 substances have been identified in cigarette smoke. Many of these produce some adverse effect(s) in the body. About 40 of these have been determined to cause cancer, to promote the development of cancer or to speed up the growth of cancer once it develops. The impressive association between cigarette smoking and the development of lung cancer was well documented by Doll in his ten years of studies on British physicians, published in the British Medical Journal in 1964.[7] These findings have been confirmed many times over by studies of numerous other researchers. The very pronounced synergistic action that is seen between cigarette smoking and asbestos may be due in part to the cilia-toxic effect of cigarette smoke. It paralyzes ciliary action and increases mucus production, thereby significantly impeding the clearance mechanism in the lung.

Cigarette smoking also causes cancer of the mouth, larynx and esophagus. Alcohol consumption accelerates the development of these cancers. Cigarette smoking has been identified as an important contributor to the production of cancer of the stomach, pancreas, kidney, bladder and cervix. The carcinogenic and mutagenic chemicals from cigarette smoke have been found in both rine and the mucus on the cervix.[8,9,10] About one-half of cancers in the urinary bladder are the result of cigarette smoking. With smoking cessation the lung cancer risk decreases over a 5 to 10-year period to near that of a non-smoker. The reduction in the incidence of the other pulmonary diseases depends upon the extent of the damage done prior to quitting.

Aside from cancers, cigarette smoking causes emphysema, bronchitis and chronic obstructive lung disease, and contributes to the development of osteoporosis. It is one of the major contributing factors in the development of coronary artery disease and heart attacks. These problems surface at a much younger age in heavy smokers than they do in a non-smoking population. Similar changes occur in the other arteries throughout the body, and an increased incidence of stroke is seen in smokers. After 1 to 2 cigarettes even chronic smokers experience an increase in heart rate, elevated blood pressure and hand tremor. The activation of enzyme systems in the liver by nicotine makes necessary higher doses of pain medications and sedatives in smokers. Those exposed to passive smoke over a prolonged period experience the same respiratory and cancer risks as do smokers. Children who live with smoking parents experience an increased incidence of respiratory diseases as well.

SOME HARMFUL COMPONENTS OF CIGARETTE SMOKE

SUBSTANCE	HARMFUL EFFECTS
Acetaldehyde	Irritant, toxic to cilia
Acrolein	Irritant, toxic to cilia
Ammonia	Irritant, toxic to cilia
Arsenic	Carcinogen
β– Naphthylamine	Carcinogen
Benzo[a]anthracene	Carcinogen
Benzo[a]pyrene	Carcinogen
Carbazole	Cancer promoter
Carbon monoxide	Deprives cells throughout the body of oxygen; promotes atherosclerosis
Catechol	Cocarcinogen
Cresol	Cocarcinogen and irritant
Formaldehyde	Irritant, toxic to cilia
Hydrazine	Carcinogen
Hydrogen cyanide	Irritant, toxic to cilia
Indole	Cancer promoter

Nickel	Carcinogen
Nicotine	Stimulant to nerves throughout body, including heart. Increases mucus production.
Nitrogen oxides	Irritant, toxic to cilia
Nitrosamines	Carcinogen
N–Nitroso-nornicotine	Carcinogen
Phenol	Cocarcinogen and irritant
Polonium 210	Carcinogen
Vinyl chloride	Carcinogen

Carcinogen causes cancer. Cocarcinogen assists another substance to cause cancer.

Individuals who smoke 20 or more cigarettes per day have twice the risk of cataract formation in the lens of the eye.[11,12,13,14] The carboxyhemoglobin level in the blood from the carbon monoxide produced by smoking cigarettes is about 8 to 10 times normal in people who smoke this quantity. The cataract formation may reflect this abnormal exposure, or it may reflect the compromised blood circulation that produces such other dramatic effects as those seen during pregnancy. The chronic carbon monoxide exposure is known to play a part in the atherosclerosis and coronary artery disease that occurs in smokers. See also Chapter XV for a discussion of tobacco use.

ANABOLIC STEROIDS

Anabolic steroids are substances that have been used in medicine for many years to restore a "positive nitrogen balance" in chronic wasting and deficiency diseases. That is the basic definition of "anabolic." The term steroid is an imprecise term, in its strictest sense referring to any one of a number of compounds that contain a specific chemical "steroid" nucleus. Included in this group are testosterone (and related compounds), estrogens, progesterone, the adrenal hormones, cholesterol and many other substances. Cholesterol is the common intermediary for all of these agents.

In the 1950s it became popular for androgens to be used by athletes for the purpose of bodybuilding. This practice continues to this day, and indeed has spread to the high school level. No sincere effort to discourage this dangerous practice has been undertaken by organized, professional sports organizations. The group of drugs taken includes many different analogues of testosterone, some of which are effective when taken by mouth (testosterone must be given by injection). Some of these are useful in some chronic diseases in that they induce an increased RNA directed protein synthesis where there has been a deficit in this activity.

In mature males the sites responsible for the building of muscle mass are already saturated with an adequate supply of androgen. It is not a simple matter of adding more fuel. In reality, however, these agents, when taken in excessive doses, do increase the lean body mass in some people. In addition football players cite increased aggressiveness as a benefit. These psychiatric side effects are not always well controlled off the field; they cannot be turned on and off. An increased aggressiveness when socializing in the local bar is not always desirable. It may lead to jail time, especially if someone's neck is broken. There are few arenas in our society today where we need an increased level of aggressiveness.

More recently the practice of anabolic steroid abuse has spread beyond the sports arena. In a study in 1991, ninety-six percent of the respondents to a survey stated that they were using the steroids to improve their physical appearance. Other reasons included physical conditioning, personal enjoyment and increased self-esteem. Increased sexual performance has also been given as a goal. Most of these individuals were in their mid 20s and use of steroids was over a prolonged period.

When administered by physicians for these anabolic effects, serious side effects must be kept in mind. As discussed earlier, no drug has a single effect; it is not possible to administer a drug, obtain a beneficial effect, and expect no other unwanted effect. With these agents, even in reasonable therapeutic doses, undesirable side effects occur. In the massive doses used for muscle development the side effects are greater in number and more severe. These substances are taken in doses that are 10 to 100 times the accepted, approved therapeutic dose. These individuals also commonly use veterinary anabolic steroids that are not approved for use in humans.

Laws to effectively deal with any physician irresponsible and unethical enough to provide these substances for other than legitimate use have long been on the books. They are more than adequate, if applied. No physician can logically defend the practice of prescribing anabolic steroids for the purpose of increasing athletic performance. Aside from the criminal penalties imposed by the statutes, defending a civil suit engendered by the serious and permanent side effects of these drugs would be a formidable task. Several states have taken action on their own, in an effort to control the illicit traffic in steroids. Some states have enacted legislation to put these agents in the same classification as cocaine and other abused substances. These laws are completely illogical and will prove to be about as effective as all of their predecessors.

There are also serious legal problems with this approach of classifying anabolic steroids in the same legal category as narcotics and drugs of abuse. In view of the inability to legislate away the abuse of cocaine and other drugs, it is difficult to see how new legislation will solve the problem. As workplace drug testing has reduced the incidence of the problem on the job, so appropriate testing in athletics should help to reduce the problem in that arena. All efforts at education should be made, but not with unrealistic expectations. Young people simply do not believe all of the scary things that we old people tell them. It is also much easier to simply close your eyes to things that you do not want to see when you are young.

Any discussion of the customary toxicity of anabolic steroids is irrelevant in the case of abuse, where the doses are astronomical. Adverse effects with abuse include liver tumors (malignant and benign), accumulation of pools of blood in the liver, stasis of bile in the liver, other structural changes in the liver, development of an abnormal lipid profile, high blood pressure, decreased hormonal levels in the blood, sterility, testicular atrophy, impotence and enlarged breasts in men. Mood swings with rage are not uncommon, and present a significant problem when working with and relating to other people.

Twenty percent of the individuals who abuse steroids experience major depression or mania; as many as 12 percent may suffer psychotic symptoms. In women who abuse these substances we find inhibition of ovulation, hirsutism (male hair pattern), deepened voice, loss of normal hair, and acne. Chronic abuse also results in an increased susceptibility to tuberculosis in both sexes, a disease that has been increasing in incidence among the AIDS population.

At least one-half of individuals using anabolic steroids do so by injection. The sharing of needles during steroid use is common, as is the case with other forms of drug abuse. The increased risk of acquiring hepatitis B & C and AIDS through this sharing should be obvious. This risk has been almost totally ignored until recently, however. The first case of AIDS in a bodybuilder who used anabolic steroids was reported in 1984. In some studies 7 percent or more of high school males had used anabolic steroids. Most of these were not athletes, but were using these agents because friends were using them. This is admittedly a low risk population for AIDS, but for how long? Given the long incubation period for AIDS, and the fact that this population has not been screened for HIV, the magnitude of the problem may simply not have surfaced as yet.

In addition to HIV, the use of nonsterile needles and the lack of aseptic technique among injecting drug abusers lead to other infections. Infections in the heart with concomitant damage to heart valves has been common. Tetanus and wound botulism results from injection through unclean skin or from contamination of the drug being injected such as Mexican black tar heroin.[15] The incidence of this complication of drug abuse has been increasing.

In 1988 congress solved the problem, as it did with the drug abuse epidemic when it passed the Comprehensive Drug Abuse Prevention and Control Act of 1970 (PL 91-517), by passing another law, the Anti-Drug Abuse Act of 1988.

Another drug that has been promoted to body builders, although not exclusively to that group, is GHB, gammahydroxybuty-rate. This substance was marketed illicitly in the United States in 1990, and promoted not only to body builders but also for weight control and as a sleep aid replacement for L-tryptophan. It has been used as an investigational drug for the treatment of narcolepsy since about 1980, and has proven successful in that application.[16] As of November 1990 at least 57 people had presented to emergency rooms for treatment of acute poisoning with this substance,[17] and the sale of GBH was banned by the U.S. Food and Drug Administration in that year. During the subsequent decade GBH abuse resulted in 5,500 emergency room visits with 45 deaths.[18] The Date-Rape Drug Prohibition Act of 2000 reclassified GHB and its analogues as Schedule I controlled substances, which consists of drugs which have a high potential for abuse and no currently accepted medical use in the United States. This is an inappropriate classification of GHB, and is an action by Congress based upon politics and emotion rather than on facts, wisdom and logic.

GHB increases dopamine levels in the brain and causes depression as well as uncontrolled skeletal muscular movements. It produces respiratory depression that is aggravated by alcohol, a recipe for death. It does nothing to "build the body", but it does take your mind off of the perceived problem until you recover. GHB has become a popular "party drug" and many cases of coma, respiratory depression and death have occurred, some when the substance was slipped into a person's drink without his knowledge. As with the amphetamines it can be produced at home or in illicit laboratories, and contamination with sodium hydroxide during these processes results in increased toxicity. It is one of the more serious and sinister of the so-called "date rape" drugs.[19] For anyone to knowingly take GHB as a "party drug" is insane, to slip it into another person's drink is reprehensible, and deserves serious punishment.

Erythropoietin, although not a drug in conventional pharmaceutical terms, is another substance that is abused by athletes. This substance is a glycoprotein that is produced normally in the kidneys, and it stimulates the production of red blood cells in the bone marrow. In chronic kidney disease the production of erythropoietin is diminished, and a chronic anemia develops. The erythropoietin gene has been cloned, and recombinant human erythropoietin (EPO) is now available to stimulate red cell production where a deficiency exists, as in chronic kidney disease.

Some athletes have utilized EPO to boost their blood count above normal levels in an effort to increase their athletic prowess. Deaths have resulted from this practice, however, because every drug has its downside, as has been amply demonstrated. The undesirable side effects of EPO are that it can aggravate hypertension and precipitate thrombosis, or clotting. In treating chronic kidney patients these side effects must be kept in mind and watched for. The risk of thrombosis is less in a patient who is greatly deficient in red cells than it is in an individual who is attempting to pack more red blood cells into arteries than they were designed for.

CAFFEINE

Caffeine is another substance that is widely consumed by man and never considered to be a drug. Fortunately its use is fairly innocuous, although dependence does develop. Habitual consumption of as little as 3 to 4 cups per day can result in withdrawal symptoms. The most common symptom of withdrawal, which can occur during a trip away from home, is headache. This can be avoided when coffee is unavailable by carrying No-Doz® tablets, or a similar generic product, in your travel kit. A 100 mg tablet, or one-half of a 200 mg tablet is usually adequate to prevent a headache, which can be severe.

The dependence associated with caffeine is similar to that seen with cigarette smoking. It is not to be confused with the addiction that develops with the opioids and other drugs of abuse. Withdrawal from the latter can result in severe, life-threatening symptoms. These terms have been used so loosely by the general public and corrupted by the politicians to such an extent that their true connotation has been obscured. This tends to confuse the relative risks involved, which is the goal of those who wish to further erode our liberties and assign greater power to government agencies that have only made the problems worse. We have learned nothing from the lessons of prohibition.

Caffeine is a potent stimulant of the central nervous system, relieving drowsiness and fatigue, and facilitating a clearer thought process. This stimulant activity has its limits, however, and is nowhere near as potent as that of the amphetamines. At higher doses the value of these actions during study or driving is compromised by the nervousness and anxiety produced. One to three cups of coffee containing 85 to 100 mg of caffeine each is normally the functional range. As with any drug it should be consumed in moderation. Keep in mind also the many other sources of caffeine, some of which are listed in the table below.

There have been many studies undertaken to link caffeine intake to carcinogenesis, mutagenesis and teratogenesis. These have been prompted by observations of inhibition of DNA repair mechanisms by caffeine in plants and in some cell cultures. This activity occurred only at doses much in excess of that consumed in beverages, however. There is no evidence that caffeine, in doses normally consumed in beverages (200mg per day), contributes to the production of cancer, birth defects or low birth weight in infants.

CAFFEINE CONTENT OF COMMON SUBSTANCES

SUBSTANCE	CONTENT, mg.
Coffee, 8 oz	100 to 200
Decaff coffee, 8 oz	5
Tea, 8 oz	40 to 80
Green tea	30
Coca-Cola, 12 oz	34
Pepsi-Cola, 12 oz	37
Mountain Dew, 12 oz	52
Chocolate bar	25
No-Doz tablets	100, 200
Vivarin tablets	200
Excedrin	65

1. This quote from Theophrastus Bombastus von Hohenheim Paracelsus has been couched in varying phraseology by different authors, perhaps reflecting variations in translation. In all, however, the accuracy and profundity of this observation is retained. Born near Zurich, Switzerland of a learned physician, he was one of the great minds of medicine of the 16th century. His many contributions to medicine of the time included the introduction of mercury salts for the treatment of syphilis, which was engulfing Europe at the time. He discarded the inaccurate dogmas of past eras and advocated experimentation and observation, in other words scientific research, as an avenue to knowledge. The author.

2. Time–Life Books, Inc. *Time Frame 1800–1850 AD, The Pulse of Enterprise.* Alexandria, VA; 1990:117.

3. Hardman J, Limbird L, Molinoff P, Ruddon R. *Goodman and Gilman's The Pharmacological Basis of Therapeutics*, Ed. 9. McGraw-Hill, Columbus, OH 1995.

4. Kramer C, Tawney M. A fatal overdose of transdermally administered fentanyl. *JAOA* 1998;**98**(7):385-86.

5. Morris K. *Ecstasy users face consequences of neurotoxicity. Lancet* 1998;**352**:1913.

6. Blaylock R. *Excitotoxins: The Taste That Kills.* Health Press, Santa Fe, NM, 1994.

7. Doll R., Hill A.B. 1964. Mortality in relation to smoking: Ten years observation of British doctors. *Br Med J* **1**: 1399.

8. Kier LD, Yamasaki E, Ames BN. Detection of mutagenic activity in cigarette smoke condensates. *Proc Nat Acad Sci USA* 1974;**71**(10):4159-4163.

9. Yamasaki E, Ames BN. Concentration of mutagens from urine by adsorption with the nonpolar resin XAD-2: Cigarette smokers have mutagenic urine. *Proc Natl Acad Sci, USA* 1977;**74**(8):3555-3559.

10. Donahue EV, McCann J, Ames BN. Detection of mutagenic impurities in carcinogens and noncarcinogens by high-pressure liquid chromatography and the Salmonella/microsome test. *Cancer Research* 1978;**38**:431-438.

11. Hankinson SE, Willett WC, Colditz GA, et al. A prospective study of cigarette smoking and risk of cataract surgery in women. *JAMA*;**268**:994–998, 1992.

12. Christen WG, Manson JE, Seddon JM, et al. A prospective study of cigarette smoking and risk of cataract in men. *JAMA*;**268**:989–993, 1992.

13. West S, Munoz B, Emmett EA, Taylor HR. Cigarette smoking and risk of nuclear cataracts. *Arch Ophthalmol*;**107**:1166–1169, 1989.

14. Leske MC, Chylack LT, Wu S-Y, et al. The Lens Opacities Case–Control Study: risk factors for cataract. *Arch Ophthalmol*;**109**:244–251, 1991.

15. CDC. Tetanus among injecting-drug users — California, 1997. *MMWR* 1998;**47**:149-151.

16. Scharf MB, Lai AA, Branigan B, et al. Pharmacokinetics of gammahydroxy butyrate (GHB) in narcoleptic patients. *Sleep* 1998;**21**(5):507-14.

17. CDC. Multistate outbreak of poisonings associated with illicit use of gamma hydroxy butyrate. *MMWR* 1990;**39**(47):861–863.

18. Nordenberg T. The death of the party. All the rave, GHB's hazards go unheeded. FDA *Consum* 2000;**34**:14-19.

19. CDC. Gamma hydroxy butyrate use — New York and Texas, 1995-1996. *MMWR* 1997;**46**:281-283.

XIII

HAZARDS OF CHEMICALS

True science teaches us to doubt and, in ignorance, to refrain.
— Claude Bernard

During the past century our civilization has been inundated by thousands of new chemicals, virtually all man made. This plethora of new compounds has made life much easier for us, and has provided us with marvels that we could not even dream of fifty years ago. Medical science has eliminated some diseases and controlled others with the vaccines, antibiotics and chemotherapeutic agents that have been produced by the scientists during this revolution. The development of a large array of pesticides has greatly increased food crop yields and delivered a better product to the consumer. These agents have also greatly assisted the science of medicine in controlling the arthropod borne diseases such as those from mosquitoes, which have killed more humans than all of the wars in history did.

These products have also delivered a number of disasters to us, however. The mass poisoning of the residents in Bhopal, India by methylisocyanate, and the exposure of more than 36,000 people in the vicinity of Seveso, Italy to a toxic cloud of TCDD (dioxin) are two examples (see Chapter XIV). Not all such poisonings result from man-made chemicals, however. The epidemic of St. Anthony's fire in France in 590 A.D. resulted from ergot poisoning.

Ergot is an alkaloid that is produced on rye by a fungus, *Claviceps purpura*. It produces a profound constriction of the arteries that frequently results in gangrene of the fingers and toes. In the pregnant female it so interrupts the blood flow to the fetus that malformations, stunted growth and death are common. These disastrous effects in pregnant women were recorded as early as 300 B.C. Many episodes of ergot poisoning have been recorded throughout history both before and after that epidemic in France in 590 A.D.

Several valuable medicines have been developed by various chemical modifications of ergot in the laboratory. Bromocriptine has been used extensively in the treatment of Parkinson's disease, to control lactation (milk production) after childbirth and in certain pituitary disorders. Other preparations are used to stimulate contraction of the uterus after obstetrical delivery to control bleeding. Ergotamine has been very useful in relieving migraine headaches, and indeed was the first truly effective medicine in that distressing disorder.

Perhaps the best known of the ergot derivatives is LSD, lysergic acid diethylamide. When its psychedelic effects were discovered in 1943 it evoked excitement in the scientific community. There was great hope that through this drug some of the mysteries of mental illness could be resolved. This research was aborted, however, by the subsequent widespread abuse of the drug by the lay public.

Other naturally occurring drugs that are as potent as any man-made substances are mescaline from the peyote cactus and psilocybin from mushrooms. The natives of Mexico and the Southwestern United States were using these when the Spanish arrived. Poisoning from the oleander plant, which contains several glycosides that stimulate the heart including ouabain and digitalis, has occurred from using the branches in barbecuing. Many of the chemicals that we manufacture and find useful today are merely duplications of or modifications of naturally occurring substances that are more efficiently and economically produced in the laboratory.

Literally billions of dollars have been wasted in the irrational war against all man-made pesticides. In fact, as Ames has shown, 99.99 percent of all of the pesticides that we consume in our diet are natural pesticides from plants.[1] All plants produce toxins to ward off disease-causing microorganisms and insects. Those plants that man has domesticated to improve yield and flavor have in the process lost some of their ability to produce these toxins. They are thus more susceptible to disease and insect predators. This fact is what prompted the search for synthetic pesticides in the first place.

In many instances, researchers in essence have backtracked to develop more resistant strains of various plants. In some cases where they have succeeded they have discovered that the product that they come up with produces these toxins too well. People become sick when they eat them. This was the case with a new potato that was developed at a cost of millions of dollars. The product had to be withdrawn from the market because of its toxicity. The levels of the toxic alkaloids solanine and chaconine in the normal potatoes in our diets are not far below those that are toxic to humans. Potatoes that have turned green as a result of light exposure, or those that are diseased or bruised contain much higher levels of solanine and are more likely to cause illness in humans.

Few people would believe that the ubiquitous potato could poison anyone. It has, however, on many occasions. It happens less frequently in our society than has been true in some others, chiefly because of our highly developed and efficient food storage and distribution systems. Nonetheless, poisoning by solanine is still seen in the emergency centers in the United States. Solanine is present in the sprouts, leaves, berries and seeds of the potato plant. It is also present in the leaves and stems of tomato plants, in bittersweet and the nightshade plant.

Solanine is very toxic, producing nausea, vomiting, diarrhea, mental confusion, delirium and acute respiratory and cardiac depression. These symptoms result from the fact that solanine is a cholinesterase inhibitor, with a very narrow safety factor (six), a feature that it has in common with some of the man-made pesticides. Few people would consider eating the sprouts from potatoes, and most people carve out their "eye" and discard it. This practice reduces the risk of toxic reactions.

Virtually none of the naturally occurring toxins have been subjected to the scrutiny for mutagenesis and carcinogenicity that their synthetic counterparts have. One exception is the psoralens (coumarins) that occur naturally in celery and parsley. The psoralens, which readily penetrate the skin, are potent photosensitizers to long wave ultraviolet light (UVA) and are carcinogenic when combined with ultraviolet light (sun) exposure (see Chapter VIII). A new variety of pest resistant celery that was developed and marketed contains almost 8 times the level of carcinogenic psoralens as regular celery. This fact was revealed after a nationwide epidemic of skin rashes occured in people who handled the celery and then were exposed to sunlight.

Many young people in Africa die each year from liver cancer that is related to both the hepatitis B virus and aflatoxins. Neither of these agents is man-made. Aflatoxins are a product of mold growth on groundnuts (peanuts), a staple in the diet in Africa. The relationship between exposure to some naturally occurring chemicals and the subsequent appearance of disease in man was recorded as far back as 370 B.C. when Hippocrates described abdominal colic in a worker who mined lead.

In the first century A.D. Pliny the Elder (23-79 A.D.) described the serious consequences of occupational exposure to asbestos, as well as arsenic and mercury. Arsenic accompanies copper and tin in geologic strata, and poisoning resulted from the extraction of those valued and widely used metals. Most of the commercial arsenic produced in the United States today is recovered from the chimneystacks of smelters where metallic ores are processed. Georg Agricola in his treatise *De Re Metallica*, published in 1556 A.D., documented the toxic effects experienced by workers mining arsenical cobalt. Arsenic, which is carcinogenic, remains a serious occupational hazard in many settings today.

Recorded examples of poisoning from environmental agents dates back at least to biblical times. During the second year of the 40 years during which Moses led his people in the wilderness following their departure from Egypt, their dissatisfaction with their diet of manna became intense. They yearned for meat, and so stated in bold and bitter terms. The Lord responded with a strong wind that drove hundreds of quail from the sea to the campsite. The people gathered hundreds of bushels of the birds and spread them out in the sun to dry, content in the knowledge that they would not be without meat for a long period of time. But before they could enjoy their bounty "the Lord smote the people with a very great plague" in response to their lack of faith and complaining. Many people who had so craved for the meat died (the actual numbers are not recorded) and were buried on that site that was thus named Graves of Craving or Greediness (Numbers 11:31-34).

One scholarly explanation for this plague is that the quails had feasted on various poisonous berries, including the hemlock plant in Africa prior to their migration north.[2,3] These berries contain coniine, a poisonous alkaloid that causes paralysis of muscles. The people died of paralysis of the respiratory muscles. This poison does not affect quail even though it accumulates in their tissue. Perhaps the modern day parallel to this episode would be the mass poisonings of people in Iraq and other countries after they had eaten birds that had consumed seed grain. The seed grain was treated with methyl mercury as a fungicide to prevent rot.

Emergency room physicians treat thousands of patients each year who are poisoned by consuming "natural" products. Many of these victims are children and that issue is discussed in Chapter III. Adults are not spared, however. In some instances the poisoning is innocent, as with the solanine in potatoes discussed above. In other cases the poisoning results from taking a "medicine" such as herbal or folk remedies, discussed in Chapter XV. Occasionally the culprit is something as simple as licorice, which contains glycyrrhizin, an aldosterone-like substance that exerts mineralocorticoid activity, and can cause sustained hypertension. When consumed in adequate amounts it can cause a sustained elevation in the blood pressure, and irregular heartbeats. The latter is mediated through a low serum potassium level that is also caused by glycyrrhizin. No studies have been done to establish a safe level of consumption of licorice, but it has been documented that serious symptoms can result from the consumption of 100 g of licorice per day. One of the main sources of licorice ingestion in the United States is chewing tobacco. Wisdom would dictate moderation, as with all things.

THE ORIGINS OF CANCER

One of the greatest challenges that we face today is to identify those chemicals that cause or contribute to cancer so that we can minimize our risk. A great deal of study has already been invested toward reaching this goal. Much time and effort has been invested in studies to determine which substances pose a threat, and the mechanisms by which cancer develops. Drs. James and Elizabeth Miller at the University of Wisconsin have been pioneers in this effort and have contributed much knowledge to the mechanisms of carcinogenesis. They have published the results of their studies on several occasions since 1970.

Dr. Bruce Ames, of the Department of Biochemistry at the University of California at Berkeley, made a major contribution in 1976 when he developed a simple and inexpensive test to screen substances for potential mutagenicity. This test, which carries his name, can also identify and differentiate between direct acting carcinogens and those that require metabolic activation. The latter have been designated procarcinogens. The Ames test provides data on both man-made and naturally occurring substances, with the exception of the metals. It does not have predictive value even in the case of metals that are known to produce cancer in humans, such as arsenic, nickel and chromium.

Chemicals exert their influence on the development of cancer in different ways. Virtually every substance that is taken into the body is bio-transformed to a different substance. Most of this activity takes place in the liver by a number of enzyme systems that produce oxidation, phosphorylation or some other chemical reaction. One of the most important, and thus most studied, of these enzyme systems is the Cytochrome P-450. A direct acting carcinogen, one capable of inducing neoplastic changes in cells in its natural form, might be transformed into a less active compound by these enzyme systems. A procarcinogen, on the other hand, which has no capacity to influence such changes, might be transformed into a more active form, and thus one that possesses the capacity to induce neoplastic changes. Cocarcinogens, on the other hand, do not produce neoplastic changes by themselves. Rather they are agents that increase the effect of a carcinogen by a direct local effect on the cells, thus enhancing the conversion to neoplastic cells. Confused?

• Direct acting carcinogen: can induce cancer in its natural form, if it is not transformed in the body to a less active compound.

• Procarcinogen: does not cause cancer unless changed to a more active, carcinogenic form by metabolic activity in the body.

• Cocarcinogen: does not cause cancer by itself but can, through its chemical action in a cell, enhance production of cancer by a pre-existing carcinogen.

Most of the chemical carcinogens in our environment fall into the classification of cocarcinogens, requiring biotransformation to an active substance. These are chemically stable for the most part, and thus persist in the environment. Most of the direct acting, or primary carcinogens, on the other hand, are chemically reactive (electrophilic) and thus do not persist for long periods in the environment.

Chemicals that are classified as promoters or enhancers are agents that facilitate the growth of dormant neoplastic cells into tumors. The cells where neoplastic changes have been induced may have been held in check by the body's homeostatic systems. This is a much-simplified description of chemical carcinogenesis, sparing you the more detailed discussions in the works published by the Millers and others.

Studies over the years have demonstrated that chemicals as well as physical agents (ultraviolet radiation, ionizing radiation as with X-rays) exert their action by altering the genetic component of the cell, the DNA (deoxyribonucleic acid). This damage to the DNA is felt to be the initial biochemical alteration that ultimately leads to pathologic change, whether it is cancer, mutagenesis or teratogenesis. The alteration of the DNA may result from physical action as with ionizing radiation and UV radiation, or it may result from highly reactive chemicals attaching to the DNA, thus altering the message conveyed when the cell divides. The latter is the mechanism by which aflatoxin B_1 produces cancer. This change is not significant until that cell divides, which fact accounts for the latency period.

In the meantime, the body has repair mechanisms, just as it does in the case of injuries and illnesses. These processes within the cell may repair the damaged DNA. If the cell divides before the repair has been made, however, the new cells will be altered because the DNA is responsible for carrying the code that defines the structure and function of the newly divided cells. It is thus that cancers are born. This danger is the greatest in those cells within the body that divide most frequently, as in the reproductive system. This danger is also greater in children who are still in the growth phase, and especially in the fetus during the first three months. This is the period of most rapid development of the fetus, and many substances introduced into the mother's body during this period produce defects in development of the various organs of the fetus. Some of these are tragic, many are gruesome and most are avoidable.

If a cancer promoter or enhancer is introduced into the cell with the altered DNA before repair has taken place, it may stimulate the production of a cancer that might otherwise have been avoided. It is known that several different types of viruses produce cancer. Some of these enter the host cell, and transfer their RNA (ribonucleic acid) to the host cell DNA, thus altering its genetic code. It is through this mechanism that these viruses are able to multiply. They also include a code that speeds up the multiplication process, inducing the cell to divide when it would not otherwise do so.

Some viruses have specificity, invading only certain types of cells within the body. This is believed to be the mechanism through which some viruses produce cancer.

CHEMICALS ASSOCIATED WITH CANCER

There are many chemicals that are known to cause cancer in humans. Some of the exposures to these occur through occupational activities. Others are chemicals that are used as medicines, chiefly in the treatment of leukemia and other cancers, ironically.

One of the earliest documentations of an occupational exposure to chemicals and the development of cancer was the association between the collection of soot and coal tars on the clothing of young chimney sweeps, and the subsequent development of cancer of the scrotum at a very young age. Sir Percivall Pott described this association in 1775 (see Chapter X). The fact that cancer developed at the site where coal tars were applied to the skin was confirmed by subsequent research. Several components of the tar were isolated and found to cause cancer individually. Benzo[a]-pyrene, which is produced on your charcoal grill, and dibenz[a,h]-anthracene were two of the earliest of these polynuclear aromatic hydrocarbons to be isolated and studied. They remain important occupational carcinogens today.

In the late 1800s Rehn documented the occurrence of tumors of the urinary bladder in workers in the coal tar dye industry in Germany. In 1937 this association was demonstrated in laboratory animals by Hueper using 2-naphthylamine, another substance that remains on the list of chemicals to most avoid. Today literally scores of related chemicals have been shown to produce cancers in the urinary bladder, including various aniline and benzidine dyes. Benzidine itself is no longer manufactured, but a long list of derivative compounds remains as important industrial and commercial products. In addition many other substances that are totally unrelated have been identified as carcinogens.

SOME SUBSTANCES KNOWN TO CAUSE CANCER

Acrylonitrile
Aflatoxins
4-Aminobiphenyl
Arsenic compounds, inorganic
Asbestos
*Azathioprine
Benzene
Benzidine
Beryllium
Bis(chloromethyl)ether
Coal tar pitch
*Chlorambucil
*1-(2-Chloroethyl)-3-(4-methylcyclohexyl)-1-nitrosourea
Chromium & certain chromium compounds
Conjugated estrogens
*Cyclophosphamide
Diethylstilbestrol
Erionite (alumino-silicate)
Hardwoods (beech & oak)
*Melphalan
Methoxsalen with Ultraviolet A
*Mustard Gas
*Myleran
2-Naphthylamine
Nickel subsulfide
Phenacetin
§Radon
Thorium Dioxide (radioactive)
Uranium
Vinyl Chloride
Zinc chromates

*Cancer chemotherapeutic agents.
§Added to Seventh Annual Report on Carcinogens, only for high exposures i.e. mining.
References: Report on Carcinogens, Ninth Edition, 2000. Includes only substances to which residents of the United States are exposed. American Conference of Industrial Hygienists (ACGIH), TLVs and BEIs, 2001; IARC Monograms on Cancer.

In addition to the substances listed in the above table, over 200 additional substances are listed "which may reasonably be anticipated to be carcinogens."[4] Some substances such as radon present a cancer risk only at high levels of exposure.

NATURALLY OCCURRING CARCINOGENS

While the environmental extremists have garnered all of the headlines with their protestations against all of the man created cancer causing chemicals, the existence of a far greater number of carcinogenic chemicals that are produced in nature has been totally ignored. Dr. Bruce Ames, who has been in the forefront in identifying chemical carcinogens, pointed out this paradox in 1987 in an effort to put the issue in perspective.[5] As he stated, tobacco is responsible for about 30 percent of all cancer deaths in the United States, and every case is avoidable. It is responsible for an even greater number of deaths from cardiovascular and other diseases. Excess alcohol consumption also is responsible for many deaths from liver and cardiovascular diseases.

Even more extensive is the field of dietary factors that influence cancer either in their absence or in excess, but this field has not been fully explored. The overwhelming majority of carcinogens in our environment occur in our foods naturally with no help from man. As Dr. Ames points out there are more known carcinogens in a cup of coffee than there are in the pesticide residue on food that one consumes over a period of one year. He has also found substances in potatoes, pears, parsnips, broccoli, brussels sprouts, basil, mangoes, mushrooms and mustard that are carcinogens as defined by the Environmental Protection Agency. All of these natural carcinogens are totally ignored by the government bureaucrats and the lunatic special interest groups who have lost all contact with reality in their obsession to rid the world of all man-made chemicals.

Carcinogens are found naturally in many different foods. In studying the high incidence of cancer on Guam it was discovered that the flour made from the cycad nut contained a potent carcinogen, cycasin. It causes cancers in the liver, kidney and digestive tract in laboratory animals. The substance can be removed by appropriate washing of the flour before consumption. The people of Japan also use this nut as food. The Japanese include another plant carcinogen, bracken fern, in their diets. Their practice of immersing the bracken in hot water reduces the carcinogenicity but does not eliminate it. Bracken causes bladder tumors in cows and is passed on in the milk, as are most chemicals. In addition to causing cancer, bracken is suspected of containing a mutagen that might be responsible for birth defects when pregnant women consume it.

In addition to its poisonous properties the Senecio plant (Golden Ragwort, Squaw Weed), that is used for making tea in some cultures, contains pyrrolizidine, which is toxic to the liver. It also produces liver cancer in rats and is thought to play a role, in conjunction with mycotoxins and viruses, in the production of cancer of the liver in humans. It has caused poisonings and deaths when cereals were contaminated with it. The alkaloids found in the Senecio plant are mutagenic and teratogenic as well as being carcinogenic.

Sassafras oil, which is extracted from the bark of the roots of the sassafras tree (laurel family), was long used not only as a folk remedy, but also as a flavoring agent for toothpaste, root beer, sarsaparilla and chewing gum until the early 1960s. At that time the Food and Drug Administration banned its use in the United States because of its safrole content. Safrole and related compounds have been found to be mutagenic as well as carcinogenic in laboratory rats. Safrole also has produced liver cancer in laboratory animals, albeit at a low incidence. Even black pepper, which also contains these compounds, produces tumors in mice.

The practice in some Asiatic countries of chewing betel nuts leads to a high incidence of cancer in the mouth. This may result from the transformation of one of the ingredients to a nitrosamine, which is known to occur. An increased incidence of cancers of the esophagus and stomach in other cultures has spurred the search for carcinogens in the herbs that are used by the various societies.

Another naturally produced chemical that enjoys wide distribution is benzo[a]pyrene. Charcoal broiled meats contain large quantities of this substance. It is one of 15 polycyclic aromatic hydrocarbons (PAH) known to produce cancer in animals. In addition to charcoal broiled foods, smoked and barbecued meats, and many other foods, are found to contain small quantities. Other sources of exposure are the exhaust of autos, trucks and busses, creosote, asphalt and road tar. Burning of wood and coal and cigarette smoke also provide exposures to it. Many occupational exposures to benzo[a]pyrene exist (see Chapter X).

Furocoumarins (psoralens) that are found in celery, parsley and related plants are mutagenic and carcinogenic, as discussed previously. They penetrate the skin and are incorporated into the DNA in these cells. Exposure to UV-A in sunlight then induces further bonding, a certain recipe for trouble. Solanine in the sprouts of potatoes, while not possessing any of the gene altering characteristics of the substances mentioned above, does cause an unpleasant illness in humans.

Aflatoxins are a group of toxins produced by the fungus *Aspergillus flavus*. These toxins were discovered in 1960 during an investigation into the death of some 100,000 turkeys in Great Britain. The turkeys had been fed a peanut meal that was discovered to be contaminated with *Aspergillus* mold. Examination of the turkeys revealed extensive liver necrosis and aflatoxins were determined to be the cause. A similar poisoning of ducklings in Uganda resulted from the feeding of peanut meal that contained aflatoxins.

Subsequent studies revealed aflatoxins to be the most potent cancer-causing substance known to man. Very small doses could produce not only necrosis in the liver but cancer as well. One part per billion in the diet produces cancer in susceptible animals such as the rat and trout. Cancers in the kidney, colon and lung have also been produced in laboratory animals. The only safe level is probably a zero level.

Peanuts (groundnuts) are a dietary staple in large populations in Africa. The high incidence of liver cancer, and its occurrence in young populations (age 20 to 30 years) is thought to be associated with aflatoxin intake. A positive correlation between aflatoxins in food and the development of liver cancer has been established in Uganda, Swaziland, Thailand, Kenya, Mozambique and China. The dietary intake of aflatoxins in these countries is measured in parts per million, however, contrasted to the 15 parts per billion or less in the U.S.[6] Hepatitis B is also endemic in the same populations in Africa and this is believed to be a synergistic factor in the production of the liver cancers seen there. In the southeast United States, however, where a high intake of aflatoxins in the diet has been noted, a higher than normal incidence of liver cancers has been observed also. Aflatoxins in our food is discussed in chapter V.

Ochratoxin A is another mycotoxin that is produced by *Aspergillus* and *Penicillium* species. It causes liver and kidney tumors in rats and mice, but such an association in man has not been demonstrated. An association between Ochratoxin A and chronic kidney damage that is common in Bulgaria and Yugoslavia has been shown, and is presumed to be associated with the contamination of cereals and bread with the mycotoxin that is also common in that area. Like the aflatoxins, Ochratoxin A is a common contaminant of corn, peanuts and grains in storage, but it is also found in decaying vegetation and moldy bread, flour, coffee beans, cereal and all grains. Residues have been found in meat from animals slaughtered after consuming contaminated feed. It appears to be much more widely distributed than the aflatoxins and human exposure is common. The significance of this exposure, especially relating to the significant incidence of chronic kidney disease in the United States, has not been determined. Greater care to prevent mold growth in all animal feed would seem to be prudent.

Some of the naturally occurring substances that cause cancer are listed below:

NATURALLY OCCURRING CARCINOGENS

SUBSTANCE	COMMENTS
Adriamycin	Produced by molds
Aflatoxins	Produced by molds (Aspergillus flavus)
β asarone	Flavoring agent
Betel nut	Chewing of causes cancer in mouth & stomach
Bracken fern	Bladder cancer in cattle; in milk
Cycasin	Plant on Pacific islands; potent carcinogen
Mushroom toxins	Chemical structure of some not yet identified
Nitrosonornicotine	Found in tobacco
Ochratoxins	Produced by Aspergillus, Penicillium and other molds
Phorbol esters	Chemical family of potent tumor promoting agents*
Pyrrolizidine (Senecio)	Used as tea

| Safrole | Used as flavoring agent |
| Radon | Radioactive gas released from certain types of geologic strata |

* Example is croton oil

RADON

Radon is a naturally occurring gas that is released from deposits of uranium that are present throughout the soils and rocks of the earth. It becomes important when it occurs in significant concentrations, as is the case in the Reading Prong, a geologic formation that extends from Berks County, Pennsylvania through northern New Jersey. The parent uranium (U^{238}) is constantly breaking down into other radionuclides, chiefly radon and polonium. (All radioactive substances disintegrate spontaneously, yielding heat and light in the process). The half-life of radon gas (Rn^{222}) is 3.8 days. This decays into polonium, Po^{218} with a half-life of 3 minutes, and Po^{214} with a half-life of less than one second. These compounds adhere to dust particles and are inhaled into the lungs where they emit alpha particles. Alpha particles are highly effective in causing changes in the DNA of the cells that line the bronchi, and this leads to bronchogenic cancer of the small cell variety.

Cigarette smoking is a synergistic factor in the cultivation of lung cancer by radioactive particles, and in fact cigarette smoke itself contains polonium, a breakdown product of radioactive lead in the phosphate fertilizer used to grow tobacco. It is obvious from their half-lives that these substances do not hang around for long. They are able to produce mischief only where a constant emission is contained sufficiently to provide a constant source of exposure. This occurs in tightly constructed houses that are built over the appropriate geologic strata, or houses that are built from radioactive materials, such as the waste tailings from uranium or phosphate mines. Visiting these houses does not present a risk. Long term occupation of a house with an elevated level might, especially for a cigarette smoker.

Uranium mines provide constant exposure to these radioactive particles among those working in the mines, and this is where most of our data and knowledge on the production of lung cancer originated. It is obvious that radon is another naturally occurring element over which we have limited control. It would be prudent to map out the areas where it might be encountered, and to take appropriate precautions in building houses in these areas (these are discussed in Chapter VI). We could ban the mining of uranium and eliminate that occupational exposure, but the people displaced from jobs would be unhappy. Uranium mining takes place for many reasons other than the production of bombs. Appropriate engineering controls and personal protective devices can limit exposure to radon. This would seem to be a more rational approach to the problem.

VIRUSES

When I took my cancer courses in 1952 it was suspected that viruses in some vague way played a hand in the development of cancer. Today an impressive list of viruses are known to play a role in a variety of different cancers, and something is known of the way in which they exert their influence. Several of the 63 known strains of human papillomaviruses (HPV) play a role in the development of cancer of the cervix, vulva, genital mucosa and anus. HPV types 6 and 11 cause genital warts, which are generally benign. Types 16 and 18, however, cause dysplastic lesions that lead to anal and genital cancers. The herpes simplex virus has also been associated with cancer of the cervix.

Hepatitis B is endemic in Africa and Asia, and the chances of developing liver cancer is 100 times greater in those who have had this viral infection than in those who have been spared. Aflatoxin, which is produced by the fungus *Aspergillus flavus* in peanuts (see Chapters V and XIII), seems to increase this risk even more. The Epstein-Barr virus (cause of infectious mononucleosis) is associated with Burkitt's lymphoma in central Africa as well as other malignancies. Most of the people in the United States experience infection with the Epstein-Barr virus by adulthood, but, although it remains resident in the body, the immune system keeps it in check. Burkitt's lymphoma is thus uncommon in the United States except with suppression of immune function.

Viruses are classified as DNA or RNA viruses. In DNA viruses the nucleic acid core is composed of deoxyribonucleic acid, whereas in RNA viruses the core is composed of ribonucleic acid. The genetic information necessary for replication is encoded in this nucleic acid core. The viruses discussed above are DNA viruses. The RNA viruses that cause cancer in humans include the human T-cell lymphotrophic virus (HTLV-1) which causes leukemia/-lymphoma, and the human immunodeficiency virus (HIV-1) which causes AIDS and Kaposi's sarcoma. The latter used to be an uncommon cancer but it is seen invariably with AIDS, and thus it is being seen with increasing frequency. These RNA viruses alter the genetic code in the DNA of the cells resulting in aberrations when the cells divide. There is no way to eliminate these viruses from the body. The immune system suppresses them, as long as it functions normally. One of the consequences of infection of cells in the body by certain viruses is a derangement of the karyotype (the full chromosome set of the nucleus of a cell). Breakage, fragmentation, rearrangement of the chromosomes, abnormal chromosomes and even changes in the number of chromosomes may occur. The identification of viruses that alter the genetic code in various diseases is in its very early stages. We still have much to learn.

A major problem in studying viruses is that they often cannot be seen and are difficult to grow in culture. The light microscope was being used by the late 1600s to study bacteria, which are in the order of 0.3 to 0.5 micron. Viruses on the other hand are 0.01 to 0.02 micron, and could not be seen until the invention of the electron microscope in the 1930s. Magnification of no more than 1000 times can be achieved by the light microscope, whereas the electron microscope permits a magnification of 7,000 times. Even today we know that there are viruses that we have not yet identified. A valuable new tool that permits identification even where the organisms cannot be visualized is the polymerase chain reaction (PCR) technique that identifies the DNA and RNA of viruses. During the past decade it has become possible to map the entire structure of these minute entities. (See also AIDS in Chapter XI)

All of nature's exposures are not dark and sinister, however. Many substances that are taken into the body work to prevent disease, and even cancer. Vitamin E and beta-carotene (vitamin A precursor) are two such examples. Vitamins E and C (ascorbic acid) inhibit oxidative reactions that are part of the chemical processes in arteriosclerosis and the development of cancer. They prevent the formation of nitrosamines and thus reduce the risk of the production of cancer by these agents. An increased oxidation of lipids in the tissues takes place when a deficiency of vitamin E is present. Both ascorbic acid and vitamin E protect against ozone toxicity. Undoubtedly many other substances play a part in keeping our body chemistry in balance, also.

MOUSE TO MAN

Millions of dollars have been spent studying the toxicity, teratogenicity and carcinogenicity of man made chemicals. The results of these studies have then been raised as a banner in a crusade to lead us back to the days of our cave dwelling ancestors. Many of the people leading this crusade are individuals with no credentials, who initiate or join an organization that is based purely upon emotional appeal, formulating a name to match, and proceeding to create hysteria nationwide. This is much easier than working for a living, but ultimately the scam should become apparent to most astute individuals. In the meantime, however, great harm is being done and the public is wasting hundreds of millions of dollars.

What has had no press coverage is the toxicity and carcinogenicity of naturally occurring substances. Not only are we exposed to a far greater number of these natural toxins, they also are for the most part more potent toxins and carcinogens than their man-made cousins. This has been demonstrated in laboratory animals, but this subject has received little attention. This point has been made several times by Dr. Ames, as described above, and more recently in *Phantom Risk* [7], which I highly recommend that you read. Dr. Ames also points out, as have others, the futility of attempting to extrapolate laboratory data on mice to humans.

Humans are a far more sophisticated chemical factory than is the rat. Humans are less susceptible to damage, have more sophisticated enzyme systems and possess more elaborate repair mechanisms. Another problem with animal testing is that it is customary to apply massive doses in these tests, doses that are always toxic and sometimes fatal, quantities far in excess of what would ever be experienced in the real world. This is done partially because the researcher does not want to wait a lifetime to see what results might occur. Another reason is that the researcher can be more certain that he will have something to write about that will arouse the readers, and be more certain of achieving acclaim by peers and academic promotion and tenure committees. Achieving spectacular and alarming results from research projects also is the only way to assure the continuation of the billions of dollars that are doled out by the various federal bureaucracies in grant money. Following these guidelines, death in humans can be achieved by the simple administration of excessive quantities of water, thus proving the toxicity of water.

The regulatory actions that have been taken by government against cyclamates, nitrites, various pesticides and other substances have all been taken under the authority delivered by the Delaney Clause. Congress passed this addition to the Pure Food and Drug Act in 1958. As with all similar actions taken by Congress the Delaney Clause was motivated by politics and a passion for establishing one's name in the halls of fame (witness Kefauver), rather than by facts and good judgement. Not surprisingly, all such actions have created great mischief and yielded no benefit. This law requires that any food additive that causes cancer in any animal at any dose be banned. It does not, however, provide for a similar banning of far more potent carcinogens that occur in food without addition by man, such as aflatoxins in peanut butter.

During the years since the passage of the Delaney Clause, the fallacy of its premise has become more and more apparent. It should have been repealed years ago, but such logical corrective action is never taken by Congress. This same Congress still subsidizes the growth of tobacco, the single most common carcinogen in our society today. Similarly, rather than encouraging people to shun the practice of deliberately soaking up carcinogenic ultraviolet rays to excess, they prefer to concentrate on wasting billions of dollars in a mythical campaign to "save the ozone" by banning chlorofluorohydrocarbons. A law banning tanning parlors would seem far more logical and certainly would be more productive.

Deliberately destroying our current system of refrigeration, for such a nebulous goal, will produce great grief for us and cost us needless millions of dollars. Such policies are destroying industries that provide jobs, that have given us our current high standard of living, our current level of health and longevity, and have reduced the incidence of all cancers except those caused by cigarettes and excess exposure to the sun. The risk of skin cancer from sun exposure has increased fifteen-fold in the past fifty years simply because of the increased leisure time that we enjoy as part of the improvement in our standard of living. It has had nothing to do with any change in the ozone layer.

TOXICITY OTHER THAN CANCER

The role of chemicals in producing cancer has had the most publicity, but of greater importance are the other toxic hazards from chemicals, both natural and man made. Most people are aware that the consumption of the "wrong" mushroom can easily be fatal. Some of these very potent poisons have not been identified yet. A table listing some of the known hazards of mushrooms and the suffering that they inflict is included at the end of this chapter.

Our food supply delivers many toxic substances to us, some deadly, some that only make us deadly sick. Fugu, a genus of the Japanese puffer fish, and a delicacy in Japan, contains a very deadly toxin that results in approximately 100 deaths each year in Japan. Scombroid poisoning results when scombroid fish (tuna, mackerel, sardines, skipjacks and bonitos) are not properly iced down after harvesting. Under these conditions histamine is produced from histidine in the muscle tissue. Another substance, not yet identified, contributes to the poisoning. Although the poisoning produces some pronounced and unpleasant symptoms, it is not fatal and is rarely serious.

Ciguatera poisoning occurs after eating certain species of tropical saltwater fish, bottom dwellers, or other fish that feed on them. Fish commonly involved are barracuda, groupers, snappers, surgeonfish, parrotfish, jacks and sea basses. Some 300 to 400 species of fish have been identified as having caused this poisoning at various times. Consumption of certain blue-green algae or of dinoflagellates is responsible for the presence of the toxin in the fish. There is no certain way to consume any of these species of fish and avoid the poisoning. The toxin is again concentrated to a greater degree in the internal organs. It is heat stable, which means that it is not destroyed by cooking.

All of these toxins in food are chemicals that occur naturally; they are not man-made. Although all of the food poisonings that are discussed in Chapter V are environmental hazards that are produced naturally, the carelessness of man and the neglect of basic hygiene both play a major role in some of them.

Gossypol, which is extracted from the cotton plant and is the substance responsible for cottonseed poisoning, is a very interesting naturally occurring chemical. It has been used in China since before 1978 as a male contraceptive, having been taken orally by thousands of patients.[8] It produces a pronounced decrease in sperm production by the Sertoli cell in the testicle, and reduces sperm motility. Unfortunately it produces some unpleasant side effects, including diarrhea, shortness of breath, weakness, neuritis and a decreased blood potassium level. These are the symptoms seen in cottonseed poisoning. Whether this naturally occurring substance is viewed as a medicine or a poison depends upon the viewpoint of the victim as well as the dose. Its toxicity precludes the use of cottonseed meal in animal feeds.

As man's inhumanity to man continues unabated as it has throughout the ages, at least ten nations, including the United States, have active research programs to develop both chemical and biological weapons. The most worrisome of these are the efforts to biologically modify pathogenic microorganisms so that they are not only more destructive, but also resistant to all of the antibiotics and chemotherapeutic agents that we possess. The most popular chemical agent among the terrorist perverts is currently sarin (GB gas), an organophosphate chemical that was used by Iraq against Kurdish villages in northern Iraq in 1988, and by terrorists in Japan in 1994 and in 1995 (see Chapter XIV). There is also evidence that American troops, as well as those of Great Britain and other countries, were exposed to this and other agents during the Gulf War in 1991. The United States government has steadfastly attempted to cover up this exposure and the illnesses that have ensued in thousands of personnel.

CS gas, which is widely used in conjunction with capsaicin (pepper gas), was used by the FBI and the BATF in the slaughter of 86 people, including 24 children, at Waco, Texas in 1993. This gas, ortho-chlorobenzylidine malonitrile, had been banned by international treaty, but over 400 canisters of it were hurled into the closed compound where these people had taken refuge. This agent had caused many deaths prior to the Waco incident, and several studies have demonstrated serious toxicity from it. A few cases of permanent reactive lung disease following exposure to CS gas and capsaicin, used in riot control, have been reported.[9] These studies have been done for the most part on exposures in the open, where concentrations are relatively low. No studies have been done on victims who are exposed to the massive concentrations used at Waco. The use of these agents is inhumane and uncivilized, behavior typical of tyrants.

A weapon equally as sinister has been developed to deliberately blind people. This is a laser weapon that can be carried on the shoulder or mounted on a helicopter so that anyone who looks up has his retina destroyed. There is currently an effort to gain international agreement to ban the use of this weapon, but such a ban has not prevented the development and use of chemical and biologic weapons. Even if an international agreement to ban its use is reached, this does not prevent governments from using it on their own people, as was demonstrated at Waco.

METALS

Arsenic, nickel and **chromium** all have produced many cancers among workers exposed to these metals and their salts in various occupational settings. These cancers were documented as long ago as 1556 A.D. In addition to the cancers produced, chromium produces severe damage to the tubules in the kidneys, nickel is a common cause of dermatitis, and arsenic produces toxic changes in virtually all of the body systems, including the brain. These are all naturally occurring elements and we cannot avoid these risks even by leaving them in the earth. Even if we made it illegal to mine or smelt these ores we would still have environmental exposures.

Serious health hazards face those who live in the regions surrounding the mining and smelting of copper and lead, which produces arsenic fallout. Children who lived in the communities surrounding Anaconda, Montana were found to have urinary arsenic levels seven times as high as children in communities that are outside of the fallout area do. This reflects ingestion of contaminated soil during play, a practice that is common in young children. Children are also exposed to arsenic through skin contact with and splinters from treated lumber in decks and playground furniture. Chromated copper arsenate is the chemical used as a preservative in this lumber. Contact with this lumber through hands and bare feet results in arsenic absorption by the skin, a clear cancer hazard.

Splinters from the wood inject the arsenic into the skin more efficiently. (See also Chapters I and III).

Mercury: One of the most insidious and destructive of all of the naturally occurring poisons is mercury. It attacks the nervous system, particularly the brain, destroying sight, speech and control of muscles. Mercury in its natural liquid form has produced these symptoms in many workers mining or smelting it, virtually throughout recorded history. The damage ensuing from these occupations was documented by several writers of the fifteenth and sixteenth century (see Chapter X). The dramatic and tragic consequences of exposure to mercury were demonstrated very graphically by the character the *Mad Hatter* in Lewis Carroll's 1865 work, *Alice's Adventures in Wonderland*.

In view of all of the documented observations of mercury's destructive effects on the brain and the most vital of bodily functions over a period of almost two thousand years, how can we be shocked and surprised at the repeated tragic poisonings such as occurred at Minamata, Japan in 1953, and in Iraq in 1971-1972? The ravaging of minds and bodies by mercury resulted from naturally occurring forms for the first two thousand years, but man has improved the poison.

Organic mercury salts proved to be invaluable when applied to seed grain to prevent rot. This resulted in an increase in crop yields and a reduction in crop diseases. Even though the grain was clearly marked with a pink dye, and a clear, large warning label was on the bag, it was consumed as feed, either for animals or directly by humans. The results were the same in both cases. In Iraq when the contaminated wheat was made into flour instead of being planted, 6,000 victims were hospitalized, and more than 500 died. In New Mexico a farmer fed grain that had been treated with methyl mercury to his hogs, even though it had a clear label warning against this use. When the family ate the meat from the hogs, his four children suffered the tragic and predictable nerve and brain damage.

There has been much publicity about the health hazard of the mercury in dental fillings. Many people have had their money extracted from their wallets through the misconception that these fillings should be replaced with a safer material. There is no better or safer material for dental restorations than the silver-mercury amalgam. It is stable and the mercury bound in this amalgam is not released into the body. This is and has been the firm position of the American Dental Association. A study by the National Institutes of Health concluded in 1992 that the mercury in dental amalgam presents no significant risk.

The mercury in dental amalgams does present a hazard when it is removed from the mouth and altered. Four adults in Michigan died from acute mercury poisoning in 1989 as a result of attempts to recover the silver in the amalgam. The amalgam had been smelted in a casting furnace in the basement of the home where the four individuals lived. Mercury fumes were distributed through the heating ducts in the home. Death ensued in spite of the diagnosis of the mercury poisoning and intensive medical treatment. With pure silver selling at less than $5 per ounce (gold was $135 at the time) this could not have been a very profitable venture, even if no deaths had ensued.

More recently concern has been expressed over the release of mercury into the environment by virtue of the process of cremation. Some mercury is released into the atmosphere during the cremation and into bodies of water or the land after deposition of the ashes. From the land it can find its way into surface water or underground aquifers. The simple process of removing the amalgam prior to cremation would eliminate this risk. It will only be a matter of time before some enterprising politician introduces such a law.

The saga of mercury demonstrates something more shameful than neglect and carelessness. It borders on stupidity on the part of people who should know better. The natural reaction of the extremists again is to ban the agent of destruction, rather than to address the problems of the one who delivered it. It seems to me that some application of wisdom and common sense would be a more appropriate reaction. We need to keep in mind that the major source of mercury in our environment is the natural degassing of the earth's crust, including landmasses, rivers and oceans. The quantity delivered to our environment through this process exceeds 100,000 tons per year. It is going to be very difficult for the environmental extremists to control this contamination, but they can undoubtedly count on complete cooperation from the news media and the Congress.

Aluminum: Since about 1975 there has been considerable interest in the role that aluminum plays in senile dementia and especially in presenile dementia (Alzheimer's disease). The question of why some people are affected while others with identical exposure are not remains unanswered. Injection of aluminum and aluminum phosphate into the spinal fluid of laboratory animals produces an encephalopathy and degenerative changes in the nerve fibers that are very similar to those found in patients with senile and presenile dementia.

A similar progressive and fatal neurological change is seen in patients who undergo long term dialysis treatments for kidney failure. The first symptom seen is a speech disorder followed by dementia, convulsions, muscle spasms and death. The symptoms begin after 3 to 7 years of treatment. The aluminum content of the brain, muscles and bone is increased in these victims suggesting aluminum intoxication. The source is believed to be the aluminum hydroxide that is commonly given to patients who are undergoing dialysis to attempt to maintain a proper calcium balance. The intravenous feeding solutions administered to premature infants routinely contains aluminum, and aluminum deposits in the brain have been found in those infants who develop neurotoxicity. Aluminum is the most common metallic element in the earth's crust, the third most common element (by weight) behind oxygen and nitrogen. It has no known biologic function, however.

Selenium: Selenium has become popular recently as a health food supplement, and serious illness has been observed as a result. Although much of selenium's activity in the body has not been mapped out, it is known to be essential to some enzyme systems. It appears to play other roles that have not been identified. Adequate supplies are obtained in food, however, since it is present in the soil in more than sufficient quantities in the U.S. and most of the world. Because of its wide distribution in nature it is found in meat, dairy products and grain in quantities that are more than adequate for nutritional needs. All of the toxic events in humans, aside from occupational exposure, have resulted from the injudicious use of selenium as a dietary supplement.

Very few regions on earth have geologic strata that is deficient in selenium. Deficiency syndromes have been seen in some regions of China and New Zealand. In other regions, such as in Colombia, where the soil is rich in selenium, malformed infants have been seen in parents with selenium toxicity. Damage to the liver and spleen as well as damage to the nervous system and loss of hair and nails occurs with excess intake. Hoof rot is seen in animals grazing in these areas. The safe range is very narrow. It has been used effectively in anti-dandruff shampoos for over 40 years in a 2.5 percent concentration for the prescription form (Selsun™). Tests in laboratory animals have demonstrated no toxic effect from this use.

Thallium: few people would even recognize the name of this metal, but it has surprisingly diverse use in the workplace, and is an extremely toxic substance. It is cumulative in the body, making occupational exposure insidious and hazardous. It is well absorbed through the skin as well as from inhalation and ingestion. It produces serious damage to the nervous system with mental confusion and death. It has been used successfully to poison humans, and while the results are not as rapid and dramatic as cyanide, it has usually accomplished its mission. The many occupational exposures to thallium as well as to the other metals, and their respective hazards are discussed in Chapter X.

Cadmium: this metal is widely distributed in nature and in industry. The many exposures in the workplace are discussed in Chapter X. Aside from the mining and smelting of lead, zinc and copper, cadmium is introduced into our environment by fuel combustion and the use of phosphate fertilizers. Food, both plant and animal, is the main source of cadmium exposure for the general population. The second most common source is the smoking of cigarettes.

Exposure to environmental cadmium by the general population results in chronic poisoning. The most serious results of this chronic toxicity are permanent damage to the kidneys, hypertension and damage to the arterial walls, and decalcification and weakening of the bones. The latter results in leg and back pain, fractures and deformities. Dietary deficiencies of iron, calcium and protein enhance the absorption of cadmium from the gastrointestinal tract. Absorbed cadmium is distributed throughout the body by the blood, and accumulates primarily in the kidneys and the liver. From these storage sites it would take the body 10 to 30 years to eliminate one-half of the amount stored. The substance thus accumulates in the body with continued exposure.

Cadmium is seldom considered as the culprit when pathology in the kidney and cardiovascular system is discovered. Its presence in the body can be detected by the presence in the urine of a low molecular weight protein (beta-2-microglobulin), but this test is not commonly ordered, and is more likely to be invoked in occupational settings. Even there cadmium is often overlooked.

LIME

Calcium oxide, known as quick lime or unslaked lime, produces serious chemical burns and is particularly damaging in the eye. Calcium oxide readily combines with water to form calcium hydroxide, or slaked lime, which is found in Portland cement and in plaster. Because of its economy it is also very useful in adjusting the pH of acidic soil. In previous times slaked lime was mixed with wheat paste to make whitewash, as used by Tom Sawyer and others on fences, barns etc. This process has been replaced by the wide availability of a multitude of economical and more durable paints.

CATARACTS:

A cataract denotes a change in the normal transparency of the lens of the eye to a translucency of varying degrees. The result is the loss of vision, the severity of which depends upon the extent of the change. Several chemicals are capable of causing these changes in the lens, including some medications. In the occupational setting inhalation or skin absorption of naphthalene vapor can produce cataracts. Acute poisoning in children has occurred from skin contact with clothes that have been stored in mothballs. Naphthalene is also a constituent of some deodorant cakes. The chemical is toxic to the retina of the eye, where damage can result in blindness.

Several hundred cases of cataracts were caused by 2,4-dinitrophenol when it was sold without a prescription as an agent for weight loss from 1935 to 1937. Passage of a law subsequently banned its use for this purpose, but it continues to be used as a herbicide. Its use as a fungicide, pesticide and miticide should have been abandoned in favor of the many more effective and less toxic agents widely available now. Medications that have the potential to induce cataracts include the long-term administration of any of the cortisone preparations, as in rheumatoid arthritis, as well as large doses of chlorpromazine over a prolonged period. Myleran used for long periods in the treatment of chronic myeloid leukemia also can produce cataracts. Individuals on any of these medications should have the same periodic examinations that are prescribed for diabetics to detect any changes early.

EMS

A new health threat delivered by a dietary substance was first described in the United States in New Mexico in October 1989. This was EMS, eosinophilia-myalgia syndrome, a disease character-ized by severe, incapacitating myalgia (muscle pain) and markedly elevated eosinophils in the blood. Deaths have occurred in up to 10 percent of the victims. The disease was caused by trace amounts of a contaminant in batches of L-tryptophan produced by one specific Japanese manufacturer.[10] L-tryptophan supplies from all other manufacturers during this period did not produce the eosinophilia-myalgia syndrome. The contaminant appeared in 1988 after changes in the manufacturing process were made. The chemical structure of the contaminant has been analyzed and has been identified as a dimer of L-tryptophan. It appears to be the product of a chemical reaction between L-tryptophan and acetaldehyde.

The risk of acquiring EMS was directly related to the dose consumed. Many milder cases occurred in people who took lower doses than did those with the more pronounced symptoms. The total number of cases that were reported in the United States through June 1990 was 1,531. The incidence of the disease dropped sharply after the FDA banned L-tryptophan from the market in 1990. No new cases have been reported subsequently.

Similarities exist in the symptoms and pathology produced by EMS and by the toxic-oil syndrome epidemic. In the latter episode 20,000 people in Madrid, Spain were poisoned in 1981 by contaminated rapeseed (canola) oil, sold illegally as olive oil. About 12,000 people were hospitalized with over 300 deaths in the first year. Serious, fatal for many, fibrosis and degenerative changes occurred in the lungs, heart and blood vessels throughout the body. In many victims the disease resembled scleroderma or systemic lupus erythematosus.[11,12] Although the contaminant that caused that epidemic has never been identified, other episodes of toxic oil syndrome have been related to aniline found in the contaminated oil.[13,14] This is chemically related to the anthranilic acid used in the preparation of tryptophan.

ETHYLENE GLYCOL

The base for all permanent antifreeze preparations is ethylene glycol, which is very toxic if consumed. When it is drained from vehicles and a puddle remains, animals are attracted to it because of its sweet taste. This same sweetness makes it attractive to children, with fatal consequences. It is metabolized to oxalic acid in the body, which is highly toxic to the kidneys. Other less concentrated sources of oxalic acid, which result in poisoning and death due to kidney damage, are the philodendron, sorrel and dieffenbachia (dumbcane) plants (see Chapter III).

Recently two companies have marketed a permanent antifreeze with a propylene glycol base, claiming them to be less of a threat to pets. It is true that this product is not sweet, and thus perhaps less likely to be consumed by animals. It is not without toxicity, however, and the same disposal precautions should prevail. It also requires a larger quantity of the product to provide a comparable protection at any given temperature.

ALAR — THE GREAT APPLE FIASCO

Moving from fact to fiction, one of the strangest dramas ever staged in the United States was acted out in early 1989. Alar (daminozide) is a chemical that was sprayed on apple trees to reduce spoilage. It also increased storage life and improved the quality of the fruit. In 1989 a self appointed environmental group, with absolutely no scientific credentials, the Natural Resources Defense Council (NRDC), launched a carefully contrived public campaign to convince the public that Alar was a dangerous chemical that was causing cancer in children. To accomplish their goal they paid Fenton Communications more than $180,000 a year to promote the lie. They produced a study, later shown to be fraudulent, that stated that "as many as 5,300 children may contract cancer from their preschool exposure to UDMH" (Alar). In fact not a single child ever has. The NRDC was joined in the conspiracy by many members of Congress, led by Senator Christopher Dodd of Connecticut who chaired a committee that promoted the false allegations through the media.

Widespread coverage of the lies was guaranteed by the appearance of a Hollywood actress, Meryl Streep, and the staged questioning of her by members of Congress who were zealous to garner as much press coverage as possible. The theme throughout these staged and widely publicized hearings was that the children of the United States were being poisoned by apples and applesauce, that they contained a dangerous cancer-causing chemical. In fact this was a deliberate lie, and everyone involved knew that it was a lie. An EPA Scientific Advisory Panel had ruled in 1985 that there was no evidence that Alar caused cancer. The British government, as well as the World Health Organization and the UN Food and Agriculture Organization all concluded in 1989 that Alar did not cause cancer and was safe in human foods.[15]

The result of the staged congressional hearing, *60 Minutes* broadcast and national news coverage was a nationwide panic, resulting in an avalanche of calls to physicians. Apples were removed from school cafeterias and from grocery stores. The resultant collapse of the market for apples forced many small growers into bankruptcy. The financial loss to growers is estimated at between $60 million and $140 million.

Unfortunately the smear campaign was given support by corrupt bureaucrats at the EPA, who were miffed at being rebuffed by a panel of scientists who reviewed the data on Alar. These studies had shown that Alar posed no toxic threat, and was not carcinogenic. The EPA then ordered that the dose of Alar in these tests be raised to at least twice the toxic level. The animals finally died of toxic overdose. The news media, in spite of the evidence to the contrary, continued to give wide national coverage to the campaign to convince the public that Alar was a carcinogen. Never was the public told that less than 15 percent of the apples marketed were treated with Alar. This unprecedented demonstration of irresponsibility by the media cost the American people hundreds of millions of dollars in addition to the loss by the growers, to say nothing of the needless anxiety imposed on the public. Many family growers, processors and packers went bankrupt.

Predictably, the company that marketed Alar withdrew it from the market, not because it posed any danger, but because the

560

media campaign had succeeded in painting it as a dangerous product. This is a pattern that has been repeated many times in the past two decades. Lawsuits with no credibility prompt companies to withdraw products rather than sustain the risk of great financial loss. This has been particularly common and unfortunate in the health care field. We have been deprived of many safe and useful products by these tactics. We have permitted a small number of corrupt, very vocal individuals to stampede us by lies and distorted propaganda into taking actions based upon emotion and hysteria rather than on facts and sound judgement. Repeated studies by both government and private laboratories have demonstrated that there is no measurable residue of pesticides in fruit and vegetables reaching the market.

The trial lawyers struck gold on an even grander scale with the issue of silicone breast implants. Their campaign pattern followed that of Alar, which had proven the effectiveness of waging a nationwide propaganda campaign to scare the public. With breast implants it succeeded beyond their wildest dreams, and they have harvested billions of dollars in fees for a claim that subsequently has been disproved. After studies reporting no association between the implants and the connective tissue disorders that they were purported to cause were published, the attack lawyers unleashed an unprecedented, vicious attack against anyone associated with these reports, including the Mayo Clinic and a sympathetic editor at the *New England Journal of Medicine*.[16]

Their accusations included corruption and greed, even "scientific money laundering." Talk about the pot calling the kettle black. In this fiasco they were again aided by the usual cast of disreputable characters; Connie Chung launched the big scare on her CBS show in 1990, Ralph Nader and Dr. Sidney Wolfe of Public Citizen spread the lie and profited by selling kits to make it easier to file lawsuits. Even Dr. David Kessler of the FDA contributed to the massacre by withdrawing the implants from the market, giving the impression that he concurred with the lawyers. His later statements that his action was not provoked by any known risk, but rather legal technicalities, was universally ignored by the media, the lawyers and the courts.

Dow Corning was put out of business, suffering the fate of the AH Robins Company (the oldest ethical pharmaceutical company in the U.S.) in the intrauterine device fiasco previously. These undertakings add to the wealth of lawyers, but they certainly are not in the best interests of the American public. Corruption and greed can be expected in the legal profession, and they have been joined by some physicians who in essence are selling their services in these schemes. In the final analysis, however, the awards are being made by the Americans serving on the juries, demonstrating a remarkable stupidity and irresponsibility. Successful self-government requires self-discipline, as well as honesty and integrity.

POISONS IN MUSHROOMS

TYPE OF POISON	SYMPTOMS
Intestinal irritant	Vomiting, diarrhea with dehydration and shock.
Muscarine, not destroyed by cooking	Profuse sweating, nausea, vomiting, abdominal pain and blurred vision.
Psilocybin	Hallucinations
Ibotenic acid (muscimol) (Amanita mushrooms)	Delirium, manic behavior.
Coprine	Antabuse-like alcohol reaction.
Monomethylhydrazine. Gyromitra (morel like)	Headache, vomiting, abdominal fullness, malaise.
Amatoxins from Amanita phalloides. Toxin not affected by cooking.	Causes almost all fatalities from mushrooms. Resembles acute hepatitis. Kidney damage may occur late.
Cortinarius species. Toxin not identified yet.	Severe kidney damage (renal tubular necrosis).

Other species cause toxic reactions but source has not been identified as yet.

Many species of fungi other than mushrooms produce toxins. The aflatoxins and ochratoxins are the only groups known to cause cancer in man, but illness can result from the toxins of others. These are listed in the table below.

MYCOTOXINS

FUNGUS	TOXIN	PRODUCT
Aspergillus flavus	Aflatoxins	Peanuts, corn other grains
Penicillium	Patulin	Apples, applejuice, apple-sauce
Fusarium, Cephalosporium, Trichoderma, others	Trichothecenes group	Cereal grains, corn
Fusarium	Zearalenones	Corn, other grains
Aspergillus & Penicillium	Ochratoxins	Cereal grains, corn
Penicillium citreoviride	Citreoviridin	Rice
Penicillium rubrum	Rubratoxins	Corn
Penicillium urticae	Griseofulvin	Grains
Penicillium cyclopium	Penicillic acid	Grains

All of the above listed toxins have the potential to cause serious illness in humans. That this occurs uncommonly in the U.S. is due to the precautions taken in harvesting and storing crops. This may be motivated by a profit incentive more than an interest in public health, but the benefits are the same. Where crops are left standing in the field over the winter, as occurred in wartime, the fungi have an opportunity to multiply and produce their respective toxins. Poisoning of the populace has been seen on these occasions, and this occurs periodically in other parts of the world as well.

1. Ames BN, Profet M, and Gold LS. 1990. Dietary pesticides (99.99% all natural). 87 *Proc. Nat. Acad. Sci.* 7777–7781.

2. Hall RL. *Proceedings of Marabou Symposium on Foods and Cancer.* Caslan Press, Stockholm, 1979.

3. Klassen CD. *Casarett and Doull's Toxicology.* Ed. 5. McGraw-Hill, Columbus, OH 1996.

4. U.S. Department of Health and Human Services, Public Health Service, National Toxicology Program. *Report on Carcinogens*, Ninth Edition, 2000.

5. Ames BN, Magaw R, Gold L. Ranking possible carcinogenic hazards. *Science* 1987;**236**:271–280.

6. One part per million is equivalent to three tablespoonfuls in the contents of an 8,000 gallon railroad tank car. One part per billion is equivalent to three tablespoonsful in the total contents of 1,000 of those cars.

7. Ames BN and Gold LS, 1993. Environmental pollution and cancer: some misconceptions. In Foster KR, Bernstein DE and Huber PW, eds. *Phantom Risk; Scientific inference and the law*, 153-181. Cambridge Mass: MIT Press.

8. During a 1979 visit to the University of California at Berkeley School of Public Health, Dr. Liu Kuo-chen of the Department of Urology, Capital Hospital, Chinese Academy of Medical Sciences, Peking (Beijing), China presented his experience with 5,000 patients who had taken gossypol as a male contraceptive. The author attended this presentation.

9. Roth VS, Franzblau A. RADS after exposure to a riot-control agent: A case report. *J Occ & Env Med* 1996. **38**:(9)863-64.

10. Philen RM, Hill RH. 3-(Phenylamino)alanine—a link between Eosinophilia-Myalgia Syndrome and Toxic Oil Syndrome? *Mayo Clin Proc* 1993;**68**:197-200.

11. Toxic Epidemic Syndrome Study Group. Toxic Epidemic Syndrome, Spain, 1981. *Lancet* 1982;**2**:697-702.

12. Kilbourne EM, Rigau-Perez JG, Heath CW Jr, et al. Clinical epidemiology of toxic-oil syndrome: manifestations of a new illness. *N Engl J Med* 1983;**309**:-1408-14.

13. Tabuenca JM. Toxic allergic syndrome caused by ingestion of rapeseed oil denatured with aniline. *Lancet* 1981;**2**:567-8.

14. Mayeno AN, Belongia EA, Feng Lin, et al. 3-(Phenylamino)alanine, a novel aniline-derived amino acid associated with Eosinophilia-Myalgia Syndrome: a link to the toxic oil syndrome? *Mayo Clin Proc*; **67**:1134-1139, 1992.

15. Marshall E. A is for Apple, Alar, and...Alarmist? *Science* 1991;**254**:20-22.

16. Angell, Marcia,MD. *Science on Trial:The Clash of Medical Evidence and the Law in the Breast Implant Case*. WW Norton, New York, 1996.

XIV

HAZARDS OF PESTICIDES AND HERBICIDES

Wisdom can come only through knowledge, experience and rational thought.
— DEW

PESTICIDES

Those of us who are in our fifth or sixth decade can well recall the fly-laden screens of our homes when we were growing up. Keeping these pests out of the house was a constant and frustrating task. This was a particularly urgent problem in the 1940's since flies were considered to be one of the chief vectors of poliomyelitis, a prevalent and dread disease of the time. Then came DDT to the rescue. DDT was discovered to be an effective insecticide by Paul Müller, a chemist in Switzerland working for Geigy, in 1939. Müller was awarded a Nobel Prize in 1948 for his work. DDT was effective against virtually all insects, and was relatively harmless to mammals. DDT in a 10 percent powder was used during World War II to dust entire populations in cities that were liberated by the Allies in order to control lice and diseases such as plague and typhus, which could have invoked death and destruction upon our troops, as had been the rule in all prior wars. It was a godsend to our troops and to our war effort.

After the war, I recall vividly the war surplus jeeps fogging the neighborhoods in my hometown with DDT, and the flies (and mosquitos) disappeared. Although DDT was to fall into disrepute, it was a great blessing at the time. The era of chemical control of pests that transmit disease and destroy our crops was thus ushered in. These weapons are, of course, a two edged sword. They cannot be used indiscriminately with impunity, and careless handling and application have resulted in illness among humans. Fortunately most of these instances in the United States have resulted in temporary illness and few fatalities. Far more serious incidents have occurred elsewhere.

More than a hundred people died in India after eating wheat that had been contaminated with parathion from spillage during shipping. Fewer deaths occurred, but more than four thousand people were poisoned by hexachlorobenzene (discussed later in this chapter) in Turkey after they ate seed grain that had been treated with this fungicide. Numerous similar tragic incidents have occurred worldwide from eating seed grain treated with organic mercurial compounds and other fungicides.

Experience in the United States has demonstrated that these chemicals can be utilized with relative safety if handled and applied with intelligence and care. Significant risk exists during the handling and application of chemicals. The individual who loads the materials aboard aircraft for aerial application of pesticides, and the flagman on the ground who marks the flight path and signals the end of the row to the pilot are especially at risk. Agriculture in general is the area where the greatest risk exists, and particularly in commercial agriculture.

The organophosphate pesticides, which in general are limited to commercial and farm use, are by far the most frequently involved in poisoning. This group of chemicals was first synthesized in Germany in 1937. The Nazis subsequently developed the more toxic of these agents for use as nerve gases, and at least one of these (cyclon-B) was used to kill victims at Auschwitz. Some of these agents remain in the stockpiles of governments today. This fact and the continuing research for more potent substances and more effective delivery systems is flatly denied by all of the involved parties. At least one of these substances, sarin (GB gas), was used by Iraq against Kurdish villages in northern Iraq in 1988,[1,2] and evidence suggests that it was also used against Iran during its war with Iraq. Sarin is the substance used in an attack in Matsumoto, Japan in June 1994 that poisoned about 600 people, killing seven, and in the Tokyo subway attack in March 1995 that killed 11 people and injured an additional 5,000.

Although all of the organophosphate chemicals that have been developed for use as pesticides were derived from nerve gases (soman, sarin and tabun), current agents are at least four generations of development removed from the original nerve gasses, and are much less toxic. Parathion, introduced in 1944, although far removed from the toxicity of the nerve gases, remains the most toxic of the organophosphate pesticides to humans, and has been largely supplanted by safer compounds. It replaced the much less toxic DDT in the 1950s after DDT was banned, and a series of fatal poisonings followed.

While the organophosphates are among the most potent toxic pesticides in existence, good treatment for poisoning is available if it is administered promptly. Most of these agents should not be used in or around the home. Regulations controlling their application are designed to minimize residual on fruits and vegetables. Washing of all fruits and vegetables before consumption is always advisable, however.

There is little excuse for events such as the poisoning of over one thousand individuals in 1985 when aldicarb (Temik) was illegally applied to melons commercially grown in California. The Centers for Disease Control reported that poisoned individuals who ate these melons were seen at medical facilities in Alaska, Arizona, Colorado, Hawaii, Idaho, Nevada, Oregon and Washington and in two provinces in Canada.[3] This case clearly demonstrates the potential widespread consequences of irresponsible use of pesticides. Several previous episodes of poisoning resulted from consumption of cucumbers and mint that had been treated with aldicarb.

Aldicarb, which is a very effective systemic pesticide, is taken up by the plant and stored in the fruit or vegetable. It is not licensed for such application. During the period when these poisonings occurred its use was limited to citrus groves and potato fields. Its use is currently limited to greenhouse applications. Even in that setting it must be handled with great care because it is absorbed through the skin. It is very toxic through this route as well as by ingestion. Deaths have occurred from such skin contact among workers in the field. Poisonings also have occurred where Aldicarb was sold illegally as a rodenticide. These cases (at least twenty-five) have been seen primarily in New York among emigrants from the Dominican Republic, where the substance can be purchased legally as a rodenticide.[4] Aldicarb is capable of causing sickness and death at the lowest concentration of any registered pesticide in the United States. Fortunately, poisoning is amenable to treatment if medical care is sought promptly. Deaths have occurred, however. Individuals who have other medical conditions or who are on certain medications are at an increased risk. No long-term harmful effects are known, and it is not a suspected carcinogen.

Much progress has been made in the development and control of pesticides during the past forty some years. Much more needs to be done, particularly in the education of the general public. These substances have produced great benefits to us, both in the reduction of disease and in increased crop yield. Every precaution must be taken, however, to prevent entry to the body through breathing, eating or application to the skin. They should never be mixed or handled in the kitchen, even though that may seem to be a convenient place for a laboratory. Shoes that are worn while applying chemicals to the lawn should be removed before entering the house. Wearing canvas shoes that can be laundered will help prevent these chemicals from gaining entrance to the house.

Many chemicals that are applied to the lawn or grounds can be tracked into the house on shoes for weeks afterwards. These chemicals also can be carried on dust by the shoes or the wind. House pets are a particular problem. Any chemical that you apply to pets, even if applied outdoors as should be the practice, will be brought indoors with them. You should not, therefore, use any chemical on them that you do not want inside the house. The same rule applies to houseplants. These should be treated outdoors also.

Several categories of pesticides exist. DDT belongs to the group classified as chlorinated hydrocarbons. Also in this group are methoxychlor, chlordane, aldrin, dieldrin, endrin, toxaphene, heptachlor, kepone, mirex, benzene hexachloride (mixed isomers) and lindane (gamma isomer). These compounds as a group are more persistent in the environment than most other pesticides, because they are resistant to breakdown. They thus tend to accumulate in the soil and in the beds of lakes and streams. This is less characteristic of DDT, however, and it has been shown in more recent studies that it does degrade both in humans and in the environment. Intestinal bacteria, especially *Aerobacter aerogenes*, have been shown to degrade DDT to several metabolites.

Because of the persistence of the chlorinated hydrocarbons they have fallen into disfavor. As a class they have less acute toxicity than the organophosphates or carbamates, but a greater potential for chronic toxicity. They are poorly absorbed through the skin and are most efficiently absorbed by ingestion. On the other hand they pass readily through the chitinous exoskeleton of insects. They are not very soluble in water. They are therefore commonly formulated in petroleum distillates, such as kerosene, so vomiting should not be induced following ingestion.

DDT

Dichlorodiphenyl-trichloroethane was first introduced for commercial use in the United States in 1947. It was the most effective of all of the synthetic insecticides, and the least costly to produce. As mentioned previously, it was widely used during World War II to control lice, and thus typhus, by dusting humans with a ten percent powder. It is poorly absorbed from the skin (unless formulated in petroleum distillates). In spite of many studies no evidence has emerged to date that any harmful effects resulted from this application to people. On the other hand our troops were spared the disease and pestilence that could reasonably have been expected. In Naples, Italy in January 1944, during a typhus epidemic, over one million civilians were dusted with ten percent DDT, and the incidence of the disease fell sharply. Subsequently thousands of troops and refugees were dusted to protect against typhus and other diseases. The results were dramatic, preventing any outbreak of typhus in these populations. In contrast thousands of cases of typhus occurred among soldiers in other theaters of the war and among persons in prison camps. Millions of people had been victims of typhus in previous wars.

There is no evidence of any fatal poisoning, or other adverse reaction, in humans from DDT in spite of such widespread and intimate application. In fact all recorded attempts at suicide where DDT was used failed. Workers at the Montrose Chemical Company absorbed 400 times as much DDT as the average American, but not a single case of cancer was reported.[5]

Virtually everyone who lived in that era, and indeed since, has demonstrable residues of DDT in the body fat tissues. Elimination from these stores is slow. The biologic half-life of DDT in cattle is 335 days. During the 1960s when DDT was widely used, levels of 5 ppm were found in human fat tissue. By the late 1960s, after the reduction in the application of DDT and the eventual ban, these levels were down to 2 ppm. By 1982 only trace levels were found in human adipose tissue.[6]

In spite of this evidence of widespread exposure and long term storage, no adverse health effects have ever evolved. DDT was reported to cause liver tumors in laboratory animals (rats and mice) as early as 1947. Then a nationwide hysteria followed the publication of Rachel Carson's book, *Silent Spring* in 1962, in which she labeled DDT a dangerous chemical that might be causing cancer in humans. Experience and scientific studies have proven her wrong. Carson, who was a vegetarian, blamed DDT for her own breast cancer. She was wrong again. Carson resorted to the distortion of facts in her book in a campaign to condemn DDT.[7]

Many others took part in this conspiracy. In EPA testimony that was published in *Science* Dr. Samuel Epstein reported that mice that were fed DDT developed cancer. He withheld the fact that the mice that were not fed DDT developed more cancers than those fed DDT (83 vs 68 in the DDT fed mice). In reality long term studies of large numbers of people have demonstrated no evidence that DDT caused cancer or otherwise shortened the lives of people exposed to it.[8,9] Extensive use of this pesticide worldwide ever since that time has failed to demonstrate any significant adverse effects in humans. DDT remains the safest and most effective pesticide ever developed.

Fish are very sensitive to the toxicity of DDT, as they are to most chemicals including soaps and detergents, and to temperature and pH. People who have tropical fish tanks are well aware of this sensitivity. Behavioral changes were among the most obvious evidence of accumulation of DDT in fish. Widespread publicity was given to claims in the 1960s that the survival of certain species of wild birds was threatened through the thinning of their eggshells. This was blamed on DDT. In reality bird populations increased significantly after DDT was introduced.[10] It was later learned that studies that were done to prove eggshell thinning were fraudulent. The study birds were deliberately malnourished and calcium was withheld, conditions known to produce eggshell thinning.

When Bitman repeated this experiment (*Nature* 1969;224:44, *Science* in 1970 and *Poultry Science* 1971;50:657-659) with appropriate calcium in the bird's diet there was no thinning of eggshells. Subsequent studies have also suggested that other industrial chemicals such as polychlorinated biphenyls (PCBs), which have been widely used in electrical transformers, may have played a part in the observed eggshell thinning. [11] Furthermore the bald eagle had been on the verge of extinction in the 1920s long before DDT. Eagles were shot for bounties and for their feathers.

An epidemic of Newcastle Disease (avian influenza) during this period also decimated some bird populations.

DDT, as well as chlordane, PCBs and PBBs, are all stored in the fatty tissues of fish and most animals including humans. The environmental zealots claimed that the higher up the food chain that these stores of chemicals were consumed, the greater would become the concentration stored in fat. They again turned to fraudulent studies to prove their claims, selecting only tissue samples that they knew would produce the desired result. In reality honest studies disproved their biomagnification claims.

On June 14, 1972 William Ruckelhaus, Administrator of the EPA, as a result of political pressure from environmental extremists, made a one man decision to ban the use of DDT in United States, a move that was illegal. He took this action ignoring 8,300 pages of testimony and the findings of the hearing examiner and most scientists and in the absence of any honest substantiating science. He subsequently refused to comply with requests made under the Freedom of Information Act and defied the National Environmental Policy Act by refusing to file an Environmental Impact Statement on the disastrous consequences of his decision. After he left the EPA Ruckelhaus affixed his name to letters soliciting membership in the Environmental Defense Fund, the organization that led the fight to ban DDT.[12]

The pesticides that replaced DDT, such as dieldrin and aldrin, are far more toxic, and have been responsible for many deaths. Because of the low cost of DDT and the absence of equally effective substitutes with low toxicity, it continued to be used internationally. When huts were sprayed with DDT only 3 percent as many mosquitoes entered as compared with the most widely used alternative.[13] This effectiveness lasted for six months or more, a feature not matched by alternative pesticides that cost three times as much.

Great pressure has been exerted on those countries to discontinue its use. In some countries such as Sri Lanka, spraying programs that had virtually eliminated malaria were terminated. As a consequence the number of cases of malaria in that country rose to 2.5 million in 1968 and 1969.[14] More than 100,000 people died as a result of malaria epidemics in Swaziland and Madagascar in the mid-1980s after house spraying with DDT was stopped. Since the early 1970s the UN and the WHO have blackmailed developing countries, through the withholding of financial aid, to force them to discontinue the use of DDT. The result has been an upsurge in the number of cases of malaria. The South African government has reported that the annual number of deaths from malaria there have risen from 20,000 to 350,000 since the ban on DDT. Malaria currently kills about two million people each year, and the number is rising.

DDT was used in Ethiopia in 1991 to control a major epidemic of louse-borne relapsing fever among the hundreds of thousands of soldiers in refugee camps.[15] As had been the case in World War II, it was highly effective in controlling the human body louse that transmits the *Borrelia recurrentis* of relapsing fever. Millions of lives have been saved by the control of mosquitos, flies and lice that transmit such diseases as malaria, yellow fever, dengue fever, filariasis and plague. Many residents of West Africa were spared the ravages of river blindness (onchocerciasis) when DDT killed the insect vector (black fly) carrying the filaria for this disease. All of this progress is now threatened by UN politicians who are either totally ignorant of the facts or dedicated to population reduction.

METHOXYCHLOR

Methoxychlor is a chlorinated ethane, the same chemical class as DDT, and it is the designated hitter for DDT in the United States. It is virtually nontoxic to mammals and demonstrates little persistence in the environment or in animals. It is stored in body fat at about 0.2 percent the extent of DDT. The half-life in the rat is about two weeks compared with six months for DDT. It is not as effective as DDT, however, and cannot be substituted universally in the control of the diseases mentioned above. It is somewhat effective against fleas, ticks, flies and mosquitoes, but malathion and chlorpyrifos are more commonly used for these pests today. Methoxychlor is commonly incorporated into home orchard sprays.

LINDANE

Lindane has been the mainstay in the treatment of head and body lice as well as scabies. It is absorbed through the skin and is toxic to the brain and other sections of the nervous system, however. It is also toxic to the liver. Although it remains the most widely used drug for lice and scabies, it should never be used on infants and young children, where convulsions have been associated with its use. Crotamiton, which is also very effective, has been substituted in young patients who have these parasites.

More recently the development of the synthetic pyrethroid permethrin (Nix) has provided an effective agent of low toxicity for the treatment of head and body lice (see pyrethroids later in this chapter). Fatal cases of aplastic anemia due to skin absorption have resulted from prolonged use of lindane in adults. The directions for the use of lindane instruct the user that it should be left on for a specified period of time, then washed off thoroughly. Significant absorption can occur during the time that it is in contact with the skin, however. Repeated applications carry an even greater risk, and this practice is discouraged.

ALDRIN, DIELDRIN, ENDRIN

These are all closely related chemical substances whose use has been markedly restricted due to their toxicity and suspicions of carcinogenicity. Subsequent studies regarding carcinogenicity have yielded conflicting reports, as is frequently the case. Dieldrin has been shown to cause liver cancer in mice, but the extrapolation of such data from mice to men has never been clearly established. This continues to be the subject of intense debate. Endrin has been shown to cause serious birth defects in the offspring of hamsters that were fed a single dose.

There is no dispute about the toxicity of these three compounds, however. Several incidents of accidental ingestion of endrin from contaminated flour have been reported, and these events have resulted in severe convulsions and many deaths. In 1956 forty-nine people became ill after eating bakery foods prepared with flour that had been contaminated with endrin. The bags of flour had been shipped in a railway car that had previously been used to ship leaking containers of endrin. Several instances of this type of contamination of food products with toxic chemicals have occurred worldwide. Over 1200 cases of illness with 45 deaths were recorded as a result of consumption of food contaminated with endrin in Wales, Quatar, Saudi Arabia and Pakistan prior to 1970.

In 1988 six residents of Orange County became acutely ill

after eating frozen taquitos, all purchased from the same store during the same week. Five of these individuals suffered multiple seizures. One seventeen–years–old boy was diagnosed as having epilepsy and was placed on anticonvulsant medication until the true cause of the seizures was discovered. Examination of the remaining taquitos from the first family revealed endrin contamination of several them. Samples taken from the store and tested by the U.S. Department of Agriculture were negative for endrin. The USDA also inspected the plant where the taquitos were produced and found no evidence of pesticide. It is suspected that the packages were deliberately contaminated somewhere in the distribution chain.[16]

Dieldrin was incorporated into aerosol sprays for home use and was available after DDT was banned. In contrast to DDT, aldrin, dieldrin and endrin are all absorbed through the intact skin, increasing the risk to individuals involved in their manufacture and handling. They also are very persistent in the environment, and they undergo bio-magnification in the food chain, as was the case with DDT. Ingestion of solutions of dieldrin can result in severe convulsions and death if not treated promptly and aggressively. Children are particularly at risk given their propensity for drinking just about any substance regardless of its taste. A number of fatalities have been attributed to these agents and the use of aldrin and dieldrin was banned in the United States in 1974.

CHLORDANE

This potent and effective pesticide was introduced for commercial use in 1945 and gained widespread use in agriculture, in the household and in the garden. Being in the same chemical classification as aldrin, dieldrin and endrin (cyclodienes), it shares most of their properties and toxicity. Abnormalities reflecting its toxicity to the brain and nervous system in general are among the most serious. It is readily absorbed through the intact skin, making its handling and application hazardous. The use of adequate and proper clothing and skin protective devices during application is imperative. Any contaminated clothing must be removed immediately and the skin should be cleansed carefully.

Chlordane is also readily absorbed when ingested or inhaled. One fatality occurred when a worker spilled chlordane on his clothing and did not remove the clothing immediately. Convulsions

575

ensued forty minutes later, followed by death. Recovery can be effected following such exposure if prompt and vigorous treatment is instituted.

Chlordane has served a very valuable role in the control of ants and termites. No other substance has proven as consistently effective over an extended period of time. Because of its toxicity its use has been restricted to licensed exterminators since 1975. Surface application is not approved even by licensed personnel; it must be injected into the soil. Its persistence in the soil for as long as five years enhances its usefulness in this application. Recently it has been linked to illness in homes where it was improperly applied to interior surfaces, or where it leaked into the home through cracks in the foundation. In some instances it found its way into heating and ventilating ducts.

The marked reduction in the usage of chlordane has been accompanied by a concomitant decrease in manufacturing facilities, so that at present less than 100 employees are engaged in its production in the United States. As a result of the strict control measures that have been maintained since 1979, no health problems have been identified in this group of workers. Its was banned for use in agriculture and most general applications effective in 1976. Its use for the control of termites was exempted from that ban.

HEPTACHLOR

This substance is closely related to chlordane chemically, and shares many of its properties and toxicity. It is only slightly less persistent in the environment. The half-life of chlordane is one year, and that of heptachlor about nine to ten months. Both have been shown to cause liver cancers in mice, and both have been tested in the National Cancer Institute's carcinogen program, not only for this reason but also because of their resistance to degradation. Heptachlor was included with chlordane in the EPA ban in 1976.

MIREX

This substance is closely related to **kepone**, and probably is degraded to kepone in the environment. It has been used extensively to control the fire ant in the southern United States. Mirex and kepone are very toxic and are carcinogenic. They are bioconcentrated in the food chain several thousand fold. This is a matter of grave concern in the Chesapeake Bay area. Gross contamination of the soil surrounding a kepone manufacturing plant in Hopewell, Virginia in 1978, and the subsequent run-off into the James River resulted in the curtailment of fishing and shellfish harvesting in this area. This contamination has extended to the Chesapeake Bay, an important commercial fishing body. This substance has been deposited in the bed of the James River and the Chesapeake Bay in significant concentration. No means of decontamination has been devised.

Whereas many pesticides undergo degradation by bacteria in water and soil, mirex and kepone show little or no such tendency. They are very persistent in the environment, and will remain in these bodies of water for decades, contaminating the shellfish and other aquatic life. They are very toxic to the liver and nervous system and are carcinogenic. This incident, one of the most serious and most irresponsible by an industry in the United States, resulted in serious illness in seventy-six workers.

ORGANOPHOSPHATES
This group of pesticides blocks the enzyme cholinesterase that maintains the normal balance at the nerve endings throughout the body. This causes an excess accumulation of acetylcholine in the nerve endings, not only in the muscles throughout the body, but in the heart and nervous system as well. The result is a tightness in the chest with wheezing, increased sweating and salivation, nausea, vomiting, diarrhea, severe cramps, slowing of the heart, headache, anxiety, insomnia, nightmares, confusion, slurred speech, tremor and convulsions. This blockade tends to be persistent, in some cases lasting for days. The onset of symptoms occurs rapidly, usually within two to three hours, in less time with heavy exposures. Death can occur in an acute exposure within twenty-four hours if untreated, usually from asphyxia as a result of respiratory paralysis.

Treatment of these disorders of the nervous system is available at medical centers that are equipped for such poisonings. Measurement of the pseudo-cholinesterase level in the red blood cell helps to confirm the diagnosis, but a base line level should be established prior to exposure in workers. A more ominous finding has been the delayed neurotoxic effects of some of these compounds. This is a degeneration of nerve cells that is sometimes permanent, with a resultant weakness in the muscles of the legs. In most of the cases these problems begin insidiously, becoming progressively worse, then subsiding. Recovery is not always complete. An electromyogram and muscle biopsy will reveal the pathology.

The organophosphate compounds are readily absorbed through the intact skin as well as by inhalation, which fact makes them more hazardous. Re-exposure is possible from contaminated shoes and clothing days after the original exposure. Several instances of significant poisoning of pet groomers and handlers from organophosphate flea dips have been reported.[17] Health officials have only become aware of these events since about 1986, and the full extent of the problem is not known. Certainly some residual pesticide is carried home on the pet and transferred to the carpet and furniture. No infant or young child should be permitted to play where this has taken place.

It is from this group of compounds that most of the commercially applied insecticides are selected. Parathion was the first organophosphate to be utilized as an insecticide (1944) and it continues to be used extensively in commercial agricultural applications. It is the pesticide most frequently involved in fatal poisonings, partly due to this widespread use and partly due to its toxicity. It is ten to two hundred times more toxic than most of the commonly used organophosphate pesticides. Parathion should not be used around the home. Its use on the farm carries a significant risk. They should be used only after a thorough study and awareness of their properties and toxicity.

Other organophosphates include **abate**, the least toxic agent in this group, and **malathion**, a substance with very wide application, frequently incorporated into home orchard sprays. Malathion is also seen in lawn and shrub sprays, and has been utilized in aerial application to control fruit flies and mosquitos, even in populated areas. No toxic reactions have been observed in these applications. Malathion carries one of the lowest toxicity levels of all of the organophosphates, including skin contact. It may be used outside around the home with relative safety.

In spite of the relatively low toxicity, when applying malathion, as with all pesticides, clothing should cover the entire body. A

578

washable cap should cover the head, and all clothing should be well laundered when application is completed. If clothing should become contaminated during application through spillage or wind drift, it should be removed immediately and the skin should be carefully cleansed by showering. Thorough showering and shampooing should, of course, be completed as soon as possible after any application of pesticides.

Dursban (chlorpyrifos), another organophosphate, has been used in neighborhood mosquito control programs. It is also used in products sold to control fleas and ticks on dogs, both as an application to the pet and as a spray for the carpet. In these applications it carries a risk to the inhabitants and to pets. It has been marketed recently in a polymer base to prolong its effectiveness in flea control on dogs to a period of weeks. The binding of Dursban in the polymer is presumed to render it less toxic by decreasing the amount released at a given time. Unfortunately the fascist bureaucrats at the EPA covertly and unilaterly mandated that chlorpyrifos could no longer be manufactured after the year 2000.

Diazinon, which is widely used to control ants and grub worms in lawns, belongs to the same chemical family as Dursban, phosphorothioates. They carry a toxicity when applied to the skin that is about ten times less than parathion. Malathion, on the other hand, is about 220 times less toxic than parathion through the skin. It is apparent that malathion carries much less risk to animals and humans. Others in this group with a relatively high toxicity include **disulfoton (Di-Syston)** and **mevinphos (Phosdrin)**.

CARBAMATES

Unlike the organophosphates, MOST of the carbamate ester insecticides have a very low toxicity when applied to the skin. **Carbaryl (Sevin)**, in particular, has developed widespread use around the home in the control of aphids, gypsy moths, leaf miners and Japanese beetles. It is useful and effective on shade trees, ornamentals and flowers. It is also effective in controlling fleas. These agents do not share the broad spectrum of the organophosphates, however, and some household pests such as the house fly and cockroach may not succumb following their application. Bees on the other hand are extremely sensitive, and their populations suffer from the application of this as with most pesticides. This occurs particularly when pesticides are applied to fruit trees and other honey producing crops. The pesticidal activity of the carbamates is enhanced by the addition of pyrethrin or piperonyl butoxide.

In 1995 the use of carbaryl on humans for the treatment of lice was restricted in the United Kingdom on the basis of its alleged carcinogenicity. Ethyl carbamate (urethan) does indeed induce tumors in mice, especially in conjunction with promoters such as phorbol esters. Carbaryl, however, is a methyl carbamate (1 naphthyl N-methylcarbamate) and this group does not produce cancers. The difference appears to lie in the fact that metabolism of the ethyl carbamates produces vinyl carbamate, a known direct carcinogen, whereas the metabolism of the methyl carbamates does not.

At the other end of the spectrum, **aldicarb** (Temik), which is structurally different from the other carbamates, has an extreme toxicity when ingested or applied to the skin. The poisoning of over one thousand individuals when this substance was inappropriately used on melons, was described previously. Its use is restricted to applications in greenhouses, and skin contact must be restricted. The relative toxicity of some of the carbamates is shown in the table below, in order of toxicity.

Ld 50, rat, mg/kg	ORAL	DERMAL
Propoxur (Baygon)	83	>2400
Carbaryl	850	>4000
Mobam	150	>2000
Temik (Aldicarb)	0.8	3
Zectran	37	1500-2500

From the above it can be seen that it takes more than 850 times as much carbaryl to produce toxicity as it does aldicarb. The mode of action of the carbamates, like the organophosphates, is the inhibition of acetylcholinesterase. This effectively paralyzes respiration in the insect. The symptoms of exposure in humans are salivation, tearing, contraction of the pupil, convulsions and death in the extreme. The carbamates are the substances that were being manufactured in Bhopal, India when the release of a toxic cloud of **methylisocyanate** (MIC) resulted in the tragic suffering and death in that community. This disaster was not caused by the pesticide, but by the MIC that was being used in its production.

PYRETHROIDS

Commercial preparations of **Pyrethrum**, an extract from chrysanthemums, were available as early as the mid-1800s. Large quantities of the powder were used during the construction of the Panama canal to control the mosquito population. The incidence of malaria was consequently reduced, and the last death from yellow fever occurred in 1906. Control of these two diseases was a major factor in the successful completion of the canal.

The insecticidal properties of pyrethrum have been recognized and utilized commercially in the United States since the 1930's. It possesses a low order of toxicity for humans, except for allergic reactions. These include a contact dermatitis that can be severe, as well as respiratory reactions after inhalation, including hay fever and asthma. Ragweed sufferers are particularly sensitive. It can also cause photosensitivity. Several synthetic pyrethroids have been developed in an effort to create substances more stable to heat and light than the naturally occurring pyrethrum. These seem to evoke less allergic response, but still precipitate symptoms of asthma and bronchitis in sensitive individuals. Caution should be exercised in spraying these substances indoors in the presence of sensitive individuals.

Permethrin (Nix), which has been marketed for the treatment and control of head and body lice, is even less sensitive to breakdown by light and heat than the other synthetic pyrethroids, which include **allethrin, cypermethrin, fenvalerate, phthalthrin, resmethrin and tetramethrin**. These substances are the common ingredients in aerosol sprays marketed for the control of insects such as flies and spiders in the home. They are effective and relatively safe, but they should not be used in the kitchen or around food, drink and utensils. Permethrin also has been marketed recently for use as an aerosol to spray onto clothing for protection against ticks. It has proven virtually 100 percent effective when used along with DEET and the proper clothing (see also chapter VIII).

We are currently in our third generation of these synthetic analogues. As the efforts to create more potent insecticides progresses, so will their toxicity increase. Individuals with known allergies or asthma should be particularly careful to avoid breathing the aerosol spray from any of the pyrethroids. None of these substances should be sprayed in the home indiscriminately, and none should be inhaled. Aerosols generally remain airborne for approximately twenty minutes, so no one should be in the room for about a half-hour after spraying in order to minimize any health risk. A fly swatter entails even less risk, and a smaller cash outlay.

ROTENONE

Rotenone is also a plant extract, derived from the roots of plants such as **derris**. It is more toxic than pyrethrum, particularly when applied as a powder. The dust causes irritation of the eyes and skin, and inhalation causes irritation of the lungs. It has been used in garden applications in the past, but has been largely supplanted by other agents today. It was "discovered" by the Indians of South America, who would spread it on the waters of likely fishing spots, then harvest the immobilized fish.

NICOTINE SULFATE

This ancient garden spray has been used to control insects on vegetables and flowers alike. It is one of the most toxic of all of the insecticides, and has been supplanted for the most part by the newer agents. Nicotine is absorbed through the skin as well as by ingestion and inhalation, and has a rapid onset of symptoms. Death usually occurs within four hours. Many unpleasant symptoms are produced in the interim. It has been responsible for many human deaths through accidental ingestion or suicide attempts. Nicotine sulfate is occasionally used in a futile effort to control moles. It has been the classical treatment for lice in chicken houses, but the pyrethroids or malathion are a safer substitute. Unfortunately, from a public health standpoint at least, most of the nicotine in cigarettes is destroyed by the heat of burning, and the smoker is spared most of the more extreme side effects of this drug.

COPPER SULFATE

Bordeaux mixture is a one to two percent mixture of copper sulfate that has been used as a spray in vineyards to control mildew growth. Some workers developed a granulomatous pneumonitis, which could be diagnosed by finding copper in the lung lesions or the mediastinal lymph nodes. These individuals had a high incidence of lung cancer also. Copper sulfate has also been used in herbicides.

PIPERONYL BUTOXIDE

This substance will be found on the label frequently, particularly with the pyrethroids and carbamates. It is not an insecticide of itself; rather it inhibits the metabolism of the pyrethroids and carbamates in insects, thus increasing the effectiveness of the insecticide. It accomplishes this role by inhibiting the oxidative enzyme in the insect that normally inactivates the pesticide. It enhances the effectiveness of the pyrethroid insecticides by a factor of 10 to 300. It has a similar effect on liver enzymes in humans, and thus it influences the metabolism of many drugs. This is a classic demonstration that even though a substance may not be particularly toxic of itself, it can nonetheless have significant effects on the body, and should not be inhaled casually.

HERBICIDES

These chemicals are weed killers, used not only to keep our lawns beautiful, but also to control weeds and undesirable plants along highways and railways and on the farm among crops. They exert their effect by accelerating the growth of the plant, thus compressing its life span into a few days rather than weeks. The most widely used herbicides are the chlorophenoxy agents, **2,4-D** and **2,4,5-T**. These substances previously were felt to pose no hazard to man, and indeed the pure compounds without contaminants are still known to be of low toxicity.

Considerable interest has been aroused by the widespread claims of Vietnam veterans of serious health hazards resulting from exposure to **Agent Orange**. This substance, which was a mixture of equal parts of 2,4-D and 2,4,5-T, was widely used as a defoliant in the jungles of Vietnam. Some troops were sprayed during aerial application. Many health problems that have subsequently evolved in these veterans and in their offspring have been blamed on this previous exposure.

Retrospective studies on exposed veterans have not substantiated any increased incidence of nervous system disorders, heart, liver or kidney disease, sterility or birth defects among offspring. These studies included those who loaded the substance on the planes and thus suffered the heaviest exposure. A study by the Veterans Administration of 13,496 Vietnam era veterans revealed no increased incidence of soft tissue sarcomas (cancers) among those individuals serving in Vietnam or among those exposed to Agent Orange. Similar studies with similar results have been done on other exposed populations.

The agent 2,4,5-T was first marketed for commercial use in 1948. In 1949 a plant manufacturing this substance in Nitro, West Virginia experienced an accident that resulted in illness among the workers who were cleaning it up. The symptoms initially were irritation of the skin, eyes, nose and throat. These symptoms subsided by the end of two weeks. Nervousness, irritability, muscle pain and general weakness persisted, and chloracne developed. Enlarged livers and abnormal liver function tests were also noted. The enlarged liver and abnormal function tests returned to normal. This group of workers was monitored and by 1953 all of the symptoms had cleared except for chloracne.

In 1957 it was discovered that **TCDD (tetrachlorodibenzo-dioxin)** had been produced as a contaminant in the manufacture of 2,4,5-T, and that it was the substance that was responsible for the production of chloracne. Such contamination occurs when the 2,4,5-trichlorophenol used to produce 2,4,5-T reacts with itself to produce TCDD. At that time virtually nothing was known about the health risks of exposure to TCDD. Since then, considerable data has been collected in the laboratory, and we now know that it is very toxic substance. We know that it is a potent carcinogen, mutagen and teratogen in laboratory animals. It is known to have been present in Agent Orange in significant quantities.

References to "dioxin," which has become almost a household term, frequently evoking near hysteria, invariably mean TCDD. TCDD is only one of some seventy-five chlorinated dioxins, but it is of far greater significance than all of the others are because it is one of the most toxic substances known. It is important, therefore, to make this distinction between TCDD and "dioxin".

In 1979 a study was undertaken of some two hundred workers from the plant in Nitro, West Virginia who had been exposed during the manufacture of 2,4,5-T from 1948 to 1969. This group of exposed workers was compared to a control group of 163 individuals who had worked at the plant during the same period, but who had had no exposure to TCDD. No evidence of birth defects, cancer, nervous system disorders, heart, liver or kidney disease or sterility was found among the exposed workers. Chloracne was found in approximately one half of the exposed group, and none was found in the control group. Evidence of an increased susceptibility to ultraviolet radiation (sun) damage in the form of elastosis of the skin was present in those who demonstrated chloracne.

A far more extensive and more serious accident occurred in 1976 in Italy. An explosion at the ICMESA plant near Seveso sent a toxic cloud into the air spreading TCDD over an area of about 700 acres. The plant was manufacturing 2,4,5-trichlorophenol for use in making both the herbicide 2,4,5-T and hexachlorophene, a surgical bactericide. The contaminated area included parts of the towns of Seveso (population 17,000), Meda, Cesano Maderno and Desio. Seveso, which was to gain worldwide notoriety, is about twelve miles north of Milan. Two hundred fifty acres were sealed off and seven hundred people were evacuated. No human fatalities occurred, but thousands of animals, including rabbits, chickens and birds, perished. The trees and vegetation over a wide area were destroyed. The entire plant was contaminated. Workers who were in the plant during and shortly after the accident were found to have abnormal liver function tests, but these had returned to normal two weeks later.

The Italian authorities took prompt and decisive actions. The area surrounding the plant was divided into three zones, based upon the concentration of TCDD found in each zone. A fourth zone, outside of the area of contamination and thus with no TCDD exposure, was added to serve as a control population. The residents of the three zones contaminated with TCDD, a population of over 36,000 people, were examined thoroughly throughout the period from 1976 to 1985.

Over 30,000 blood samples were collected and measured for TCDD during this period. The only significant abnormal finding in this exposed population has been the development of chloracne. This has occurred in only a small percentage of the population, as contrasted to the cleanup workers following the plant accident in Nitro, West Virginia. There was a higher incidence of chloracne among the maintenance workers at the ICMESA plant subsequently.

TCDD has a strong association with the production of chloracne and porphyria in humans. It appears to have a relatively low toxicity in man otherwise, compared to certain species of animals, especially the guinea pig. In the guinea pig it is an extremely toxic chemical, causing degenerative changes in the liver and thymus gland and fetal abnormalities. It also suppresses the immune system, and non-Hodgkin's lymphoma is known to occur more frequently in immuno-deficient states in humans. This relationship has prompted several studies to establish a relationship between exposure to TCDD and the subsequent development of lymphomas. No such association has been seen in the populations who have had significant exposure. Furthermore, TCDD is a potent animal carcinogen, inducing cancer in the lung, nose, mouth, tongue, liver, thyroid and skin in the guinea pig. No such propensity has been shown for 2,4-D in animals.

The accident at Seveso provided a large population of people who had been exposed to significant levels of TCDD. The health authorities have monitored and carefully evaluated this population. Valuable data has been collected on the impact of acute exposure of humans to high levels of TCDD. The TCDD levels in the blood collected from these people are the highest ever reported in humans. No adverse health effects other than the chloracne have been found. Not all of the individuals with a high blood level of TCDD developed chloracne. Those who did develop this skin problem appear to be at increased risk of skin damage following ultraviolet (sun) exposure. No increased incidence of skin cancer has evolved as yet. Since TCDD persists in the body tissues for many years, these individuals will need to exercise great care to avoid exposure to the sun.

It is true that TCDD is a very toxic chemical, but its production is not limited to the industry of man. Chlorinated dioxins such as TCDD are produced in natural circumstances where combustion takes place in the presence of chlorine, such as in forest fires, in wood burning fireplaces and on the grill whenever steaks are prepared. They have been with us at least since fire was discovered. In spite of acute toxic episodes where humans were exposed to large doses, no evidence of cancer, mutagenesis or teratogenesis has appeared. In this respect it appears to cause less harm in humans than the nitrosamines that are produced when grilling meat. Recent advances in analytical techniques permit us to measure substances that are a thousand times weaker than what we could measure just a few years ago. In those days we didn't know that they existed. We may have been better off for the ignorance. The fact that a chemical is toxic in animal studies does not automatically mean that it produces serious harm to humans. The human organism is a far more sophisticated creature physiologically than the animals that we study in the laboratory. Toxic effects seen there cannot be directly extrapolated to humans. These findings should provoke thoughtful study, but not panic.

A Kansas study suggested that farmers who spent more than twenty days per year applying 2,4-D experienced a six fold increase in the incidence of non-Hodgkin's lymphoma. No such risk was found in exposures of lessor length. A Swedish study yielded similar findings. The possibility that a toxic contaminant existed in the 2,4-D used by these farmers earlier (1946) has been postulated. Several other investigators have criticized the findings of the Swedish studies after evaluating them, however. No similar risk following exposure to 2,4-D has been seen elsewhere in spite of worldwide use.

Aside from the industrial accidents, poisoning resulting from use of the chlorophenoxy herbicides has been rare. Both 2,4-D and 2,4,5-T that has not been contaminated with TCDD during manufacture have a low order of toxicity for all animals including humans. Use of 2,4-D in particular appears to be reasonably safe for the control of broad leaf weeds such as dandelions, plantain and chickweed on lawns, parks, campuses, golf courses and among crops. Skin contact should be avoided as with all pesticides and herbicides. These substances in themselves do not accumulate in animals and thus pose no threat to the food chain. In 1979 the Environmental Protection Agency banned 2,4,5-T from use around homes, in parks and around most food crops because of the past contamination by TCDD. It had been totally banned in Italy in 1970.

BIPYRIDYL COMPOUNDS

Paraquat is the best known and most widely used substance in this group of herbicides. Unfortunately its use is expanding. It is used in harvesting cotton by spraying the cotton plant to eliminate the leaves prior to processing. It is extremely toxic to the lungs whether ingested or inhaled, resulting in acute pulmonary edema and death by respiratory failure. These dire consequences do not require massive or repeated dosing. A single dose has preceded most of the deaths that have resulted from smoking marijuana that had been contaminated with this substance. Even with low levels of contamination, pulmonary fibrosis may occur over time. Several hundred deaths have occurred as a result of accidental or suicidal exposures. Numerous deaths have resulted from smoking contaminated marijuana.

Paraquat has been the herbicide used by the United States authorities to spray illicit marijuana fields in an effort to control the use of this drug. Approximately twenty percent of the marijuana in the Southwestern United States has been found to be contaminated with this agent. This practice by the authorities has been strongly criticized because of the serious consequences and the fatalities that have resulted.

Agricultural workers who have been exposed to paraquat spray over extended periods of time have developed irritation and inflammation of the mouth, throat and lungs with a resultant cough. Skin and eye irritation has also been noted, as well as damage and deformity of nails, even the loss of nails in some instances. Minimal skin absorption occurs, but even these small quantities can produce serious damage to the lungs and kidneys. Additionally, workers in the field frequently have minor scratches on the hands and arms that permit significantly greater absorption. One worker who mistakenly took a mouthful from a container, and immediately spit it out, nonetheless developed severe dyspnea and cyanosis fourteen days later. Survivors of acute lung reactions from paraquat exposure may develop chronic obstructive lung disease and respiratory failure later in life. Studies in laboratory animals regarding the inhalation of dust from soils that had been sprayed with paraquat were unable to demonstrate any harmful effects from this exposure.

DIQUAT

This related compound does not produce the acute toxic effects in the lung that are seen with paraquat, but both compounds produce serious destruction in the liver and kidney.

PENTACHLOROPHENOL

This substance is used as a herbicide, as well as a fungicide and as a wood preservative, to protect against termites and other wood-boring insects. It also provides protection against wood rot caused by fungus. Wood pulp used in the production of paper and paperboard is treated with pentachlorophenol to prevent the growth of slime producing organisms. It is also used to defoliate plants prior to harvest. It is readily absorbed through the intact skin and it accumulates in the body. A number of cases of acute poisoning in man have occurred, including a number of deaths. Cattle have also suffered poisoning as a result of rubbing against timbers that had been treated with this preservative. Twenty infants in a hospital nursery were poisoned as a result of diapers that had been contaminated with pentachlorophenol in the laundry where it had been used as a fungicide. Two of the infants died.

Some commercial pentachlorophenol has been discovered to be contaminated with dioxins other than TCDD, and with dibenzofurans, both of which are toxic substances. These substances produce chloracne and liver damage, including porphyria. Even when pure, pentachlorophenol is toxic in its own right. The use of pentachlorophenol as a soil fumigant and wood preservative in structures in contact with the ground has resulted in contamination of surface and drinking water in some locations. This has raised serious concern about the health threat produced by the toxicity of pentachlorophenol as well as the chlorinated dioxins.

AMINOTRIAZOLE

Amitrole (aminotriazole) produces cancer in animals, even though it is lacking in acute toxicity. It is a very potent antithyroid agent, suppressing the function of the thyroid gland, and it can produce goiter. This substance provides an important lesson for us in that an agent that does not demonstrate acute toxicity nonetheless can invoke significant harm in humans through other mechanisms. Many of the pesticides and herbicides have an influence on the function of the enzymes, particularly in the liver. These alterations are not always apparent, and they are not readily discovered by the studies commonly performed in most laboratories. A Swedish study suggested that railway workers who had been exposed to amitrole experienced an increased incidence of cancer. Few other studies regarding this risk have been completed. Amitrole is not permitted as a herbicide on food crops.

DINITROPHENOL

This group of compounds includes several different substances that are very toxic. They interfere with cellular metabolism producing anoxia in the cells (lack of oxygen) even though abundant blood and oxygen are present. Death or recovery usually occurs within twenty-four to forty-eight hours. They are marketed for the control of weeds.

Dinitro-orthocresol (dinitrophenol) causes cataracts in some individuals subjected to chronic exposure. It was sold without a prescription from 1935 to 1937 as an anti-obesity agent. Cataracts developed in several hundred of the people who tried this remedy. Interestingly, cataracts do not show up in studies on laboratory animals, except for rabbits. Acute poisoning may produce a marked increase in metabolism, with temperature elevation and death due to hyperthermia. Chronic poisoning produces anxiety, sweating, thirst and weight loss. The risk is much greater in hot weather.

Nitrocresol compounds have similar uses and similar toxicity. All contact with these substances should be avoided.

CARBAMATE DERIVATIVES

These substances are less commonly used but have a relatively low order of acute toxicity. Propham is a typical example. (See previous discussion of carbamate pesticides) Barban is somewhat more toxic than propham and is a potent sensitizing agent, provoking skin rashes and other allergic reactions.

ORGANOPHOSPHATES

Some agents in this class have been used as herbicides in special application. **Merphos** and **DEF** (**S,S,S-tributylphosphorotrithioate**) are used as defoliants to facilitate the harvesting of cotton. These are usually applied through aerial spraying, and the greatest risk is to the mixers, pilots and especially the flagmen. These agents carry the customary risks of the organophosphates, and additionally the delayed neurotoxic effects, both of which have been discussed previously under the pesticides.

TRIAZINE:

Atrazine and **Simazine** are marketed as herbicides and for weed control. They also have a low level of toxicity, but are not as widely marketed to the general public.

DINITROANALINE

Trifluralin and **benefin** possess a low toxicity and have demonstrated no ill effects in dogs and rats in laboratory studies.

ARYL ALIPHATIC ACIDS

Dicamba is a pre-emergence weed control and has a low order of toxicity. Some of the other substances in this category that are used to control vegetation such as ivy require more caution in handling. Some of these are used in commercial farming, where the residue is of some concern, specifically as to any potential for a cancer risk. Some of these substances have not been carefully studied.

DALAPON

2,4-dichloropropionic acid has been proposed as a substitute for some of the more toxic herbicides described above because it has a low order of toxicity for all animals, including humans. It, along with trichloracetic acid, has been used in the control of perennial weeds, but they are of limited usefulness.

In summary, 2,4-D is the only herbicide commonly sold for general use by the public to control dandelions and other broadleaf weeds in the lawn. There is no TCDD or any other dioxin in 2,4-D. It can be used with relative safety if skin contact is avoided. The major risk to health from the remaining herbicides resides in their application in agriculture, where residues in foods such as rice pose a threat. It must be kept in mind also that walking through areas where these substances are used to control weeds and brush growth carries a very real risk of skin and clothing contamination. In general, people will be unaware of such contact, unless a rash occurs. Even with the occurrence of a rash the association is seldom made.

RODENTICIDES

These are substances marketed to control mice, rats, gophers and sometimes rabbits. Rat poisons have produced numerous deaths in man, and these lethal products are still available. Fortunately, however, the most widely used agent today, **warfarin,** carries little risk for man or pets unless consumed as a regular diet, for it requires repeated dosing. This does not rule out children as victims, of course, since they have repeatedly demonstrated that they will consume many improbable substances. Warfarin destroys rodents by inhibiting blood-clotting mechanisms and thus causing internal hemorrhage. Repeated feeding is necessary before an adequate blood level is reached to accomplish this event. Hopefully, when the animal takes his last meal he will retire to quarters well removed from the household.

The difference in dosages, based upon animal weight, required to produce fatal bleeding is used in South America to control vampire bats. Warfarin can be safely fed to cattle, but the vampire bat, after extracting a sufficient quantity of blood, succumbs due to internal hemorrhage.

The **indandiones** are similar in action to warfarin, producing hemorrhage by interfering with Vitamin K metabolism in the production of prothrombin. This group of agents has an advantage over warfarin in that they are water soluble, and thus are easier to formulate in baits without arousing the suspicion of the dinner guest. Other products in this category are marketed under the following names: **Diphacin, Fumarin, Pival, PMP, Valone, Pindone** and **Triban.**

Bleeding in humans who had handled bait containing these substances has occurred after repeated skin contact and the resultant absorption. Individuals who are on cimetidine and other ulcer medications are particularly sensitive to this risk. Since most substances can be absorbed through the intact skin to varying degrees, such contact should be avoided when handling toxic agents. Appropriate gloves can help avoid this risk.

FLUOROACETATES

These are among the most potent rodenticides and are highly toxic to humans. Poisoning can occur not only by ingestion but also by absorption through the skin and by breathing the dust. There have been a number of fatalities in humans as a result of contact with these agents. Convulsions and heart irregularities leading to cardiac arrest are the usual causes of death. Their use is for the most part restricted to licensed pest control personnel, and extreme caution is required in handling them.

RED SQUILL

The bulbs of this plant, known as sea onion, have been used as a rodenticide for many years. They kill mainly by inducing irregularities in the heart with resultant cardiac arrest. The bulbs also contain a substance that induces vomiting in animals other than the rodent, a fact that contributes to its relative safety in humans. The inability of the rat to vomit accounts, in great measure, for the effectiveness of this product.

PHOSPHORUS

Used as a paste, this substance is spread on bread for rats, and it has poisoned man on several occasions. Because of its severe toxicity to humans safer and more selective substances have supplanted it.

THALLIUM

This metallic element is extremely toxic and is absorbed through the intact skin. The powder is toxic when it is inhaled. It resulted in poisoning of hundreds of individuals, including many fatalities, until its use as a rodenticide was banned in the United States in 1955. At first its use was restricted to licensed personnel, but it is no longer available even to these individuals. It is very effective for that purpose however, and continues to be widely used in Mexico, South America and abroad. Serious cases of poisoning continue to appear among immigrants who obtain it from relatives or other sources in those countries. Emergency physicians in Texas and other regions with an immigrant population from Mexico or South America see cases of poisoning by thallium.

Other than these imported cases, toxicity in the United States occurs chiefly as a result of exposure in industry, where thallium compounds are widely encountered. The symptoms of thallium poisoning and its diagnostic challenges are discussed in Chapter X.

STRYCHNINE

Known as extract nux vomica, this substance is derived from the nuts of the strychnine tree, which grows in Australia and southeastern Asia. This and arsenic are perhaps the most widely known poisons. It has been used as a rodenticide since the sixteenth century, and continues to be marketed as bait (on peanuts) for gophers and moles. It produces severe convulsions in man, leading to death by asphyxia. Symptoms of muscle stiffness and excitability may occur as soon as fifteen to thirty minutes after ingestion. No effective treatment is available.

ARSENIC

Arsenic compounds were used as insecticides in the sixteenth century, and continued to be mainstays into the 1940s. Even in the 1950s enormous quantities of lead arsenate were used every year to spray orchids and other crops to control insects. Paris Green (copper arsenite) was used for the control of beetles in the late 1800s, and was still in use when I left home for the U.S. Navy in 1943. Calcium arsenate and lead arsenate were other arsenicals that were dusted and sprayed on fruit and vegetables to control pests. These were replaced by the development of modern pesticides, such as DDT, which fortunately was available to control typhus during the war.

The arsenical pesticides were toxic, as can be attested to by Joe Foss, the World War II Marine fighter pilot ace and later governor of South Dakota. While filming a segment for his television series *Outdoorsman* in Nebraska he reverted to an old habit of his youth of chewing on corn stalks. As it turned out the corn had been treated with an arsenical pesticide for the corn borer. Foss developed serious arsenic poisoning and was close to death

594

before the cause was finally identified. It took him about a year to recover, even after the diagnosis was made.

HYDROGEN CYANIDE

This gas, with the smell of bitter almonds, is a potent rodenticide and pesticide, and is used to fumigate ships and buildings. Its severe lethality has had wide publicity in recent years through deliberate contamination of food and drugs by sick and perverted individuals. It is readily absorbed by all routes and death can occur a few minutes after ingestion of a small quantity. Cyanide is released when certain plastics used in furniture (i.e., polyurethane) are burned. Fires on airplanes and in public buildings have resulted in numerous deaths. Efforts are underway currently to substitute safer materials. Needless to say, plastics should not be burned in the fireplace, backyard or around the campfire.

Amygdalin, the chief ingredient in **Laetrile**, releases cyanide in the intestinal tract through the action of bacteria. Several instances of human poisoning have resulted from this "therapy." Amygdalin occurs naturally in apricot and peach pits as well as in sweet almonds.

HYDROGEN SULFIDE

This well-known sewer gas is occasionally used by exterminators. It produces symptoms similar in almost every respect to cyanide. It is present in some natural gas deposits and in volcanic gases. It is produced by the putrefaction of organic matter. Numerous deaths have occurred among workers in sewers. In 1983 a worker in the City of Omaha waste treatment plant was found unconscious after he had gone to collect routine samples from the area where the wastewater enters the plant. He subsequently died from hydrogen sulfide exposure as a result of an excessive level of accumulation of the gas.

Rat poisons have produced considerable morbidity and mortality in man. As a general rule, any substance applied by professional exterminators for the purpose of eliminating rodents must be considered to be very toxic, and it should not be permitted to come in contact with food, utensils and certainly not the skin. The need for extermination can be greatly reduced by storing garbage and pet food in rat proof containers. Traps provide a much safer alternative to poisons in the control of rodent populations around residences.

The control of rats is a significant public health imperative. No other creature has contributed so greatly to the demise of populations. During the fourteenth century, plague transmitted by the rat flea killed half of the population of England and one-fourth of the entire European population. In the United States the risk of plague transmission currently resides more with the ground squirrel. The fleas of these animals carry the potential for disease in man in southern California and Arizona. The risk has been compounded by the expansion of housing into the hills where the squirrels have their burrows. Efforts to control the disease in this area center more on ingenious devices to dust the animals with a pesticide to eliminate the fleas, than in the destruction of the squirrels.

FUNGICIDES

This is a diverse group of agents, used on plants, seeds and produce, to control fungus diseases. One or the other of these agents is usually incorporated into home orchard sprays and is customarily added to pesticide sprays for roses. They also have been used in formulations for housepaints and stains to inhibit mildew formation. **Captan** is frequently incorporated with the insecticides malathion and methoxychlor in home orchard sprays. It is structurally similar to thalidomide and is known to produce birth defects in animals. **Folpet,** another common fungicide, is incorporated into rose sprays along with insecticides. It also has structural similarities to thalidomide, and has been shown to produce birth defects in some animal species.

Mercury, a metal which is liquid at room temperature, and its compounds are effective fungicides and have been widely used to treat seed grains to prevent rot. These compounds also have been used in paint and stain formulations to prevent mildew. They are extremely toxic and are potent teratogens. The organic mercurials such as methyl mercury and ethyl mercury are particularly dangerous. Several large poisoning events have resulted from the consumption of food that had been contaminated by mercury compounds. Most of these cases involved fish or seafood and grain that had been prepared for use as seed. These mercury compounds are severely toxic to the brain and nervous system as well as to the kidneys.

The poisoning episodes have been particularly tragic in the cases where the contaminated food was consumed during pregnancy and severely retarded and defective infants were born. Organic mercury compounds such as methyl mercury cross the placenta into the fetal circulation. They also appear in the mothers milk, as do virtually all drugs and chemicals that gain access to the woman's body (See also mercury in Chapter V).

DITHIOCARBAMATE

This group of fungicides includes **ziram**, **ferbam** and **maneb**. They have been widely used in agriculture and have a low level of toxicity in all animals. There have been no significant reports of toxic effects or of human illness following exposure to them. The breakdown of some of these compounds during cooking to substances which suppress the thyroid gland and may be carcinogenic, mutagenic and teratogenic mandates that a minimal residue in food be assured.

HEXACHLOROBENZENE

Hexachlorobenzene is a fungicide with serious toxic properties. Like DDT it bioaccumulates in the fatty tissues of the body, and is slow to breakdown in the environment. It produced more than 4000 cases of acquired toxic porphyria in Turkey between 1955 and 1959 when seed grain that was prepared for planting was treated with this substance and subsequently consumed as food following crop failure. In addition to the classic skin lesions and liver damage some individuals developed a suppurative arthritis, osteomyelitis and osteoporosis in the bones of the hands. Eighty percent of those afflicted were children. Ninety percent of nursing infants who acquired the substance through their mother's milk died. Hexachlorobenzene also has caused illness where it has been used as a disinfectant. This toxic substance should not be confused with lindane, which is frequently called gamma benzenehexachloride, but is more accurately described as hexachlorohexane.

PENTACHLOROPHENOL

Commonly called penta, this substance is used as a wood preservative, as an insecticide and herbicide as well as a disinfectant. Its action in protecting wood is similar to creosote, which is a mixture of phenols. Several instances of poisoning, both in man and in cattle, have occurred, including the deaths of several infants in a hospital nursery from inappropriate use, as described previously. (See p.566) This is a substance that should not be permitted to contact the skin, since it is readily absorbed and is toxic. In handling lumber and fence posts treated with it the worker must be aware that it will penetrate most gloves customarily used for such work.

CREOSOTE

This mixture of phenols is derived from wood or coal by distillation. It is retained in treated wood for over twenty-five years. It has a similar action and toxicity as pentachlorophenol. Wood treated with either of these substances, or indeed any of the pressure treated wood that contains products such as copper arsenate, should not be burned. Serious illness has resulted from burning these products in fireplaces or stoves. Vapors from creosote are irritating and produce burning of the nose, throat and eyes. Corneal scarring has been reported among exposed workers. Caution also should be taken when sawing treated wood. The sawdust should not be permitted to come in contact with the skin.

BIS

Bis{tributyltin}oxide is an organic tin compound sold in a 25 percent solution to be added to paint as a mildewcide. It was previously incorporated into marine paints to inhibit the growth of marine life on boats. This use has been discontinued due to its potent toxic effects and the dispersion of the compound into the marine environment. This substance and some other organic tin preparations, notable triethyltin, are very toxic when ingested producing serious central nervous system (brain) symptoms. They are also readily absorbed through the intact skin with the same risk of brain damage. Skin contact should be avoided, from both the compound and the subsequently treated paint. Pronounced irritation can occur, even if washed immediately.

598

Great care should be exercised when adding this substance to paint. BIS should be used as an additive only to exterior paints. Serious poisonings of families have occurred when it was added to interior latex paint. Since 1988 the labels on the bottles of this compound include the stipulation that they are for exterior use only. Paint treated with BIS should be applied only with adequate ventilation and only in areas where no risk of human poisoning exists. The many cases of lead poisoning that have resulted from the lead pigments in paints should be warning enough to avoid applying this or any treated paint in the house. Whereas removal of lead from the body can be facilitated, no such remedy is available for these tin compounds.

1. Black RM, Clarke RJ, Reid RW, Reid MTJ. Application of gas chromatography-mass spectrometry and gas chromatography-tandem mass spectrometry to the analysis of chemical warfare samples, found to contain residues of the nerve agent sarin, sulphur mustard and their degradation products. *J Chromatogr A* 1994; **662**:301-21.

2. Macilain C. Study proves Iraq used nerve gas. *Nature* 1993;**363**:3.

3. CDC. Aldicarb food poisoning from contaminated melons—California. *MMWR* 1986;**35**:254-258.

4. CDC. Poisonings associated with illegal use of Aldicarb as a rodenticide — New York City, 1994-1997.

5. *Arch Environ Health*, 1967;**15**:766-775.

6. Klassen CD, Amdur MO, Doull JD. *Casarett and Doull's Toxicology*, ed 5. McGraw-Hill, Columbus, OH 1996.

7. Rachel Carson quoted Albert Schweitzer as saying, "Man has lost the capacity to foresee and forestall. He will end by destroying the earth." Carson made it appear that he was referring to pesticides, and DDT in particular. She knew that he was referring to nuclear weapons and atomic warfare. In fact, in his autobiography he wrote "How much labor and waste of time these wicked insects do cause us...but a ray of hope, in the use of DDT, is now held out to us." (p. 262)

8. Austin H, Keil JE, Cole P. A prospective follow-up study of cancer mortality in relation to serum DDT. *Am J Pub Health* 1989;**79**(1):43.

9. Key T, Reeves G. Organochlorines in the environment and breast cancer. *Br Med J* **308**(1994):1520-1521.

10. Bird counts in 1960 (after DDT) vs. 1941 yielded 12 times more robins, 21 times more cowbirds, 38 times more blackbirds and 131 times more grackles.

Diseases of birds carried by mosquitos were eliminated, and food supply and protective cover were increased by DDT.

11. Edwards JG. DDT effects on bird abundance and reproduction, in Lehr JH (ed) *Rational Readings on Environmental Concerns*. New York: Van Nostrand Reinhold;1992:195-216.

12. Lee Ray D, Guzzo L. *Trashing the Planet*. Regnery Gateway, Washington, DC 1990.

13. Research by Dr. Don Roberts, Uniformed Services University of Health Sciences.

14. Green, MB. *Pesticides — Boon or Bane?* Boulder, CO: Westview Press, 1976.

15. Sundnes K, Haimanot A. Epidemic of louse-borne relapsing fever in Ethiopia. *The Lancet* 1993;**342**:1213-1215.

16. CDC. Endrin poisoning associated with taquito ingestion — California. *MMWR* 1989;**38**:345-347.

17. Ames RG, Brown SK, Rosenberg J et al. Health symptoms and occupational exposure to flea control products among California pet handlers. *Am Ind Hyg J* 1989;**50**(9):466-472.

XV

HEALTH MAINTENANCE: REDUCING HAZARDS

To find health should be the object of the doctor. Anyone can find disease.
— Andrew Taylor Still, M.D. [1]

Good health is one of life's many blessings that we best appreciate only after it has passed us by. Most of us come into this world with healthy bodies and all of the opportunities that we need to maintain them that way. The destruction of health is almost always self-inflicted, as are most of our woes. The concept of the body as a temple provides an excellent guide to the preservation of health. If we keep it clean, provide the proper nutrition and adequate rest that are essential to the body and avoid abuse of all substances, including food, we can be reasonably well assured of good health and longevity. If we ignore these simple guidelines we can expect to pay the consequences ultimately with impaired health and suffering.

NUTRITION

Good nutrition is one of the prime requisites for good health. In the United States this mandate is much more frequently deviated from in the extreme than on the short side. Moderation in all things is wise counsel in nutrition as with most other aspects of life. Unlike so many of the developing societies, the wealth and abundance in the United States kills far more individuals than does starvation. Obesity and excessive consumption of animal fats and refined sugars deliver many people to an early grave, and much suffering along the way. Some of the adverse consequences of obesity are:

• The incidence of diabetes mellitus is three times greater in overweight individuals. The prevalence of diabetes in the United States has increased by 33 percent in the past decade,[2] and three-quarters of these patients who have Non-Insulin Dependent Diabetes are obese. Obesity promotes insulin resistance.

• The incidence of hypertension is three times greater in obese individuals.

• An increased incidence of left ventricular hypertrophy with a greater risk of congestive heart failure and sudden death.

• Elevated triglycerides and lower high-density lipoprotein levels.

• Respiratory disorders, including chronic hypoxemia (low blood oxygen).

• An increased incidence of varicose veins with thrombophlebitis and pulmonary embolism.

• Sleep apnea is common in severely obese individuals; weight reduction frequently results in improvement.

• Post-menopausal breast cancer is more common in obese women.

• Endometrial cancer is two to three times more common in obese women.

• Obese individuals suffer a higher incidence of osteoarthritis and degenerative joint disease, particularly in the weight bearing joints such as the knees, hips and low back.

• Obese individuals suffer a higher incidence of gallstones, with resultant gallbladder surgery. The incidence of complications at surgery is increased in these people.

• Obese individuals have a high incidence of abnormal liver function tests.

• Obese individuals have a higher mortality rate due to coronary heart disease, stroke, diabetes, digestive diseases and cancer.

Our society has been experiencing an epidemic of gross obesity since the 1960s, and a significant percentage of these individuals will be burdened with these and many other health problems. The fact that large numbers of teenagers and young adults have cultivated this excess weight is especially tragic, for although they may be able to reduce weight they will not be able to remove the excess fat cells later in life.

Our bodies require certain raw materials in order to perform the essential tasks of growth and repair, and the warding off of disease. These raw materials include meat to provide the eight essential amino acids that the body cannot manufacture from other sources. Also required is a small quantity of fat to provide the body with the essential fatty acids that it cannot synthesize, as well as cholesterol. Cholesterol is the raw material for the production of the various hormones in the body. In addition to protein and fat, carbohydrates are needed to supply the balance of calories needed for energy and metabolic processes. Besides these three basic groups, certain vitamins and minerals are required.

All of this can be accomplished by the ingestion of approximately 1500 to 1800 calories per day of a properly balanced diet for most people. The exact requirement depends upon the individual's ideal body weight and level of physical activity. Active individuals might require 2000 to 2500 calories to meet these requirements. Many people, even sendentary individuals, consume well in excess of 3000 to 4000 calories daily. Radical surgical procedures to passively limit the quantity of food that these people can eat have become popular. Cosmetic surgery is then required to remove the excess skin. All calories in excess of those required by the body for these essential functions are converted to fat in the storage depots. (You know where these are.)

PROTEIN: Neglect of any of the essential basic materials carries the risk of developing a variety of disorders. The most efficient and the only reliable source of complete protein is meat, eggs and milk. Protein from animal sources provides the body with the eight essential amino acids. All of the legumes are lacking in one or more of these essential materials. With a careful balance of legumes it is possible to come close to providing a complete balance of essential amino acids, but the only source of cholesterol, which is essential for the production of all of the hormones in the body, is animal fat.

Grains similarly are not complete proteins; wheat and rice, for instance, have a low level of the essential amino acid lysine. In cultures where animal intake of proteins is inadequate, supplementation of the basic wheat diet with lysine resulted in an increased height, weight and skinfold thickness and improved blood hemoglobin values.[3] Where mixtures of plant sources of protein are utilized to compensate for the amino acid deficiencies of each, it is essential that they be consumed together. Unlike fats, the body does not store protein for subsequent needs. Since there is no mechanism for the storage of amino acids in the body, consuming one group of incomplete protein one day, and the balance the next day will not meet the needs of the body; they must be available at the same time.

In reality such a careful balance seldom is achieved among vegetarians, and some supplement their diet with eggs to assure against a deficiency of these essential nutritional elements. This remedy is deferred by others because of the cholesterol content of eggs and the widespread campaign to convince people of the evils of this vital substance. Where there is excess cholesterol in the diet (unlikely in a reasonable diet) this presumed disadvantage can be avoided by consuming only the egg white. Contrary to the current hype of many faddists, in order to maintain good health it is essential to consume 6 to 7 ounces of lean meat daily.

Diets that are deficient in proteins, choline, methionine, vitamin B_{12} and folic acid result in fatty deposits in the liver and predispose to the development of cirrhosis. Extensive studies of individuals on vegetarian diets demonstrated low levels of stored iron and a deficiency of zinc. This results in a loss of taste for meat, which further aggravates the deficiency. Also found were low levels of sodium and potassium, with a corresponding elevation of calcium and magnesium levels, a pattern associated with diminished adrenal and thyroid output. Another finding was copper imbalance. All of these distortions adversely affect many enzyme systems in the body, with a resultant compromise of health and feeling well.

A dramatic example of the damage that may result from nutritional neglect is the case of the 33-year-old man who developed a marked loss of vision (less than 20/400 in both eyes) as a result of a strict vegetarian diet.[4] He had initiated the diet for "improved health" at the age of 20 years. The loss of vision was permanent and irreversible. A study in Sidney, Australia revealed that individuals with diets that are deficient in protein, niacin, thiamin, riboflavin and vitamin A are more likely to develop nuclear cataracts (a cataract of the central portion of the lens).[5] Another study revealed that men whose diet was largely tofu demonstrated brain atrophy and cognitive impairment.[6] This may well explain some of the widespread incompetence and aberrant behavior apparent in our society today.

Much attention has been focused recently on elevated levels of homocysteine in the blood as a risk factor for atherosclerosis and heart disease. Homocysteine is an intermediate chemical step in the conversion of the amino acid methionine to cysteine. The liver uses the amino acid cysteine to detoxify many substances, including alcohol. Inadequate diets and aging impede this conversion, resulting in abnormally high levels of homocysteine. Adequate amounts of folic acid and vitamins B6 and B12 facilitate the conversion to cysteine, helping to reduce the level of homocysteine in the blood. Recent studies have demonstrated that supplementing the diet with at least 400 mcg daily of folic acid reduces elevated homocysteine levels. This amount of folic acid is now included in most therapeutic strength multivitamin preparations. Folic acid is also vital during the earliest days of pregnancy to prevent birth defects (see Chapter IV).

Protein and specifically the essential amino acids are the building blocks that the body uses in the manufacture of all of the protein substances in the body, including blood and some of the elements of the immune system that protect the body from disease. Neglect of this component of the diet can result in increased susceptibility to infections in general. In addition to being building blocks, some amino acids serve as neurotransmitters. Others such as the essential amino acids phenylalanine and tryptophan are precursors of hormones, enzymes and other vital substances.

Another suggestion of potential serious consequences of a deficiency of the essential amino acids has evolved from recent studies linking sleep disorders with a reduction in the production of melatonin from tryptophan in the pineal gland (see Sleep below). Protein, along with carbohydrates, also provides fuel for energy. The amount needed depends on many factors, including illness or the state of health, and whether or not growth is still progressing. For the average adult the intake of fifty grams of protein daily balances the protein that is used up in metabolic activities in the body. This assumes that a proper balance between protein, fat and carbohydrate exists.

COMPLICATIONS OF PROTEIN DEFICIENCY

IMMUNE SYSTEM: both cell mediated and humoral immunity (antibodies) are diminished. The T lymphocytes, the polymorphonuclear leukocytes and the complement system are all depressed. The B lymphocyte function may be impaired. The result is an increased susceptibility to infections; infections then worsen the existing malnutrition through loss of appetite.

CHILDHOOD AND ADOLESCENCE: Incomplete development of the immune system with an increased susceptibility to infections. Growth is retarded with a failure to achieve normal height and weight. Puberty and thus menstruation may be delayed.

PEM (protein-energy malnutrition) is common in the less-developed countries. PEM is present when insufficient protein is available to meet the metabolic needs, and results in the impairment of many physiologic processes. In the U.S. in the Ten State Survey of the National Health and Nutrition Survey 20 to 30 percent of the children in low income families demonstrated retarded growth. A significant reduction in birth weight and length has been observed in multiple studies of famine, not only in the less developed countries but also during wartime in Holland and during the siege of Leningrad. Malnourished, protein deficient patients suffer from increased fatigability and decreased mental alertness. When these patients go to surgery they have an increased incidence of post-operative infections and delayed healing.

SEVERE PEM: in more severe cases of protein deprivation muscle wasting is present, as evidenced by atrophy of the interosseous muscles of the hand. There is also a loss of subcutaneous fat and muscle mass generally, and decreased elasticity of the skin resulting in a wrinkled skin. Decubitus ulcers are common. The hair becomes sparse and dry, loses its sheen and can be pulled out easily. The color of the hair may change to a reddish or dull brown. Lethargy is common. Gastrointestinal complications include constipation, and difficulty ingesting normal size meals due to early satiety and vomiting. The heart rate, blood pressure and core temperature may be subnormal. This condition is commonly seen in Africa and other underdeveloped countries where the name kwashiorkor has long been applied to it.

HYPOPROTEINEMIC PEM: occurs when there is an inadequate intake of protein but total caloric intake is not severely restricted. In this condition the liver may be enlarged and tender, and fatty liver develops. The serum LDL and VLDL are subnormal, and the degree of fatty infiltration of the liver correlates with the degree of depression of these lipoproteins.

MARASMIC PEM: marasmus is a condition that occurs mainly during the first year of life. It is characterized by retardation of growth and progressive wasting of muscle and subcutaneous fat. It results when there is an inadequate intake of both protein and total calories. Edema is absent in this condition, as contrasted to pure protein malnutrition. In kwashiorkor where there is a deficiency of both protein and calories the term marasmic kwashior-kor is applied.

FAT: A minimum amount of fat is also vital to provide the body with the three essential fatty acids that it cannot synthesize. These are linolenic, linoleic and arachidonic acids. The latter is a precursor of the various prostaglandins that play a vital role at the cellular level in virtually every organ in the body. Fat has had a bad press recently, and it is true that many people have consumed far too much of it. We do, however, need about 25 to 30 percent of our daily calories in fat in order to provide these essential fatty acids. At that reduced level we are minimizing the risk of arterio-sclerosis. A deficiency of the essential fatty acids shows up as a dry and scaly skin, and in infants and children in a deficiency in growth as well.

DO NOT consume any of the recently developed nonabsorb-able fats that are promoted to permit us to consume as much of the junk foods as we wish without penalty. Currently these synthetic fat substitutes are marketed primarily in snack foods such as the various chips. In a short time however they will be incorporated in every food that contains oils and fats, including cereals, bread, cookies and all baked goods. It will become very difficult to avoid consumption of these very dangerous products. These artificial fats will prevent absorption of the fat-soluble vitamins, A, D, E and K. The FDA has also given approval to a new drug that prevents the body from absorbing fats, which will have the same side effects. These products will cause a return to a serious health problem that was common in medicine in a past era when mineral oil was commonly used as a laxative. In addition they will result in a deficiency of the essential fatty acids discussed above. In spite of the economic potential for these products they should never have been approved.

"Fat free foods" is a hoax that has been perpetrated on the American people by the food industry, with the aid of federal food regulators. By their definition these foods may contain monoglycer-ides and diglycerides, but not triglycerides. This is nonsense, for the body metabolizes all three in essentially the same way. People are led to believe that they may eat these "fat free" foods with impunity, when in reality they are increasing their caloric intake and accomplishing nothing, except to gain weight.

The remainder of the daily caloric intake that is not supplied by fat and protein comes from carbohydrates, mainly starches and sugars. There have been several sweetener substitutes introduced to the market place over the past fifty years, so that we might have our cake without penalty. It has been suggested that an excess consumption of refined sugar in our society might be a contributing factor in the high incidence of diabetes. The chief motivation for sugar substitutes, however, has been to simply permit us to reduce calories without pain. The objective is the same as with the fat substitutes, and similar complications accompany these products. One of the most successful substitutes was cyclamate, but it was removed from the U.S. market after massive doses caused bladder tumors in beagles. It is still marketed throughout the rest of the world, and no adverse effects have been seen from it there.

Unfortunately cyclamate was replaced by another discovery, aspartame, which has become widely used as a sweetener in food, deserts and soft drinks. It has been recognized by many experts to be an excitotoxin. Reactions to aspartame that have been reported in thousands of individuals over a long period of time include headache, irritability, decreased mental acuity, memory loss and depression. Studies have associated these symptoms with the permanent destruction of nerve cells in the brain. Both aspartic acid and glutamic acid (from MSG or monosodium glutamate) induce the influx of an excess of calcium into the cells of neurons in the brain. This influx results in an excess of free radicals in the cells, which kills them.[7]

The extent of cell death is related to the quantity of excito-toxins consumed and to the length of time of the exposure. The effect is increased when multiple agents are consumed at the same time, as would be the case with drugs, alcohol and certain dietary substances. This damage from excitotoxins has been associated with the development later in life of Parkinson's disease, Alzheimer's dementia, Huntington's disease and Amyotrophic Lateral Sclerosis. Dr. John Olney reported the development of brain tumors in rats that were fed aspartame in 1987. This association had been noted in the original studies reported to the FDA by the G.D. Searle company, but the company obfuscated these events in follow-up studies. Studies by others have confirmed it subsequently, however. From 1973 to 1990 brain tumors in people over the age of 65 increased by 67 percent.[8] The introduction of aspartame into the food chain has been suggested as a plausible explanation for this increase.[9]

Neuron damage in the developing fetus has been shown to result from the consumption of these agents during pregnancy.[10,11,12] This may account for some of a variety of neuro-developmental abnormalities seen in newborn infants and children. Whereas most developmental abnormalities that result from chemical exposures occur during early pregnancy, the excitotoxins can destroy cells in the brain at any time during pregnancy, up to the time of delivery. In spite of a large number of complaints over a considerable period of time, and numerous studies demonstrating the deleterious effects of these substances, there has been a great reluctance to acknowledge any harmful effect from consuming aspartame, chiefly because of the massive economic market involved.

Saccharin has had the longest history as a sugar substitute, and although it is known to be an effective promoter (see Chapter XIII) for bladder cancers in rats at very high doses, it has not produced these results in humans. Being a derivative of benzoic acid it does, however, invoke toxic reactions if consumed in excessive doses. The only reason that saccharin is marketed in the United States while cyclamate is not is because the U.S. Congress passed an exemption for saccharin that permitted its use. Xylitol and sorbitol, both of which are sugar alcohols, are also permitted as food additives and are used as sweeteners in gum as well as food. These substances can cause an osmotic diarrhea even with modest consumption, such as ten sticks of gum daily. Even though they are approved as food additives the National Toxicology Program of the U.S. Department of Health and Human Services lists saccharin, sorbitol and xylitol as carcinogens.

Stevia, a plant that yields the glycoside stevioside, is 300 times sweeter than table sugar, and contains neither calories nor food value. It has been used as a noncaloric sweetener in soft drinks, candy, and foods in Japan since 1970, and has demonstrated no toxic effects. After intensive testing it was ruled safe by the Japanese authorities. It would appear to be the ideal sweetener, especially for diabetics, but the collusion of industry and the FDA has deprived the American public of this product.

The official position of the American Medical Association has been that, given a normal, adequate diet, supplemental vitamins are not necessary. Under ideal circumstances and with good discipline this would be true. Few societies have either. It is not easy, for instance, to assure an adequate intake of vitamin C (ascorbic acid) in northern climates in the winter. The usual sources, citrus juices, cannot be relied upon if they have been allowed to thaw and then refrozen during shipment, as is often the case. Ascorbic acid is readily oxidized by heat and by zinc in the coatings of some containers and strainers. The ideal material for strainers is stainless steel, and these are widely available now.

Fruit that reaches the table is seldom "tree ripened" and thus the vitamin C content is questionable. Ascorbic acid is easily synthesized and is reasonably inexpensive. A tablet containing 250 milligrams taken once or twice daily carries no risk, if taken with food to protect the stomach, and assures that the minimum daily requirement for vitamin C is met. This vitamin cannot be stored in the body, so a daily intake is necessary.

Taking one therapeutic strength vitamin from a reputable manufacturer (such as Theragran-M®) daily does not carry a risk for the average individual. Such a practice insures that the minimum daily requirement of virtually all of the vitamins and minerals is met. One should be cognizant of the fact, however, that vitamins A and D can be overdosed, with potentially serious consequences. Both of these vitamins are routinely added to several foods such as bread, milk, cereals and other foods and drinks, increasing the risk of excessive consumption. It is important to limit the routine intake of therapeutic strength vitamins to not more than one daily.

Vitamin D carries a smaller margin of safety than most of the other vitamins, and presents a risk of overdose, with potential damage to the eyes and kidneys. The current recommended daily dose is 400 to 800 units, with the average adult in the United States ingesting about 100 to 150 IU daily from dietary sources. It is routinely added to milk, bread and margarine and is found naturally in egg yolk, liver and salt water fish. Absorption of vitamin D takes place in the ileum (small intestine) and requires bile salts. Impaired function of the gallbladder therefore can reduce absorption, as can increased motility in the intestine and fat malabsorption syndromes. The ingestion of mineral oil or the recently introduced dietary fat substitutes such as Olestra® also interferes with absorption of not only vitamin D, but all of the fat-soluble vitamins, A, D, E, and K. Another product that was introduced recently to combat obesity, Orlistat®, also interferes with the absorption of all of the fat-soluble vitamins. It works by decreasing the absorption of fats from the gastrointestinal tract.

Aging of the individual decreases the absorption of vitamin D by about 40 percent, especially after the age of 65 years. These factors should be considered when deciding upon an optimal level of supplementation. Overt toxicity is usually seen only with ingestion of 60,000 IU or more daily over an extended period. One of the complications of this toxicity, however, is the formation of kidney stones, a consequence best avoided. The precise level at which this becomes a risk has not been determined.

Vitamin D is also formed in the body as a result of exposure of the skin to the sun's ultraviolet irradiation. The application of sunscreens, and the deposition of melanin in the skin with tanning both diminish this production. Production is also diminished in the elderly. Deficiency of vitamin D contributes to the development of osteoporosis. It is included in many calcium supplements, but women taking these should utilize the products that do not contain vitamin D. Otherwise significant overdosage of this vitamin can occur.

Excessive doses of vitamin A can result in damage to the eye, including hemorrhage, blurring of vision and double vision, as well as loss of eyebrows and eyelashes. Loss of appetite, dry, fissured skin, brittle nails, hair loss, inflammation of the gums and mouth, overgrowth of bone, liver damage and nervous system disorders are other side effects. Much larger doses of this vitamin are required to produce toxic effects than is the case with vitamin D; thus some less risk is involved. Sources of vitamin A include milk, butter, margarine, liver, carrots, sweet potatoes, other yellow vegetables and tomato juice. A number of cases of yellowing of the skin (carotenemia) have resulted from consuming excessive quantities of substances containing vitamin A, such as carrot juice.

Vitamin A in the form of its precursor beta carotene and vitamin E have been suggested to have benefits in inhibiting carcinogenesis in several target organs. Studies in laboratory animals have demonstrated that there is an increased binding of carcinogenic chemicals to the DNA of the cells lining the lungs in the absence of vitamin A precursors. Other studies have shown that individuals who have an adequate intake of vitamin A experience a lower incidence of lung cancer than do those who have a deficiency in their diet.

Ascorbic acid and alpha tocopherol (vitamin E) have been shown to protect against ozone toxicity and to inhibit atherosclerosis through their influence on lipid metabolism. These effects are mediated through the antioxidant activities of these two vitamins. Oxidative reactions at various chemical, enzyme and cellular levels in the body contribute to the aging process as well as to cancer production. Vitamin C and E also prevent formation of nitrosamines, thus reducing the risk of cancer formation in the liver, stomach and respiratory tract. If both of these are taken twice daily, vitamin E as 200 international units of alphatocopherol, vitamin C as 250 mg at the noon and evening meals, along with intelligent dietary measures, many of the adverse effects of premature aging might be delayed or avoided.

Calcium is an essential mineral that is commonly deficient in our diet. In children (through adolescence) it is needed for the formation of both bone and teeth. For the entirety of our life it plays an essential role in cellular and other metabolism in the body, and it is essential in maintaining the bony integrity of our skeletal systems. Very often leg cramps at night or in the early morning reflect a deficiency of calcium in the muscle cells. The safest and most efficient supplement is oyster shell calcium (calcium carbonate), without added vitamin D. Taking calcium supplements that combine vitamin D run the risk of overdosage of that vitamin. Dolomite as a source of calcium should be avoided. It provides calcium as well as magnesium, but may also be contaminated with lead and talc, both of which can cause serious harm.

Iodine is essential for the production of thyroid hormone, which is vital for normal growth, development and everyday metabolism. Deficiency of iodine in soils, and thus in foods, in the Great Lakes region resulted in many goiters until the practice of routinely adding iodine to table salt was instituted. Iodine deficiency is still a serious problem in some parts of the world, and the World Health Organization has experimented with various means of dietary supplementation in those areas. A less dramatic low level dietary deficiency is even more widespread.

A simple home test for iodine deficiency that has been proposed is to paint a 3-inch square of skin on the thigh or abdomen with 2 percent tincture of iodine. If the yellow stain disappears in less than 24 hours this indicates a deficiency of iodine in the body. Repeat of this procedure at different areas on the thighs or abdomen after the stain has disappeared, until the stain persists for 24 hours will bring the iodine level in the body up to normal.[13] Iodine deficiency can be remedied by consuming foods rich in iodine, such as kelp and seafood, and by using iodized salt. Where salt restriction is indicated, as in individuals with hypertension and during pregnancy, a supplement may be needed. For those on thyroid supplements the dose of these must be cut back before iodine is added in any form.

Osteoporosis is very common in post-menopausal women, and is very tragic when it results in deformity of the spine. Cigarette smoking plays a very significant role in this pathology by decreasing the blood circulation to bone. Calcium deficiency plays an important role even in non-smokers, however. Maintaining the integrity of bone requires hormone (estrogen), protein (meat), calcium and weight bearing. Physicians observed fifty years ago that the development of osteoporosis was prevented in women who were treated with estrogens for the other symptoms of the menopause. This issue has been very controversial in the intervening years, partially because of the fear of the role that estrogens might play in the production of cancer.

It is now universally accepted, however, that proper administration of estrogens in a cyclical pattern (first three weeks of the month only), balanced with progesterone taken the 15th to the 25th day of the cycle, does help prevent the development of osteoporosis. This program also reduces the risk of heart attacks and ameliorates other problems associated with aging. In spite of these facts a study in 1997 revealed that only 24 percent of American postmenopausal women use hormone replacement therapy. Only 47.4 percent of postmenopausal women doctors take advantage of it.[14]

Just as important in maintaining bone integrity is calcium, and it too must be started very early before bone loss begins. No substance and no program have proven successful in rebuilding bone once it has been lost. For this reason it has been recommended that women supplement their diet throughout their life with oyster shell calcium in doses of 500 to 1000 mg daily, depending upon the quantity received from the other sources in the diet. The total daily intake should be 1200 to 1500 mg, and this level is seldom reached, especially in the teen years. Oxalic acid combines with calcium to form calcium oxalate, which is not absorbed. Taking calcium supplements with foods that contain oxalic acid therefore may not provide the expected quantity of calcium to the body. Some of these foods are spinach, beets, cocoa, tea, dried figs, beans, tomatoes, almonds, cashew nuts and most berries.

Adequate protein in the form of 4 to 6 ounces of lean meat daily is also essential. This meat should be beef for the most part because of its higher biologic value. Recent studies have demonstrated that 0.625 mg of conjugated estrogens is the appropriate and effective dose of that hormone. Less is inadequate to prevent osteoporosis; more produces no more benefit but does increase the incidence of side effects. In women with no family history of breast or uterine cancer there is no increased risk at the 0.625 mg dose, especially when balanced with progesterone as it always should be. Unfortunately the majority of women who were placed on hormone replacement therapy in the fifties and sixties were given the classical pill that contains 1.25 mg. The re-education of physicians in using the appropriate dose was a slow process. This balanced hormone replacement therapy should be continued throughout life. The administration of estrogen to women with a significant family history of breast or uterine cancer is not recommended.

Christiansen (Denmark) reported a 50 percent reduction in fractures in postmenopausal women who were treated with this regime beginning at or before menopause. Full benefit is realized only with long-term therapy, however. Some benefit is realized even where hormone replacement therapy is delayed until after the menopause. Christiansen's study also showed the need for 1000 mg of calcium daily, 500 mg if the diet was adequate, a rare occurrence. Cigarette smoking must also be eliminated, however, and this cannot be stressed enough. Dr. Robert Wilson discussed some of the other benefits of hormone replacement therapy in his book, *Feminine Forever*, in 1966. The changes that are alleviated include not only the hot flushes and night sweats, but insomnia, mood swings, memory loss, loss of skin elasticity and vaginal dryness. The onset of these changes typically begins during the forties in conjunction with the fall in the level of estrogens produced in the body. The benefit of reducing the risk of heart attacks is also significant and has had considerable publicity.

Several metals and trace elements are essential dietary components but these are toxic in excess, and excess is very easy to achieve with some. Serious illness has been observed as a result of selenium supplementation, which has gained popularity recently as a health food supplement. Although much of selenium's activity in the body has not been mapped out it is known to be essential to some enzyme systems. It has recently gained attention as an antioxidant, along with vitamins A, C and E and zinc, as a preventative of atherosclerosis and age related macular degeneration (eye). Adequate supplies of selenium are obtained in food, however, since it is present in the soil in more than sufficient quantities. Because of this presence it is found in meat, eggs, dairy products and grain.

Very few regions on earth have geologic strata that is deficient in selenium. Deficiency syndromes have been seen in some regions of China and New Zealand. In other regions such as in Colombia, where the soil is rich in selenium, malformed infants have been seen in parents with selenium toxicity. Damage to the liver and spleen as well as damage to the nervous system and loss of hair and nails occurs with excess intake. Growth retardation has been observed even with moderate excess selenium in the diet.[15] The safe range is very narrow, and the maximum supplementation for most residents in the United States on a normal, balanced diet should not exceed 20 to 30 μg per day. Some vitamin supplements such as Theragran-M® now contain 21 μg in each tablet, which is an adequate daily supplementation for most people.

Chromium, another metal, is important in several enzyme systems in the body. It has been used also to improve glucose intolerance in some elderly patients and to reduce insulin requirements. Chromium produces destruction of the tubules in the kidneys, however, and supplementation requires caution. Molybdenum can produce an anemia through poorly understood mechanisms. In 1967 several deaths from heart failure resulted from the addition of cobalt to beer to enhance foam formation.[16] This practice has been discontinued. Iron, copper, magnesium, manganese and zinc are more forgiving but nonetheless can produce ill effects.

A normal, well-balanced diet that includes cereals, nuts and meats will easily provide an adequate supply of all of these minerals except for iron. Iron is cheap and easy to acquire, since no prescription is required. It must be taken with prudence, however, for iron overload is possible, with toxic results. Many children have lost their lives due to ingestion of iron tablets that were left within their reach.

Zinc has been promoted as a preventative for prostate disease for several years now. There are some authorities who believe that the incidence of prostate cancer could be reduced if all males took zinc supplements regularly throughout their lifetime. The prostatic enzyme acid phosphatase has a high zinc content. More recently zinc supplements have been prescribe as a preventative for age related macular degeneration, which can cause blindness.

Serious illness in infants due to zinc deficiency or malabsorption is sometimes seen, due chiefly to dietary deficiency caused by the feeding of cow's milk alone. In infants thus deprived of the normal meat, grain and vegetable dietary components, significant iron deficiency anemia is present. Although these infants are usually fat, their pallor reveals their true nutritional status. Zinc is normally distributed in the tissues throughout the body, and as with other trace elements, has a complex metabolism.

Parasitic infestations, poor nutrition and a number of elements in the diet interfere with normal absorption and metabolism of zinc. Isoniazid and some antibiotics such as penicillin interfere with absorption. Zinc is present in most foods and in water, so significant deficiency is uncommon. Seafood, meats, nuts, whole grains, dairy products and legumes are high in zinc content. Excess intake can occur from consumption of foods that are left in galvanized containers. Although the body tolerates a wider range of zinc intake than of selenium, supplementation should be undertaken judiciously. Daily supplementation probably should not exceed 15 to 30 mg of elemental zinc.

Periodically, contaminants in health food supplements produce poisoning in people who consume them. Sometimes large numbers of people are involved, and sometimes tragedy is invoked. Such was the case in October 1989 when EMS, eosinophilia-myalgia syndrome, was first reported in New Mexico (see Chapter XIII). Severe, incapacitating myalgia (muscle pain) and a markedly elevated number of eosinophils in the blood characterized this syndrome. Deaths have occurred in up to 10 percent of the victims.

The eosinophilia-myalgia syndrome was caused by a contaminant in certain batches of L-tryptophan that were produced by one specific manufacturer. L-tryptophan from all other manufacturers during this period has not yielded the syndrome. The risk of acquiring this disease was in direct proportion to the quantity of the contaminated L-tryptophan consumed. Many milder cases have occurred in people who took lower doses than did those who exhibited the more pronounced symptoms.

NATURAL MEDICINE

There has been a remarkable, explosive interest in so called "natural medicine" in recent years. This subject has even attracted many physicians to the cause. In the past, fear of ostracism by the American Medical Association or local colleagues would have tempered the enthusiasm that is expressed, even promoted in advertising by some physicians. While it is wise and commendable to keep an open mind on every subject in medicine, one should be very careful to not mislead people, however innocently. The consequences can be devastating. The most basic and sacred mandate of the practice of medicine is "first do no harm."

It is true that many of our modern medicines had their origins in botanicals, and some still do. During the Middle Ages the absence of scientific, effective remedies led people to seek help from individuals who offered brews and concoctions for every purpose from abortion to fertility to murder. As is the case today, where physicians could offer no remedy, people sought help where it was available. Some remedies were helpful but some were deadly. Wormwood (absinthe) was used as a remedy for intestinal worms, gout, kidney stones and jaundice, and to stimulate menstruation. We know today that it is not effective for any of these problems, and we also know that it seriously damages the nervous system, including the brain, and the heart (see Chapter XII).

It was from a local English herbal practitioner that William Withering, one of the ablest and most respected clinician of his time (1741-1799),[17] learned in 1776 that foxglove is useful in treating dropsy (heart failure). The digitalis preparations derived from this plant remain the most effective remedies for strengthening the failing heart muscle to this day. Tablets made from the ground leaves of the foxglove plant (*Digitalis purpurea*) remained in use through the 1950s. However it was discovered that two glycosides, digitoxin and digoxin, could be extracted from the raw product. These preparations produce more precise products that enabled more accurate dosing and fewer side effects.

This has been the pattern in virtually every medicine of plant origin. Thus when we need aspirin, we no longer brew a tea from willow bark; rather we take a tablet of acetylsalicylic acid that has been produced and standardized in a modern pharmaceutical plant. Using a purified product that provides the desired action in the body without the undesirable side effects of the whole plant has delivered a more scientific approach to the treatment of disease. One can still relieve dropsy and the shortness of breath of heart failure by chewing the leaves of *Digitalis purpurea*, but the use of one of the purified derivatives is more efficient, and produces less risk of toxic side effects. In the sixteenth century when a medicine was needed there was no alternative to the natural source.

An exception is quinine and its optical isomer quinidine, which are still derived solely from the bark of the cinchona tree of S. America and Indonesia. They can be synthesized, but the process is complex and costly. Quinine was essential to prevent and treat malaria during World War II, and when Indonesia fell into Japanese hands it was necessary to manufacture the drug. Several other drugs have been developed for treating malaria, but quinine has regained importance as resistance to the newer drugs developed in the malaria parasite. It also is used in treating nocturnal leg cramps. In some cases these may be relieved by drinking a small quantity of tonic water, which contains quinine, at bedtime. Serious toxic effects, which include visual disturbances, ringing in the ears and kidney damage can result from consuming too much quinine. Quinidine is an important medicine in treating heart irregularities.

Certainly we should continue to investigate plant sources for effective medicines. It seems foolish, however, to abandon the labors of and knowledge imparted by all of the many scientists throughout history who devoted their lives to isolating the most effective ingredients of the various plants, laying the groundwork for the production of purified and safer medications. When a plant source is found to produce beneficial effects, the active compound should be identified, purified and standardized. In this manner the desirable actions will be harvested without damaging body organs or causing death.

It is common practice in the promotional material for natural remedies to refer to them as "homeopathic," as though this identifies them as innocuous, desirable and without potential harm. This is completely inaccurate and misleading. The philosophy of homeopathy was conceived in Germany in 1810 by Hahnemann. It was an extension of a doctrine expressed by Paracelsus (c.1540) that "like cures like." The theory held that an illness in an individual should be treated with drugs that produce in a well person the symptoms expressed in the illness. Hahnemann theorized that the dose for a given substance should be the smallest one required to produce like symptoms in a well person. Homeopathic practitioners continue to believe that remedies become more potent with greater dilution. This lowering of the dose also reduced the incidence of adverse reactions and deaths from medicines, which may account for the great popularity that homeopathy achieved. Hahnemann died a millionaire in Paris in 1843.

A wide diversity of health food products are promoted for the purpose of bestowing better health, better sleep or increased longevity. Many of these are natural products, and many natural products are toxic, some even poisonous. One of these products is chaparral, which is advertised as a "free radical scavenger." This is an attempt to capitalize on the antioxidant benefits recently described for vitamins C and E. The product is made by grinding the leaves of an evergreen desert shrub known as the creosote bush, and it is indeed an antioxidant. It also produces toxic effects in the body, however, including a very pronounced toxic hepatitis.[18]

Several other natural products that are promoted in capsules or as a tea that are known to be toxic to the liver include germander, Senecio, skullcap, senna, Symphytum, Heliotropium, Crotolaria Phorandendron, mistletoe and sassafras (see Chapters III and XIII). Deaths have occurred in some of the cases of toxic hepatitis produced by these natural supplements. Many of those individuals who do survive have to live with the sequelae of chronic hepatitis. The many claims of the medicinal and curative value of sassafras tea, highly popular for generations in the United States, have never been substantiated. It has been determined also that the safrole in sassafras causes liver tumors in laboratory animals and it has been banned under the Delaney clause.

In 1988 a large number of individuals in Texas (93 were tested and evaluated) consumed an illegal pharmaceutical product known as "chuifong tokuwan" and sold as "The Miracle Herb— Mother Nature's Finest." Manufactured by a company in Hong Kong it contained a mixture of diazepam, indomethacin, hydrochlorothiazide, mefenamic acid, dexamethasone, lead and cadmium.[19] The latter two substances are serious poisons that permanently damage the brain, kidneys and lungs. The other ingredients are an improbable and unrelated potpourri of various drugs, somewhat like picking one pill from each bottle on the shelf in the hopes of curing whatever symptom is present for the day. You should never find lead or cadmium in any pill on the shelf, however. Such inclusion should be considered criminal misconduct.

Numerous other incidents of poisoning from herbal or illegal medications have occurred. Three children with serious life-threatening poisoning that resulted from the ingestion of Jin Bu Huan tablets (for pain and insomnia) were treated in hospitals in Colorado in 1993.[20] In July and August 1993 three women in Los Angeles were treated for acute hepatitis that resulted from taking Jin Bu Huan tablets.[21] The package listed the plant *Polygala chinensis* as the source, but an analysis revealed that the chemical in the tablets came from other genera of plants. Any product that produces the serious liver inflammation experienced by these women should be avoided.

Several incidents of serious organ damage resulting from Chinese herbal medicines that were discovered to contain botanicals other than those specified on the package for the medicine have been reported. In some instances the botanical had a digitalis-like effect on the heart. In one study of Asian medicines from retail herbal stores 32 percent contained pharmaceuticals that were not listed as ingredients.[22] In one report from Brussels, Belgium, women who had been placed on a slimming regime that included Chinese herbs suffered terminal renal failure from herbal components that were toxic to the kidney.[23] The Chinese preparation contained *Aristolochia* species, which contains aristolochic acid, known to be toxic to both the liver and kidneys, and to be carcinogenic.[24,25,26,27,28] Approximately 100 additional cases were identified subsequently. About one-third of these women also developed valvular heart disease.[29] Although these herbal medicines are widely used by the Chinese population in the United States there has been no established protocol to identify and regulate the toxic ingredients. The American species, *Aristolochia serpentaria*, or snakeroot, has been prescribed as an aphrodisiac.

Lead poisonings from aphrodisiacs and from Chinese herbal medicine were first reported in the United States in 1977 and 1978, and these continue to the present. There has been an ongoing enthusiastic search for an effective aphrodisiac throughout history. Lead poisoning also occurred among Hmong children in immigrant families from Southeast Asia in 1983. During a one-year period in 1992 the California Department of Health received reports of 40 children who had elevated blood lead levels as a result of ethnic remedies.[30] These remedies included azarcon and greta (laxative) from Mexico, paylooah from Southeast Asia, surma from India and ayurvedic from Tibet. In one study, 24 of 260 Asian products collected from California herbal stores contained a median of 30 ppm of lead.[31] There is no place for any quantity of lead in medicines.

These "remedies" result in permanent brain damage and impaired learning in children. The great tragedy of these cases is that rather than the health benefits that the people thought they were getting, they had permanent, irreparable damage to the brain and other body organs inflicted upon them. It is unwise to consume any product promoted as a safe natural health food supplement unless its safety has been assured by competent authority. The products in the instances listed above were not tested or approved by any agency, government or private. The toxicity of most natural plants is well known from the many cases that appear in emergency rooms and poison control centers. The deliberate inclusions of such serious poisons as lead and cadmium cannot be, and would not be, anticipated. In some cases the source of the lead has been a red dye used to color the products. Red and yellow dyes and pigments commonly include lead and cadmium respectively.

In 1996 residents of border communities in Texas and Arizona suffered mercury toxicity from a cosmetic cream that was manufactured in Mexico. The cream contained calomel (mercurous chloride) which was absorbed through the skin.[32] The use of this serious poison in a skin cream is not only irrational but also irresponsible.

Another very toxic substance that is found in herbal medications, particularly in Chinese preparations, is aconite. This common flowering plant, also known as monkshood, blue rocket and wolfsbane, causes serious heart irregularities and death. It was used in China as a poison for arrows in previous eras. Poisoning occurs when children eat it or when the plant is mistaken for horseradish. Life threatening heart and lung complications occur with small doses and there is no antidote for the poisoning. The preparation is also widely available from Chinese herb stores.

Gelsemium, or yellow or Carolina Jasmine, has been used in the past as an antispasmodic and to combat neuralgia, and has resulted in poisoning and death. All parts of the plant contain a poisonous alkaloid, gelsemine, which has been likened to hemlock. Although it was formerly listed in the U.S. Pharmacopeia it has been discontinued due to its narrow and unpredictable safety range.

The pharmacological effects of mahuang (Chinese ephedra) was first noted in 1595 by Shi Cheng Li, and its active ingredient, the crystalline alkaloid ephedrine, was introduced to modern medicine in 1887 by Nagai. It (and the stereoisomer pseudoephedrine) continues to be used as effective bronchodilators in asthma and bronchitis as well as in decongestant products. In the United States and most other industrialized countries, these products are synthesized rather than being extracted from the plant. A more pure and standardized product can be produced in this manner. Interestingly, the several species of North American ephedra bushes, also known as Mormon tea, do not contain any ephedrine.

Mahuang was recently marketed in the United States as a natural remedy for the suppression of appetite, but it is not effective in that role. The rationale, if there is any, presumably is that ephedrine belongs to the same general pharmacological class as the amphetamines. Since the latter are on the untouchable list from the federal bureaucracy, mahuang might seem a logical substitute to someone with little or no knowledge of pharmacotherapeutics. As of this writing there have been at least 17 deaths and more than 800 adverse reactions, including heart irregularities and infarctions, strokes and seizures from the use of mahuang. Some studies suggest that other as yet unidentified substances from the plant might contribute to its toxicity.[33] There is widespread interest in substances that might help control appetite and weight, but unfortunately the only people who will benefit from this product are those who market it.

Licorice, which has been used as a flavoring in candy for generations, and which was used in Chinese medicine for headache, can cause serious illness and death. The roots of the wild licorice plant, *Glycyrrhiza*, which is found in the United States, contain glycyrrhizin, which has an action similar to aldosterone. It causes retention of sodium and depletion of potassium. This results in muscle weakness, a sustained elevation in the blood pressure, irregularities of the heart beat and death. A number of patients with these symptoms have been hospitalized as a result of excessive consumption of licorice candy, and deaths have occurred. Another common source of licorice in the United States is chewing tobacco where it is used for flavor.

Glycyrrhizin is fifty times sweeter than sugar, and unlike most sugars it quenches thirst rather than increasing it. As has been the trend in copying Chinese herbal medicines, licorice is now sold in the United States as a nutritional supplement. It is also incorporated in many of the fountain of youth cocktails being promoted to the public, and more recently in a mixture of herbs from China promoted to treat prostate cancer. The latter preparation has caused deep vein thrombosis and pulmonary embolism.[34] Thus another serious hazard has been added to the health food grab bag.

Khat (*Catha edulis*) which is a shrub that is cultivated in the Middle East for its leaves and buds that are a source of an habituating stimulant when chewed or used as a tea is discussed in Chapter XII.

Many plants do provide useful and safe products. Peppermint and spearmint are widely used as flavorings and as carminatives. European pennyroyal, however, can produce serious poisoning, and it grows wild in the United States. Seeds of dill, fennel, anise and caraway, all members of the carrot family, produce flavorful essential oils (oils that retain the flavor or odor of the plant). These also have been used as carminatives. Other essential oils are clove (eugenol), nutmeg (isoeugenol) vanilla and thyme (thymol). Gum Arabic (acacia) is harvested from certain African acacia trees, and is widely used as a stabilizer and to maintain texture in products such as ice cream and jellies.

Recently studies have confirmed that Ginkgo biloba does indeed improve memory in some people, even in some who are suffering from Alzheimer's disease. Individuals suffering from various degrees of "senile dementia" benefit the most. Echinacea has been shown to boost the immune system, an effect that could be beneficial in combating infections, but could be harmful to individuals who suffer from rheumatoid arthritis or other autoimmune diseases.

St. John's Wort (*Hypericum perforatum*), which has become very popular as a mood elevator recently, was awarded its name by virtue of the fact that it is in bloom during the summer solstice, or about the time celebrated as the birth date of St. John the Baptist (June 24). It contains hypericin, a photosensitizer that may cause sunburn and skin damage with subsequent exposure to the sun. The plant has caused significant skin damage in livestock, especially sheep. Few other serious adverse effects have been noted during the use of St. John's Wort. It does lower the serum concentration of some drugs such as digoxin and theophylline, however, while increasing the toxicity of selective serotonin reuptake inhibitors (SSRI) such as Prozac, Paxil and Zoloft. It's action as a mood elevator is mediated through the same mechanism as the conventional antidepressant medications, namely through inhibition of uptake of the neurotransmitters serotonin, norepinephrine and dopamine. St. John's wort should not be taken in combination with any of these medications. The term "wort" was the old English word for "plant."

Capsules and creams containing the steroid substance *diosgenin* from yams, on the other hand, are of no value because the human body does not have the enzyme necessary to convert the diosgenin to pregnenolone, the raw material for all of the hormones in the body. This conversion can be accomplished in the laboratory, and the body then can utilize the resultant pregnenolone. These products are fraudulently promoted as a "natural progesterone." It has also been proposed that the lower than expected birth rate among some peoples, such as certain Mexican Indians, can be attributed to the consumption of yams as a staple in their diet. This thesis is contradicted by the absence of the enzyme mentioned above.

A very thorough reference for the natural medicines may be found in *Herbal Medicine*.[35]

EXERCISE

Adequate and appropriate exercise is essential for the maintenance of muscle tone, to maintain bone density and to keep the heart and lung in good working order. Exercise need not be demanding or extreme. Walking one to three miles daily, or at least every other day, is adequate for an individual of average activity. Some added benefits of running have been demonstrated for the heart, lungs and blood pressure, but again there is no added benefit beyond running one to three miles every other day. Running presents an added risk of disorders of the feet, knees and hip joints. This is particularly true for those individuals unfortunate enough to inherit a proclivity toward arthritis.

Swimming is excellent exercise, with virtually no risk or adverse effect (other than the risk of drowning), but it is not as readily available as is running or walking. Well-designed exercise bicycles provide good exercise for the cardiovascular system. These have the advantage of being available regardless of the weather. For winter season exercise, both downhill and cross country skiing provide not only good aerobic exercise, but add considerable pleasure to life. This is particularly welcome later in life when some of the other pleasures have deserted us.

Two practices that present risks to the cardiovascular system are long sitting and crossing the legs. The latter is an extremely common practice, seemingly an innate behavioral trait. It damages the veins in the legs, however, encouraging the development of varicosities and thrombophlebitis. It is a habit that should be resisted. During long airline flights or jobs that require sitting, the individual should get up and walk up and down the isle periodically. The greater risk from thrombophlebitis that develops from prolonged sitting is a pulmonary embolus, which can be fatal.

WEIGHT

Maintaining the body weight as close to ideal as possible will deliver not only the greatest longevity, but also the minimum amount of grief. Many of our serious diseases, as outlined previously, are brought on earlier and are made worse by being overweight. William Banting in 1863 wrote his *Letter on Corpulence* in which he outlined a cure for obesity by a general reduction in food intake, including exclusion of fats and carbohydrates. Not much has changed since then except the propaganda and promotional hype for quick fixes.

Ideal body weight simply means having as little excess fat stored as possible. This can be determined by measuring lean body mass by immersion techniques, but the classical insurance tables give a good ballpark estimate. Collecting the abdominal wall between the thumb and index finger also gives a good estimate, and these tools are with us at all times. A more recent method for calculating ideal weight is the Body Mass Index (BMI), arrived at by dividing the weight in kilograms by the square of the height in meters. (Weight in pounds x 0.455 = kilograms. Height in inches x 0.0254 = meters) Health risks and premature mortality increase as the index rises above 25.

Weight can be maintained close to the ideal by eating the essential nutrients and avoiding all of the surplus foods that we can live without (I never said it would be easy). Throw in the exercise that you have to get to keep your motor tuned up and half the battle is won. This effort needs to be ingrained as a daily habit. The classical Framingham studies suggested, among other findings, that fluctuations in body weight led to a shorter life span and an increased risk of coronary heart disease. It is neither necessary nor desirable to be compulsive about weight. Some variation produces no harm, but wide swings in weight should be avoided. That is the pattern that many people settle into, unfortunately.

SLEEP

Requirements for sleep vary some from one individual to another, but generally fall in the range of seven to eight hours nightly, with the majority of people requiring the latter. Individuals who require nine hours or more to feel rested most likely have a deficiency of thyroid function. In mild cases this is difficult to measure by current laboratory methods. Sleep deprivation results in impaired thought and reasoning, aggravation of depression and other psychiatric disorders, and impaired motor skills that may adversely affect driving and job performance, and thus lead to an increased incidence of accidents.

The process of sleep is not completely understood, but studies in recent years have revealed that it is divided into stages, and that body functions perform in a distinctive fashion during each stage. It has been observed that the first four stages of sleep are characterized by the absence of eye movement, and thus are classified as non rapid eye movement (NREM) sleep. The first of these four stages is a transitional stage, the second is a light sleep stage, the third and fourth stage are classified as delta sleep, the deepest and most restful stages of sleep. During this deep sleep stage the heart and breathing rate slow, the blood pressure is lowered and there is very little muscle activity. The level of metabolism drops as all body functions are lowered to a basal level. This is reflected in the lowering of the body temperature, and a decrease in thyroid function correlates with a decrease in the production of TSH (thyroid stimulating hormone). All of these changes are similar to the hibernation that takes place in some animal species, albeit for a much shorter period in the human sleep cycle.

The next stage of sleep is REM or rapid eye movement sleep, a period when bodily activity more closely approximates the awake state. This stage is characterized by rapid scanning movements of the eyes. REM sleep follows the four stages of NREM sleep, and it is during this period that dreaming takes place. It has been theorized that during this period the mind is processing the information and data encountered during the day, including experiences that involve conflict or that require resolution. Some studies have suggested that REM sleep is an integral part of the learning process, a process that has been demonstrated to be impaired following sleep deprivation. A technique of simulating this rapid eye movement has been used in the treatment of post traumatic stress disorders, most notable with servicemen from the Vietnam War, with some success in conflict resolution.

There are four or five cycles of these stages of sleep each night in a young person, NREM sleep accounting for about 80 percent of the total sleep. Each stage is important and although deep sleep is the most restful it is essential that adequate REM sleep occur also. It seems that the deep, restful sleep is necessary for recovery and rejuvenation of the physical and physiological/-biochemical body functions, whereas the REM stage is necessary for the processing and ordering of data at the cerebral level. In order to restore all of these body functions to normal there must be a continuity of uninterrupted sleep.

Sleep is only one of several biologic activities that operate on a circadian cycle of 24 hours. The timing center or biologic clock for the sleep cycle is in the suprachiasmatic nuclei in the hypothalamus. It is set by light mediated through a nerve connection from the retina of the eye, and must be reset each day. It is disruption of this system that accounts for the symptoms associated with jet travel. This circadian pacemaker can be reset within a period of 2 to 3 days by properly timed exposure to light of sufficient intensity. The many other biologic clocks that maintain various bodily functions on a 24-hour cycle, such as metabolism, are not influenced by light in this manner.

Some of the more common problems that interfere with sleep are light, pain from any source, indigestion or other gastrointestinal problems such as gastroesophageal reflux, stress and anxiety, noise, alcohol abuse and menopausal symptoms. A cough from asthma or bronchitis is another common interference with sleep, although during deep sleep the cough reflex is suppressed. Hormone replacement therapy relieves the interference with sleep that frequently accompanies the menopause. Carrying a sleep mask when traveling provides protection when trapped in a hotel room that does not provide adequate protection from light. Similarly, earplugs should be in the travel kit for noisy motels, although these do not eliminate the vibration of sound that is transmitted through the bones of the skull. Taking a comfortable pillow from home provides additional protection from allergens such as feathers and dust mites that may be lurking in the communal pillows in motels.

Chronic neglect of sleep adversely affects us both physically and emotionally. Cerebral functions such as thinking, reasoning and planning are impaired, resulting in the inability to make decisions readily and react promptly. Exhaustion and diminished efficiency set in at an earlier point. The impaired ability to deal with stress and the diminished neuromuscular coordination that result from sleep deprivation have been clearly demonstrated among troops and pilots under combat conditions. Also documented is an increased activity of the gastrointestinal tract, as is seen with stress in general. This is manifested by an increase in the frequency of stools, a stool of smaller caliber and perhaps a watery stool. Bloating and an increase in the amount of intestinal gas may be noticed along with this. It also may be accompanied by pain and cramping in the abdomen, or pain in the lower back. A stomach or duodenal ulcer may develop after protracted periods of stress. Recent studies have also shown that the immune system is depressed following sleep deprivation, increasing the susceptibility to infections.

An individual can ascertain his own sleep needs by simple observation. If a person feels tired and worn out throughout most of the day, and very sleepy in the early afternoon, it is likely that inadequate sleep has been experienced. This assessment should be made over a period of several days, for anyone can have a restless night, especially if severe thunderstorms pass through or a barking dog serenades all night long. As stated above, most people will require about eight hours each night in order to function efficiently.

Sleep disorders in the elderly has been a topic for discussion and investigation for many years. In the past it was felt by some that older people required less sleep. This belief evolved from the observation that people in their fifties and sixties and beyond have more difficulty sleeping, spend less time in deep, slow wave sleep, and are more readily awakened by sounds that previously would not have interfered with their sleep. The fact is that those older people who experience inadequate sleep suffer the typical symptoms of sleep deprivation.

It was demonstrated in 1988[36] that the amount of melatonin produced at night decreases with aging. Recent studies have shown that those older people who suffer from inadequate sleep clearly demonstrate a reduced level of melatonin production. Melatonin is a hormone that is synthesized in the pineal gland from the essential amino acid tryptophan and secreted at night. It is interrelated with the quality of sleep, and the various stages of sleep. Melatonin production is turned off by exposure to light, so it is important to maintain a dark environment for sleep.

Experiments have been conducted that demonstrate that supplementation of controlled-release melatonin improves the sleep patterns in those individuals with sleep disturbances. Some studies suggested that controlled (sustained) release products or repetitive dosing is necessary because one-half of the melatonin in the blood is excreted in less than an hour. Others have found that a single bedtime dose yielded improved sleep patterns. These beneficial results were observed even where the sleep pattern had been altered by drugs such as beta-blockers and sleeping medication. The role of melatonin in sleep disorders that result from daytime napping, a common problem, is yet to be determined. The best solution to this problem is to take a walk in the afternoon rather than napping.

While all of the studies conducted to date have concentrated on the administration of exogenous melatonin, no one has attempted to determine if the basic underlying problem in some individuals is in reality a dietary deficiency of tryptophan, the basic material from which the melatonin is produced. Eating habits of elderly people are notoriously poor, and their diets are especially deficient in meat. It is possible that the inclusion of adequate high biologic value protein might resolve the melatonin deficiency in some of these people. The studies of melatonin production may also help to explain the success that tryptophan supplements had with sleep disorders, before they were removed from the market after the outbreak of the eosinophilia-myalgia syndrome discussed above and in Chapter XIII. Tryptophan supplementation might provide the raw material from which the pineal gland can synthesize an adequate level of melatonin.

ALLERGIES

An allergy is an exaggerated response of the body's immune mechanisms to a foreign protein, such as pollens. It occurs only after the body has been sensitized by a previous exposure to that protein. It may occur after the second encounter with the foreign protein, or it may not occur for many years. The most common allergies are those affecting the respiratory tract; the nose, sinuses, bronchi and lung. Asthma, of course, is the extreme form of these allergies. The eyes (conjunctiva) are commonly affected at the same time. The incidence of allergies in the general population seems to have increased significantly in recent years.

There are many agents in our environment that can precipitate allergic reactions. Many different weeds, trees and grasses contain protein substances (pollens) that can sensitize people. These reactions can be very uncomfortable and annoying, but at least they are seasonal. Similar substances in the home plague us throughout the year. Various types of agents can cause symptoms in the home, but most have in common the feature of being airborne. This suggests the measures that can be taken to minimize the exposure.

Dust in the home (see Chapter VI) should be kept to a minimum. Carpets and drapes collect dust, and these need to be cleaned frequently. For people who have serious problems with allergies carpeting should be eliminated wherever possible, especially in the bedroom. Draperies should be made of material that can be laundered frequently. The bedroom should be kept as free of offending agents as possible. Pets should not be kept in the home at all, but certainly not in the bedroom. Pets, particularly cats, are one of the most common offending agents for people with allergies. This is especially true of asthma.

Mattresses, box springs and pillows should all be encased in a sealed impervious cover. Bed covers should be selected for easy laundering and freedom from lint. Frequent laundering of bedclothes in hot water with adequate detergent helps to keep the dust mite population down. A high efficiency (HEPA) filter of adequate size placed in the bedroom helps reduce the dust level. These filters can reduce the circulating dust particles by as much as 70 percent. Lint on clothing (especially flannel shirts) and bedding, as well as toilet tissues all contribute to household dust. Lint free tissues have been available in the scientific world for years, but these have not been made available to the general public, as they should be.

All of the above presupposes that the house in general is kept as free of dust and offending agents as is possible. Measures to accomplish this are discussed in Chapter VI. The only vacuum cleaner in the house should be a central unit exhausted to the outside. Conventional vacuum cleaners do collect most of the dirt and dust in the home, but they also re-disperse much of it in the air. The filters on household vacuum cleaners permit the passage of a significant quantity of particulate material back into the room air. Industrial vacuum cleaners with HEPA filters are available, but at greater cost. The Japanese custom of removing shoes when entering the house may seem bothersome, but it makes good sense from a cleanliness and hygienic standpoint. It is a lot more difficult and time consuming to attempt to remove the dirt after it is tracked in.

The table below lists some of the substances in the home that evoke or aggravate respiratory allergies.

AGENTS IN THE HOME THAT INDUCE ALLERGIC REACTIONS

Cat dander	Dust mites, cockroaches
Cigarette smoke	Fireplaces, wood burning
Cleaning fluids, other chemicals	Fungi, various
Cosmetics, perfumes	Oven fumes
Dog dander	Pesticides
Dried flower arrangements	Plants, house
Dust (lint from clothing, bedding, carpets, tissues)	Potpourri

HYGIENE

Cleanliness and personal hygiene are equally as important as nutrition in maintaining good health. Adequate nutrition provides the raw materials that the body needs in order to manufacture the various elements in the immune system and the other defense mechanisms. Cleanliness and good hygiene lessen the demands on these defense mechanisms by reducing the number of microbial agents that gain entrance to the body. In many instances these measures prevent serious disease-causing organisms from gaining entrance to the body altogether. This frequently makes the difference between health and disease, particularly in the case of organisms that the body is less able to ward off.

In the case of viral hepatitis, for instance, careful hand washing after handling soiled diapers may protect a person from contracting this disease from an infected baby. It will also help to avoid spreading it to other members of the family. A review of foodborne diseases in Chapter V will reinforce the importance of hand washing in the prevention of illness.

Hand washing mechanically removes disease-causing microbial agents from the hands. This is an particularly important practice to cultivate if your business practices lead you to shake hands with others. This custom, which is deeply imbedded in Western culture, is an archaic and unwise practice. As the number of and the resistance of emerging (and perhaps cultivated) microorganisms grows, hand contact with others becomes ever more risky. Using a hand soap that contains an effective germicide such as triclocarban (Dial®, Safeguard®) enhances the removal of bacteria and fungi. Liquid soaps contain triclosan rather than triclocarban. Some people develop sun sensitivity when using these products, so this must be watched for. Use of Betadine skin cleanser (used by physicians in surgery, available in pharmacies) when handling fecal or infectious, contaminated material is even more effective, and should be used in cases of hepatitis. The use of a germicidal soap is very useful after changing diapers, as mentioned above. Disposable gloves should always be used for this procedure. Some disease-causing bacteria have been found to survive on bar soap, even on those containing a germicide. Bar soaps should not be shared with members of the family who have communicable illnesses. Public rest rooms should be equipped with liquid soap dispensers, never bar soap.

The hands can never be rendered sterile (that is why we wear gloves in surgery), but contaminating microorganisms that present a threat of disease can be removed by washing well with Betadine®. Studies have demonstrated that pathogenic bacteria, viruses and eggs of parasites are harbored in the dirt under fingernails. Keeping nails closely trimmed and scrubbing with a nailbrush will help to minimize this risk. This is especially important after changing diapers or caring for people who are ill with communicable diseases. The latter would include conjunctivitis and other infections that are transmissible from one person to another. An investigation of the cholera epidemic in Trujillo, Peru in 1991 revealed that the water in the storage containers in homes became contaminated rapidly with fecal organisms from hands, and became progressively more so with the passage of time. The disease was being spread in the homes.[37]

Washing the hands before eating is a mandate that dates back to biblical times, but it seems to have been forgotten in our reliance on miracle drugs. The limitations of these drugs are periodically demonstrated to us in dramatic fashion, and should serve to remind us that "an ounce of prevention is worth a pound of cure." When Moses was leading his people through the wilderness, he had no antibiotics. The rules for hygiene and a clean campsite that he mandated were vital to survival. These are clearly delineated in Deuteronomy where it was mandated that a place outside the campsite was to be designated for the deposition of human excrement. A paddle that was carried with the weapon was to be used to dig a hole for such deposition, and the excrement was to be covered afterwards (23:12-13).

Moses wrote all of the very detailed rules of sanitation as well as the laws governing social, civil and criminal behavior into a book just before he died. He delivered these laws to the Levites as the *Lord's statutes and His commandments,* and commanded that they be placed at the side of the Ark of the Covenant. Every seven years, when all of the people of Israel were gathered, they were to be read as a reinforcement to all (Deut. 31:10). The people were further commanded to build a stone wall after they crossed over the Jordan into Canaan, and to write these laws on that stone wall. The significance of these statutes resides in their essential role in the survival of that, and indeed any society, and to avoid chaos and anarchy. With this task completed, Moses could *lie with his ancestors.*

With all of our modern medicines, equipment, systems and knowledge, we are much more fortunate. Our modern sanitary systems and public water supplies provide us with protection against disease with no effort on our part, other than paying our taxes to support them. The arrogance and ignorance that has prompted the current level of complacency in cleanliness is ill advised, however. Many individuals in our society die as a result of infections each year in spite of the best efforts of medicine and miracle drugs. We tend to dwell upon our strengths and to ignore our weaknesses. Periodically, as with the ancient Hebrews, we are sent a message of remembrance, and occasionally it is a forceful one.

Hand washing and personal hygiene were considered a basic part of the curriculum in elementary school when I was growing up. I was given a firm indoctrination at home by a mother who had received a limited formal education. The commandments of Moses were apparently passed to her through the generations by her family. This was in evidence in both of my parents, in their teachings not only of personal hygiene, but also of the rules of social and economic responsibilities. This is another of the basic responsibilities of parents that has been abdicated by many in our society. These skills and these values should be taught to children virtually from birth, but we are much more diligent about potty-training and shoe tying.

There is also a widespread conviction in our society today that these responsibilities lie elsewhere, with the public schools for instance. This abdication of parental responsibility has been reinforced by some bureaucrats, and encouraged by even some school officials in their lust for more power. Some school officials firmly believe that they know best what and when our children should be taught about sex and sociology.

It is especially distressing to observe the common practice of food handlers in restaurants returning to their posts after a trip to the rest room without washing their hands. Many cases of diarrhea and other food-borne diseases are suffered by people each year because of this irresponsible behavior. More than 3 million people each year suffer from rotavirus diarrhea alone. Some 65,000 children are hospitalized with this infection. Hundreds of thousands of cases of infection of the gastrointestinal tract occur each year that could be avoided by simple attention to hygiene. Take note on your next trip to a public rest room of how many people walk out without washing their hands. Take particular note of your waiter/ waitress. Infections acquired from food as a result of careless hygiene are discussed in more detail in Chapter V.

DISEASES OF HUMANS TRANSMITTED BY THE FECAL-ORAL ROUTE[§]

Ascariasis (intestinal roundworm)	Enterotoxigenic E. coli
Amoeba (dysentery)	Enteroviruses (several strains)
Cholera	Giardia (intestinal parasite, diarrhea)
Clostridium (diarrhea, enteritis)	Hepatitis A and E
Coxsackie virus (enteritis)	Norwalk virus (epidemic diarrhea, also Snow Mountain, Marin County viruses)

Cryptosporidiosis (intestinal parasite)	Rotavirus (gastroenteritis)
Cysticercosis (Taenia solium, pork tapeworm)	Salmonella (foodborne infection other than typhoid)
Echovirus (enteritis)	Shigella (foodborne infection)
Enterobius vermicularis (pinworm)	Typhoid fever

§ Transmitted by the transference of fecal material to the mouth of one's self or to others, usually by hand contamination of food, vegetables or water. Some may also be transmitted on dust particles. In some foodborne infections such as staphylococcus the organism is transmitted directly from the hands and does not require fecal contamination.

Sanitary systems designed for the collection and processing of human waste were developed for the purpose of preventing the spread of disease. Although we tend to think of these systems only in terms of their aesthetic value, the necessity of isolating human waste from any food or water supply in order to prevent disease was well understood by civilizations in the past. Moses established laws to accomplish this and protect his people in their nomadic life, as described above. Most civilizations since that time have had similar codes and regulations.

Modern sewage processing facilities have the added advantage that they destroy many of the pathogenic organisms as well as isolating them from our food and water supplies. The blessings of these systems are better appreciated when one looks at the rates of disease transmission in countries where they are lacking. This has been tragically demonstrated during the recent Cholera epidemic in South and Central America and Mexico. Over 600,000 people have acquired this serious disease in the first cholera epidemic in this region in the 20th century.

Peru and many other countries throughout the world use raw wastewater for crop irrigation. This is especially true in areas where water is scarce. This practice readily spreads diseases such as cholera and hepatitis by contamination of vegetables, especially cabbage and other leafy crops. Even where crude efforts are made to "treat" the sewage effluent in lagoons, it has been shown that the cholera organism is not suppressed, and in fact it may multiply in these lagoons. With the recent emergence of cryptosporidium outbreaks from water supplies and swimming pools, this disease also can be expected to be spread by such recycling of sewage.

The widespread outbreak in the U.S. in 1996 of *Cyclospora* infections from raspberries imported from Guatemala (see Chapter V) is an example of another disease that is spread by contamination of crops with sewage water. Hepatitis A long has been endemic in China at least in part because of the practice of using human excrement for fertilizer on food crops. In March 1997 hundreds of people in six states in the U. S. were exposed to Hepatitis A through the consumption of strawberries that had been imported from Mexico. At least 153 cases of active hepatitis A were reported in Michigan alone.[38]

Sharing of towels and washcloths is another violation of basic hygiene that frequently leads to the sharing of illnesses. This is especially risky when one member of the family has an overt infection, such as conjunctivitis (pinkeye). This bacterial infection is readily transmitted from one person to another. Other infections that may be transmitted in this manner may be less obvious, but may be even more health threatening. Of particular importance is viral hepatitis, which is much more prevalent today than it was twenty years ago. There is a serious risk of spreading hepatitis A through the communal sharing of towels and washcloths.

The Mosaic laws, as delineated in the first five books of the bible and the Pentateuch or Torah, isolated all people with obvious infections from the remainder of the community, generally for a period of seven days. The practice of incinerating the clothing and other contaminated objects, the scraping of the walls of houses, or destroying the house by fire are also documented. These are among the first recorded descriptions of terminal disinfection (Lev. 13-15).

In 1986 in a case reported to the Centers for Disease Control a three–year–old boy was diagnosed as having hepatitis B. This disease is unusual in children under the age of fourteen years. Investigation by health authorities revealed evidence of hepatitis B infection in ten other family members. Nine family members shared four toothbrushes, and this appeared to be the means of transmission of the disease. The role that the sharing of towels and washcloths played in this episode cannot be separated from that of the toothbrushes. Sharing of razors and other toilet articles carries the same risk of transmission of disease, the most serious of which would be hepatitis A, B, and C, as well as AIDS. Many barbers have discontinued the practice of using a razor during haircuts, and you should make certain that your barber has. Public health laws should ban the practice everywhere.

One of the most basic goals of personal hygiene is the prevention of the transmission of disease-causing organisms from one person to another. It is not necessary for the donor to be ill in order to transmit a disease. Many people are carriers of streptococci and other pathogenic organisms with no apparent sickness. Frequently people who have recovered from an acute bout with giardia, or a host of other pathogenic organisms, continue to shed organisms capable of causing disease in other people.

Sixty years ago it was common practice to hang a communal tin cup on the pump at the well to be used by all. Even today a communal water jug in the refrigerator is shared in some families. These practices could have been excused before the germ theory of disease was advanced in 1855, but their continuation today can be attributed only to ignorance of the very basics of the cause and transmission of disease. Enlightenment is the solution.

In some investigations, repeated tonsil and other mouth infections have been traced to contaminated toothbrushes. This can be prevented by soaking the toothbrush in a solution of household chlorine bleach for thirty minutes. One tablespoonful of bleach in a glass of water is sufficient for most bacterial pathogens such as streptococci. Twice that amount of bleach is needed for resistant spores of other organisms. This should be done at least on a weekly basis to control these infections. Some studies have suggested that a much higher concentration would be required to inactivate the AIDS virus, perhaps two ounces (four tablespoonsful) in an 8-10 ounce glass of water. While the Human Immunodeficiency Virus is inactivated in the laboratory by both fresh chlorine bleach (1:10) and rubbing alcohol, they are much less effective in practice where organic material such as blood is present.

The household bleach must be fresh, since it is not stable and loses strength over a period of time. This means that if your jug has been sitting around for a while, it should be tossed and replaced with a fresh one. You also should make your purchases at a store where there is a high enough rate of turnover to assure freshness.

In addition to regular brushing and flossing to remove impacted food particles, the WaterPik® is invaluable, especially for those who have full crowns, loosening of the gums or inflammation of the gums. Even after the most careful brushing and flossing this device will remove demonstrable food particles.

Dentures should be scrubbed daily to remove adhered debris and microbial growth. They then should be soaked in a solution of household bleach, one tablespoonful in eight ounces of water for thirty to sixty minutes. This will control the yeast and bacterial organisms that tend to grow on these appliances (see above remarks for AIDS virus). This practice is especially important for diabetics and for everyone after eating foods containing sugar. Dentures give the appearance of being impervious. In reality microorganisms readily set up shop on their surfaces and in the many crevices that are present.

Frequent (and adequate) laundering of towels, washcloths, bed linen, clothing and even pillows also serves to reduce the risk of and frequency of infections and illness in general. This may be required after one usage if soilage occurs. Pillows are a particular problem, but those constructed of synthetic materials can be laundered. It is inevitable that pillows will accumulate dust mites, and possibly other pathogenic microorganisms. This fact as well as allergies to feathers makes it wise to carry your own pillow for visits to hotels. It should be kept in mind that, as with the washing of hands, laundering becomes much more urgent after soilage by fecal material or by secretions from an obviously infected source, such as a family member with hepatitis. In order to accomplish the destruction of disease-causing microbes, hot water and an effective laundry detergent, in adequate concentration, are needed.

Badly soiled loads will need a larger measure of detergents than the same quantity of clothing that is less heavily soiled. Skimping on detergent defeats the purpose of laundering. Hot water is also essential to destroy microorganisms, parasites and dust mites. The trend in recent years to lower the temperature in the water heater in order to conserve energy seriously compromises the effectiveness of laundering in preventing disease. The minimal cost savings are not worth the resultant risk.

In dealing with clothes or bedding that have been contaminated by materials with the potential for causing disease, household bleach is very effective in killing most bacterial and fungal organisms. The organic matter, such as blood and feces must be removed by laundering first to assure effectiveness. Clothing and bed linen that are soiled by blood or feces by a family member who is suffering from a communicable disease such as hepatitis should be laundered with adequate detergent and hot water to remove this soilage. They then should be run through another wash cycle with detergent, hot water and bleach, whenever the fabric will tolerate the latter.

Chlorine bleach and most antimicrobial agents will not work in the presence of organic material such as blood and feces. Products based upon phenols or liquor cresolis compound USP (a mixture of cresols in a linseed oil soap) in a 5 percent solution (see table below) are effective in destroying virtually all microbial agents even in fecal contaminated materials. Diapers that have been contaminated by a patient who has hepatitis may be soaked in this solution for sixty minutes prior to laundering in order to inactivate the virus. Disposable surgical gloves should be worn when handling any contaminated diapers or bed linen. Contamination underneath fingernails is very difficult to remove, and gloves help to prevent the collection of infectious material there.

An ortho-phenylphenol compound has been readily available in every grocery store and pharmacy as Lysol® since the early 1900s. Tragically in 1996 the company that markets Lysol changed the formulation to a quaternary ammonium compound, even though the labelling remains virtually identical, with the same claims of efficacy. This action was taken reportedly under intimidation from the U. S. Environmental Protection Agency (personal communication with company representative). Thus the consumer is unknowingly purchasing a product that is, as a cationic detergent, weakly effective against bacteria, but ineffective against viruses. In the face of the spreading epidemic of AIDS, hepatitis and tuberculosis, at the very time that we desperately need this one effective germicide it has been taken from us. Such arrogance and abuse is being seen more and more frequently by those public officials who have assumed power never granted by the Constitution. Their elimination of safe, effective agents in the field of public health and in controlling disease transmitting insects is foolish and irresponsible.

Phenol (carbolic acid) has been considered the most effective germicide since Lord Joseph Lister's research on surgical infections in 1865-1867.[39] Lister, a surgeon, and the first medical person to be named to the House of Lords, demonstrated that the infections that universally complicated surgery in those days could be prevented by the use of a carbolic acid spray to destroy bacteria that were contaminating wounds. This practice revolutionized surgery and became the standard of care. Phenol subsequently became the standard against which all antibacterial agents were measured (the phenol coefficient).

The cresols, which are chemical relatives of phenol, are five times more potent than phenol as germicides. Lysol®, in the original ortho-phenylphenol formulation, was also more powerful than plain phenol. Organic matter does not interfere with the germicidal properties of these agents; thus they are very useful in the presence of blood, pus, sputum and feces.[40] They are invaluable in caring for patients who have serious illnesses such as hepatitis, tuberculosis and HIV infections. There is no comparable substitute for them, certainly not what is now sold as Lysol®. There also is no rational reason to remove them from the market. Part of the tragedy is that most people will continue to purchase the product that they have had confidence in but they will not have the protection that was previosly provided. This is arrogance and ignorance at its worse.

Some of the agents that are effective for disinfecting various objects are listed in a table at the end of this chapter.

In no area of the house is cleanliness more urgent than in the kitchen. Frequent hand washing is a must with food handling. It should be done as often as is needed, after handling anything that might be contaminated with *Salmonella* or other disease causing organisms, such as eggs or poultry (see Chapter V). The household cook should wash her hands immediately after handling poultry or any raw meat, and wash the faucet handles. This may seem obsessive until you have suffered through an acute *Salmonella* diarrhea.

Keeping all counter tops, handles (refrigerator, stove, microwave) and tables clean and free of food residues is also essential in the prevention of illness. Bacteria multiply rapidly in these residues, particularly at room temperature. (Whether or not an individual succumbs to a bacterial diarrhea frequently depends upon the number of organisms ingested.) We are fortunate in that the hand and dishwashing detergents (and detergents in general) that we have available to us today are very effective in destroying disease causing organisms. They are much more effective surface-active agents than the soaps that were formerly available, and thus are more effective in disrupting the bacterial capsules. This renders the organisms incapable of reproducing and causing disease.

Proper refrigeration of food (see Chapter V) cannot be stressed too strongly. Those who had the dubious privilege of living with iceboxes and winter window storage boxes should have a deep appreciation for the modern refrigerator and freezer that most people take for granted. Food cannot be left sitting at room temperature after it has been prepared or after a meal without risking illness. Some bacteria multiply rapidly at room temperature, increasing the risk of foodborne illness. Other bacteria produce potent toxins at room temperature, causing serious and very unpleasant illness.

Adequate cold temperatures diminish these bacterial activities. Additionally, rapid cooling of some disease-causing bacteria can destroy up to 90 percent of the organisms. Effective refrigeration requires a maximum temperature of 38 to 40 degrees Fahrenheit. Freezers should be kept at a temperature of zero degrees Fahrenheit or below. For most refrigerators that are manufactured for home use, this will require a setting in the upper three-fourths of the dial. If liquids such as milk tend to freeze or form ice crystals, the temperature will have to be raised slightly. Every refrigerator should have an accurate thermometer in it to monitor the temperature. Manufacturers frequently installed these in the past.

One of the most effective means of spreading disease is by coughing or sneezing. The photograph of a sneeze that has been published in books for many years is a dramatic demonstration of this potential. The disease containing droplets are disseminated over a wide area, to be deposited into the innermost reaches of the lungs of anyone breathing the contaminated air. The most notorious disease spread in this fashion is tuberculosis, but it is not alone. Many bacterial and viral infections can be spread from person to person in this manner. It is suspected that the HIV virus may also be spread in this manner. Although no studies have been undertaken to specifically prove such transmission, it is a reasonable hypothesis.

Older people, people with chronic illnesses and people with suppressed immune systems are particularly vulnerable to infections from airborne infectious agents. Covering the mouth and nose with a tissue to prevent this air borne dissemination is another common sense practice that seems to have fallen by the wayside. Many of the cases of colds, influenza and bronchitis that are suffered each year result from this carelessness.

It seems that virtually every household in the United States incorporates pets as members of the family. As affluence has grown, so too has the number of pets in the home. Thirty percent of families currently have cats, 38 percent have dogs. In my neighborhood, I believe that the percentage is closer to 98. Any pet kept indoors introduces health hazards, and these are discussed in Chapter VII. Pets in the home add considerably to the needs for cleanliness and attention to hygiene. Monitoring the hygienic practices of children is a full time job at best, but it becomes much more urgent and demanding when pets are present. Cleaning and vacuuming must be done more frequently and both dogs and cats must be bathed weekly. Diseases ranging from parasitic infestations to meningitis from the pet licking the child in the face (see Chapter III) have increased in incidence with the growth in the pet population.

Pimples, or more accurately furuncles or folliculitis, are red, hard, tender nodules that progress to a pus "point" if not arrested. They are infections that are most commonly caused by a staphylococcus strain that is acquired from another individual. The buttocks and the back of the neck are the most common sites for these to occur. Toilet seats are an obvious source of the former, and the latter can occur after a visit to a barbershop where the instruments and linens have not been adequately sterilized. Sharing of clothing can also be a source for infection. Other sources include bed clothing, tubs and contaminated ointments and cosmetics.

When furuncles occur repeatedly, especially at other sites of the body, diabetes and/or a chronic infection in the teeth or tonsils should be suspected. If furuncles are detected when they first appear they can usually be aborted by the prompt application of tincture of iodine (USP 2%) with a cotton applicator, repeating after six hours. For those who are sensitive to iodine, plain rubbing alcohol (70%) applied by holding a saturated cotton ball on the furuncle for about a minute, repeating three times daily until resolution is noted, is usually successful. When the infection has progressed to an advanced stage, or where multiple furuncles have developed, a systemic antibiotic may be necessary. In view of the widespread cultivation of strains of staphylococcus that are resistant to antibiotics, this will require sensitivity testing and careful selection of a suitable agent. Cleansing of public toilet seats with a cleansing pad prior to use is an appropriate prophylactic measure.

HEPATITIS

Viral hepatitis is an acute infection of the liver, produced by one of several viruses, five of which have been identified and classified. Hepatitis A is spread from human to human almost exclusively through the fecal–oral route. This means that fecal material of an infected individual reaches the mouth of another individual in some fashion. This most commonly occurs when an individual with the disease makes a trip to the bathroom, then returns without washing his hands. The contaminated hands then transmit the virus to food, ice or eating utensils, or to any substance or object that may find its way to the mouth of a non-infected individual. When the infected individual is a food handler (cook, waiter/waitress) in a restaurant they are provided the opportunity to share this disease with many other persons.

While it is hard to believe that anyone involved in the processing and serving of food to others would be so sloven and careless in personal hygiene, such behavior has become very common, unfortunately. Obviously virtually all such transmission of Hepatitis A by this means could be avoided by the simple measure of adequate hand washing with soap and warm water. Hepatitis A accounts for about 30 percent of all hepatitis cases in the United States.

Hepatitis A has a delayed onset, usually 14 to 50 days from the time that the virus is contracted. Symptoms usually include fever, loss of appetite, nausea, abdominal discomfort and jaundice. The disease typically lasts about six weeks, although the acute symptoms subside much before that. It can be prevented in those who are exposed to an individual with the disease by the administration of gamma globulin within two weeks after exposure. This is of no benefit, however, if administration is delayed. In the past gamma globulin has been given as a prophylactic measure to those traveling to areas where hepatitis A is endemic, to prevent infection.

Three types of vaccine have been under development, one of which has been in use in Switzerland. In 1995 an inactivated viral vaccine became available in the United States, and in 1996 a second similar vaccine was licensed. These vaccines provide a more certain and sustained protection and have replaced gamma globulin in those traveling to areas of risk. Although a booster dose is recommended 6 to 12 months after the initial dose, the level of protection following the first dose surpasses that of gamma globulin. Natural infection normally confers a life-long immunity, but the ultimate duration of the protection provided by these vaccines has not been determined as yet. Neither vaccine can be administered to children under two years of age.

About 24,000 cases of hepatitis A are reported to the Centers for Disease Control each year. Many cases are not reported and some estimates place the true number at 100,000 annually, with about 100 deaths. Every case is preventable. If all sewage were properly treated and if everyone practiced good personal hygiene such as careful hand washing, we would not have this large number of cases. Hepatitis A is commonly spread to others within households and in institutions such as nursing homes when a case is present. It is most commonly spread by contamination of food, or by sharing towels or toilet articles in these circumstances.

Hepatitis A is also spread by contamination of water, milk and shellfish. All of the shellfish that is harvested from the coastal waters in the regions near the larger cities, especially along the eastern seaboard, the Gulf of Mexico and in Mexico, must be suspected of being contaminated. This contamination has come about as a result of the widespread practice of dumping untreated sewage into the coastal waters of our continent. Only the waters along the northern New England coast, and other sparsely populated areas, where such dumping does not occur, are free of this hazard.

Although exposure to blood clotting factor products has been linked to hepatitis A infections in Europe, such transmission had not been observed in the United States until 1996. At least four cases of hepatitis A among hemophiliacs resulted from treatment with clotting factor that had been treated with the solvent-detergent method of viral inactivation. This method is considered effective for lipid enveloped viruses such as hepatitis B and C, and for HIV, but it is not effective for non-enveloped viruses such as hepatitis A. Similar outbreaks of hepatitis A from blood products occurred in Europe during the previous four years, and several manufacturers there had added a sterilization process of high temperature terminal dry heat (HTTDH). This process, utilizing temperatures of 80-100°C, not only inactivates the hepatitis A virus, but most other infectious agents as well. It should be used routinely in the manufacture of factor VIII.[41,42]

The existence of Hepatitis A in our society at present levels is a national disgrace. It is a graphic demonstration of the deterioration in our public health and personal hygiene practices. Many cases of hepatitis A occur each year in the United States as a result of eating improperly cooked oysters and clams from sewage contaminated regions. Although recovery without serious sequelae is the rule in most healthy people, this is a significant illness that restricts activity for about six weeks. There is no antibiotic or other direct remedy for it. There is no carrier state for hepatitis A and there is little apparent residual damage to the liver in most cases. Nevertheless, it is prudent to avoid any infection in the liver, or any other vital organ of the body, to the greatest extent possible.

Hepatitis B used to be a relatively uncommon disease in the United States, but it has reached epidemic proportions recently among select populations. It increased by about 37 percent from 1979 to 1989, with between 200,000 and 300,000 new cases each year. The number of cases reported has since diminished to about 10,000 yearly. The sharing of needles by IV drug users, the sexual revolution and the AIDS epidemic all played a part in this development. About 50 percent of all cases of hepatitis reported in the U.S. are hepatitis B.

Hepatitis B is a more serious disease in that it has a far more severe impact upon the liver. A significant percentage of individuals suffer a chronic stage that can result in death. Some people suffer a particularly severe case of acute hepatitis B that results in death in a matter of a few months after the initial infection. A pathogen that has been labeled the Delta agent causes some of these cases. It has been identified as an incomplete or defective virus that can replicate only in the presence of the hepatitis B virus. This hepatitis D virus utilizes and is dependent upon the envelope of the hepatitis B virus. It occurs either as a co-infection with or as a superinfection of established hepatitis B. This is a much more serious disease, with a higher incidence of death. As with hepatitis B the Delta agent is spread primarily by needles, and is limited to individuals who are exposed to blood and blood products. It has thus become very common among IV drug abusers. Many hemophiliacs have been infected with it through contaminated factor VIII.

There is a carrier state with hepatitis B, and these individuals can transmit the disease to others throughout their lifetime. Ninety-five percent of newborns who are infected become chronic carriers because of the immaturity of their immune systems.[43] By contrast thirty percent of children who are infected between the ages of one year and six years remain carriers. Cancer of the liver is another complication of chronic hepatitis B infection. About 90 percent of the people infected with hepatitis B recover. The course is more prolonged and more severe in the elderly however, and in those with underlying disease such as diabetes, anemia and heart disease.

Currently, the most common method of transmission of hepatitis B is through contaminated needles. Since the advent of disposable needles over twenty years ago, such transmission does not occur through legitimate needle use, except for accidental needle sticks to doctors and nurses. Body piercing and tattooing carries a risk of transmission of hepatitis B and C, as well as other blood borne diseases. The explosive growth of drug abuse as a recreation in our society, and the concomitant sharing of contaminated needles, accounts for the great majority of cases today. At least one-half of individuals using anabolic steroids do so by injection. The sharing of needles during steroid use is common, as is the case with other forms of drug abuse. This presents a risk of acquiring hepatitis B and C and the human immunodeficiency virus (AIDS) as well. This risk has not been recognized until recently. In some studies seven-percent or more of high school males had used anabolic steroids. (See Chapter XII for a discussion of drug abuse). With the passage of time the true risk and implications of this practice will become more apparent.

The other primary method by which hepatitis B is spread is through sexual transmission. Unlike hepatitis A, hepatitis B is not spread through the feces because of the nature of its lipid envelope. The semen and saliva are infectious, however, and sexual contact with people who either have active disease or who are carriers presents a very real risk of contracting the disease. Similarly, sharing a razor, toothbrush or eating utensils with an infectious individual can result in the transmission of Hepatitis B.

Hepatitis B is also spread from the mother to the infant through the placenta. Most infants born to mothers who have active disease or who are chronic carriers will acquire the disease. Ninety percent of these infants will become carriers of the virus and about 25 percent of these will die in adulthood of cirrhosis or cancer of the liver. All infants who are born to mothers who test positive for the hepatitis B virus should receive both immune globulin and hepatitis B vaccine immediately after birth to prevent these tragic sequelae.

The first vaccine that was developed for hepatitis B was derived from whole blood, which evoked concern in many people. It was fully safe for adults, however, and effective. It provided protection for many people for several years. More recently a bio-engineered recombinant vaccine has been developed that has no association with blood. This is produced by cloning part of the virus gene into yeast cells, which in turn produce the antigen for the vaccine. This product is equally as effective and is more acceptable to those worried about AIDS transmission. The vaccine derived from blood is no longer marketed in the United States. Those individuals who are at risk for hepatitis B should receive vaccine protection. This includes all health care workers as well as those who come into contact with blood and blood products. Others who are at risk should make their decision in consultation with their family physician.

Although lifetime immunity customarily follows infection with hepatitis B, the antibody level produced by the administration of hepatitis B vaccine begins to wane in some individuals after about 5 to 7 years. About one-half of those who demonstrate an antibody response after receiving the vaccine will have no detectable antibodies 12 years later. The CDC believes that this antibody level would be boosted again if the body were challenged with an infection, and thus currently does not recommend either periodic testing of antibody level or subsequent booster doses. They acknowledge that the need for booster doses will need to be re-assessed as more data is collected.[44] For those who are at risk of hepatitis B it would be prudent to obtain a serum antibody level five years after receiving the vaccine, and if the titre has fallen below 10, to receive a booster injection. If the titre has not fallen, it should be monitored at two-year intervals thereafter. This is especially important in health care workers and those who are exposed to blood. With the passage of time, and the collection of additional data, it may indeed be safe to conclude that a program of monitoring and booster doses is not needed. Unfortunately all of the vaccines for both hepatitis A and B are expensive. (See Chapter III for hepatitis B immunization of newborns)

People who are at a high risk of contracting hepatitis B include:

- Spouses, household and sexual contacts of individuals with acute hepatitis B or carriers of the disease
- Sexually promiscuous individuals
- Homosexual men
- Health care workers exposed to needles or blood products
- Individuals who receive transfusions
- Users of illicit injectable drugs
- Hemodialysis patients
- Infants born to mothers with positive hepatitis B test
- Hemophiliacs, through blood products (newer high purity products that eliminate this risk have been available since 1989 but have not been used universally).
- Residents and staff of institutions: prisons, nursing homes, mental institutions
- Staff of day care centers with an attendee who has hepatitis B or carrier status.

Hepatitis B is not transmitted through gamma globulin or through Rhogram (for Rh negative pregnant women). The processing of these products inactivates the virus. Unfortunately this has not been the case for whole blood and some of the blood products. Since 1989 higher purity factor VIII and IX products, agents that are essential to hemophiliacs, have been available. In spite of this, hepatitis A continued (through late 1995) to be transmitted to hemophiliacs because of the improper treatment of these blood products (see Chapter XI). The universal use of properly treated products would eliminate this risk of hepatitis for hemophiliacs.

Interferon alpha, which boosts the natural immunologic response of the body, has been shown to be an effective treatment in about 40 percent of adults with hepatitis B. It is most likely to clear the infection in those who have had the infection no longer than 5 to 10 years. It has a much lower success rate in those who acquire the infection at birth, and in those who have had the disease longer than 10 years. There are also serious side effects with this agent that necessitate reduction in dose or discontinuation in a significant percentage of patients.

Physicians have known for years that a small percentage of cases of hepatitis are caused by agents other than the viruses that cause types A and B. These cases had been classified as non-A, non-B hepatitis in the past. The Chiron Corporation finally identified the hepatitis C virus in 1987 through molecular biological techniques, and the genetic structure of the virus has since been mapped. It is an RNA virus that belongs to the same family of viruses that cause dengue fever and yellow fever, the flaviviruses. Other members of this family cause hog cholera and bovine diarrheal disease. It was determined that this virus has been responsible for about 80 percent of the cases of non-A, non-B hepatitis in the United States.

Hepatitis C is now known to be a common disease. It is the most common chronic bloodborne infection in the United States (it has accounted for 90 percent of the cases of hepatitis that developed after a blood transfusion in the past. Approximately 3 million people receive transfusions in the United States each year. Patients who undergo heart surgery have received as much as 42 units of blood during this procedure,[45] greatly increasing their risk of acquiring the diseases transmitted in blood. Since 1994 the risk from transfusion has been greatly reduced because of the development of screening tests. Prior to that about 170,000 people per year developed acute hepatitis C as a result of transfusions. Currently most cases are acquired through injecting drug abuse (sharing needles).

According to the Centers for Disease Control nearly 4 million Americans had hepatitis C as of October 1998, with about 30,000 new infections each year. In addition to being the most common chronic blood-borne infection in the United States hepatitis C is the most common cause of chronic viral hepatitis (and chronic active hepatitis). Chronic hepatitis develops in eighty percent and cirrhosis in twenty percent of those who acquire hepatitis C. Heavy alcohol consumption greatly increases the risk of developing cirrhosis. Six percent progress to liver failure, and four percent develop liver cancer. The mean interval between blood transfusion and the diagnosis of hepatocellular carcinoma is 29 years. About four percent of individuals who are infected with HCV will die as a result of the disease. In the next decade (2001-2010) deaths from this infection will triple.[46] Chronic liver disease caused by hepatitis C is the most frequent indication for liver transplants in the U.S. Even after liver transplant the hepatitis C virus infection recurs in the new liver in virtually every case because the virus remains in other tissues of the body. Hepatitis C causes an estimated 8,000 to 10,000 deaths each year.[47] Among the remaining unknown agents causing hepatitis, two new flaviviruses have been identified recently.[48]

Over 85 percent of patients with acute hepatitis C develop persistent infection. Chronic hepatitis, with characteristic histologic features, develops in 70 percent. The carrier rate is 10 times that of hepatitis B. Cirrhosis of the liver develops in about 20 percent of those with chronic hepatitis C. The risk of developing liver cancer is increased about 100 fold with both hepatitis C and hepatitis B. Hepatitis C is a much more serious form of hepatitis than hepatitis B.

The discovery of the hepatitis C virus was followed by the development of an antibody test. In May, 1990 this test was approved by the FDA to screen blood donors for hepatitis C. Prior to that there was no reliable means of detecting this virus either in donors or in donated blood. An improved second-generation test was approved in March 1992, and all hospitals and blood collection centers began using it. Individuals receiving transfusions of blood after that time should not have acquired hepatitis C by that route.

Even with this progress, in 1993 and 1994 an immunoglobulin product (Gammagard®) that did not include a specific viral inactivation step transmitted hepatitis C to 200 patients worldwide who had received it. The product was withdrawn from the market in February 1994.[49,50] In May 1994 a solvent-detergent treatment designed to inactivate contaminating viruses was instituted for Gammagard® and other intravenous immunoglobulin products. A more definitive confirmatory test for hepatitis C — RIBA (recombinant immunoblot assay) — is currently available, but it may not become positive in an individual suffering the disease until about twenty weeks after the onset. Several enzyme-linked immunoassay (ELISA) tests also became available by 1999. These tests detect the presence of antibodies (anti-HCV) to the virus in the serum. A newer polymerase chain reaction (PCR) test that actually identifies the virus itself in the blood is also currently available. The use of the PCR test will eliminate about 90 percent of the cases of post transfusion hepatitis. There remains another, much less common virus in the blood supply that has not been identified yet, however.

Although the hepatitis C virus is present in semen and sexual transmission of it has been reported, the risk seems to be less than with Hepatitis B. Those with multiple sex partners are at increased risk, however, and sexual partners of HCV positive individuals should be tested. Hepatitis C is transmitted primarily by needle stick or other blood exposure. The most common route of transmission currently is through injecting-drug use. Up to 80 percent of intravenous drug users have acquired the disease within 6 to 12 months of adopting their drug habit. As with hepatitis B it can be transmitted by body piercing and tattooing. It has also been transmitted by human bites and by organ transplantation. A hepatitis C infected pregnant woman can transmit the disease to her fetus. In studies done in Japan in regions with a high incidence of hepatitis C it was determined that transmission was not occurring as the result of sexual activity or childbirth, but rather was associated with acupuncture needles.[51] The same prohibitions against sharing razors and toothbrushes listed for hepatitis B apply to hepatitis C. As with hepatitis B the virus has a lipid envelope that precludes its transmission through the fecal-oral route.

Interferon alpha, which is licensed for treatment of hepatitis C, can completely clear the virus from the liver in 10 to 20 percent of the cases of hepatitis C if treatment is continued for 12 months. It produces some improvement in about one-half of the patients with chronic disease after six months of treatment. Serious side effects associated with interferon alpha do not always permit this duration of treatment, however, and one-half of these chronic cases relapse when the treatment is discontinued. A combination regime adding oral ribavirin was approved by the FDA in June 1998, and is now the treatment of choice for chronic hepatitis C.[52] Both drugs are expensive, costing about $7,000 for six months of combined therapy. Only about 30 percent of patients in the U.S. exhibit a sustained response to the combined treatment. Interferon has been found to worsen the liver disease in chronic HCV infection, and deaths have resulted. This appears to be one of several autoimmune diseases seen with interferon therapy.

One of the problems in treating hepatitis C is that the viral infection in the liver may smolder at a low level for years before it is detected. The incubation period for newly acquired infections averages six to seven weeks, but may be as long as six months. Most of these newly infected individuals (60 to 70 percent) do not display symptoms of hepatitis and very few develop jaundice. The infection may be associated with vague and nonspecific symptoms such as loss of appetite, fatigue, abdominal pain and joint aching. Liver function tests (serum aminotransferase) are variable and do not correlate with the severity of the disease and the prognosis.

Chronic liver damage and cirrhosis occurs in many of these patients before the diagnosis is made and liver cancer develops, as with hepatitis B, in an unknown percentage. As with all types of hepatitis the consumption of alcohol increases the risk of complications. It is very important for all patients who have had hepatitis B or C to have their liver status monitored by serum enzyme tests. Because these tests are more variable in chronic hepatitis C, a liver biopsy should be considered to ascertain the degree of inflammation and the amount of fibrosis. The frequency and duration of such monitoring must be determined for each individual. Glomerulonephritis also develops in some patients with hepatitis C as a result of vasculitis.

No vaccine has been developed for hepatitis C, and the outlook is not promising. Like other retroviruses, the hepatitis C virus mutates frequently during replication, resulting in subspecies even within an individual. These are not recognized by the antibodies that developed in response to the initial infection. This results in a persistent infection that is not inhibited by the body's immune defenses. For the same reason lifetime immunity is not conferred by infection with hepatitis C. There are six distinct genotypes of the hepatitis C virus worldwide. Genotype 1 is the most common (70 percent) in the United States, and this genotype is less responsive to therapy than the other genotypes.

A second virus that causes non-A, non-B hepatitis was identified in 1989 and has been labeled the hepatitis E virus. It is similar to hepatitis A in many respects, being transmitted by the fecal-oral route. It causes a self-limiting disease that does not result in chronic hepatitis or a carrier state. It does produce a 20 percent fatality rate when it is acquired in the third trimester of pregnancy. Hepatitis E is endemic in India, Nepal, Afghanistan, Bangladesh, Borneo, Burma, China, Mongolia, Pakistan, Russia, Mexico, Africa and several countries in the Middle East. It has caused outbreaks of hepatitis in all of these regions. An outbreak in New Delhi, India in 1955 that resulted from fecal contamination of the city water supply is now known to have caused hepatitis E in 29,000 people. The risk in these regions is especially great during times of flooding. Pregnant women should avoid travel to these regions, at least until a vaccine that is currently under development is marketed.

Between 1989, when the first test for hepatitis E became available, and 1992, six people who had traveled outside the United States were identified as having contracted hepatitis E. Two of these were individuals who had taken all of the proper precautions, but then swam in the Ganges River, a certain recipe for infection. Another woman contracted the infection during a visit to Mexico. The immune globulin injections that were given in the United States to protect against hepatitis A during foreign travel provided no protection against hepatitis E. In order to avoid contracting hepatitis E it is necessary to adhere strictly to the guidelines for consumption of food and water during travel. A polymerase chain reaction (PCR) test is now available for the hepatitis E virus, at least in research labs and at the Centers for Disease Control in Atlanta.[53,54]

The third virus transmitted through blood transfusions and blood products that was identified as causing non-A, non-B hepatitis is the hepatitis G virus, HGV. It was identified in early 1996 through the polymerase chain reaction (PCR) technology. HGV belongs to the same family as HCV, the flaviviruses. It also has been reported to have been transmitted from infected women to their newborn infants, and to patients through dialysis. Early studies suggest that it may be a less serious threat than hepatitis B and C.

It appears to be cleared from the blood in many cases, and thus is less prone to develop a chronic infection. This may be due to a difference in the composition of the viral envelope. More recent studies have revealed that it is a lymphotrophic virus that replicates primarily in the spleen and bone marrow. The implications of this are yet to be established, but some studies suggest that it does not cause hepatitis. In 1998 yet another transfusion-transmitted virus (TTV) was identified and studied using PCR techniques. It has been found to be common among blood donors, to be present in blood products such as factors VIII and IX, and to be a cause of post-transfusion hepatitis.[55] This agent needs further study and documentation. There remain other agents causing hepatitis that still have not been idendified.

TOBACCO

Second only to imprudent eating and drinking practices, cigarette smoking is the single most damaging behavior in our society. The destruction of health from this widespread practice includes not only lung, bladder and cervical cancer, but also osteoporosis, emphysema, chronic obstructive lung disease, heart disease and other vascular disease. The risk of developing pneumonia or meningitis from pneumococci that are commonly present in the respiratory tract of healthy individuals is increased significantly by cigarette smoking. Cigarette smoke not only impairs mucociliary action in the lungs, but also diminishes cellular and humoral defense mechanisms, and increases the permeability of the cells lining the respiratory tract. This increases the susceptibility to viruses and other pathogens.

Smoking can also double the risk of cataract formation and contributes to the development of osteoporosis. Menopause normally occurs at age 50 to 51, but premature menopause occurs prior to age 40. In the absence of surgery this is most frequently seen in association with cigarette smoking. Psychological and emotional symptoms and sleep disturbances are more pronounced when menopause is experienced prematurely.

The tobacco plant contains cancer-causing agents such as nitrosonornicotine and related compounds even before burning. This is attested to by the significant incidence of mouth cancer associated with the use of smokeless tobacco, even in young men.

The death in recent years of a high school athlete as a result of the use of smokeless tobacco is a grim testimonial to this danger.

Tobacco smoke contains an even more diverse complex of carcinogens, cancer accelerators and cancer promoters. About forty of these agents have been identified. These include several polycyclic aromatic hydrocarbons and phenolic compounds. The great increase in lung cancer in men since 1930 is associated with the introduction of manufactured cigarettes in 1915. Women picked up the smoking habit in earnest in the early 1940's, during World War II, and the lung cancer incidence in women related to this cigarette smoking began to increase in 1960. They are now approaching parity with men. The serious consequences of smoking, and of the use of smokeless tobacco, have gained widespread recognition in recent years. Significant progress has been achieved finally in reducing the incidence of this health hazard. See Chapter XII for a more detailed discussion of the health hazards of smoking and a table of the harmful components of cigarette smoke.

SCABIES

The "seven year itch" is caused by the female of a species of mite that burrows underneath the skin. There it deposits large eggs, 2 to 3 daily, for thirty to sixty days. Sensitization to the mites and their excrement, which is manifest about 30 to 40 days after infestation, causes an intense, severe itching that is worse at night and after a hot bath. The most common sites for these burrows, and the first to appear, are between the fingers on the back of the hand and on the inner surface of the wrists. Other sites that may be involved include the axilla, male genitalia and women's breasts.

As the infestation progresses it spreads to other areas of the body. The face and head and the palms of the hands are usually not involved in adults but may be in children. Larva from the hatched eggs mature to adults on the skin surface in about two weeks and then these continue the cycle. Individuals with poor personal hygiene habits suffer heavier infestations than do people who are more fastidious in their bathing and laundry habits. The infestation is also more persistent in immunocompromised individuals such as AIDS patients.

Scabies is transmitted from person to person, frequently as a result of sharing beds and clothing. Mere skin contact with an infested person is enough to contract the disease, as many derma-tologists can attest to. It is also transmitted through fomites such as hand pumps at public water sources in developing countries. Epidemics occur in long term care facilities for the elderly. This disease, as with all of the diseases that are caused by mites that feed on man, is directly related to low levels of hygiene and cleanliness. It is more common in regions with a hot climate where water is scarce. Frequent and regular laundering of clothing and bedding with detergent and hot water destroys the organism and reduces the frequency and intensity of the disease.

In ancient times the clothing and bedding would have been burned. Modern laundering techniques with hot water and deter-gents make it possible to salvage these contaminated items. During the past twenty to twenty-five years scabies has spread from an uncommon disease among the "middle class" in the United States to the status of a disease that is seen regularly by physicians. Secondary bacterial infections result from scratching, and strepto-coccal infections thus acquired have caused serious kidney damage in a number of individuals.

Scabies of course does not persist for seven years, at least not if it is treated adequately, and if the sources for re-infestation are eliminated. A five-percent permethrin cream, which is much less toxic, has replaced the classic one percent lindane or crotamiton treatment of scabies. It is just as effective as lindane and more effective than crotamiton. It must be applied to the entire body and left on for 12 to 14 hours before being washed off. One application is sufficient if all of the clothing and bedclothing are treated properly. This is a big if, however, for as with head lice, it is difficult to motivate some people to invest the necessary time and effort.

In these unmotivated cases a single oral dose of ivermectin has been shown to kill the scabies mites.[56] Ivermectin may also be more successful in institutions and in homeless populations where compliance can be a problem. Ivermectin cannot be used in children under the age of five, however. This new medication, which has been used to control heartworm in dogs since 1980, is also effective against other round worms in humans such as *Ascaris*, pinworm (*Enterobius*) and whipworm (*Trichuris*). It is less effective against hookworm (*Necator* and *Ancylostoma*), but these are seen primarily in warm climates where human excrement is deposited on soil or sand where people walk barefoot.

The itching of scabies may persist for several weeks after the destruction of the parasites, and should be treated with antihistamines. Repeated application of lindane or crotamiton will not relieve the itching and it may lead to the development of sensitization to the medication. Such practice should be avoided. Topical cortisone cream may spread any secondary bacterial infection that has developed and should be avoided also.

Everyone in the household who harbors the parasite, every sexual contact, everyone who shares a bed with the victim, must be treated at the same time. Even individuals who have had only casual physical contact with the infested person may need treatment. All clothing and bed linen must be well laundered with detergent and hot water. Fabrics that cannot be laundered must be dry-cleaned. Re-infestations are common as a result of failure to follow these dictums, and this is one disease that no one wants to repeat.

PEDICULOSIS

Three varieties oflice are seen in humans, and all are transferred from one human to another. They feed on the blood of man, thus acquiring the pathologic agents from infected individuals, and transmitting them in their feces to non-infected persons. When the infected feces is rubbed into the bite or any other break in the skin, infection ensues. The louse dies within two weeks after becoming infected with some agents such as *Rickettsia*; otherwise it lives out its thirty-day life cycle. If the victim providing the blood dies and thus loses normal body temperature, or if fever results from infection, the louse departs in search of a more hospitable host. Body lice are seen primarily among the homeless and individuals of extremely low levels of sanitation. They live in the seams of clothing that is worn next to the skin, and lice and their ova can be seen there. Laundering the clothing with adequate detergent and hot water will destroy both. Head lice, which are seen predominately among school children, are about two to three millimeters in length.

Pubic or crab lice are most commonly a sexually transmitted disease (see Chapter XI), although they can be acquired readily from infested clothing and bedding. When they are acquired sexually the possibility of any of the other sexually transmitted diseases exists, and these should be tested for. Pubic lice are about five millimeters in length and almost as wide. As with scabies, all clothing and bed linen must be laundered thoroughly, unless you prefer to burn them. Heating to about 160 to 170° F for 30 minutes will destroy lice and their eggs on clothing and bedding. Your wash water will not quite reach this level, particularly with the low settings of water heaters that are popular today. It has become common practice to set water heaters at 140° F. or lower to "save energy." Destruction of disease-causing microorganisms is accomplished more efficiently with settings of 160° F. or higher. Obviously caution must be exercised at kitchen and bath faucets with water that hot. The use of an adequate amount of detergent will help make up the difference in the laundry if the temperature of the wash water is only slightly lower.

It may be necessary to run an extra rinse cycle to eliminate the detergent, unless your machine has two rinses as an option. It is important not to abbreviate the laundry as many people do. The 15 to 20 minutes built into the timers on modern machines is barely long enough for routine laundering. It would be wise to allow the clothing to soak for at least twenty minutes, with hot water and detergent, before starting the wash cycle. At least 20 to 30 minutes in the dryer on the hot cycle will help complete the task. With some clothing dry-cleaning is the only option, even though it is less effective.

A hot iron will also destroy lice and their eggs in the seams of clothing. Malathion and DDT are both effective, especially in eliminating lice from furniture and other elements of the environment that cannot be placed in the washing machine. These products are no longer available in the United States, however. Benzyl benzoate powder, marketed as Acarosan® to eliminate dust mites from carpeting, should be effective also against any lice in the carpet.

Boiling in water will disinfect combs and hairbrushes. These human infestations can be eradicated by carefully following the physician's instructions for using lindane (Kwell®) in adults, but not on children. Pyrethrum extract from chrysanthemums with piperonyl butoxide added (Rid®) is still marketed, but 1% permethrin (Nix®), one of the synthetic pyrethroids is more effective in all forms of pediculosis.[57] It is poorly absorbed through the skin and presents less risk of toxicity to the nervous system than does lindane. Directions must be followed, leaving the shampoo or lotion on for the specified time period, then washing it off carefully and completely. The nits on the hair shafts must be removed by a special fine tooth comb, otherwise they will hatch and the infestation continues. All hats, caps, scarves, and bed linen must be sanitized adequately. Thorough vacuuming, especially of the bedroom, is also important. Inadequate attention to these onerous details is what has accounted for most of the failures to eliminate infestations in schools in the past, not failure of the medication. Carelessness and neglect in treatment regimes has encouraged the development of resistance to the current medication by the mites.

After resistance developed as a result of failure to completely follow directions, 5 percent permethrin cream (Elimite®) applied to clean, dry hair, covered with a shower cap, and left on for 8 to 12 hours usually effected a cure. Recently, however, studies carried out in the Czech Republic and Israel have demonstrated that at least some strains of head lice have developed a resistance to even the stronger 5 percent concentration of permethrin.[58] The Israeli studies indicated that malathion remains fully effective, but this product is not approved in the United States.[59] This latter study also showed that permethrin remains effective against body lice. Studies have shown that malathion in an aqueous preparation is not absorbed through the skin and is thus safe to use in treating head lice.[60]

We have had the technology and knowledge to eliminate these scourges of mankind completely, but that would require cooperation and cleanliness on the part of all. We had the same opportunity to eliminate syphilis and gonorrhea from the face of the earth after World War II, when both diseases were easily cured with penicillin. Gonorrhea has since developed widespread resistance to not only penicillin but other antibiotics as well. One might conclude that man is his own worst enemy.

Body lice transmit epidemic typhus, relapsing fever (see Chapter VII) and trench fever. Trench fever, so named because of its prevalence among troops during wartime, is endemic in Russia, Poland, Tunisia and Mexico. It had not been recognized in the United States until 1990 when it was found in a specimen of blood from an HIV-infected patient.[61] In 1993 trench fever was diagnosed in homeless people in Seattle who were not infected with the HIV.[62] In 1997 an outbreak of trench fever among homeless people in Marseilles, France was associated with body lice. It was discovered that some of the homeless were chronically infected even though they had no symptoms.[63]   The causative agent of trench fever, *Bartonella quintana*, a bacterium that the louse transmits from an infected human to a non-infected person through its feces, was identified by special laboratory techniques, including PCR.   The organism lives in and reproduces in the gut of the louse for the thirty-day life of the louse.   In addition to trench fever this bacterium causes liver tumors and damage to heart valves.   Trench fever cannot exist without lack of cleanliness and hygiene among human populations.

TICKS

With the emergence of Lyme disease and its rapid spread throughout most of the continental United States, a safe, effective and prompt method of removal of ticks that have attached themselves to the body has become a matter of considerable urgency.   It is important to avoid removing the body and leaving the head by traction that is too aggressive.   If the head is left behind, infection may ensue.   More important, the head can continue to burrow deeper into the skin where it will develop a granuloma, creating the need for surgical removal.   The previously popular techniques of applying a burning cigarette or a noxious liquid to force the tick to release its grasp results in regurgitation by the tick, with resultant injection of its infectious contents.   This technique is now condemned.

A technique that has proven successful and safe is the application of a shampoo that contains permethrin and piperonyl butoxide.   These products are marketed for the treatment of head lice and are available without prescription.   They are particularly useful for the removal of very small ticks, such as seed ticks and *Ixodes dammini* of Lyme disease.   Seed ticks are the first stage larvae of the hard ticks that transmit Rocky Mountain spotted fever, tularemia, Lyme disease and babesiosis in the United States.   They may appear to be insect bites, being about 0.6 mm in diameter, and are not recognized as ticks without magnification, or when they are observed to move.   Magnification will reveal that they have six legs instead of the eight legs found on the next two stages of the tick, the nymph and adult. This characteristic may cause them to be misidentified as lice.

Children can become infested with large numbers of these ticks from the grass or shrubs in their yards. It does not require a stroll through the forest. The risk of acquiring an infection from these arthropods was not great in most parts of the country in the past, but that risk has changed dramatically. It is necessary to be alert for ticks at all times during the warm months of the year, especially with children. The permethrin shampoo described above is particularly useful when children acquire many ticks.

BEDBUGS

These are wingless insects, about four to five millimeters in length, that hide in the mattress seams, furniture or even wallpaper during the day, and feed on humans at night. Sensitivity to the saliva may develop in some individuals and this produces itching. Batbugs belong to the same family (*Cimicidae*) and genus (*Cimex*) as bedbugs, and have similarly attacked humans when a colony of bats nested in a house.[64] This should serve as a caution to those who explore caves and other nesting sites of bats.

In the past it has been assumed that bedbugs did not transmit disease. Viral hepatitis is a known exception. If these arthropods can transmit viral hepatitis it is only logical to conclude that they are also capable of transmitting the human immunodeficiency virus of AIDS. In both cases the transmission is purely a mechanical one, caused by contamination of the mouthparts when feeding on an infected host. The virus does not undergo a replication cycle in the arthropod. In one study the AIDS virus was found to persist in bedbugs for up to 8 days after feeding on infected blood. Since the virus does not replicate in the insect some authorities have concluded that the risk of transmission of AIDS is low.[65] It may indeed be low, but there is no doubt that such transmission can occur. How often it occurs is unknown, and a study to make this determination would be very difficult to undertake. There appears to be little or no interest in such an investigation.

Anemia can also result from persistent feeding of bedbugs. Bathing and proper laundering of both clothing and bed linen on a regular basis can help to eliminate these creatures. Good hygiene, along with modern plumbing and appliances, has given us great freedom from this bane of mankind.

Sulfur dioxide fumigation through the burning of sulfur was a popular remedy in past years. It was a very effective means of eliminating the bugs, but the fumes (sulfur dioxide) are toxic to humans and must be avoided. Professionals also used fumigation by hydrocyanic acid (HCN) in the past. It is very effective but is dangerous to handle or even to be around. These techniques have been supplanted by the pesticides, several of which are effective. The organophosphates, such as 2 percent malathion, are effective but they cannot be taken to bed with you. These are even more effective when used in conjunction with the pyrethrins, which act as an irritant and force the bedbugs from their hiding places.

DDT in a five percent emulsion proved to be very effective in eliminating bedbugs, but this product is no longer available in the United States. The mattress and bedroom can be sprayed with an aerosol containing pyrethrin and piperonyl butoxide, making certain that you stay out of the room for at least thirty minutes after spraying. A plastic mattress cover and a freshly laundered cloth mattress cover will then help to prevent skin contact with the pyrethrin. Even this relatively non-toxic group of pesticides (pyrethroids) cannot be used by those who are sensitized to them. Individuals with eczema and asthma in particular should exercise caution.

DUST MITES

Dust mites have escaped scrutiny as a health problem until relatively recently. In recent years it seems that there has been an effort to make up for lost time, judging from the number of studies published. These mites are a common offending agent in asthma as well as in bronchitis, eczema and nasal allergies. Both the body of the mite and the fecal pellets that they distribute in the bedding and carpeting cause allergic reactions. Many different species of mites (Acari) can cause an intense irritation and dermatitis in humans. This is a problem commonly seen in individuals who handle grain, cottonseeds, beans and especially straw. Grocer's itch and baker's itch from handling grain products such as flour results in severe itching. The mite that has burrowed into the skin can be killed by application of dilute phenol (Campho-Phenique®) or 5% permethrin cream (Elimite™). The house dust mite (Dermatophagoides) does not burrow into the skin but it does produce the most potent allergen of all of the mites.[66] Inhalation of the mite or its fecal pellets can provoke asthma or bronchitis in susceptible individuals. These mites feed on shed human skin cells.

Studies have shown that a reduction in the population of dust mites through the use of an acaricide (Acarosan®) produces a remarkable improvement in symptoms of asthma, eczema and nasal allergy.[67] Acarosan is a moist powder that is sprinkled on the carpet, distributed evenly and allowed to dry for 1 to 3 hours. It is then vacuumed up, removing the dust mites and their excreta. This product has been marketed in the United States only since about 1990. It contains benzyl benzoate, in a rather low 4.6 percent concentration. Benzyl benzoate was the original treatment for the scabies mite prior to the development of lindane (see scabies above). In that application it was applied to the entire body in a 25 percent lotion.

Benzyl benzoate is relatively harmless, although the precautions on the package should be observed. As with any chemical, it should not be carried to the mouth by the hands when eating, drinking or smoking. This is another instance where hand washing is required. Other agents that are effective in killing the mites include permethrin, resmethrin, tetramethrin and other synthetic pyrethroids. These can be sprayed on the carpet prior to vacuuming to help reduce mite populations. Use only aqueous preparations that are designed for use in the household. Even these must be used with caution around individuals with asthma, hay fever or allergies to chrysanthemums.

Several other studies have demonstrated that the single most successful means of reducing the numbers of dust mites (not eliminating them) is by thorough vacuuming of the carpet, furniture and room in general. This should be done weekly. The allergens from dust mites do not remain suspended in the air for long because of their relatively large sizes (20 microns compared to 2-10 microns for cat allergen, which does remain suspended). They do become suspended with any activity in the bed or bedroom, however. Frequent and adequate laundering of bedding and draperies also helps to keep the mite population under control. Keep in mind that hot water and adequate detergent must be used to be effective. Dust mites also have been found to thrive and proliferate on the scalps of children,[68] so cleanliness must extend to personal hygiene. All of these measures will need to be attended to more stringently where dust mites are causing allergic problems, as is frequently the case.

OTHER INSECT VECTORS OF DISEASE

Flies, gnats, cockroaches and other insects have been important agents in the transmission of disease throughout history. They transmit typhoid fever, cholera, *Salmonella*, *Shigella*, amebiasis, viruses, various worms, and indeed virtually all of the organisms that cause foodborne infections and diarrheal disease. Flies are especially important in the transmission of shigella where only a minute inoculum is required to produce diarrhea. Flies are strongly attracted to both feces and garbage and to food in homes. This provides an efficient means of anal-oral transmission of disease.

Control of flies is a major element in the prevention of trachoma, an eye infection that has resulted in blindness in an estimated 7 million people worldwide. Trachoma is caused by the bacterium *Chlamydia trachomatis* which is deposited on the lids of the eye when the fly feeds. Poor personal hygiene is also a contributing factor. Although the disease is rare in the United States an estimated 500 million people suffer with trachoma worldwide.

Organized and effective public health systems in the United States, with weekly garbage pick-ups, control of refuse and pesticide applications have greatly reduced the fly population. Modern very tight homes with screening and very effective yet safe pesticides for residential use serve additionally to protect the public from disease (see Chapter XIV). Obviously our homes and kitchens should be kept free of all of these insect vectors of disease. A much greater problem in control of flies exists on farms where organic material is abundant in the barnyard and elsewhere. Broader applications of pesticides, and pesticides of greater toxicity are both needed. Flytraps that include baited pesticides are also essential. The problem is no less urgent on the farm, just more difficult.

Cockroaches present a much more difficult challenge. Studies over the past 30 years have demonstrated that the residue from cockroaches is a powerful allergen, stimulating asthmatic attacks in sensitized individuals, especially children.[69,70,71,72] They have been notoriously resistant to all of the pesticides that we have developed. Bait traps containing hydramethylnon are claimed to be effective in killing roaches. Cockroaches have been considered to be the most successful survival experts of the past 2 or 3 thousand years. In addition to food they find nourishment from starch and glue. A mixture of equal parts of cornstarch and plaster of Paris sprinkled in their path is claimed to destroy them by binding up after they ingest the mixture. Sprinkling boric acid under the sink in their path has proven to be a useful control. To be effective it must be placed where the cockroach will contaminate its legs with it. It must never be placed near any food, dishes or other eating utensils because of its toxicity to humans. It is a very dangerous substance to have in the home.

Very recently allopurinol has been reported to be effective in eradicating cockroaches. This is one of the medications that have been used for many years in the control of gout. I do not know the mechanism for its application in controlling cockroaches, but I presume that it would be similar to boric acid. Finding a source of supply for the powder might be difficult however.

CONTACT LENSES

The loss of sight is one of the greatest tragedies that can befall a person. This happens far more often than it should as a result of neglect of proper care among diabetics and patients with glaucoma. The extremely widespread popularity of contact lenses has given us an additional risk that is causing loss of vision unnecessarily. This loss is unnecessary because it can be prevented in every instance if instructions are followed and if lenses are properly cared for.

These precautions are frequently neglected because they require a significant investment in time and effort on a daily basis. No one should decide to acquire contact lenses until after they have thoroughly reviewed the procedures that are mandatory for the maintenance and care of these devices. After having reviewed these procedures and precautions consideration of contact lens use should be abandoned unless the individual is committed and willing to follow these procedures diligently. No parent should permit a teenager to get contact lenses until these requirements are reviewed, and until the parent feels certain that the child will comply with them.

The chief risk entailed in wearing contact lenses is damage to the cornea, the clear covering over the center of the eye. Scratching the cornea during insertion of the lens can cause damage, but more frequently corneal damage is caused by deposits on the contact lens. The hemoglobin in blood serves as an efficient system for the transport of oxygen to all of the living tissues of the body, except for the cornea. The cornea is provided with no circulation, no blood vessels, and no hemoglobin. Every living tissue requires oxygen, and the cornea is no exception. It must obtain the oxygen that it requires from the air, through the tears, and it must expel carbon dioxide the same way. This latter substance renders the surface of the cornea acidic, which is damaging to contact lenses. A buffering solution is inserted with these lenses to protect them from this acidic environment.

The cornea actually uses oxygen at a fairly rapid rate, making this method of oxygen transport all the more remarkable. The original hard lenses interfered with this function seriously, and that feature accounted for most of the problems that wearers experienced with them. If this oxygen deprivation continues long enough, neovascularization, a growth of blood vessels into the cornea, can occur. This can result in impairment of vision. Soft contact lenses have a water content of as much as 80 percent, and thus they carry oxygen to the cornea much more efficiently. This eliminated many of the problems that were associated with hard lens use.

The down side of this feature of soft lenses is that the high water content results in the retention of many different chemicals in the contact lens. This includes those chemicals that are used for cleansing and disinfecting. It also provides a better media in which microorganisms can multiply. These soft lenses are further characterized by the buildup of protein deposits from the tears. These deposits cause irritation of the cornea and sensitivity reactions in the inner lining of the upper lid. For these reasons, cleansing and purging of the lenses becomes even more urgent.

Soft contact lenses must be cleaned daily. The deposit of protein materials begins almost immediately after insertion of the lens. In addition to the irritation of the cornea and the sensitivity reaction of the lids, these deposits can ruin the contact lens. A daily cleaner solution is designed to remove these protein deposits, but it does not disinfect the lens. This requires a second step. Prior to progressing to the second step it is essential to remove all of the cleaning solution by thorough rinsing. If this is not done, the daily cleaner solution that is retained in the contact lens can irritate the cornea and damage the contact lens.

After rinsing the lens thoroughly, disinfection is then carried out. Classically this has been accomplished by boiling for thirty minutes, which effectively destroys all of the microorganisms that have accumulated in the lens. It is important to clean and disinfect the lens case also; otherwise the lenses will become contaminated again when they are placed in the case.

Chemical disinfectants have become popular as a replacement for boiling. While less troublesome, they are not as effective as boiling. Hydrogen peroxide has enjoyed popularity in the past, and is fairly effective. Standard hydrogen peroxide loses its strength on the shelf, however, and for this reason stabilized solutions have been developed. It is important to use only fresh 3 percent hydrogen peroxide solution sold for this purpose, or a similar stabilized solution. It is fairly effective in sterilizing contact lenses, if they have been thoroughly cleansed of organic deposits. Hydrogen peroxide is totally ineffective as an antiseptic in wounds because it is decomposed and inactivated by the tissue enzymes almost immediately. If this occurs while disinfecting your lens, there is no way for you to know, unless you do a culture.

Hydrogen peroxide has the advantage of not leaving a residue build up in contact lenses. It must be thoroughly rinsed out of the lens, however, or a painful eye will result. Other chemical disinfectants are being investigated currently. Poly-amino-propylbiguanide has been marketed, and others will follow. One hindrance to the development of new agents is the cost of investigation and approval by the Food and Drug Administration. This process takes years in addition to the high cost. The other obstacle is the same one that has prevented the use of many effective germicides in medicine in general. Many substances that kill microorganisms have similar deleterious effects on the tissues of the body. Phenol, while very effective in destroying bacteria, cannot be used in the eye. The same can be said about tincture of iodine.

Some preservatives in the various solutions also cause irritation of the eye. Thimerosal was commonly used in some saline and other solutions for a long time. Although it was effective it frequently caused irritation of the eye due to the development of sensitivity to it. This problem was compounded by the fact that the contact lens takes up and retains the thimerosal. It has been replaced by sodium borate, sorbic acid and ethylenediaminetetra-acetic acid. The latter substance is usually abbreviated to EDTA or to edetate sodium. There is a possibility of sensitization with EDTA, however.

An enzyme cleaning solution is used weekly to remove any residual protein deposits that are not removed by the daily cleaner. Porcine pancreatic enzyme is commonly used, replacing papain, which caused sensitivity reactions. For all of these processes and for all of these solutions, the directions from the manufacturer should be read carefully and adhered to strictly. Only the solutions that are specified for your lenses should be used. Most are not interchangeable. Ignoring this caveat risks damage to the contact lens, the eye, or both. Efforts to conserve solutions and money have led many people to mix their own saline solution from salt tablets. This practice has led to serious infections in the eye.

Any infection in the eye is a very serious matter, but the infections that result from home brewed saline solutions involve *Acanthamoeba*. This is a protozoan that has not been associated with eye infections previously. This organism is widespread in soil and in water all around us, including the water from your faucet. It does not cause disease ordinarily. Heat sterilization as described above will kill this organism and its cysts. Other means of sterilization will not assure the destruction of *Acanthamoeba*, however.

Infections by *Acanthamoeba* are particularly worrisome because we have no medication that is effective in destroying the organism. Antibiotics are effective in controlling most bacterial infections, but we do not have comparable agents for infections caused by protozoa. *Acanthamoeba* also can be acquired by wearing contact lenses in the swimming pool, in hot tubs and by placing the lenses in the mouth. The mouth and saliva are far from sterile and saliva makes a poor wetting agent. These infections threaten blindness or even the loss of the eye. Random testing has demonstrated that every sample of homemade saline solution that was examined was contaminated by bacteria, fungi or *Acanthamoeba*.

The water that comes from your faucet is not sterile. Neither is the distilled water that you buy in the supermarket.

Only sterile saline solutions should be used in caring for contact lenses. Hands should always be washed carefully before handling lenses, not only to avoid contamination of lenses with microorganisms, but also to remove all hand cream, cosmetics and other greases. Some soaps leave a residue of lanolin or other oleaginous substances on the hands that then contaminates the contact lens. There is generally no way to salvage lenses contaminated by these oils. This financial disaster can be avoided by using only a pure soap such as Ivory® or Neutrogena® before handling lenses. People who wear contact lenses should inspect the ingredients of hand and bath soaps carefully before purchasing them. The oils in hair conditioners and hair rinses can also destroy contact lenses. Eye doctors who examine contact lenses see such contamination frequently.

During the past decade new materials have been developed for hard lenses that permit the transportation of oxygen through them to the cornea. These are called rigid gas permeable lenses. The newer polymers for these lenses are also more resistant to protein deposits than previous materials, and much more so than soft lenses. These lenses still require a longer period of adaptation than do soft lenses. Since they lack the high moisture content of soft lenses they do not dry out and change shape, as soft lenses tend to do. Visual correction may be better as a result. These lenses are also easier to keep clean, and they last longer. They are much more expensive, however, and they require more care and expertise in fitting. They also require different solutions for care and maintenance than those used with soft lenses.

Individuals with allergies are destined to have more problems with contact lenses than do people who are not thus plagued. Contact lenses also cannot be worn in certain occupational settings, such as dusty atmospheres and in laboratories where chemical vapors are encountered. Most people can discipline themselves to not wear their lenses at work where they know that a risk exists. It is a great temptation to forget about contact lenses when sawing or grinding jobs need to be done in the home workshop, however.

Soft contact lenses should not be worn when working with household ammonia, oven cleaners or wall and tile cleaners either.

Any cleaner that gives off vapors that irritate the nose, throat or eyes may collect in the contact lenses. This risk is less with the soft contact lenses that are 38 percent water. Many still contain 55 percent water, however, and some 70 percent. In view of the risk of irritation of the cornea, and the cost of the contact lenses, it would be wise to play it safe. This is less of a risk with the new gas permeable lenses. Any irritation or problem that is not readily resolved by removal and cleaning of the lens, or any problem that recurs when the lens is reinserted, should be taken to the doctor for examination.

Visitations to high altitudes such as are encountered when skiing may also result in more problems from contact lenses. The reduced oxygen content of the air results in even less oxygen being available to the cornea. In addition the increased loss of fluid by the body that results from the low humidity of the ambient air and the reduced atmospheric pressure also produces greater drying of the lens and the cornea. Periodic moistening of the lens and cornea with an acceptable wetting agent will minimize this problem. Contact lenses will require more attention during these visitations.

COSMETICS:

Congress passed the Food, Drug and Cosmetic Act in 1938 to protect the public from foods, drugs and cosmetic products that are "injurious to health." The intent of the law is to provide the same protection to the public for cosmetics as is accorded to the food and drug supply. Manufacturers do not have to obtain prior approval before marketing cosmetic products, however. Manufacturers hastily withdraw any product that causes widespread acute reactions, but such actions are less prompt where the results are subtler. A major concern has been the various dyes, since previously marketed agents, as with food dyes, have been permitted to remain on the market pending further studies.

Two red dyes in lipsticks have been removed from the market, one because of cancer fears and the other because of the numbers of cases of sore throat provoked by it. Aside from these cases, the majority of health problems from cosmetics have arisen out of their propensity to cause allergic reactions. Most of these reactions have been provoked by the chemical agents added to the cosmetics to inhibit the growth of microbial organisms.

These substances include thimerosal, methylparaben, propyl-paraben, hexachlorophene, EDTA (ethylenediaminetetraacetic acid), formaldehyde and benzalkonium chloride. These compounds are invariably listed on the label, but you will need your bifocals to read them. Whenever a rash occurs you should discontinue the use of any product that you have been applying. Even skin creams and lotions cause a rash in some people, usually due to the paraben preservatives.

As is the case with foods and medications, preservatives have a limited effectiveness in preventing infections. Infections have resulted from the sharing of cosmetic applicators, such as with mascara, on many occasions. This causes great concern, for as has been the case where microbial pathogens have shown up in other products containing agents to inhibit their growth, we are usually faced with organisms that are very resistant to our medications. One such organism is *Pseudomonas*, and this has been found in mascara. Sharing of any utensil that is inoculated with the organisms from another person is a recipe for trouble. Most of the people who share cosmetic applicators would be aghast at any suggestion that they share a toothbrush.

Talc is a hydrated magnesium silicate. It is similar to asbestos, which is a series of minerals composed of silicates of iron and magnesium. Talc also contains up to 5 percent of silica, which causes silicosis. An increased incidence of chronic obstructive lung disease from the use of talc in rubber workers has been documented. Use of this product on infants or adults in a manner that permits inhalation introduces the risk of this serious and permanent lung disorder. The fine particle size of powders ensures that they will become airborne and will be inhaled. Talc was universally used in baby powders in the United States for many years, but fortunately it is being slowly replaced by an old standby, cornstarch. As of this writing containers of baby powder that appear identical, from a major supplier, sit side by side on the shelf, one containing talc, the other only corn starch. In order to avoid talc you must read the ingredients carefully. Zinc oxide and zinc stearate are acceptable, but talc is not. In spite of its usefulness and benefits, talc is a product that should be avoided.

Studies also have incriminated the use of talcum powder on the female genitalia and sanitary napkins in the development of ovarian cancer. Women who use it daily have a threefold increase in the incidence of this serious malignancy. Those who use it intermittently still demonstrated twice the incidence as do those women who did not use it. In some studies talc particles have been found imbedded in over 70 percent of human ovarian cancer tissue samples, demonstrating that the mineral indeed does migrate through the uterus and tubes. Even talc that is not contaminated with asbestos is known to produce a severe inflammatory reaction. This was discovered in surgery over fifty years ago. Starch and other substances have been substituted for dusting gloves since that time.

IMMUNIZATION

The latter half of the twentieth century witnessed the virtual elimination of epidemics of infectious diseases that formerly were common in the United States. In the previous generation virtually every child experienced measles, mumps and chickenpox, sometimes sharing them with their parents. Measles is a disease with very serious implications for any female who is or might become pregnant (and for her offspring). It is completely preventable. Diphtheria has been virtually eliminated in the United States by routine immunization of infants. More than 200,000 cases were reported in 1921, but only 20 cases were reported in the first half of the 1980's. Several large epidemics have occurred since then due to neglect of immunizations. Everyone is aware of the success of the polio vaccines, but we still have occasional outbreaks of poliomyelitis in populations that are not adequately immunized.

Most of these disease outbreaks occur because of human complacency. Only about one half of the children in the United States are properly immunized by the age of two years. Politicians blame the cost of vaccines for this neglect. However parents find the means to get their children immunized when they are forced to by regulations requiring it for entry into school. Immunizations are available free of charge to all children in every state at public health clinics. The cost of the vaccines is borne by the taxpayers. Of the $21.00 cost of DTP vaccine, $18.00 is a federal tax to defray the cost of lawsuits. The cost of the vaccine itself is a small part of the total price to the consumer or taxpayer. This is just one of many examples of hidden costs imposed upon the public by government, which then publicly blames the manufacturer.

The widespread malady of parental neglect seen in our society in recent years is reflected in this area of disease prophylaxis, as well as in many of our other social problems. It is not cost that is responsible for the failure to immunize our children. Rather it is complacency, lack of responsibility and misplaced priorities. The time and effort required to acquire the protection offered by immunization is minuscule compared to the grief experienced by failure to make the investment.

The most desirable type of immunization is active immunization, where the body is prompted to develop antibodies to fight off the disease. This is accomplished by the injection of killed or attenuated microbial agents. This takes some time, however, and does not afford the immediate protection that is needed in some instances after exposure. Passive immunity, on the other hand, is conferred by injecting immune globulin, which affords some degree of immunity sooner. This immunity is short lived however. A list of diseases that are preventable by immunization is presented at the end of this chapter.

In some instances both active and passive immunization are advisable, as when immediate protection is needed after exposure. This is frequently the case after a bite by a rabid animal and with many tetanus prone injuries. Some immunizations are advisable only when a risk is likely to be encountered, as with travel to regions where exposure is likely, and in laboratory workers. The risk of some diseases for which we have no immunization may also be lessened by chemotherapeutic agents, as is the case with malaria. Here again, however, many of the malaria parasites have become resistant to all of the medications that we have available.

INFLUENZA

Influenza is a highly contagious acute respiratory illness caused by one of several strains of three different types of viruses, A, B and C. Whereas influenza B and C viruses customarily infect only humans, influenza A viruses, the most common group, infect many different animal species, including birds, swine, horses and sea mammals. Minor changes in the surface antigen of the virus are constantly taking place, and because of this, nationwide epidemics of type A occur about every 3 years. Typically more than 10,000 additional deaths occur in the United States during these epidemics.

Many of these deaths result from pneumonia caused either by the influenza virus itself, a secondary bacterial infection or a mixture of the two. In temperate climates outbreaks occur during the winter months, whereas in tropical regions activity may continue through the year. Major genetic shifts in the virus occur about every 10 to 15 years, producing a strain to which the public has little or no immunity. Pandemics (a worldwide epidemic), which have occurred in 1957, 1968 and 1976, ensue during these periods. The new strain responsible for all three of the recent pandemics originated in southern China, so this region is being monitored yearly.

In the great pandemic of 1918 more than 20 million people world wide died, 548,000 in the U.S. alone.[73] This was a greater number of deaths than occurred in all of the battles of World War I together. The virus, which was a particularly virulent strain, was probably transmitted from China in March of 1918 during World War I by Indo-Chinese troops landing in France.[74] The "swine flu" epidemic of 1976 was caused by a strain of virus antigenically similar to the one that caused the pandemic of 1918-1919, but apparently was not as virulent. Influenza B is less common, producing an epidemic about every 5 years, but seldom a pandemic.

Influenza is spread by aerosol of respiratory secretions, and also by articles contaminated by these secretions. Considerable morbidity and mortality result during epidemics of either type. It is especially important for those individuals over 65 years of age and everyone with any chronic illness to avail themselves of influenza immunization each October. During an epidemic a significant number of people in these categories are hospitalized for pneumonia, heart failure or exacerbation of chronic lung disease, and many deaths occur. Outbreaks in the United States typically occur during the winter months, usually beginning in December and lasting for 2 to 3 months. The vaccine composition has to be adjusted each year to accommodate any changes in the viral strains that are circulating. Epidemics resulting from new strains result in far more serious illness due to the lack of immunity in the population.

It has been suspected for over twenty years that southern China serves as the epicenter for influenza epidemics worldwide, and for the development of new strains. Various studies have added credence to this hypothesis, demonstrating a reservoir of influenza

A virus in pigs, ducks and migratory waterfowl. This has led to the suggestion that new strains of the influenza A virus result from man living in close proximity to animals, particularly pigs and fowl. Studies have shown that the subtypes that have produced epidemics reside throughout the year in domestic ducks in southern China and in pigs. Whereas the virus cannot be transmitted from ducks to man, or vice versa, the virus can be transferred from both to pigs. Mutations can then take place in the pig to produce a more virulent strain. This can then be transmitted to man. It is a common custom in southern China is to have living quarters in the upstairs of a dwelling, keeping the animals on the ground floor. It has been suggested that such proximity facilitates a genetic rearrangement in the virus, producing new strains for which we have not developed any immunity.

The virus for the pandemic of 1968 emerged from southern China through Hong Kong, thus its label "Hong Kong flu". Influenza outbreaks in China typically occur during the summer, which permits the CDC to determine the strain(s) that we can expect when our season arrives. This will be especially important when a new strain for our next pandemic appears. If it proves to be as virulent as the 1918 strain was there would likely be far more deaths than resulted from that pandemic.

BACK DISORDERS

One of the most common and most enigmatic health problems in the United States is the variety of disorders that afflict the back. These are a particular problem for employers, both because of the frequency with which they occur and the difficulty in dealing with them. An experienced physician can expose the many cases of malingering, but the majority of cases involve injury with inflammation of the muscles, ligaments, joints or a combination thereof. These present a problem because they take time to resolve, and the type of work that precipitated the injury is likely to lead to a delayed recovery, or even a repeat injury.

Anyone can suffer a torn muscle or pulled ligament, but individuals who are born with anatomical variations are much more susceptible to injury. These individuals generally should not be employed in jobs that require lifting or bending. Unfortunately these conditions are usually diagnosed only after an injury, because the basic problem can be seen only with an x-ray, CAT scan or MRI. The most common such problem is an imperfection in the formation of one or more of the lumbar vertebra. An increase in the angle of the sacrum, which is the base for the lumbar vertebra, is another problem that predisposes to back injuries. In some cases of congenital malformation the fifth lumbar vertebra, which sits on the sacrum, actually slips forward, adding to the strain.

Much more common but less serious are cases where lateral (side to side) curvatures of the spine result from a slanted sacral base due to a difference in the lengths of the legs. Lack of symmetry is common throughout the body, but it has far less significance in the arms than it does in the legs. With the sacrum slanted to one side the lumbar spine also tilts in that direction. In an effort to keep the head in the midline the spine develops compensatory curves. On the convexity of these curves the muscles are stretched beyond their normal relaxed state. This can result in fatigue and aching in these muscles, but equally as important is that these muscles are more susceptible to strains and tears with lifting.

The problems associated with the curvatures of the spine from unequal leg length are easily corrected in most cases by simply building up the heel of the shoe on the short side. This requires accurate measurement by x-ray, however, for the problem can be made worse unless modification is made in the correct direction and of the proper magnitude, and done in acceptable increments. There are several basic fundamentals that need to be followed in treating this problem. This is not a complicated procedure, but few physicians are trained in the specifics, and even fewer are concerned with the problem.

Regardless of whether or not there exist any underlying anatomical variations, there are some common fundamentals that apply to every back. First and foremost is good muscle tone. Even in an individual who exercises and keeps in good shape generally, there are some specific exercises that will tone up the muscles that support the spine and that are involved in lifting. Leg raising exercises and sit-ups are two examples that require no special equipment. Of equal importance is excess weight, which places additional stress on every joint that bears that weight. A protuberant abdomen pulls on the spine, abnormally increasing its forward curvature, placing it under stress and rendering it more susceptible to injury. This has been amply demonstrated in millions of women during pregnancy. Their problem lasts only for nine months. A beerbelly usually lasts for a lifetime.

There are proper techniques for lifting that can minimize the risk of injury to the back. Employers generally make an effort to educate employees in these techniques where lifting is part of the job. The most important of these techniques is to keep the back straight, using the knees to lift objects. Wide banded waist supports to help protect the back are also widely used now, and these have been shown to reduce the incidence of injuries. It should also be remembered that the back, like any machine, has its limits. Any weight beyond about 35 pounds increases the risk of injury.

This discussion is placed in this chapter because this problem is a personal one, only incidentally related to the job. As many or more back injuries occur outside of the workplace as on the job, and all of the measures outlined above should be undertaken by every individual, where indicated, as a part of the general health program.

PREVENTATIVE MAINTENANCE

During our youthful years few of us give much thought to living to a ripe old age. By the time we start thinking about it, it's pretty late in the game to undo all of the harm that we have done. For those of us who are blessed with good health at birth (the majority of us), we could exceed the life expectancy norm by following moderation in all things. Eating intelligently, maintaining our weight close to the ideal, resting our minds and bodies regularly and adequately, exercising regularly, avoiding smoking and all of the other hazards to health outlined previously. This is not really asking a lot in the way of sacrifices. We can still have our cake and eat it too, just not every day, and not in huge amounts.

We do inherit proclivities toward some diseases. It is wise to be cognizant of these and behave appropriately from the earliest possible moment. High blood pressure is one of the most common such inheritance in our society, and this mandates avoidance of salt, control of weight and regular exercise throughout life. Diabetes is also common in our society, and the same behavior is essential to avoid its complications. In addition to self-discipline, a scheduled program of preventative maintenance is important to detect these diseases at their earliest onset, and take appropriate actions.

Fortunately we have very effective medications currently for both hypertension and diabetes when they become necessary.

A proclivity to develop some cancers is also inherited. Everyone should be familiar with the health history of their parents, grandparents and aunts and uncles. Where there is a pattern of a cancer such as breast or uterine cancer, more frequent and more careful scrutiny should be instituted. Women who have not had children by their early thirties are at greater risk of developing breast cancer than are women who have had children. Women who elect to have an induced abortion increase their risk of developing breast cancer by up to fifty percent. The breast self-exam becomes even more urgent for both of these groups, as does regular professional exams by a physician and mammography.

The following outline provides general guidelines for the majority of the population. Where there exists a positive family history for such problems as heart attacks at an early age, breast or uterine cancer, high blood pressure or diabetes some of these tests need to be instituted at an earlier age and rechecked more frequently than indicated. Your family physician should be your consultant and your guide. This schedule assumes appropriate pediatric evaluations and treatment up to age 18 years.

AGES 19 TO 39:
- Physical examination with basic blood count and blood chemistry profile* every three years.
- Electrocardiogram at age 39 for assessment and future reference.
- Pelvic exam with Pap smear and breast exam yearly (start earlier when sexually active, when the activity begins). More frequent if Pap report is abnormal.
- Mammogram at age 35 for baseline. Breast self-exam monthly.‡
- Dental exam yearly.
- Vision screen every two years if history of myopia (near sighted) in family.
- Hearing screen every two years, especially with noise exposure (see Chapters VIII and X).

AGES 40 TO 50:
- Physical examination with basic blood count and blood chemistry profile* every one to three years.
- Pelvic exam with Pap smear and breast exam every year, more frequent if abnormal.
- Endometrial cytology at age 45 or menopause, then yearly in women at risk.§
- Mammogram every one to two years. Breast self-exam monthly.‡
- Dental exam every six months to yearly.

- Vision screen with ophthalmoscopic exam at age 40, then every one to two years as indicated.
- Hearing screen every two years, more often with noise exposure or hearing loss.
- Prostate exam with occult blood test every year.

AGES 50 TO 65:
- Physical examination with basic blood count and blood chemistry profile* every one to three years.
- Pelvic exam with Pap smear and breast exam every year, more frequent if ab normal.
- Endometrial cytology every year in women at risk.§
- Mammogram every year, more frequent if family or personal history of cancer. Breast self-exam monthly.‡
- Dental exam every six months to yearly.
- Vision screen with ophthalmoscopic exam every one to two years as indicated.
- Hearing screen every two years, more often with noise exposure or hearing loss.
- Prostate exam with occult blood test yearly.
- Sigmoidoscopy at age 50, then every three years if negative.

OVER AGE 65:
- Physical examination with basic blood count and blood chemistry profile* every year.
- Pelvic exam with Pap smear and breast exam every year, more frequent if abnormal.
- Endometrial cytology every year in women at risk.§
- Mammogram every year, more frequent if family or personal history of cancer. Breast self-exam monthly.‡
- Dental exam every six months to yearly.
- Vision screen with ophthalmoscopic exam yearly.
- Hearing screen every year, more often with noise exposure or hearing loss.
- Prostate exam with occult blood test yearly.
- Sigmoidoscopy every year.

* Basic blood count should include RBC, Hb, Hct, Sed rate, MCV, MCHb, WBC, differential. Blood chemistry profile should include glucose, cholesterol, triglycerides, sodium, chloride, potassium, CO^2, total protein, albumin, A:G ratio, total bilirubin, alkaline phosphatase, BUN, creatinine, uric acid, sugar, CO_2, liver enzymes and lipids.

§ Women at risk for uterine cancer include obesity, diabetes, hypertension, estrogen therapy, cigarette smoking, history of chronic anovulatory cycles and family history of uterine cancer.

‡ The risk of breast cancer is increased significantly in women who have not had children by their early thirties. The estrogen level in the breast tissue of these women is higher than in women of the same age who have had children. This increases cell division and thus the risk of cancer. Regular, careful breast examination is vital.

The Pap smear (George Papanicolaou, MD) for screening for cervical cancer came into widespread use in the late 1950s, and has been a very valuable contribution in the battle against cancer. The incidence of cervical cancer prior to regular Pap screening was 30 per 100,000 woman years. In the year 2001 that incidence has been reduced to 3 per 100,000 woman years as a result of the routine use of the Pap smear. Some symptoms and events that require an immediate assessment by the family physician regardless of the results of the past exams and tests include:

• Any unexplained bleeding.
• Coughing up blood.
• Onset of a persistent cough.
• Unexplained weight loss.
• A change in bowel habits.
• Development of persistent or repeated headaches, awakening with headache.
• Persistent pain in any organ of the body.
• Change in size or color of a mole or other skin lesion.
• Development of hoarseness or difficulty swallowing.
• A lump in or discharge from the breast.
• Development of lumps anywhere on the body.
• A sore anywhere that does not heal.

The importance of proper nutrition in maintaining good health cannot be over emphasized. Too many calories and the wrong foods are significant causes of death and suffering in our society. An obsession with losing weight by sacrificing good nutrition can produce just as much harm, however. The people of the United States are bombarded daily with medical and nutritional advice, most of it inaccurate. Even some of the so-called experts deliver bad advice. There is no magic involved in nutrition. The basic nutritional needs have not changed in the past 50 years; only the propaganda and the hype have.

All of the previous discussions have dealt with the physical needs of the human body. It would be a great mistake to neglect the spiritual and social needs as well. The stress that results from anxiety and a lack of inner peace has a deleterious effect on all of the vital organs of the body as well as on the efficiency of decisions and performance. It also impairs interpersonal relationships, thus adding to the stress and tension, and robbing individuals of happiness and fulfillment.

It is not popular in our society today to talk of faith and morality. This reality is reflected in the sickness that pervades our government and our society. Interestingly, the words and writings of all of the Founding Fathers, as well as our early presidents, routinely admonished us to seek guidance and counseling from God. His Commandments were to be the basis of our society. These writings are available for all to read, but they are commonly ignored, significantly so in our courts, in our government and in our schools. I fear that we have become yet another lost civilization.

Dr. Maurice Rawlings, in his book *To Hell and Back*, confesses his annoyance when a patient, during resuscitation, requested that he pray for him. (He later developed a greater appreciation for the patient's request.) I had never thought much about how physicians separate themselves from the role of the ministry. In reality the two roles are closely intertwined. In all of my years in the practice of medicine I never felt that I carried on my work isolated from God. Quite the contrary. If a patient had asked me to pray for him I would not have felt offended, but I would have felt that he had made a poor choice of a spokesman. I recommend that you read Dr. Rawling's book for his great insight, as well as for his research into clinical death experiences.

So neither ought you to attempt to cure the body without the soul; and this is the reason why the cure of many diseases is unknown to the physicians of Hella, because they are ignorant of the whole, which ought to be studied also. For this is the great error of our day in the treatment of the human body, that physicians separate the soul from the body.

—— PLATO c. 429— 347 B.C.

This statement is as relevant today as it was in the days of Plato.

SOME DISEASES PREVENTABLE BY IMMUNIZATION

ACTIVE IMMUNIZATION §	PASSIVE IMMUNIZATION §
Diphtheria	Hepatitis A (immune globulin)
Pertussis (whooping cough)	Hepatitis B (immune globulin)
Tetanus	Tetanus
Measles (rubeola)	Rabies
Mumps	Measles
Rubella (German measles)	Rubella
Hemophilus influenza type b	
Polio (paralytic, three strains)	
Varicella (chicken pox, zoster)	
Hepatitis B (vaccine)	
Hepatitis A (vaccine introduced in 1995)	
Influenza	
Pneumococcal pneumonia	
Rabies (human diploid cell)	
Meningococcal meningitis	
Yellow fever	
Typhoid	
Cholera*	
Varicella (vaccine introduced in 1995)	

§ Active immunity involves the production of antibodies in the body after administration of a vaccine. This immunity persists for long periods, for life in some cases. Passive immunity involves injection into the individual of antibodies previously produced. These remain for a short period of time. They confer immediate, but short lived, immunity.

* Only the oral vaccine, currently being tested, is effective. The injectable vaccine is ineffective and is no longer recommended.

IMMUNIZATION SCHEDULE FOR ADULTS IN THE U. S.

VACCINE	SCHEDULE
Diphtheria and tetanus toxoids, combined	Every 10 years and after injury. (Assumes primary immunization completed earlier)
Live measles	One dose if no history of previous infection or immunization, if born in 1957 or later.
Live mumps	One dose if no history of previous infection or immunization.
Live rubella	One dose for all females with negative blood titre.
Influenza, tailored for current year	All adults age 65 and over; all adults with any chronic illness. Given yearly, generally in October.
Pneumococcal	One dose for all adults with chronic illness and other adults at age 65
Hepatitis B	Three doses for individuals at risk (see section on hepatitis).
Hepatitis A	A single injection, followed by a booster in 6-12 mo.
Inactivated polio	Non-immunized adults with children receiving vaccine; Non-immunized health care workers.
Varicella	Series of two doses for adolescents and young adults lacking antibody titre or history of chickenpox.

See Chapter III for immunization recommendations for children.

CHEMICALS FOR DISINFECTING

PREPARATION	APPLICATION
* Household (chlorine) bleach, one cup per 10 gal of water to sanitize, one Tbs per 10 gal for the road.	Potable water storage tanks and containers.
* Household (chlorine) bleach, 1 cup per quart of water for bacteria and fungi (1:4 solution	Toilet seats, table & counter tops, dishes (after removal of food and organic matter).
§* Phenolic compounds such as liquor cresolis USP, 5%, two tablespoons or 1 oz. per pint of water	Same as above. Not on eating surfaces unless washed well afterwards to remove residue. Diapers prior to laundry.
Soaps with triclocarban or triclosan (Safeguard®, Dial®)	Washing contaminated hands and skin.
Betadine® skin cleanser	Washing contaminated hands and skin.
Tincture of iodine, USP (2%)	Application to animal bites and skin injuries.
Silver sulfadiazine (Silvadene®)	Application to burns with sterile dressing covering.
Miconazole (Micatin®) 2% cream	Fungal infections of skin, including candida.
Bacitracin-polymyxin-neomycin ointment (Betadine ointment is preferable)	Infected wounds, abrasions of skin.

* Protective gloves should be worn when applying these agents as with all chemicals.

§ Formerly available as Lysol, but which has been reformulated (see text above).

Individuals with known sensitivities to any of the above should avoid contact with them.

1. Still, Andrew Taylor; *Philosophy of Osteopathy*. A.A. Still, Kirksville, MO, 1899.

2. *Diabetes Care* 2000;**23**:1278-83.

3. Burton BT, ed. *The Heinz Handbook of Nutrition*. New York, McGraw-Hill, 1965.

4. Milea D, Cassoux N, LeHoaug P. Blindness in a strict vegan. *N Engl J Med* 2000 Mar 23;**342**(12):897-898.

5. Blue Mountain Eye Study. *Ophthalmology*, **107**(3):450-456, March 2000.

6. *J Am College Nutrition*, April 2000.

7. Blaylock R. *Excitotoxins: The Taste That Kills*. Health Press, Santa Fe, NM, 1994.

8. National Cancer Institute.

9. Olney JW, Farber NB, Spitznagel E, Robins LN. Increasing brain tumor rates: is there a link to aspartame? *J Neuropathol Exp Neurol* 1996 Nov;**55**(11):1115-23.

10. Bradbury J. How drugs might damage developing brains. *Lancet*,1999;**353**:-126.

11. Olney JW. *Glutamate, A Neurotoxic Transmitter. J Child Neurology* **4**(1989):218-225.

12. Roberts HJ. *Aspartame (Nutrasweet®) Is It Safe?* Charles Press, Philadelphia, 1990.

13. Surbeck J. *Health Journal*, Summer, 1997, Price-Pottenger Nutrition Foundation, California.

14. McNagny S, *Ann Int Med* 1997;**127**:1093-1096.

15. Thorlacius-Ussing O, Flyvjerg A, Esmann J. Evidence that selenium induces growth retardation through reduced growth hormone and somatomedin C production. *Endocrinology* 1987;**120**:659-663.

16. Morin Y and Daniel P: Quebec beer-drinkers cardiomyopathy: etiological consideration. *J. Can. Med. Assoc.*, **97**:926-931, 1967.

17. Garrison FH. *An Introduction to the History of Medicine*, ed 4. Philadelphia: WB Saunders 1929.

18. CDC. Chaparral-induced toxic hepatitis — California and Texas, 1992. *MMWR* 1992;**41**:812-813.

19. CDC. Cadmium and lead exposure associated with pharmaceuticals imported from Asia — Texas. *MMWR* 1989;**38**:612–614.

20. CDC. Jin Bu Huan toxicity in children — Colorado, 1993. *MMWR*1993;**42**:-633-636.

21. CDC. Jin Bu Huan toxicity in adults — Los Angeles, 1993. *MMWR* 1993;**42**:920-922.

22. Ko RJ. Adulterants in Asian patent medicines. *N Engl J Med* 1998;**339**:847.

23. Vanherweghem J-L, Depirreux M, Tielemans C, et al. Rapidly progressive interstitial renal fibrosis in young women: association with slimming regimen including Chinese herbs. *Lancet* 1993; **341**:387-91.

24. Lord GM, Tagore R, Cook T, et al. Nephropathy caused by Chinese herbs in the UK. *Lancet* 1999;**354**:481-82.

25. Vanherweghem JL. Misuse of herbal remedies: the case of an outbreak of terminal renal failure in Belgium (Chinese herbs nephropathy). *J Altern Complement Med* 1998;**4**:9-13.

26. Cosyns JP, Jadoul M, Squifflet JP, et al. Urothelial lesions in Chinese herb nephropathy. *Am J Kidney Dis* 1999;**33**:1011-17.

27. Vanherweghem JL. Aristolochia sp and chronic interstitial nephropathies in Indians. *Lancet* 1997;**349**:1399.

28. Lord GM, Cook T, Arit VM et al. Urothelial malignant disease and Chinese herbal nephropathy. *Lancet* 2001;**358**:1515-16.

29. Vanherweghem J-L. Association of valvular heart disease with Chinese-herb nephropathy. *Lancet* 1997;**350**:1858.

30. CDC. Lead poisoning associated with use of traditional ethnic remedies — California, 1991–1992. *MMWR* 1993;**42**:521-524.

31. Ko, RJ. Adulterants in Asian Patent Medicines. *New Eng J Med* 1998;**339**:-847.

32. McRill C, Boyer LV, Flood TJ, Ortega L. Mercury toxicity due to use of a cosmetic cream. *JOEM* 2000;**42**:4-7.

33. Lee MK, Cheng BW, Che CT, Hsieh DP. Cytotoxicity assessment of Ma-huang (Ephedra) under different conditions of preparation. *Toxicol Sci* 2000 Aug;**56**(2):424-30.

34. *The Medical Letter*, New Rochelle, New York, February 19, 2001.

35. Blumenthal M, Goldberg A, Brinckman J. *Herbal Medicine; Expanded Commission E Monographs*. Integrative Medicine Communications, Newton, MA, 2000.

36. Waldhouser F, Weiszenbacher G, Tatzer E, et al. Alterations in nocturnal serum melatonin levels in humans with growth and aging. *J Clin Endocrinol Metab* 1988;**66**:648-52.

37. Swerdlow DL, Mintz ED, Rodriguez M, et al. Waterborne transmission of epidemic cholera in Trujillo, Peru: lessons for a continent at risk. *Lancet*

1992;**340**:28–33.

38. CDC. Hepatitis A associated with consumption of frozen strawberries — Michigan, March 1997. *MMWR* 1997;**46**:288-295.

39. Garrison, FH. *An Introduction to the History of Medicine*, ed 4. Philadelphia: W.B. Saunders Co., 1929.

40. Birkeland, J. *Microbiology and Man*, ed 2. Williams & Wilkins, Baltimore, 1949.

41. McCarthy M. Hepatitis A linked to clotting factors in USA. *Lancet* 1996;**347**:251.

42. Haller JD. Blood sterilization with high temperature terminal dry heat. *Lancet* 1996;**347**:827-28.

43. Lee WM. Hepatitis B Virus Infection. *N Engl J Med*. 1997;**337**:1733-1745.

44. CDC. Immunization of health care workers: Recommendations of the Advisory Committee on Immunization Practices and the Hospital Infection Control Practices Advisory Committee. *MMWR* 1997;**46** (No RR-18)

45. Nelson K, Donahue JG, Muñoz A, et al. Transmission of retroviruses from seronegative donors by transfusion during cardiac surgery: a multicenter study of HIV-1 and HTLV-I/II infections. *Ann Intern Med*. 1992;**117**:554-559.

46. Fauci AS, Braunwald E, Isselbacher KJ et al; *Harrison's Principles of Internal Medicine*, ed 14. McGraw-Hill, Columbus, OH, 1997.

47. CDC. Recommendations for prevention and control of hepatitis C virus (HCV) infection and HCV-related chronic disease. MMWR 1998;47(RR-19):1-12.

48. Simons JN, Pilot-Matias TJ, Leary TP, et al. Identification of two flavivirus-like genomes in the GB hepatitis agent. *Proc Natl Acad Sci* U S A. 1995;**92**:3401-3405.

49. Yu MW, Mason BL, Guo ZP, et al. Hepatitis C transmission associated with intravenous immunoglobulins. *Lancet* 1995;**345**:1173-74.

50. Outbreak of hepatitis C associated with intravenous immunoglobulin administration — United States, October 1993–June 1994. *MMWR* 1994;**43**:505-509.

51. Nakashima K, Ikematsu H, Hayashi J, et al. Intrafamilial transmission of hepatitis C virus among the population of an endemic area of Japan. *JAMA*. 1995;**274**:1459-1461.

52. Interferon plus ribavirin for chronic hepatitis C. *The Medical Letter* 1998;**41**:June 4,1999.

53. CDC. Hepatitis E among U.S. travelers, 1989–1992. *MMWR* 1993;**42**:1–4.

54. Chauhan A, Dilawari JB, Kaur U, et al. Hepatitis E virus transmission to a volunteer. *Lancet* 1993;**341**:149–50.

55. Simmonds P, Davidson F, Lycett C, et al. Detection of a novel DNA virus (TTV) in blood donors and blood products. *Lancet* 1998 Jul 18;**352**(9123):191-195.

56. Meinking TL, Taplin D, Hermida JL et al. The treatment of scabies with ivermectin. *N Engl J Med* 1995;**333**:26-30.

57. Rid® contains pyrethrum extract plus piperonyl butoxide. Nix® contains 1% permethrin. The latter is one of the latest synthesized pyrethroids and is very stable and effective. A generic preparation of permethrin is also available at a lower cost.

58. Rupes V, Moravec J, Chmela J, et al. A resistance of head lice (Pediculus capitis) to permethrin in Czech Republic. *Cent Eur J Public Health* 1995. Feb;**3**(1):30-32.

59. Mumcuoglu KY, Hemingway J, Miller J, et al. Permethrin resistance in the head louse Pediculus capitis from Israel. *Med Vet Entomol* 1995. Oct;**9**(4):427-432, 447.

60. Dennis GA, Lee PN. A phase I volunteer study to establish the degree of absorption and effect on cholinesterase activity of four head lice preparations containing malathion. *Clin Drug Invest* 1999;**18**:105-115.

61. Welch DF, Pickett DA, Slater DN, et al. *Rolachimaea henselae* sp., a cause of septicemia, bacillary angiomatosis, and parenchymal bacillary peliosis. *J Clin Microbiology* 1992;**30**:275-280.

62. Spach D, Kanter AS, Dougherty MJ et al. *Bartonella (Rochilamaea) quintana* bacteremia in inner-city patients with chronic alcoholism. *N Engl J Med* 1995;**332**:424-428.

63. Brouqui P, Lascola B, Roux V, Raoult D. Chronic *Bartonella quintella* bacteremia in homeless patients. *N Engl J Med* 1999;**340**:184-189.

64. Whyte A S, Garnett P A, Whittington A E. Bats in the belfry, bugs in the bed? *Lancet* 2001;**357**:604.

65. Webb PA et al. *J Infect Dis*, Dec 1989;**160**(6):970-7.

66. Manson-Bahr PEC, Bell DR. *Manson's Tropical Diseases*, 19th ed. Bailliere Tindall, London, 1987.

67. Brown HM, Merrett TG. Effectiveness of an acaricide in management of house dust mite allergy. *Ann Allergy*, Jul 1991, **67**(1):25-31.

68. Naspitz CK, Diniz C, Rizzo MC et al. Human scalps as a reservoir of domestic mites. *Lancet* 1997;**349**:404.

69. Schulaner FA. Sensitivity to the cockroach in three groups of allergic children. *Pediatrics* 1970;**45**:465-466.

70. Kang B, Sulit N. A comparative study of prevalence of skin hypersensitivity to cockroach and house dust antigens. *Ann Allergy* 1978;**41**:333-336.

71. Sastre J, Ibanez MD, Lombardero M,et al. Allergy to cockroaches in patients with asthma and rhinitis in an urban area (Madrid). *Allergy* 1996;**51**:582-586.

72. Rosenstreich DL, Eggleston P, Kattan M, et al. The role of cockroach allergy and exposure to cockroach allergen in causing morbidity among inner-city children with asthma. *N Engl J Med* 1997;**336**:1356-63.

73. The World Almanac and Book of Facts, 1993. Pharos Books, New York.

74. Garrison FW. *History of medicine*, ed 4. Philadelphia, WB Saunders 1961.

GLOSSARY

Acaricide — a substance that kills mites.

Acarina — an order of the Class Arachnida which includes ticks and mites.

Acarus — a genus of small mites. They act as external parasites on the body. Various members cause itch, mange and other diseases.

Acute — of sudden onset, relatively short duration and usually severe.

Adsorbed — clinging to the surface only, as opposed to absorbed, in which the substance is taken up and distributed within.

Aerosol — very small solid or liquid particles that remain suspended in the air for some time.

Alkaloid — one of a large group of organic, basic substances found in plants. They are usually bitter to taste. Examples: atropine, caffeine, coniine, morphine, nicotine, quinine and strychnine.

Allotropism — the existence of a substance in two or more distinct forms with distinct physical properties, e.g. graphite and diamond, allotropic forms of carbon.

Amalgam — an alloy of mercury with another metal.

Amino acids — the basic structural groups of which proteins are composed.

Anaerobic — absence of oxygen.

Analogue — a chemical compound with a structure similar to another but differing in one component.

Antioxidant — a substance that inhibits oxidation.

Arachnida — a class of the Arthopoda that includes spiders, ticks, mites and scorpions.

Arbovirus — a contraction for arthropod borne virus. These are diseases that are transmitted by mosquitoes and ticks. Over 250 distinct members have been identified.

Arthropoda — a phyllum of the animal kingdom composed of organisms having a hard, jointed exoskeleton and paired, jointed legs. It includes Arachnida and Insecta. Many species serve as parasites of man, or transmit to man organisms that cause disease.

Arteriosclerosis — thickening and hardening of the walls of the arteries.

Arthropod — a group of organisms that includes the arachnids (spiders, ticks, mites, scorpions) and insecta (flies, midges, mosquitoes, cockroaches, bees, wasps, ants, beetles, moths, butterflies).

Atmosphere — the layer of gases that surrounds and moves with the earth, about 22,000 miles high.

Bednar's aphthae — small ulcers on the hard palate of infants; thought to result from the pressure of the nipple during nursing.

Body Mass Index — the weight in kilograms divided by the square of the height in meters. Health risks increase as the index increases above 25.

Borrelia — a genus of bacteria under the order Spirochaetalis, family Treponemataceae.

Brass — an alloy of copper and zinc.

Bronze — an alloy of copper and tin.

Calcine — to reduce to a fine powder by heat.

Carcinogenic — causing cancer.

Catalyst — an agent which either speeds up or slows down a chemical reaction without itself being changed.

Caveat — a warning. Let him beware.

Caveat emptor — let the buyer beware. One buys at his own risk.

Central Nervous System (CNS) — the brain and all of the nerves extending from it to the skeletal muscles and the senses; hearing, seeing, pain, temperature, touch and speech.

Chronic — persisting for long periods.

Cicutoxin — a poisonous higher alcohol found in Water Hemlock (Spotted Cowbane).

Compound — a substance that is made up of two or more chemical elements.

Conjunctiva — the membrane that covers the inner portion of the eyelids and the exposed portion of the sclera of the eye (the white portion).

Coniine — a poisonous alkaloid found in Poison Hemlock.

Croton oil — a phorbol ester derived from a shrub of the same name. A powerful irritant and cancer promoter. Used to induce mouse skin tumors.

Defoliate — to cause the leaves of a plant or tree to drop prematurely.

Denature — to modify the molecular structure of a compound (i.e. protein or DNA) by heat, acid, alkali or ultraviolet radiation and thus destroy or modify its original biologic activity.

Detergent — a surface-active chemical, other than soaps, that is capable of emulsifying dirt.

Dinoflagellate — a minute marine plantlike protozoan.

Disinfect — to eliminate pathogenic orgnisms, or render them inert, incapable of causing disease.

DNA — deoxyribonucleic acid. A substance in all living cells that is the carrier of genetic information for all organisms except for the RNA viruses.

Dysentery — a generic term applied to diarrhea accompanied by abdominal cramping, pain and blood and mucus in the stool. It may be caused by bacteria, protozoa, parasitic worms or chemical irritants. Amebic dysentery is caused by *Entamoeba hystolytica*, and bacillary dysentery is caused by various strains of *Shigella*.

Endemic — present at all times.

Enterovirus — a virus that infects the gastrointestinal tract and is discharged in the feces. Includes poliovirus, cochsackievirus and echovirus.

Enzootic — a disease which is present in an animal community at all times, but present in small numbers.

Enzyme — any of numerous complex proteins that are produced by various cells in the body for the purpose of catalyzing specific biologic functions.

Epidemic — a disease attacking many people in a community or region at one time. Not normally present, or present in small numbers.

Essential oils — oils that retain the flavor or odor of the plant.

Eutectic mixture — that mixture of two or more substances which has the lowest melting point.

Excitotoxin — a substance that induces excessive stimulation of neuronal transmitters in the nervous system.

Excrement — feces.

Excreta — waste materials excreted by the body, e.g., urine and feces.

Feldspar — a group of crystalline minerals that consist of aluminum silicates with either calcium, sodium, potassium or barium.

Fibrosis — the formation of fibrous tissue, tissue that contains fibers, replacing the normal cells.

Flatulence — gas in the stomach and intestines.

Fomite — an inanimate object such as a doorknob, handles, book, article of clothing etc. which is capable of harboring and thus transmiting bacteria, viruses and other infectious agents to others.

Fungicide — a chemical substance that kills fungi.

Gardnerella vaginalis — formerly termed *Corynebacterium vaginale* or *Haemophilus vaginalis*.

Gastrointestinal tract — the stomach and intestines.

Gum arabic (acasia) — a resinous sap from the acacia tree of northwest Africa, used as a stabilizer to improve or maintain the texture and consistency of mixed foods such as ice cream, jellies and cough drops. It is also used as a binder for medicine tablets. It was used by the Nubians (Egypt & Sudan) in ancient times as a glue for gems and colored glass. It remains useful as a glue on envelopes and postage stamps.

Half-life — the length of time required for the disintegration of one-half of the number of atoms in a radioactive element.

Hemolysis — destruction of red blood cells with the release of hemoglobin into the serum.

Heterozygous — carrying only one dominate gene for a particular trait.

HIV — human immunodeficiency virus.

Homozygous — carrying both genes for a particular trait, thus assuring expression of the trait.

Hormesis — the stimulating effect of subinhibitory concentrations of any toxic substance on any organism.

Hydrocarbon — chemical substances composed soley of hydrogen and carbon molecules.

Hygiene — the science of health and prevention of disease: cleanliness.

Hygroscopic — absorbing and retaining moisture from the air.

Infestation — the establishment of parasites on the body, usually on the skin.

Ingestion — taken into the body through the mouth.

Insecticide — a chemical substance which kills insects.

Kaolin — a fine, very pure white clay used in making porcelain, paper and textiles, and in medicine in the treatment of diarrhea. It is mixed with feldspar when making dinnerware. It is named after the hill in China where it was found.

Keratin — a tough, very insoluble protein of which hair, nails and horns are composed.

Jesuit fever — malaria

Khat (*Catha edulis*) — a shrub cultivated in the Middle East and Africa for its leaves and buds that are a source of a stumulant which is habituating. It is chewed or brewed as a tea.

Labyrinth — the inner ear.

La plus ca change, la plus ces't la même chose — the more things change, the more they remain the same.

Lectin — a group of hemagglutinating proteins found primarily in plant seeds, which bind specifically to sugar molecules of glycoproteins and glycolipids on the surface of cells. Certain lectins selectively cause agglutination of erythrocytes of certain blood groups and of malignant cells but not their normal counterparts; others stimulate the proliferation of lymphocytes.

Leishmania — a genus of parasitic protozoa of the family Trypanosoma.

Ligand — a molecule that binds to another molecule, such as an antigen to an antibody, a neurotransmitter to a receptor.

Limestone — calcium carbonate. Much of it formed by the remains of sea animals, e.g., mollusks and coral. Marble was formed from limestone by heat and pressure.

Lye — a mixture of sodium hydroxide and sodium carbonate yielded by percolating water through wood ash.

Lymphoma — malignant proliferation of lymphoid cells in various sites of the immune system, including lymph nodes, bone marrow, spleen, liver and the gastrointestinal tract.

Microbial agent — one of the microorganisms, usually one that causes disease.

Micron (symbol is μ) — a unit of measure, one millionth of a meter, one thousandth of a millimeter, 1/25,000 of an inch. A human hair is about 50 microns in diameter.

Microgram — one one thousandth of a milligram.

Microorganisms — bacteria, viruses and protozoa that can be seen only with a microscope.

Mil — one thousandth of an inch, 0.0254 millimeter; measurement of the diameter of a wire or the thickness of coatings.

Milli — one one-thousandth (10^{-3})

Morbidity — sickness. The condition of being ill.

Mutagen — a substance that induces genetic mutations in plants or animals.

Necrosis — death of tissue: decay.

Neuropathy — diminished function in a peripheral nerve, due to inflammation, degeneration or other pathology.

Nix® — permethrin 1% for head lice.

Organic compounds — substances that contain carbon in the molecular structure.

Ozone — an allotropic and more active form of oxygen containing three molecules (O_3), unstable and used as an oxidizing or bleaching agent.

Pandemic — a widespread epidemic, usually throughout a continent. Involving several countries rather than one singly.

Particulate — a very small, separate particle that remains suspended in the air. Includes fog, mist, smoke, smog, fume (welding) and dust.

Pathogenic — having the capacity to cause disease.

PCR — polymerase chain reaction; a sensitive test for detecting and identifying viruses by amplification of viral nucleic acids.

Personal hygiene — cleanliness: sanitary behavior.

pH — a symbol for the acidity or alkalinity of a substance. Derived from the French *puissance hydrogen*.

Phenolic — of or containing phenol, a strong and corrosive substance derived from coal tar. Also a substance with a chemical structure similar to phenol.

Photophobia — abnormal visual intolerance of light.

Phytoplankton — planktonic plant life.

Photoreaction — a chemical reaction produced by light.

Photosensitivity — abnormal reactivity of the skin to sunlight.

Phototoxic — increased sunburn response of the skin to ultraviolet light; not an allergic reaction.

Plankton — passively floating minute plant and animal life in water.

Porphyria — a metabolic disorder characterized by the excretion of porphyrins in the urine and by a serious sensitivity to the sun. It may be inherited or acquired by exposure to certain chemicals.

Potash — potassium hydroxide, used in fertilizers.

Protozoa — minute single celled organisms, the simplest forms of the animal kingdom.

Ptomaine — several toxins produced by bacterial action upon foods, e.g. cadaverine, muscarine and putrescine.

Replication — the process of duplicating or multiplying.

Respirable particles — particles that remain suspended in air, that are small enough to pass into the lungs when they are inhaled. Generally up to about five micrometers.

Rhizome — the underground stem of a plant (as contrasted to the root).

Ricin — a potent poison found in Castor beans, for which there is no known antedote.

Ricksettsia — nonfilterable microorganisms somewhere between the bacteria and the viruses in size, structure and organization.

Rid® — a shampoo which contains pyrethrum extract and piperonyl butoxide, for head, body and pubic lice.

Silica — silicon dioxide. Most of the earth's crust is composed of this substance, including quartz, flint, granite and sand.

Silicates — combined forms of silica, including asbestos, mica and talc.

Spirochaete — a spiral, motile bacteria. Members of this group cause syphilis, yaws, relapsing fever and Lyme disease.

Sterilize — to eliminate all microorgnaisms, or render them incapable of reproducing.

Sweetbread — the pancreas or thymus gland of a young animal, i.e. a calf.

Sweet oil — any mild edible oil, such as olive oil

Systemic — affecting the body (or plant) as a whole rather than a single organ. A systemic pesticide is taken up by the plant and distributed throughout the plant and its fruit.

Teratogen — an agent that produces physical defects in the fetus.

Toxicity — the degree of poisonous or harmfulness of a substance.

Virus — a very large group of very small infectious agents that are able to reproduce only within the living cells of other organisms. They lack the system of metabolism that is common to other living organisms including bacteria.

Vector — an animal, usually an arthropod, that transfers an infectious agent from one host to another.

Wormwood — artemisia absinthium, a flowering plant. The dried leaves and flowers produce a bitter oil, absinthin. The term wormwood is used metaphorically throughout the bible to denote a bitter calamity or sorrow.

Zeolite — any of a large number of natural hydrous aluminum silicates of sodium, calcium, potassium, barium etc. characterized by a rapid gain or loss of water of hydration. Many are capable of ion exchange, some natural or synthetic used for water softening.

Zygote — a cell formed by the fertilization of an ova by a sperm cell.

REFERENCES

• Klassen CD. *Casarett and Doull's Toxicology*, ed 5. McGraw-Hill, Columbus, OH 1996.

• Bennett JC, Plum, F. *Cecil Textbook of Medicine*, ed 20. WB Saunders, 1996.

• Fauci AS, Braunwald E, Isselbacher KJ et al; *Harrison's Principles of Internal Medicine*, ed 14. McGraw-Hill, Columbus, OH, 1997.

• Am Conf Govt Ind Hyg. *Threshold limit values for chemical substances and physical agents*;2001: Cincinnati, OH, 2001.

• Arnold HL, Odom RB, James WD. *Andrew's Diseases of the Skin*, ed 8. Saunders, Philadelphia, 1990.

• Benenson AS, ed. *Control of communicable diseases manual*, ed 16. Am Pub Health Ass; Washington, 1995.

• Blumenthal M, ed. *Herbal medicine; expanded commission E monographs*. Integrative medicine communications. Newton, MA, 2000.

• Blaylock RL. *Excitotoxins: the taste that kills*. Health Press, Santa Fe, NM, 1994.

• Roberts HJ. *Aspartame: is it safe?* Charles Press, Philadelphia, 1990.

• Cain HD. *Flint's emergency treatment and management*, ed 7. WB Saunders, Philadelphia, 1985.

• Centers for Disease Control. *Summary of notifiable diseases, United States, 1999*. MMWR 1999;**48**(No.53).

• Centers for Disease Control. *NIOSH recommendations for occupational safety and health standards*. MMWR 1988;**37**(suppl. No. S-7).

• Harris. *Patty's industrial hygiene and toxicology*, ed 5. Wiley, New York, 2001.

• Foster KR, Bernstein DE and Huber PW editors. *Phantom risk, scientific inference and the law*. MIT Press, Cambridge 1993.

• Huber P. *Galileo's revenge: Junk science in the courtroom*. Basic Books, New York, 1991. ISBN 0-465-02624-9

• Bailey R. *Ecoscam: The false prophets of ecological apocalypse*. St. Martin's Press, New York, 1993. ISBN 0-312-08698-9

• Bailey R, ed. *The True State of the Planet*. Free Press. New York, 1995

• Fumento M. *Science Under Siege*. Wm Morrow. New York, 1993.

• Baden JA. *Environmental Gore; A Constructive Response to Earth in the Balance*. Pacific Research Institute. San Francisco, 1994.

• Kaufman W. *No Turning Back*. Basic Books, New York, 1994.

• Singer SF. *Hot Talk, Cold Science*. The Independent Institute. Oakland, 1997.

• Garrison FW. *An Introduction to the History of Medicine,* ed 4. WB Saunders, Philadelphia, 1961.

• Hardman JG, Limbird LE, Molinoff PB, Ruddib RW, Gilman AG, eds. *Goodman and Gilman's the Pharmacological Basis of Therapeutics*, ed 9. McGraw-Hill, New York, 1996.

• Hiatt HH, Watson JD, Winsten JA. *Origins of human cancer*. Cold Spring Harbor Lab., 1977.

• Raffle PAB, et al. *Hunter's Diseases of Occupations*, ed 8. Arnold, London; Boston, 1994. RC 964 H8 1994.

• Brooks, GF, Butel, JS, Ornston, LN. *Jawetz, Melnick and Adelberg's Medical Microbiology*, ed 20. Appleton & Lange, Norwalk, Connecticut, 1995.

• Manson–Bahr PEC, Apted FIC. *Manson's tropical diseases*, ed 19. Baillière Tindall, London, 1988.

• Nagda NL, ed. *Air Quality and Comfort in Airliner Cabins*. American Society for Testing and Materials. West Conshohocken, PA, 2000.

• Ravel R. *Clinical Laboratory Medicine*, ed 6. Mosby, St. Louis, 1995.

• Salvato JA. *Environmental Engineering and Sanitation*, ed 2. Wiley, New York, 1972.

• USDHEW. *The Industrial Environment — Its Evaluation and Control*. Govt Print Off, 1973.

• Lide, DR. *CRC Handbook of chemistry and physics*. CRC Press, Boca Raton, FL, 2001.

• Isselbacher KJ, Braunwald E, Wilson JD, et al eds. *Harrison's Principles of Internal Medicine*, ed 13. McGraw–Hill, New York, 1994.

• Zenz C. *Occupational medicine*, ed 2. Year Book Med Pub, Chicago, 1988

• Ladou, J. *Occupational and Environmental Medicine*, McGraw-Hill, New York, 1997.

• Doll, R. and A.B. Hill. A Study of the Aetiology of Carcinoma of the Lung. *Br Med J* 1952;**ii**:1271-86.

• Doll, R. and A.B. Hill. Mortality in Relation to Smoking: Ten Years Observation of British Doctors. *Br Med J* 1964;**1**:1399.

LYME DISEASE

• Logigran EL, Kaplan RF, Steere AC. Chronic neurological manifestations of Lyme disease. *N Engl J Med* 1990;**323**:1438-44.

• McAlister HF. Lyme carditis. *Ann Intern Med* 1989;**110**:339-45.

• Spach Dh, Liles WC, Campbell GL et al. Tick-borne diseases in the United States. *N Engl J Med* 1993;**329**:936-947.

• Steere AC. Lyme disease. *N Engl J Med* 1989;**320**:586-794.

Index

704